CW00346546

Veterinary Medical Education

Veterinary Medical Education: A Practical Guide

Edited by

Jennifer L. Hodgson
Virginia Maryland College of Veterinary Medicine, VA, USA

Jacquelyn M. Pelzer
Virginia Maryland College of Veterinary Medicine, VA, USA

WILEY Blackwell

This edition first published 2017 © 2017 John Wiley & Sons, Inc.

All rights reserved. No part of this publication may be reproduced, stored in a retrieval system, or transmitted, in any form or by any means, electronic, mechanical, photocopying, recording or otherwise, except as permitted by law. Advice on how to obtain permission to reuse material from this title is available at http://www.wiley.com/go/permissions.

The right of Jennifer L. Hodgson and Jacquelyn M. Pelzer to be identified as the author(s) of the editorial material in this work has been asserted in accordance with law.

Registered Offices
John Wiley & Sons, Inc., 111 River Street, Hoboken, NJ 07030, USA

John Wiley & Sons Ltd, The Atrium, Southern Gate, Chichester, West Sussex, PO19 8SQ, UK

Editorial Office
1606 Golden Aspen Drive, Suites 103 and 104, Ames, Iowa 50010, USA

For details of our global editorial offices, customer services, and more information about Wiley products visit us at www.wiley.com.

Wiley also publishes its books in a variety of electronic formats and by print-on-demand. Some content that appears in standard print versions of this book may not be available in other formats.

Limit of Liability/Disclaimer of Warranty
The contents of this work are intended to further general scientific research, understanding, and discussion only and are not intended and should not be relied upon as recommending or promoting scientific method, diagnosis, or treatment by physicians for any particular patient. The publisher and the authors make no representations or warranties with respect to the accuracy and completeness of the contents of this work and specifically disclaim all warranties, including without limitation any implied warranties of fitness for a particular purpose. In view of ongoing research, equipment modifications, changes in governmental regulations, and the constant flow of information relating to the use of medicines, equipment, and devices, the reader is urged to review and evaluate the information provided in the package insert or instructions for each medicine, equipment, or device for, among other things, any changes in the instructions or indication of usage and for added warnings and precautions. Readers should consult with a specialist where appropriate. The fact that an organization or website is referred to in this work as a citation and/or potential source of further information does not mean that the author or the publisher endorses the information the organization or website may provide or recommendations it may make. Further, readers should be aware that websites listed in this work may have changed or disappeared between when this works was written and when it is read. No warranty may be created or extended by any promotional statements for this work. Neither the publisher nor the author shall be liable for any damages arising herefrom.

Library of Congress Cataloging-in-Publication Data applied for.

ISBN: 9781119125006

Cover design: Wiley
Cover image: Top Image: Purestock/Gettyimages
          Middle Image: Courtesy of the editors
          Bottom Image: Jose Luis Pelaez Inc/Gettyimages

Set in 10/12pt WarnockPro by SPi Global, Chennai, India

Printed in the United States of America.

10 9 8 7 6 5 4 3 2 1

This book is dedicated

To Dave and Noelle for their patience.

To the authors, for their outstanding contributions to the book and their continued dedication to improving veterinary medical education.

Finally, to veterinary students worldwide, who encourage us every day to become better educators.

Icons

To help guide readers to some of the fundamental messages in each chapter, authors have created boxes, together with their corresponding icons, which represent different themes. The boxes and themes are centered around: main points ("Key Messages"); application of a tool or process ("How To"); information supporting the chapter's theme ("Where's the Evidence"); highlighting a specific topic ("Focus On"); contemplation of themes within the chapter ("Reflections"), familiarizing the reader with educational terminology or concepts ("What's the Meaning"); alerting the reader to handy recommendations ("Quick Tips"); and describing characteristics or illustrations of concepts and theories ("Example Of").

Key messages

How to…

Where's the evidence?

Focus on…

Reflection

What's the meaning?

Quick tips

Example of…

Part I

The Curriculum

1

Curricular Design, Review, and Reform

Jennifer L. Hodgson[1] and Jan E. Ilkiw[2]

[1] *Virginia-Maryland College of Veterinary Medicine, Virginia Tech, USA*
[2] *School of Veterinary Medicine, University of California, Davis, USA*

 Box 1.1: Key messages

- Modern veterinary curricula should focus on the fundamental skills required of all graduates and incorporate the principles of learning that will achieve these.
- A curriculum should be designed to be the best fit for the purpose and context of its place and time.
- A curriculum is the totality of student experiences that occur in an educational process, including not only what is taught, but how it is taught, learned, and assessed, how the learning is managed and communicated, and the overall learning environment.

- Curriculum design, review, and reform are complex processes that should involve well-defined steps and input from a wide variety of stakeholders.
- Communication, leadership, a cooperative climate, participation by organizational members, evaluation, human resource development, and politics are all key components in the success of curricular development and reform.
- Curricular evaluation, as an ongoing process for program improvement, should be a component of curricular design and development.

Introduction

Curricular planning, design, and development have always played an important role in veterinary education, but never more so than today. The veterinary degree, perhaps more than any of the other health science degrees, poses a challenge to curricular designers due to the breadth of material that must be covered and the variety of career options available to veterinarians. Modern veterinary curricula also must adapt to a world where information is available at our fingertips, but expanding at a prodigious rate. Therefore, rather than dwelling on past models of learning and teaching, contemporary veterinary curricula must refocus on the fundamental knowledge, skills, and behaviors required of all graduates and utilize modern methods, grounded in educational theory, to best achieve this.

Curricular design can be an arena in which many battles are fought, with differing views

Veterinary Medical Education: A Practical Guide, First Edition. Edited by Jennifer L. Hodgson and Jacquelyn M. Pelzer.
© 2017 John Wiley & Sons, Inc. Published 2017 by John Wiley & Sons, Inc.

about what veterinary students should learn, how they should learn, what additional qualities we want them to develop, when and how the basic and clinical sciences should contribute to the curriculum, how long the program should take, and ultimately who owns the curriculum. Interestingly, there is no body of evidence demonstrating that there is one best choice for framing a curriculum as a whole, or any of its parts, in either medical education (Grant, 2013) or veterinary education. Instead, a curriculum should be designed to be the best fit for the purpose and context of its place and time. Further, a curriculum should be dynamic; it should be continually developing in response to curricular evaluation as well as changes in professional and societal needs.

In this chapter we have defined what a curriculum is, the factors that may influence its design, and the steps that may be undertaken in order to develop, implement, review, and reform a modern veterinary curriculum.

What Is a Curriculum? Definition and Standards

Definition

There are widely varying views regarding the term "curriculum," with the word meaning different things to different people. Some people take a narrow view of the term, as frequently found in dictionary definitions: "the courses offered by an educational institution or a set of courses constituting an area of specialization" (Merriam-Webster, 2016). From this perspective, the curriculum may be perceived as largely equivalent to content.

Other people take a wider view, where a curriculum may be broadly defined as the totality of student experiences that occur in the educational process (Wiles, 2009). In this sense, the curriculum is seen as covering not only what is taught, but also how it is taught, learned, and assessed, how the learning is managed and communicated, and the overall learning environment (Harden, 2001). This extended view of a curriculum is illustrated in Figure 1.1 and will be used in this chapter.

Standards for the Curriculum

An alternate way to define a curriculum is through the standards that accrediting agencies require. One example of these standards is that developed in the United States by the American Veterinary Medical Association's (AVMA) Council on Education (COE). Standard 9, which addresses the curriculum, is one of 11 standards outlining the requirements that colleges or schools of veterinary medicine must meet in order to become accredited (AVMA, 2014).

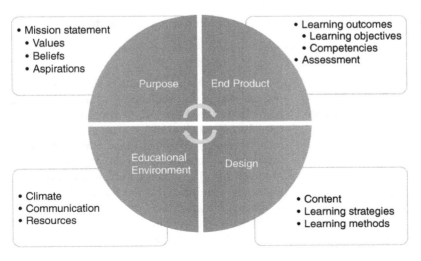

Figure 1.1 Curricular elements.

- Mission statement
- Values
- Beliefs
- Aspirations

Purpose

- Learning outcomes
- Learning objectives
- Competencies
- Assessment

End Product

Educational Environment

Design

- Climate
- Communication
- Resources

- Content
- Learning strategies
- Learning methods

Table 1.1 Factors influencing curricular design and their effects.

Factor	Specific Influence	Effect
Academic	Theories of learning	Learner-centered design (e.g., problem-based learning); integrated curricula
	Expansion of knowledge	Core and elective curricula
	Decreasing resources	Distributed clinical teaching
Professional	Veterinary practitioners	Inclusion or expansion in the curriculum for communication and business skills; emphasis on teamwork and professionalism
	Accreditation and licensure	Outcomes-based curricula; focus on competencies; changes to curricula due to changes in licensing exams, e.g., North American Veterinary Licensing Examination (NAVLE)
Societal	One Health	Multiprofessional elements
	Social values	Widening-participation curricula to address underserved areas or communities; fewer animal use courses and introduction of clinical skills laboratories
Political	Length of curriculum	Shorter curricula, or earlier entrance to Doctor of Veterinary Medicine programs, to address cost of veterinary education

Source: Adapted from Grant (2013). Reproduced with permission of Wiley Blackwell.

Standard 9 states that the curriculum in veterinary medical education is the purview of the faculty of each college, but must be managed centrally based on the mission and resources of the college. Additional points in this standard include the requirement that the curriculum extends over a period equivalent to a minimum of four academic years, with a minimum of one academic year of hands-on clinical education; the subject areas that must be covered in the curriculum are defined, but it is not prescribed as to when or how these subjects should be taught or assessed; and the curriculum as a whole must be reviewed at least every seven years. More information about this standard, and those of other agencies that accredit veterinary colleges and schools around the world, can be found in Part Five, Chapter 22: Accreditation.

Factors Influencing Curricular Design

Curricular design is a complex process and may be influenced by a variety of factors internal and external to a college or school of veterinary medicine. These factors may include academic, professional, societal, and political influences (see Table 1.1).

Some of these factors affect the content of the curriculum and others affect curricular design. For example, emerging theories on adult learning can result in different curricular models, and changing expectations of the veterinary profession may cause alterations in the content of the curriculum. As Grant observed, "At any one point, a curriculum is a child of its time" (Grant, 2013, p. 36).

Steps in Curricular Design and Development

Veterinary medical educators now appreciate that curricular design encompasses much more than a statement of the content to be covered in the course or program. Instead, curricular design is a rational, open, and accountable process that may cover all aspects of a curriculum, or may focus on a specific area where curricular revision and renewal are desired. Development of a curriculum can be a lengthy process and usually involves a team of individuals who bring to the table different expertise, such as content specialists; basic, paraclinical, and clinical faculty; students, educationalists, administrators, or managers; and external stakeholders such as veterinary practitioners.

Recently, Harden outlined a comprehensive, 10-step process used for curricular design in medical education (Harden, 2013). These steps have been employed as a framework for this chapter, as all the steps are equally relevant to veterinary education, with some modification for the different educational contexts. Further, these principles of curricular design are fundamental, yet flexible enough to yield different types of curricula in different hands, depending on the local environment in which veterinary curricula are developed or reviewed. This last point is very important, as it is not the intent of this chapter to describe a "cookie-cutter" curriculum that is suitable for all veterinary programs regardless of their location or available resources. Rather, we have included the essential guiding principles that should be applied to achieve optimal student learning outcomes and to result in veterinary graduates who are prepared for the future challenges of our profession.

Although these steps are discussed serially, in real life many of the decisions occur in parallel, or in a different order. This rearrangement is acceptable, as the steps are ultimately interdependent and the timing of their development may be a function of the college or school's needs or resources. It should also be noted that many of the items mentioned in these steps are discussed in greater detail in the chapters that follow.

Step 1: Identify the Overall Purpose of the Educational Program

The first step in curricular design should involve the preparation of a document that includes an ideological mission statement, expressing values, beliefs, and aspirations for a program. These values and aspirations should be derived from the professional, social, political, and cultural contexts of the institution (Grant, 2013). In this way, emerging local needs can be specifically identified and addressed in the curriculum, and may help counterbalance a sole focus on the requirements of national and international standards. Examples of mission statements applicable to veterinary programs can be found on the web sites of many veterinary colleges.

When approaching curricular planning, there is a temptation to assume that there is a shared understanding of the overall purpose or aim of the program. However, unless the terms that are employed are defined and are specific, misunderstandings will arise (Leinster, 2013). For example, it is unhelpful to have the stated aim of a program to be to "produce a good veterinarian," as this is too vague and begs the question of how a good veterinarian is defined!

Step 2: Determine the Specific Student Learning Outcomes or Competencies

One of the major emerging themes in medical education has been the recognition that curricular design should begin at the end (backwards design). In other words, the outcomes of the educational process should be specifically determined, then the curriculum designed to achieve these outcomes. This is in contrast to earlier approaches, where the content that faculty believed should be taught was arranged without regard for the end product. Implicit in this forward-thinking, input approach is that the focus is on the educational process regardless of the outcome.

This method utilizing backwards design began in the late 1980s, but has become more popular in the 2010s. However, there has been considerable debate regarding the definition of the end product, the most common terms being objectives, attributes, outcomes, and competencies. Specifically, people have argued about what the terms mean, how they differ, what they imply, and how they should be used. Of these terms, competencies have predominated in medical education and competency-based medical education (CBME) is now a primary driver for curricular planning (Harden, 2014). A similar movement has begun in veterinary education, and a number of competency frameworks relevant to veterinary practice have been developed in recent years (Bok *et al.*, 2011; Shung and Osburn, 2011; AVMA, 2014; RCVS, 2014).

In common curriculum parlance, a competency is a specific area of performance that can be described and measured (Sklar, 2015). Thus, the emphasis has shifted from "what the student knows" and "what the teacher does" to "what the student does" (Corbett and Whitcomb, 2004). This system has the added advantage of allowing student achievement to determine advancement, so that progression is defined by the demonstration of required competencies, rather than by time spent in a program (Prideaux, 2016).

However, CBME is not without its critics, who argue that this is a reductionist approach with a focus on the parts rather than the whole (Brooks, 2009). As a result, this educational model may have difficulty capturing the complex requirements of medical practice or the central skills of professional judgment, decision making, and clinical reasoning (Grant, 2013). Further, some critics believe that competency frameworks are too theoretical to be useful for teaching and assessment in daily practice. In response to these concerns, entrustable professional activities (EPAs) have recently been developed to work in tandem with competencies to produce a more 'holistic' basis for curricular design (Prideaux, 2016). Further information about CBME, especially how it relates to veterinary education, can be found in Part One, Chapter 2: Competency-Based Education.

Step 3: Determine the Content to Be Included

Historically, the starting point for curricular design and development was often content; that is, what faculty believed should be taught. However, there are two fundamental fallacies with this approach: teaching is not synonymous with learning, and the possession of knowledge of an area does not guarantee the ability to perform in that area (May and Silva-Fletcher, 2015). A shift to competency-based educational models

helps address this problem, as these models are based on clearly defined and measurable competencies, together with student demonstration that these have been achieved. In this way, the required competencies, rather than individual faculty expectations, drive curricular content.

This focus on competencies is particularly important in the age of the Internet and the expanding information available for learners. It is clear that curricular content can no longer include all the knowledge available in veterinary education. Furthermore, the length of time available for Doctor of Veterinary Medicine (DVM) programs (usually four years post degree, or five to six years post high school) is unlikely to lengthen given the concerns surrounding student educational debt. Therefore, the underpinning knowledge needed for students to develop the required competencies has to be identified, thus creating logical priorities for the content to be included in a curriculum.

There are a number of specific issues in relation to this point that deserve greater discussion.

Core and Elective Curricula

One model that is gaining some traction in veterinary education, and that may help with the expansion of knowledge, is a core/elective or core/tracking/elective curriculum. These curricula identify the content that is deemed to be core and that all students must acquire, then allow students to choose additional courses to gain deeper knowledge based on their personal preferences and career goals. In a tracking curriculum, the additional courses are determined by the specific track on which a student wishes to focus, for example livestock, small animal, or public corporate. Alternatively, all additional courses may be optional.

In this model, the first requirement is to determine what is core, with optional material being determined by the resources available, for example faculty interest and expertise. As discussed earlier, the core content should focus on the required competencies, but the issue remains of how to determine the competencies that should be core for all students. A number of ways have been used in medical education to answer this questions, ranging from modified Delphi processes and other formal consultations to statistical and epidemiological methods, or more informal consultation with various stakeholders (Grant, 2013). One approach that is gaining traction in medical schools is the identification of index cases or presentations that are based on the different ways in which the population comes into contact with healthcare professionals (critical incident technique; Pavlish, Brown-Saltzman, and So, 2015). The core knowledge and skills that students need within each discipline are determined by what they need to know and do in order to understand and manage these core clinical problems.

Whatever method is chosen, care should be taken that the content reflects a consensus of views, including those of specialists and generalists. Specialists alone should not be permitted to determine the core curricular content in their own discipline (Leinster, 2013). The core content should be well understood and publicized, and take into consideration the vision of the college or school and the timeframe available for delivery of the core material. Finally, this process must include consideration of accreditation requirements as well as materials that will be included in licensing exams, such as the NAVLE.

Content Overload

One of the major concepts to emerge from educational research in the last 40 years is the idea that students take different approaches to learning (Marton and Saljo, 1976). Briefly, students who take a deep approach have the intention of understanding, engaging with, operating in, and valuing the subject, while students who take a surface approach tend not to have the primary intention of becoming interested in or understanding the subject, but rather their motivation tends to be jumping through the necessary hoops in order to acquire the mark, or the grade, or the qualification (Biggs, 1999; Lublin, 2003). The enemy of deep learning in any discipline is content overload (Ramsden, 1992), which leads to the superficial acquisition

of facts, overwhelming any drive toward understanding and extracting meaning (May, 2008; May and Silva-Fletcher, 2015).

In conjunction with a competency-based approach to delineate and prioritize the core content to be included in a curriculum, the process of curricular mapping may assist with content overload. A comprehensive curricular map allows identification of material that should be included, as well as any uncoordinated rather than planned repetition, and, most importantly, redundant material that is irrelevant or not required. More discussion on curricular mapping can be found in Part One, Chapter 3: Curriculum Mapping.

"Just in Time" versus "Just in Case"

Another concept gaining increased attention in health sciences education is "just in time" teaching as opposed to "just in case". This concept acknowledges the greatly expanded knowledge available on the Internet and the important skill of information literacy, with which students are able to source and evaluate this information correctly. In this way, students can apply or adapt the information in appropriate contexts when it is needed ("just in time"). This compares to the more historical approach in transmission-focused models of veterinary education where faculty take sole responsibility for sourcing the information that they determine to be needed, verify the quality of the information, and ask students to remember it "just in case" they might one day require it. The "just in time" model still acknowledges that essential concepts are core, but these act as frameworks for knowledge sourced on a "just in time" basis in response to a specific challenge (May and Silva-Fletcher, 2015).

Step 4: Determine the Organization of the Content, Including the Sequence in Which It Is Covered

Once the content of the curriculum has been determined, the next step in curricular design is to decide how this content will be organized within the allotted timeframe. There is no absolutely correct order for courses in a veterinary curriculum, but there should be a transparent logic behind the arrangement. In addition, there may be some constraints that determine how much time may be allocated to a specific topic or subject area, and where in the curriculum it should be taught.

The first of these constraints may be the course structure of the university, which may influence how much time can be allocated to a course. For example, a university may have a credit system where a credit equates to a set number of hours of lectures and/or laboratory classes. In these situations, the subject area is allocated a number of credits that is roughly based on the content to be covered, but does not take into account the amount of time specifically required. For example, a subject may be given one credit, which might be equivalent to 15 hours, but only 10 hours may be required to cover the core material. However, with a credit system, all 15 hours would be dedicated to this subject. Such a situation may be exacerbated by systems where courses are traditionally "owned" by departments and the heads of department allocate the teaching time to members of the faculty as part of their teaching effort assignment, and the latter then fill the lecture and practical classes with material at their discretion. These courses may also be taught in isolation, without regard for the content of other courses. Taken together these processes may result in fragmented curricula, with omission, duplication, and particularly redundancy, together with non-coherent skill development.

Solutions for these issues could include larger, integrated courses, which may give more freedom for appropriate allotment of the time required for individual subjects or disciplines within a course. In addition, this process should be controlled at a college level, where a central course design team works together with discipline experts to ensure appropriate time allocation, correct sequencing of content, lack of duplication, omission, and redundancy, as well as progressive skill development. In this way, the teachers who will be delivering the curriculum still feel that they have a stake in the course and have been involved in decision-making, but

the decisions are ultimately made through a consensus process involving a multidisciplinary group.

The second issue is how the courses are organized within the curriculum, and a decision must be made whether to use a more traditional modular model, or an integrated approach. These options are not mutually exclusive, nor is one approach necessarily preferable to the other, and many curricula display elements of both depending on the resources available.

Modular Curricular Design

A module is a self-contained course or unit of study. The course should have its own outcomes or learning objectives, activities, and assessments. In most veterinary curricula, students take more than one course at a time, with the courses taught conjointly and with a logical timing and sequence. Further, the timing of the courses should be planned according to a rational progression of knowledge and skills through the curriculum, although this may also be dependent on the availability of resources. Currently, a modular design is the most common curricular model in veterinary education.

A downside to this model is that knowledge and skills may be presented in isolation, with integration of subject areas occurring later, often by the student themselves, through use of the concepts in clinical settings.

Integrated Curricular Design

One organizational model that is becoming increasingly popular in medical education is an integrated curriculum. At its most fundamental, integration is the organization of teaching material to interrelate or unify subjects frequently taught in separate academic courses or departments (Malik and Malik, 2011). This approach helps students combine the facts they have learned and develop holistic approaches to medical problems.

The adoption of an integrated model may involve either a significant or a complete reorganization of the curriculum, so decisions must be made about the framework around which the content will be integrated. Different approaches to achieving integration have been used with varying degrees of success, but the most common involve either vertical or horizontal integration or a mixture of both. These models, together with other models of integration, are discussed in greater detail in Part Two, Chapter 5: Integrated Learning. It must also be remembered that whatever the final structure of the course, integration can only take place at the level of the students' experience of learning. There is no point in integrating topics that are not coherent in their approach and level of difficulty.

Spiral Curriculum

Another organizational strategy that is frequently employed in curricular design is the concept of a spiral curriculum. The principal features of a spiral curriculum are the following:

- Topics, themes, or subjects are revisited on a number of occasions throughout the curriculum or program.
- Topics are revisited at increasing levels of difficulty.
- New learning is related to prior learning.
- The competence of the learner increases with each visit to the topic (Harden, 1999).

This spiral arrangement means that important themes are revisited, with continual development and reinforcement, over the duration of the program. Only by building a curricular structure based on increasing student challenge can progressive knowledge and skill development be fully realized (May and Silva-Fletcher, 2015).

Step 5: Determine the Educational Strategies or Learning Methods

There has been much discussion in medical education regarding the strategies that can be used in a curriculum, and the same can be said of veterinary education. In order to simplify the discussion, Harden developed the SPICES model (see Table 1.2) for planning the educational strategies to be included in a new curriculum, or evaluating those in an existing one (Harden, Sowden, and Dunn, 1984). Often the different strategies described in this model are seen as either "traditional" or "innovative," although in reality each strategy should not be seen as one or the other, but rather as a continuum.

The SPICES model includes choices between various strategies, described in what follows. An additional educational strategy, introduced by May and Silva-Fletcher, is included at the end of this section.

Student-Centered versus Teacher-Centered Learning

In student-centered learning models, students are given more responsibility for their own learning, rather than the teacher wholly deciding what they will learn. While student-centered learning is consistent with adult learning theories, teachers still have an extremely important role as facilitators of learning. Students should not be abandoned to their own learning; rather, they need appropriate guidance and support throughout the program. In this way the teacher functions as a facilitator of

Table 1.2 The SPICES model for educational strategies.

Innovative		Traditional
Student-centered	---	Teacher-centered
Problem-based	---	Information-oriented
Integrated or interprofessional	---	Subject or discipline-based
Community-based	---	Hospital-based
Elective-driven	---	Uniform (or core)
Systematic	---	Opportunistic

Source: Harden, 1984. Reproduced with permission of Wiley Blackwell.

learning, is intellectually critical, stimulating, and challenging, but within a learning context that emphasizes support and mutual respect (Grant, 2013). This shift away from teaching and toward learning is at the root of curricular models such as problem-based learning (PBL).

Inquiry-Based Learning versus Information-Oriented Learning

In order to achieve optimal learning outcomes, students should be actively engaged in their own learning. Strategies developed to try to optimize student engagement have included PBL and allied learning approaches (e.g., case-based learning, team-based learning, and task-based learning). In these learning paradigms, students explore scientific concepts in the context of clinical problems (or cases or tasks) and, rather than being provided with the knowledge (information-oriented learning), they establish their own knowledge and use it ultimately to solve clinical challenges. In this way, inquiry-based learning allows students to make connections between prior knowledge and new information, especially in the context of how they will use the information, and this facilitates knowledge storage and retrieval.

Problem-based learning, and allied strategies, may be employed in small groups, large groups, individualized learning, or with students working at a distance. The group approaches to learning are discussed further in Part Two, Chapter 6: Collaborative Learning. In addition, Harden and Davis developed 11 steps or stages that can be recognized in the continuum between inquiry-based learning and information-oriented learning (Harden and Davis, 1998).

Integration versus Subject- or Discipline-Based Learning

As discussed earlier in this chapter, medical education has moved from structuring the curriculum around the disciplines, first in basic sciences then in clinical medicine, to models where these are integrated.

In addition to integration within a curriculum between disciplines (horizontal integration) and between the basic and clinical sciences (vertical integration), there is also a move to interprofessional teaching, where integrated teaching and learning involve different health-care professionals, and where students look at a subject from the perspective of other professions as well as their own. This concept is discussed further in Part Two, Chapter 7: Teaching Interprofessionalism.

Community-Based Learning versus Veterinary Teaching Hospital

Traditionally, clinical teaching in veterinary programs has largely been conducted in veterinary teaching hospitals (VTHs) that are owned and run by a college. In these hospitals, significant emphasis is placed on specialty practice with secondary or tertiary patient care. More recently there has been a recognition that these experiences may not provide veterinary students with sufficient exposure to common or routine clinical cases and there has been a move toward primary care or community practices. These clinics may be situated within VTHs, within off-site practices owned by the college, or in practices at large that have partnered with colleges to provide this clinical learning experience.

There is more detailed discussion of the learning that may occur in veterinary teaching hospitals in Part Three, Chapter 12: Learning in the Veterinary Teaching Hospital, and that in community-based practices in Part Three, Chapter 13: Learning in Real-World Settings.

Elective versus Core

The curricular strategy involving core and elective courses has been discussed earlier in this chapter. As noted, electives are now firmly established as a valued component of the curriculum in most veterinary colleges and are important contributors to the individual student's learning outcomes. The main driving force for their development is that it is no longer possible for students to study in depth all topics in a curriculum, and elective courses offer students an opportunity to study areas of interest to them in greater detail and within the resources of the college.

Systematic versus Opportunistic Approach

This strategy refers to curricular planning in which an opportunistic approach involves faculty teaching what is of interest to them, and the cases to which students are exposed in the clinics are those that happen to be available (Harden, 2013). Once a curriculum becomes competency or outcome focused, this paradigm must shift to a more systematic approach to curricular planning to ensure that students have learning experiences that match the expected learning outcomes and that the core curriculum includes the competencies essential for graduation.

Scaffolded Active Learning in Veterinary Curricula

One curricular strategy that has been advocated to suit veterinary medical education is "scaffolded active learning" (May and Silva-Fletcher, 2015). In this model, core knowledge is provided through framework lectures, then additional knowledge is attained through context-related problem-solving, involving collaborative learning and case-based exercises, or self-directed learning. The intention of the model is that the interest stimulated by context-related problem-solving, and the associated active learning, will build on the framework knowledge, thereby allowing personal and integrated knowledge construction in a way that is similar to, but more efficient than, PBL. There are nine pedagogical principles that further underpin this

model (see Box 1.2). This model of teaching has been developed in a number of veterinary colleges and schools (May, 2008; Jaarsma, Scherpbier, and van Beukelen, 2009; Howell *et al.*, 2002).

Step 6: Determine Learning and Teaching Methods

Decisions about the learning and teaching methods to be used in a curriculum should flow from the planning of previous stages. For example, if a curriculum is to be student centered and problem based, then learning methods that encourage these approaches should be used.

It should be remembered there is no holy grail of instructional wizardry that will always provide an optimal learning outcome. In general, however, the teaching methods used in a curriculum should promote active rather than passive learning. Active learning occurs when students engage in activities that promote analysis, reflection, and problem-solving. Further, any educational method that includes an appropriate motivational context, a high degree of learner activity, interaction with peers and teachers, and a well-structured knowledge base will encourage a deep approach to learning. Conversely, any teaching or learning method, whether apparently learner centered or not, that has a heavy workload, high contact hours, excessive material, or an emphasis on coverage

---

Box 1.2: Focus on the pedagogical principles underpinning scaffolded active learning

May and Silva-Fletcher (2015) have offered a veterinary curricular model that promotes effective problem-solving, integrated knowledge, and clinical reasoning. This model is underpinned by nine pedagogical principles:

1) Outcomes-based curriculum design.
2) Valid and reliable assessments.
3) Active learning.
4) Integrated knowledge for action.
5) Tightly controlled core curriculum.
6) "Just in time" rather than "just in case" knowledge.
7) Vertical integration, the spiral curriculum, and sequential skills development.
8) Learning skills support.
9) Bridges from classroom to workplace.

expressed in the form of Miller's pyramid, with the outcome levels ranging from "knows how" to "mastery" (Miller, 1990). An illustration of Miller's pyramid is included in Part Four, Chapter 16: Performance and Workplace-Based Assessment. In curricular planning, the necessary clinical skills, as well as the expected levels, should be specified.

Step 8: Communicate the Curricular Design and Principles to All Stakeholders, Including Students

As already stated, designing a curriculum is a complex process and should involve documentation of the methodology, quality assurance, and recognition of all stakeholders. Failure to communicate the intended outcomes of the curriculum, and how the design and learning methods will achieve these outcomes, is a recipe for problems during curricular design and/or revision.

Communication may be in many forms and to a variety of stakeholders. Particular attention should be provided to communication with students, who should have a clear understanding of what the learning outcome should be at every level of the curriculum, the range of learning experiences and opportunities provided to help them attain these outcomes, how they may shape their learning experiences to suit their personal needs, and feedback as to whether they have attained the required outcomes (Harden, 2013). Documentation that may help to communicate this information can include course syllabi, course study guides, a curricular map, and a handbook of student policies and procedures that includes guidelines for academic progression.

Step 9: Include Consideration of the Educational Environment

Increasingly in medical education there is a realization that the educational environment, or "climate" in which student learning takes place, is a key aspect of the curriculum (Genn, 2001). Traditionally, a curriculum has been described through the content outlined in the syllabi and the listed topics that are covered in lectures, laboratory classes, and other learning opportunities. However, what is learned in a program is rarely solely that which is stated within an institution's documents. Rather, the curriculum may be thought of as the "taught curriculum" (what the student is taught), the "learned curriculum" (what the student learns), and the "hidden curriculum" (the student's informal learning that is different from what is taught). In particular, the hidden curriculum is influenced by the educational environment in which the learning takes place. Further information about this topic is included in Part Seven, Chapter 33: The Hidden Curriculum.

Measurement of the educational environment should be part of ongoing curricular evaluation. Tools are available to assess the educational environment, such as the Dundee Ready Education Environment Measure (DREEM; Roff, 2005), and have been validated in veterinary programs (Pelzer, Hodgson, and Werre, 2014). More information about this and other tools used to assess the educational environment is provided in Part Seven, Chapter 32: Student Learning Environment.

Step 10: Determine How the Curriculum Will Be Managed, Including Resource Allocation

With the increasing complexity of veterinary education, attention to how a curriculum is managed has become more important. This complexity includes the traditional resources that may be required to support a veterinary curriculum, such as sufficient numbers of faculty and staff with appropriate qualifications across all major species and subject areas; access to appropriate facilities, including lecture halls that are big enough to hold the entire class at one time and have appropriate information technology resources; laboratory spaces, animal handling facilities, and clinical skills laboratories; and VTHs that are either included within the college or distributed in the community. Curricula with newer modalities of teaching such as PBL may require additional resources, including increased numbers of faculty and tutorial spaces to house small-group teaching. Consideration in curricular design must also be given to the increasing pressures on faculty regarding their clinical duties, teaching responsibilities, and research commitments; growing demands and higher student numbers at a time of financial constraints; as well as increasing requirements for transparency and accountability on the part of accrediting agencies as well as the general public.

In order to manage the increasing complexity of medical programs, Harden developed a number of recommendations, which can be equally applied to veterinary programs. These are outlined in Box 1.3. Of particular importance is the central management of the curriculum, which is also mandated in the accreditation standards of the AVMA COE.

Curricular Review and Reform

As discussed in the introduction to this chapter, curricula in veterinary medicine must refocus on the fundamental skills required of all graduates and incorporate the principles of learning that will achieve these skills. Thus, most veterinary curricula in North America are presently undergoing review, followed by either modification of the existing curriculum, or redesign

and implementation of a new curriculum. Irrespective of the path chosen, this process in an academic environment is not easy, as either path will involve change. Change in medical education has been described as neither enduring nor certain (Shuster and Reynolds, 1998) and the widely used phrase "reform without change" has represented the outcome of many medical education reform efforts (Matson *et al.*, 2013).

Classically, review is defined as the act of carefully looking at or examining the quality or condition of something or someone, or a report that gives someone's opinion about the quality of something. Reform is defined as the improvement of something by removing faults or problems. When applied to a curriculum, a review is usually an in-depth evaluation of either components of the curriculum or the curriculum as a whole, with the end result being to determine what is working well and what could be improved. Generally, reform is the process that is undertaken to correct problems, in the belief that there will be a positive change. Change can be considered as the transformation of an individual or a system from one state to another, a process that may be initiated by internal factors, external forces, or both.

A widespread barrier to reform of medical education is faculty resistance, often because faculty are more vested in maintaining the

---

Box 1.3: How to implement curricular management strategies

- Ensure that responsibilities and resources for teaching are allocated at a college rather than departmental level.
- Develop a curriculum committee with faculty, staff, and student representation, which is responsible for planning and implementing the curriculum.
- Appoint a teaching dean or director of veterinary education who has a commitment to curriculum development and implementation.
- Appoint faculty with particular expertise in curriculum planning, teaching methods,

and assessment to support work on the curriculum.
- Recognize the time and contributions of faculty to teaching and learning.
- Introduce a required faculty development program involving "teaching the teacher."
- Allocate responsibility to an independent group for academic standards and quality assurance.

Source: After Harden (2013).

Figure 1.3 Curricular evaluation leading to curricular improvement.

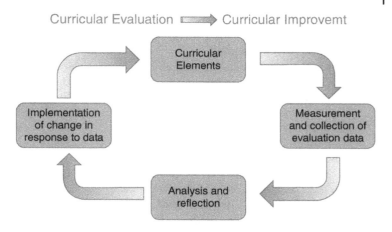

Curricular Evaluation ⟹ Curricular Improvemt

Curricular Elements

Measurement and collection of evaluation data

Analysis and reflection

Implementation of change in response to data

Lovato and Wall, 2014; Harden and Laidlaw, 2012).

Conclusion

Veterinary curricular design, revision, and reform are all complex processes requiring significant time, effort, and resources. All studies in medical education that discuss the design of new curricula, or reform of existing ones, report how difficult it is to accomplish. One such study reported: "it requires dedication, hard work, and the ability to recover when we inevitably falter. We also found that change represents a complex interaction among many elements and that individuals and chance play critical roles. Last, we learned to expect the unexpected: No matter what we anticipated, and how we prepared, we were continually surprised by the turn of events" (Krackov and Mennin, 1998, p. S3).

References

ACGME (2013) *Glossary of Terms*. Accreditation Council for Graduate Medical Education. https://www.acgme.org/Portals/0/PDFs/ab_ACGMEglossary.pdf (accessed January 24, 2016).

Anderson, L.W., and Krathwohl, D.R. (2001) *A Taxonomy for Learning, Teaching, and Assessing: A Revision of Bloom's Taxonomy of Educational Objectives*, Longman, New York.

AVMA (2014) *Accreditation Policies and Procedures*. American Veterinary Medical Association. https://www.avma.org/ProfessionalDevelopment/Education/Accreditation/Colleges/Pages/coe-pp-requirements-of-accredited-college.aspx (accessed December 31, 2015).

Biggs, J. (1999) What the student does: Teaching for enhanced learning. *Higher Education Research and Development*, **18**, 57–75.

Bland, C.J., Starnaman, S., Wersal, L., Moorehead-Rosenberg, L., Zonia, S., and Henry, R. (2000) Curricular change in medical schools: How to succeed. *Academic Medicine*, **75**, 575–594.

Bloom, S.W. (1989) The medical school as a social organization: The sources of resistance to change. *Medical Education*, **23**, 228–241.

Bok, H.G., Jaarsma, D.A., Teunissen, P.W., van der Vleuten, C.P.M., and van Buekelen, P. (2011) Development and validation of a competency framework for veterinarians. *Journal of Veterinary Medical Education*, **38**, 262–269.

Brooks, M. (2009) Medical education and the tyranny of competency. *Perspectives in Biology and Medicine*, **52**, 90–102.

Christakis, N.A. (1995) The similarity and frequency of proposals to reform US medical education. Constant concerns. *JAMA*, **274**, 706–711.

Cohen, J., Dannefer, E.F., Seidel, H.M., *et al.* (1994) Medical education change: A detailed study of six medical schools. *Medical Education*, **28**, 350–360.

Corbett, E.C., and Whitcomb, M.E. (2004) *The AAMC Project on the Clinical Education of Medical Students: Clinical Skills*, AAMC, Washington, DC.

Dannefer, E.F., Johnston, M.A., and Krackov, S.K. (1998) Communication and the process of educational change. *Academic Medicine*, **73**, S16–S23.

Frye, A.W., and Hemmer, P.A. (2012) Program evaluation models and related theories: AMEE guide no. 67. *Medical Teacher*, **34**, e288–e299.

Genn, J. (2001) AMEE medical education guide no. 23 (part 1): Curriculum, environment, climate, quality and change in medical education: A unifying perspective. *Medical Teacher*, **23**, 337–344.

Gerrity, M.S., and Mahaffy, J. (1998) Evaluating change in medical school curricula: How did we know where we were going? *Academic Medicine*, **73**, S55–S59.

Grant, J. (2013) Principles of curriculum design, in *Understanding Medical Education: Evidence, Theory and Practice*, 2nd edn (ed. T. Swanwick), Wiley-Blackwell, London, pp. 31–46.

Harden, R.M. (1999) What is a spiral curriculum? *Medical Teacher*, **21**, 141–143.

Harden, R.M. (2001) The learning environment and the curriculum. *Medical Teacher*, **23**, 335–336.

Harden, R.M. (2013) Curriculum planning and development, in *A Practical Guide for Medical Teachers*, 4th edn (eds J.A. Dent and R.M. Harden), Churchill Livingstone, Edinburgh, pp. 10–16.

Harden, R.M. (2014) Progression in competency-based education. *Medical Education*, **48**, 838.

Harden, R.M., and Davis, M.H. (1998) The continuum of problem-based learning. *Medical Teacher*, **20**, 317–322.

Harden, R.M., and Laidlaw, J.M. (2012) Evaluating the curriculum, in *Essential Skills for a Medical Teacher: An Introduction to Teaching and Learning in Medicine* (eds R.M. Harden and J.M. Laidlaw), Churchill Livingstone, Edinburgh, pp. 276–283.

Harden, R.M., Sowden, S., and Dunn, W. (1984) Educational strategies in curriculum development: The SPICES model. *Medical Education*, **18**, 284–297.

Howell, N.E., Lane, I.F., Brace, J.J., and Shull, R.M. (2002) Integration of problem-based learning in a veterinary medical curriculum: First year experiences with application-based learning exercises at the University of Tennessee College of Veterinary Medicine. *Journal of Veterinary Medical Education*, **29**, 169–175.

Jaarsma, D.A., Scherpbier, A.J., and van Beukelen, P. (2009) A retrospective analysis of veterinary medical curriculum development in the Netherlands. *Journal of Veterinary Medical Education*, **36**, 232–240.

Kassebaum, D.G., Cutler, E.R., and Eaglen, R.H. (1997) The influence of accreditation on educational change in U.S. medical schools. *Academic Medicine*, **72**, 1127–1133.

Kaufman, A. (1998) Leadership and governance. *Academic Medicine*, **73**, S11–S15.

Kotter, J.P. (1996) *Leading Change*, Harvard Business School Press, Boston, MA.

Krackov, S.K., and Mennin, S.P. (1998) A story of change. *Academic Medicine*, **73**, S1–S3.

Krathwohl, D.R. (2002) A revision of Bloom's taxonomy: An overview. *Theory into Practice*, **41**, 212–264.

Leinster, S.J. (2013) The undergraduate curriculum and clinical teaching in the early years, in *A Practical Guide for Medical Teachers*, 4th edn (eds J.A. Dent and R.M. Harden), Churchill Livingstone, London, pp. 16–22.

Lindberg, M.A. (1998) The process of change: Stories of the journey. *Academic Medicine*, **73**, S4–S10.

Loeser, H., O'Sullivan, P., and Irby, D.M. (2007) Leadership lessons from curricular change at the University of California, San Francisco, School of Medicine. *Academic Medicine*, **82**, 324–330.

Lovato, C., and Wall, D. (2014) Programme evaluation: Improving practice, influencing policy and decision-making, in *Understanding Medical Education: Evidence, Theory, and Practice*, 2nd edn (eds T. Swanwick and Association for the Study of Medical Education), Wiley-Blackwell, Chichester, pp. 385–399.

Lublin, J. (2003) *Good Practices in Teaching and Learning: Deep, Surface and Strategic Approaches to Learning*, Center for Teaching and Learning, University College Dublin, Belfield.

Malik, A.S., and Malik, R.H. (2011) Twelve tips for developing an integrated curriculum. *Medical Teacher*, **33**, 99–104.

Marton, F., and Saljo, R. (1976) On qualitative differences in learning. I-Outcome and process. *British Journal of Educational Psychology*, **46**, 4–11.

Matson, C., Davis, A., Stephens, M., and ADFM Educational Transformation Committee (2013) Another century of "reform without change?" *Annals of Family Medicine*, **11**, 581–582.

May, S.A. (2008) Modern veterinary graduates are outstanding, but can they get better? *Journal of Veterinary Medical Education*, **35**, 573–580.

May, S.A., and Silva-Fletcher, A. (2015) Scaffolded active learning: Nine pedagogical principles for building a modern veterinary curriculum, *Journal of Veterinary Medical Education*, **42**, 332–339.

MERRIAM-WEBSTER (2016) *Definition of Curriculum* [Online]. http://www.merriam-webster.com/dictionary/curriculum:Merriam-Webster (accessed December 31, 2015).

Michaelsen, L.K., Davidson, N., and Major, C. (2014) Team based learning practices and principles in comparison with cooperative learning and problem based learning. *Journal on Excellence in College Teaching*, **25**, 3–15.

Miller, G.E. (1990) The assessment of clinical skills/competence/performance. *Academic Medicine*, **65**, S63–S67.

Pavlish, C., Brown-Saltzman, K., and So, L. (2015) Avenues of action in ethically complex situations: A critical incident study. *Journal of Nursing Administration*, **45**, 311–318.

Pelzer, J.M., Hodgson, J.L., and Werre, S.R. (2014) Veterinary students' perceptions of their learning environment as measured by the Dundee Ready Education Environment Measure. *BMC Research Notes*, **24**, 170.

Prideaux, D. (2016) The emperor's new wardrobe: The whole and the sum of the parts in curriculum design. *Medical Education*, **50**, 3–23.

Ramsden, P. (1992) *Learning to Teach in Higher Education*, Routledge, London.

RCVS (2014) *Day One Competencies*. Royal College of Veterinary Surgeons. http://www.rcvs.org.uk/document-library/day-one-competences/ (accessed December 28, 2015).

Robins, L.S., White, C.B., and Fantone, J.C. (2000) The difficulty of sustaining curricular reforms: A study of "drift" at one school, *Academic Medicine*, **75**, 801–805.

Roff, S. (2005) The Dundee Ready Educational Environment Measure (DREEM): A generic instrument for measuring students' perceptions of undergraduate health professions curricula. *Medical Teacher*, **27**, 322–325.

Shung, G., and Osburn, B.I. (2011) The North American Veterinary Medical Education Consortium (NAVMEC) looks to veterinary education for the future. Roadmap for veterinary medical education in the 21st century: Responsive, collaborative, flexible. *Journal of Veterinary Medical Education*, **38**, 320–327.

Shuster, A.L., and Reynolds, R.C. (1998) Medical education: Can we do better? *Academic Medicine*, **73**, Sv–Svi.

Sklar, D.P. (2015) Competencies, milestones, and entrustable professional activities: What they are, what they could be. *Academic Medicine*, **90**, 395–397.

Wiles, J. (2009) *Leading Curriculum Development*, Corwin Press, Newbury Park, CA.

2

Competency-Based Education

Harold G.J. Bok[1] and A. Debbie C. Jaarsma[2]

[1] Faculty of Veterinary Medicine, Utrecht University, The Netherlands
[2] Faculty of Medical Sciences, University of Groningen, The Netherlands

---

 Box 2.1: Key messages

- For competency-based education to be successful, it is essential to focus on implementation strategies and faculty development.
- A learning culture facilitating the conditions and opportunities for the exchange of high-quality feedback to occur is essential in competency-based education.

- Learning outcomes should be constructively aligned throughout the curriculum.
- Performance outcomes and programs of assessment should be framed on authentic learning activities.
- In competency-based education learners need to be active agents seeking performance-relevant information.

Introduction

After graduation, veterinary professionals need to possess relevant attributes to face society's current and future needs. Therefore, designing veterinary curricula that guide students' competency development on the trajectory from novice student to veterinary professional is one of the major responsibilities of any veterinary school. In this chapter we will describe what such a competency-based training program could look like and provide some design and implementation guidelines based on our own experiences with competency-based veterinary education.

The Changing Role of Veterinary Professionals in Healthcare

Up until the beginning of the twentieth century, veterinary medicine was mainly focused on curative medicine concerning cattle and horses, relevant to transportation and agriculture. From the 1950s on, companion animal veterinary medicine became an important part of daily practice, as was already forecast by Christian Petersen in 1937 in his sculpture *The Gentle Doctor* (Prasse, Heider, and Maccabe, 2001). Due to changing societal needs and global interdependence during the last decades, veterinary professionals increasingly have been placed in a central position in the

Veterinary Medical Education: A Practical Guide, First Edition. Edited by Jennifer L. Hodgson and Jacquelyn M. Pelzer.
© 2017 John Wiley & Sons, Inc. Published 2017 by John Wiley & Sons, Inc.

feedback and better evaluate students' development over time (van der Zwet, 2014). Further information regarding giving and receiving feedback can be found in Part Four, Chapter 17: Feedback.

Student Learning

Increased attention should be paid to the crucial role that students have in self-directing their own education (Driessen, Overeem, and van Tartwijk, 2010). Therefore, students also need to be trained and informed about how to optimize their performance in competency-based veterinary education.

- Students need to be aware of the factors influencing their feedback-seeking behavior in the clinical workplace. In addition, they need to be skilled in seeking and providing feedback. As students are working in teams, peer feedback is an important aspect of daily practice.
- It cannot be overemphasized that in order for students to learn and develop into competent professionals, credible, high-quality feedback is of the utmost importance. In accordance, we underline the importance of making students aware of the fact that reflective and self-directed behavior, active

participation, and increased responsibilities are essential aspects of making a smooth transition into clinical practice. Students therefore need to be empowered to keep asking for performance-relevant information that allows them to become competent veterinary professionals.

Conclusion

Just like any major curriculum change, the implementation of a competency-based approach to learning and assessment in veterinary education has its challenges. Therefore, best practices should be shared and further research should focus on developing effective implementation strategies. In addition, the international veterinary education community should aim at developing a shared understanding of what a competent veterinary professional comprehends. Together with the guidelines and experiences described in this chapter, this would provide direction for designing undergraduate and postgraduate veterinary CBE curricula, and could enable international and interdisciplinary collaboration.

References

AVMA (2008) *One Health: A New Professional Imperative*, One Health Initiative Task Force, American Veterinary Medical Association, Schaumburg, IL.

AVMA (2014) COE Accreditation Policies and Procedures: Requirements, https://www.avma.org/ProfessionalDevelopment/Education/Accreditation/Colleges/Pages/coe-pp-requirements-of-accredited-college.aspx (accessed October 21, 2016).

Biggs, J., and Tang, C. (2011) *Teaching for Quality Learning at University*, 4th edn, Society for Research into Higher Education and Open University Press, Buckingham.

Bok, H.G.J. (2014) Competency-based veterinary education: An integrative approach to learning and assessment. PhD thesis. Utrecht University.

Bok, H.G.J., and Teunissen, P.W. (2013) Patients and learners: Time for a re-evaluation of our goals in bringing them together. *Medical Education*, **47** (**12**), 1157–1159.

Bok, H.G.J., Jaarsma, A.D.C., Spruijt A., *et al.* (2016) Feedback-giving behaviour in performance evaluations during clinical clerkships. *Medical Teacher*, **38** (**1**), 88–95.

Bok, H.G.J., Jaarsma, A.D.C., Teunissen, P.W., *et al.* (2011) Development and validation of a veterinary competency framework. *Journal of Veterinary Medical Education*, **38** (**3**), 262–269.

Bok, H.G.J., Teunissen P.W., Favier R.P., *et al.* (2013) Programmatic assessment of competency-based workplace learning: When theory meets practice. *BMC Medical Education*, **13**, 123.

Bok, H.G.J., Teunissen P.W., Spruijt A., *et al.* (2013) Clarifying students' feedback-seeking behaviour within the clinical workplace. *Medical Education*, **47** (3), 282–291.

Brown, J.P., and Silverman, J.D. (1999) The current and future market for veterinarians and veterinary medical services in the United States. *Journal of the American Veterinary Medical Association*, **215** (2), 161–183.

Carraccio, C.L., and Englander, R. (2013) From Flexner to competencies: Reflections on a decade and the journey ahead. *Academic Medicine*, **88** (8), 1067–1073.

Carraccio, C.L., Wolfsthal, S.D., Englander, R., *et al.* (2002) Shifting paradigms: From Flexner to competencies. *Academic Medicine*, **77**, 361–367.

Collins, A. (2006) Cognitive apprenticeship, in *The Cambridge Handbook of the Learning Sciences* (ed. R. Sawyer), Cambridge University Press, Cambridge, pp. 47–60.

Cron, W.L., Slocum, J.V., Goodnight, D.B., and Volk, J.O. (2000) Executive summary of the Brakke management and behavior study. *Journal of the American Veterinary Medical Association*, **217** (3), 332–338.

Dornan, T. (2006) Experienced based learning: Learning clinical medicine in workplaces. Maastricht University, Maastricht, The Netherlands.

Driessen, E.W., Overeem, K., and van Tartwijk, J. (2010) Learning from practice: Mentoring, feedback, and portfolios, in *Medical Education, Theory and Practice* (eds T. Dornan, K. Mann, A. Scherpbier, and J. Spencer), Churchill Livingstone, Edinburgh, pp. 211–227.

Durning, S.J., and Artino, A.R. (2011) Situativity theory: A perspective on how participants and the environment can interact: AMEE guide no. 52. *Medical Teacher*, **33** (3), 188–199.

EAEVE-ESEVT (2016) *Manual of Standard Operating Procedures*, http://www.eaeve.org/fileadmin/downloads/SOP/ESEVT__Uppsala__SOP_May_2016.pdf (accessed December 2, 2016).

Frank, J.R., Mungroo, R., Ahmad Y., *et al.* (2010) Toward a definition of competency-based education in medicine: A systematic review of published definitions. *Medical Teacher*, **32**, 631–637.

Frank, J.R., Snell, L., Ten Cate, O., *et al.* (2010) Competency-based medical education: Theory to practice. *Medical Teacher*, **32** (8), 638–645.

Govaerts, M.J.B., van de Wiel, M.W.J., and van der Vleuten, C.P.M. (2013) Quality of feedback following performance assessments: Does assessor expertise matter? *European Journal of Training and Development*, **37** (1), 105–125.

Harden, R.M., and Laidlaw, J.M. (2012) *Essential Skills for a Medical Teacher: An Introduction to Teaching and Learning in Medicine*, Churchill Livingstone Elsevier, Edinburgh.

Hattie, J. (2009) The black box of tertiary assessments: An impeding revolution, in *Tertiary Assessment and Higher Education Student Outcomes: Policy, Practice and Research* (eds L.H. Meyer, S. Davidson, H. Anderson, *et al.*), Ako Aotearoa, Wellington.

Heeneman, S., Oudkerk Pool, A., Schuwirth, L.W.T., *et al.* (2015) The impact of programmatic assessment on student learning: theory versus practice. *Medical Education*, **49** (5), 487–498.

Hodgson, J.L., Pelzer, J.M., and Inzana, K.D. (2013) Beyond NAVMEC: Competency-based veterinary education and assessment of the professional competencies. *Journal of Veterinary Medical Education*, **40** (2), 102–118.

Holmboe, E.S., and Batalden, P. (2015) Achieving the desired transformation: Thoughts on next steps for outcomes-based medical education. *Academic Medicine*, **90** (9), 1215–1223.

Jaarsma, D.A.D.C., Dolmans, D.H.J.M., Scherpbier, A.J.J.A., *et al.* (2008) Preparation for practice by veterinary school: A comparison of the perceptions of alumni from a traditional and an innovative curriculum. *Journal of Veterinary Medical Education*, **35**, 431–438.

Kolb, D.A. (1984) *Experiential Learning: Experience as the Source of Learning and Development*, Prentice-Hall, Englewood Cliffs, NJ.

Lave, J., and Wenger, E. (1991) *Situated Learning: Legitimate Peripheral Participation*, Cambridge University Press, Cambridge.

Lewis, R.E., and Klausner, J.S. (2003) Nontechnical competencies underlying career success as a veterinarian. *Journal of the American Veterinary Medical Association*, **222** (**12**), 1690–1696.

Lineberry, M., Park, Y.S., Cook, D.A., and Yudkowsky, R. (2015) Making the case for mastery learning assessments: Key issues in validation and justification. *Academic Medicine*, **90** (**11**), 1445–1450.

McGaghie, W.C., Barsuk, J.H., and Cohen, E.R. (2015) Dissemination of an innovative mastery learning curriculum grounded in implementation science principles: A case study. *Academic Medicine*, **90** (**11**), 1487–1494.

McGaghie, W.C., Miller, G.E., Sajid, A.W., *et al.* (1978) Competency-based curriculum development in medical education: An introduction. World Health Organization, Geneva. *Public Health Paper 68*.

Prasse, K.W., Heider, L.E., and Maccabe, A.T. (2001) Envisioning the future of veterinary medicine: The imperative for change in veterinary medical education. *Journal of the American Veterinary Medical Association*, **231** (**9**), 1340–1342.

Pritchard, W.R. (ed.) (1988) *Future Directions for Veterinary Medicine: Report of the Pew National Veterinary Educational Program*, Duke University, Durham, NC.

RCSV (2015) *Day One Competencies*, http://www .rcvs.org.uk/document-library/day-one-competences (accessed October 21, 2016).

Soanes, C., and Stevenson A. (eds) (2005) *The Oxford Dictionary of English*, rev. edn, Oxford University Press, Oxford.

Summerlee, A.J.S. (2010) Gazing into the crystal ball: Where should the veterinary profession go next? *Journal of Veterinary Medical Education*, **37** (**4**), 328–332.

Ten Cate, O., and Scheele F. (2007) Competency-based postgraduate training: Can we bridge the gap between theory and clinical practice? *Academic Medicine*, **82** (**6**), 542–547.

Ten Cate, O., Chen, C., Hoff, R., *et al.* (2015) Curriculum development for the workplace using entrustable professional activities (EPAs): AMEE guide no. 99. *Medical Teacher*, **37** (**11**), 983–1002.

Teunissen, P.W. (2009) Unraveling learning by doing: A study of workplace learning in postgraduate medical education. PhD thesis. VU Medical Center, Amsterdam.

Teunissen, P.W., and Bok, H.G.J. (2013) Believing is seeing: How people's beliefs influence goals, emotions and behaviour. *Medical Education*, **47** (**11**), 1064–1072.

van der Vleuten, C.P.M., Schuwirth, L.W.T., Driessen, E.W., *et al.* (2012) A model for programmatic assessment fit for purpose. *Medical Teacher*, **34**, 205–214.

van der Zwet, J. (2014) Identity, interaction, and power. Explaining the affordance of doctor-student interaction during clerkships. PhD thesis. Maastricht University.

Watling, C.J., Driessen, E.W., van der Vleuten, C.P.M., *et al.* (2013) Beyond individualism: Professional culture and its influence on feedback. *Medical Education*, **47** (**6**), 585–594.

Willis, N.G., Monroe, F.A., Potworeski, J.A., *et al.* 2007. Envisioning the future of veterinary medical education: The Association of American Veterinary Medical Colleges foresight project, final report. *Journal of Veterinary Medical Education*, **34** (**1**), 1–41.

3

Curriculum Mapping

Karen Dyer Inzana

Virginia-Maryland College of Veterinary Medicine, Virginia Tech, USA

 Box 3.1: Key messages

The goals of curriculum mapping should be to:

- Ensure coverage of content while identifying redundancies.
- Demonstrate alignment of curricular learning outcomes with learning activities and assessments.

- Create an avenue for communication and reflection on curricular issues.

Introduction

Pressure from accrediting agents for curricula to focus on student achievement rather than the educational process has driven curricular reform in all health professions, including veterinary medicine. Veterinary educators are currently striving for better, more effective means of developing professionals who are competent to take on the many challenges of modern veterinary practice on graduation. Curriculum mapping is a critical tool to facilitate educational reform. When used to its fullest potential, a well-designed curriculum map should ensure appropriate coverage of content, align teaching and learning with curriculum goals, improve integration across the curriculum, and facilitate demonstration of outcomes to external stakeholders and accrediting agencies (Harden,

2001; Bell, Ellaway, and Rhind, 2009). However, there are additional benefits since the process itself creates an environment for collaboration, reflection on practice, and discussion of individual and collective beliefs about not only what is being taught, but how and why it is being taught (Bester and Scholtz, 2012; Jacobs, 1997; Udelhofen, 2005; Uchiyama and Radin, 2009).

The concept of curriculum mapping was originated in the 1980s by Fenwick English as a means of documenting the learning activities occurring in elementary and high schools (English, 1980). Heidi Hayes Jacobs expanded this concept to an electronic format and has, alongside Susan Udelhofen, become a leading figure in advancing curriculum mapping in K-12 education (Jacobs, 1997; Udelhofen, 2005). While its roots are in elementary education, curriculum mapping has become commonplace in

Veterinary Medical Education: A Practical Guide, First Edition. Edited by Jennifer L. Hodgson and Jacquelyn M. Pelzer.
© 2017 John Wiley & Sons, Inc. Published 2017 by John Wiley & Sons, Inc.

medical education (Willett, 2008; Ellaway *et al.*, 2014). In fact, the Data Collection Instrument required by the Liaison Committee on Medical Education (LCME) has become so lengthy and detailed, it is almost impossible to address all the information required for medical school accreditation without an electronic curriculum map (LCME, 2015). In 1999, the American Association of Medical Colleges (AAMC) released an online curriculum management and information tool (CurrMIT) designed to facilitate curriculum data collection and reporting (Cohen, 2000; Salas *et al.*, 2003; Cottrell, Linger, and Shumway, 2004). Unfortunately, the format of CurrMIT proved too rigid to accommodate the wide variety of medical school structures so, with the help of MedBiquitous, AAMC created a newer data based called Curriculum Inventory and Reports (CIR; AAMC, 2016). Rather than being a tool to enter curricular data directly, CIR became a tool to house and compare data from different medical education programs (Ellaway *et al.*, 2014). It was designed to receive data from a variety of management systems and link individual school learning outcomes with an overarching competency framework (Englander *et al.*, 2013). CIR is able to generate a variety of reports for the LCME from the data entered, but also can compare one school's data with dozens of other programs. In the 2015 reporting year, 135 medical colleges in the United States and Canada used CIR to catalog their curriculum structure, content, and delivery methods as well as their different assessment methods, providing an unprecedented opportunity to compare approaches and benchmark best practices in medical education.

Getting Started

Step 1: Deciding on Content

The most common content elements in a curriculum map include the sequencing of courses, the course goals or objectives, the learning activities that comprise a course with the intended learning objectives attached to each of these activities, and the assessment tools used to measure these objectives. While the aim of true competency-based educational curricula is to de-emphasize time-based training (Frank *et al.*, 2010), the American Veterinary Medical Association's (AVMA) Council on Education (COE) accreditation policies and procedures require that all accredited veterinary colleges contain a minimum of four academic years of education, at least one year of which consists of hands-on clinical education. Therefore, most veterinary schools have a relatively rigid sequence of preclinical and clinical instruction. Mapping in a veterinary context typically is based on the sequence in which courses are delivered during Year 1, Year 2, and so on. Using the curriculum calendar as a starting point not only provides some organization for the map, but constitutes a critical element of how a given course content relates to both previous and future content.

Step 2: Selecting the Database

There are a number of web-based databases that have been developed for the purpose of curriculum mapping. A list of those programs that were developed primarily for medical education and integrate with the CIR is provided in Table 3.1.

It is unlikely that there is a single best curriculum management system. The choice will depend on the program budget, the availability of information technology (IT) support, as well as the need for additional features provided by the supplier. It should be noted that curriculum management software is different from a learning management system (LMS). While the terminology is still somewhat imprecise, LMSs are designed to support the delivery and administration of courses, but do not support the indexing of the multiple data sets necessary to build a curriculum map (Steketee, 2015). Common examples of LMSs are Moodle, Edmodo, Infrastructure, Canvas, and Blackboard (Fenton, 2016). However, two of the curriculum management sytems listed (TUSK and 4iQ) include many features of a traditional LMS and an additional two (Illios and Entrada) advertise easy integration with commonly used

Table 3.1 Software utilized for curriculum mapping in medical education.

Name	Web site	Notes
Illios	http://meded.ucsf.edu/tee/ilios-curriculum-management	• Non-profit, open-source MIT (management and information tool) • Integrates with online course learning management systems, include Moodle, Blackboard, and Canvas
TUSK	http://tusk.tufts.edu/about/overview	• Non-profit • Online course learning management system integrated with curriculum management
4iQ	www.4iqsolutions.com	• Commercial • Online course learning management system integrated with curriculum management
ALLOFE	www.allofe.com	• Commercial suite of programs with secure testing features, scheduling, and student data management
E*Value	www.medhub.com	• Commercial • Scheduling • Student data management
Entrada	www.entrada-project.org	• Open source or commercial • Scheduling • Student data management • Integrates with learning management systems
Knowledge 4 You	knowledge4you.com	• Commercial • Scheduling • Student data management
LCMS+	lcmsplus.com	• Commercial • Scheduling • Student data management
Medhub	www.medhub.com	• Commercial • Scheduling • Student data management
New Innovations	https://www.new-innov.com/pub/	• Commercial • Scheduling • Student data management
OASIS	www.schillingconsulting.com	• Commercial • Scheduling • Student data management
One45	www.one45.com	• Commercial • Scheduling • Student data management
OpalQM	www.opalqm.com	• Commercial • Scheduling • Student data management

LMSs. Another system, ALLOFE, features a suite of different platforms that, in addition to a curriculum management system (ecurriculum), includes a patient encounter and procedure tracking system (eCLAS), rotation scheduling (eduschedule), a document management system for items such as site agreement forms, preceptor information, and student immunization (ekeeper), a clinical and faculty evaluation platform (evaluate), and an online testing resource complete with browser lockdown and question data analytics (examn). The remainder of the programs listed in Table 3.1 are commercial programs designed to manage clinical scheduling, disseminate and collate clinical evaluation tools, and function as a curriculum management tool.

Step 3: Entering the Data

There are two approaches to how the appropriate data is entered into the curriculum management system: either individual instructors enter their own data, or data is entered via a centralized source. There are several benefits to having the individuals most familiar with the learning events enter the data. Ideally, instructors who engage with the process will not only enter a more complete set of data, but in doing so will be encouraged to reflect on the alignment of course outcomes with learning opportunities and assessment techniques. Unfortunately, this not always perceived favorably by all faculty, leaving gaps and inaccuracies within the map.

The second approach is to have a centralized person enter the data gathered from a combination of course syllabi, course artifacts housed in LMSs, and personal interviews with course instructors. This approach may ensure more consistent data entry, but is extremely time consuming. If material could be directly imported from LMSs, it would avoid redundant efforts by faculty and staff as well as maintain the most current representation of curriculum content. This would be a strong argument for platforms where the two systems are integrated, because, above all else, the map should be considered a dynamic process that is sustainable and reflects growth and change within the curriculum.

Step 4: Retrieving the Data

In most cases, when a medical curriculum is documented at the individual session level, the content will consist of a list of thousands of learning objectives. These must be organized in some manner to be useful. All the commercial curriculum management tools have the ability to search the database by key words. This can be useful when searching for specific content, such as "Where do students learn about listeria." However, developing a data set designed to answer larger questions, such as "what do we teach about poultry" or "where do we teach immunology," requires the development of institutional key words.

Key words should be carefully chosen so that they will provide useful information to a variety of stakeholders. They should also align with the overall goals and mission of the college and be able to document coverage of all outcomes required by accrediting agencies, such as the nine graduate competencies required by AVMA in Standard 11. The list of key words in Table 3.2 contains elements that would allow data retrieval in each of these competencies as well as those proposed by others, including NAVMEC, VetPro, and RCVS Day One Competencies (NAVMEC, 2010; Bok *et al.*, 2011; RCVS, 2015). However, drawing from the experiences of our medical colleagues, it would be extremely helpful if a single accepted competency framework could be developed for most colleges of veterinary medicine, to facilitate the sharing of curricular data between different institutions (Englander *et al.*, 2013).

Step 5: Analyzing the Data

Data analysis should occur on many levels: at the level of the individual, at the level of a curriculum board, and as a part of the review process for accreditation. Clearly, a curriculum map is intended for multiple stakeholders, in order to have a resource for answering individual questions about content, sequencing, omissions, and redundancies. The culture of the institution should encourage such inquiry by making the database easily accessible to students, staff, faculty, and administrators, with clear instructions on how to obtain data. Course syllabi should make explicit how that course will build on previous curricular material to help students achieve one or more competencies.

Formal review of the curriculum, including detection of omissions, duplications, and redundancies, by a college curriculum committee at least every seven years is an accreditation

Table 3.2 Key words for curriculum mapping.

Table 3.2 (Continued)

Species (from NAVLE Job Analysis)
- Multiple species
- Canine
- Feline
- Bovine
- Porcine
- Ovine/caprine
- Equine
- Camelidae
- Cervidae
- Poultry
- Pet birds
- Other small animals
  - Rabbits
  - Ferrets
  - Hamsters
  - Rats and mice
  - Guinea pigs
  - Turtles
  - Snakes
  - Iguanas
  - Primates

Systems (from NAVLE Job Analysis)
- Cardiovascular
- Endocrine
- Gastrointestinal
- Hemic/lymphatic
- Integumentary
- Multisystems
- Infectious
- Behavior
- Musculoskeletal
- Nervous
- Reproductive
- Respiratory
- Special senses
- Urinary

Foundational knowledge, paraclinical skills
- Anatomy – gross
- Anatomy – cellular
- Embryology
- Physiology
- Microbiology
- Virology
- Parasitology
- Toxicology
- Pharmacology
- Immunology
- Epidemiology
- Genetics
- Pathology – gross
- Pathology – clinical
- Nutrition

Clinical skills
- Knowledge of disease
- Animal handling
- Instrument handling
- Physical examination
- Anesthesia/pain management
- Diagnostic imaging
- Surgery
- Non-surgical medical skills
- Emergency case management
- Clinical reasoning
- Communication
- Professionalism/reflective learning
- One Health
- Collaboration
- Leadership
- Diversity and multicultural awareness
- Lifelong learning, scholarship, value of research

Purpose of the course in the curriculum
- Core
- Track
- Elective

requirement by the AVMA COE. Therefore, individual teams should be assigned to periodically review the curriculum and report to the college committee. Teams could be developed according to any of the searchable key words, such as content provided by species, or by system, or by both. Team members should draw conclusions about whether there is appropriate coverage of content and sequential development of skills in each of their areas. For example, a team may be assigned to evaluate the attributes necessary for an equine lameness exam. That team would examine the integration of anatomy, physiology, pathology, clinical disease knowledge, and clinical skill development at multiple phases in the curriculum related to the equine musculoskeletal system (Britton *et al.*, 2008).

Finally, the curriculum map must be linked to the outcome measures that each institution uses to "close the gap." For example, most veterinary colleges use a combination of surveys from students, alumni, and employers to inform them of the success of their program. Both positive and negative responses to individual survey questions can help inform curriculum design if the areas of concern can be traced back to how and where those attributes were developed within the curriculum. Direct measures of student achievement, such as those on standardized exams, should also be related to the curriculum, and the key words listed will facilitate the retrieval of curricular information related to the North American Veterinary Licensing Exam (NAVLE) reporting scheme. Similarly, in-house comprehensive assessments should have their results tagged to elements in the curriculum map, so that once again indications of poor or exemplary performance can be traced back to where and how that concept was taught and previously assessed.

Conclusion

Every phase of curriculum mapping, from data entry to establishing links, from generating reports to analyzing the data, is labor intensive. However, most institutions report that this process has made their curriculum more transparent, better aligned, and capable of continuous improvement. Curriculum mapping breaks down the silos so often created between different courses and improves communication and collegiality among faculty, staff, and students. If mechanisms can be found to share this information in a meaningful way among different institutions, we will have a powerful tool to effect change.

References

AAMC (2016) *Curriculum Inventory and Reports (CIR)*. Association of American Medical Colleges. https://www.aamc.org/initiatives/cir/ (accessed October 22, 2016).

AVMA (2014) COE Accreditation Policies and Procedures: Requirements. American Veterinary Medical Association. https://www.avma.org/ProfessionalDevelopment/Education/Accreditation/Colleges/Pages/coe-pp-requirements-of-accredited-college.aspx (accessed October 22, 2016).

Bester, M., and Scholtz, D. (2012) Mapping our way to coherence, alignment, and responsiveness. *South African Journal of Higher Education*, **26** (**2**), 282–299.

Bok, H.G.J., Jaarsma, D.A.D.C., Teunissen, P.W., *et al.* (2011) Development and validation of a competency framework for veterinarians. *Journal of Veterinary Medical Education*, **38** (**3**), 262–268.

Britton, M., Letassy, N., Medina, M.S., and Er, N. (2008) A curriculum review and mapping process supported by an electronic database system. *American Journal of Pharmaceutical Education*, **72** (**5**), 1–6.

Cohen, J.J. (2000) CurrMIT: You've gotta use this thing! *Academic Medicine*, **76** (**4**), 319.

Cottrell, S., Linger, B., and Shumway, J. (2004) Using information contained in the curriculum management information tool (CurrMIT) to capture opportunities for student learning and development. *Medical Teacher*, **26** (**5**), 423–427.

Ellaway, R.H., Albright, S., Smothers, V., *et al.* (2014) Curriculum inventory: Modeling, sharing and comparing medical education programs. *Medical Teacher*, **36** (**3**), 208–215.

Englander, R., Cameron, T., Ballard, A.J., *et al.* (2013) Toward a common taxonomy of competency domains for health professions and competencies for physicians. *Academic Medicine*, **88** (**8**), 1–7.

English, F.W. (1980) Curriculum mapping. *Educational Leadership*, **37** (**7**), 558–559.

Fenton, W. (2016) *The Best Learning Management Systems (LMS) for 2016*. PCMag UK. http://www.pcmag.com/article2/0,2817,2488347,00.asp (accessed October 21, 2016).

Frank, J.R., Snell, L.S., Ten Cate, O., *et al.* (2010) Competency based medical education: Theory to practice. *Medical Teacher*, **32** (**8**), 638–645.

Harden, R.M. (2001) AMEE guide no 21: Curriculum mapping: A tool for transparent and authentic teaching and learning. *Medical Teacher*, **23** (**2**), 123–137.

Jacobs, H.H. (1997) *Mapping the Big Picture: Integrating Curriculum and Assessment K-12*, Association for Supervision and Curriculum Development, Alexandria, VA.

LCME (2015) *Data Collection Instrument*. Liaison Committee on Medical Education, Washington, DC.

NAVMEC (2010) *Roadmap for Veterinary Medical Education in the 21st Century: Responsive, Collaborative, Flexible*. North American Veterinary Medical Education Consortium. http://www.aavmc.org/data/files/navmec/navmec_roadmapreport_web_booklet.pdf (accessed October 22, 2016).

RCVS (2015) *Day One Competences*. Royal College of Veterinary Surgeons. http://www.rcvs.org.uk/document-library/day-one-competences

Salas, A.A., Anderson, M.B., LaCourse, L., *et al.* (2003) CurrMit: A tool for managing medical school curricula. *Academic Medicine*, **78** (**3**), 275–279.

Steketee, C. (2015) Prudentia: A medical school's solution to curriculum mapping and curriculum management. *Journal of University Teaching and Learning Practice*, **12** (**4**), 1–10.

Uchiyama, K.P., and Radin, J.L. (2009) Curriculum mapping in higher education: A vehicle for collaboration. *Innovation in Higher Education*, **33** (**4**), 271–280.

Udelhofen, S. (2005) *Keys to Curriculum Mapping: Strategies and Tools to Make It Work*, Corwin Press, Thousand Oaks, CA.

Willett, T.G. (2008) Current status of curriculum mapping in Canada and the UK. *Medical Education*, **42** (**8**), 786–793.

Part II

Learning and Teaching Strategies

4

Learning Concepts and Theories, and Their Application to Educational Practice

Stephen A. May

Royal Veterinary College, UK

 Box 4.1: Key messages

- Different learning theories are "lenses" that provide different perspectives on the complex process of learning.
- Learning involves iterative interactions between the learner's social group(s) and environment and the learner's cognitive processes aimed at making meaning of their life.
- An understanding of learner development, maturity, and capacity helps those involved in educational delivery in the process of designing effective and efficient learning programs.
- Although all of us have individual learning preferences, there is little evidence that

accommodating these in educational design and delivery enhances professional knowledge and skills development.
- Emotions play a crucial part in our learning. It is important that individuals regard their learning environment as "safe" and that they trust that their teachers have the learner's best interests at heart.
- Building on prior learning so that the learner is supported in their zone of proximal development (at their "learning edge"), where they can make progress with appropriate advice and encouragement, is the best use of valuable teacher time.

Introduction

Stephen Hawking spent most of his career attempting to unify the laws of physics, particularly as they relate to the four fundamental forces, into a single, overarching theory and equation. As scientists we like order, creating periodic tables and taxonomies and preferring to regard complex systems as merely complicated, ultimately capable of reduction to their constituent elements. Therefore, it is natural,

when academics start to examine the evidence base for their teaching practice, that those with a scientific background look for some sort of classification of educational theories, or even a "theory of theories" that holds the secret to excellent teaching.

Readers who have already embarked on such a search will know that it is fruitless. The process of learning, including teaching and the teacher effect, is complex. We know that the most important factor in effective learning is

---

Veterinary Medical Education: A Practical Guide, First Edition. Edited by Jennifer L. Hodgson and Jacquelyn M. Pelzer.
© 2017 John Wiley & Sons, Inc. Published 2017 by John Wiley & Sons, Inc.

what the student does (Shuell, 1986), but a crucial factor in this is the teacher (Rowe, 2002). However, what we choose to call excellent teaching – beautifully crafted presentations and handouts, which have all the key points highlighted and are scored highly by students – does not always stimulate the highest quality of learning. The teachers who are apparently less organized and greater risk-takers (McAlpine *et al.*, 1999; Fryer-Edwards *et al.*, 2006), who "teach on the edge of chaos" (Tosey, 2002), may ultimately support the development of better learners than the authorities in their field, who deliver lectures that contain the last word in their subject area (Entwistle and Entwistle, 1992).

The aim of this chapter is to bring some sense to this apparent paradox. In accepting that learning and teaching form a complex system, we need to start to view learning theories as different and complementary "lenses" for understanding individual aspects of the system (Bordage, 2009). We will begin by looking at the nature of knowledge and its implications for learning. We will then look at the "big three theories" of learning that dominated discussions over the whole of the twentieth century. After moving on to consider learning capacity and then the complexity of learning in relation to its social and emotional dimensions, finally we will discuss the implications of all this for teaching and the teacher. My intentions in providing this framework are to highlight the relevance of learning theories to understanding our individual teaching experience, and to provide the foundations for, and act as a bridge into, other chapters that explore in greater detail each aspect of our practice. If, in the process, this chapter acts as a catalyst for further exploration by readers of learning theories themselves, this will be a bonus!

What Is Knowledge; What Is Learning?

Aristotle (384–322 BC) regarded knowledge as falling into three categories: "episteme," corresponding to scientific and theoretical knowledge, sometimes referred to as propositional knowledge; "techne" (the root of our word technical), corresponding to the practice of skills and crafts; and "phronesis," corresponding to practical wisdom that comes with experience, including ethics and reasoning. In the case of the latter, he was keen to distinguish this from the Greek concept of "sophia," often translated as wisdom, which relates to reasoning concerning universal truths. "Phronesis" is concerned with thinking and reasoning that are directly related to praxis (Schwartz, 2006; Reeve, 2010).

As practitioners and scientists, we can recognize all three categories of knowledge in our daily work. We build on an evidence base, including current theories, to advance our disciplines, and we combine this evidence base with our experience to make judgments about our actions, and also to take action in the clinic, the laboratory, and all other aspects of our professional lives. Therefore, for veterinarians, like members of all the other professions, it is vital that our educational systems support the development of all types of knowledge, and the related professional skills, both technical and non-technical, as well as the ability of graduates to continue developing throughout their professional lives.

Crucially, learning has been defined as any change in an individual that expresses itself in a relatively stable form of behavior (Bower and Hilgard, 1981). As we shall see, it is the process whereby individuals "perceive the world and reciprocally respond to its affordances physically, psychologically and socially ... the simple recall of that which was previously learned does not constitute learning per se" (Alexander, Schallert, and Reynolds, 2009, p. 186). Learning must be distinguished from "maturation, development and accidental changes in a person's capacities" (Säljö, 2009, p. 202), although motivation plays an important part in learner engagement and thus learning itself, physical development has an important part to play in our capacity to embrace concepts related to how we understand the material world. Collectively, for us as veterinary educational leaders and teachers, the behavior change that we are assessing is the ability of our graduates to work and succeed as "Day One" skilled members of our profession. Since the demands of society and the expectations of new graduates have never been higher, the better we can understand how to support learner development, the better we should be able to ensure that our charges meet these expectations (May, 2008).

The Big Three Theories of Learning

The big theories that dominated discussions in learning over the course of the twentieth century are behaviorism, cognitivism, and social constructivism. Much has been written on these elsewhere (e.g., Ertmer and Newby, 2013; Amirault and Branson, 2006), so the detail will not be repeated here. Nevertheless, it is helpful to highlight the aspects of each that are relevant to our teaching practice and the relatively recent coalescence of our understanding of the interaction of the learner's mind with their environment.

Behaviorism

Behaviorism arose from Ivan Pavlov's (1849–1936) classic work with conditioning in animals, and developed over the first half of the twentieth century through the work of John B. Watson and Edward Thorndike, and later B.F. Skinner, around 1950. Key to the theory is the way in which repetitive external stimuli and rewards can lead to physiological associations (salivation when a bell rings) and the establishment of certain behaviors (pushing a lever to obtain food). As researchers in the latter part of the twentieth century started to recognize the deficiencies of this perspective on learning, cognitivism came to prominence. However, behaviorism reminds us of the importance of external (and internal) rewards for certain types of learning, and the way in which repeated stimuli can lead to associations in our minds. Learners will quickly respond to our expectations of them, for both good and bad, if pleasing us as teachers is seen

as a desirable course of action. They will also look for patterns in their experience and make associations that will affect their future decisions, some of which may be justified and some not (Gladwell, 2006). As scientists, we like to think of ourselves as objective and rational creatures, and to a certain extent we can cognitively overcome a tendency to act irrationally. However, it is sobering to discover, as research with trick problems and playing card arrangements demonstrates, that only about 20% of participants with the highest cognitive ability are able largely to inhibit matching bias (Evans, 2006).

Cognitivism

In contrast to behaviorism, with its emphasis on the environment, cognitivism, which emerged in the second half of the twentieth century, emphasized our nature as rational thinkers, using our mental processes to make sense of our world. However, once more this was seen as inadequate, and theorists then returned to the earlier work of Lev Vygotsky (1896–1934) in order to explore social constructivism and the relationship of those around the learner with the learner's own thinking. Knowledge was viewed increasingly as collaboratively constructed, through learners collectively and individually making sense of the world, and through shared experiences and discussions, whether at the level of scientific disciplines or individual families and other social groups.

Social Constructivism

The social constructivist approach provides us with at least three important insights into learning and knowledge. Vygotsky recognized that for all of us there is a zone of proximal development that lies between what we can learn for ourselves and what, even with help, we are not currently able to comprehend (because we do not yet have sufficient foundational knowledge). This is a zone where, if our learning is "scaffolded" (a concept introduced by Jerome Bruner, building on Vygotsky's work) through the support of a teacher, we can make progress (Wood, Bruner, and Ross, 1976). In relation to small-group teaching, this zone has been described as the "learning edge" (Fryer-Edwards *et al.*, 2006) and it represents the best use of our most costly and precious resource, the teacher. Ideally, the learner's zone of proximal development continues to move forward as new knowledge is integrated and forms more substantial foundations for more advanced concepts. This highlights the way in which our knowledge and skills need to progress sequentially, so that intermediate stages are successfully navigated in order to reach the forefront of any discipline or profession. If knowledge is presented haphazardly, particularly in large amounts, there is a risk of it being memorized but not integrated. This has been described as fragile knowledge (Perkins, 1995). It may be learned on a short-term basis for paper-based assessments, but is not easily applied to practical problems and is quickly forgotten. The final insight provided by social constructivism comes from a consideration of the work of Pierre Bourdieu and his concepts of the "habitus" and the "field." Each of us negotiates a field, or various fields, the group or groups, social and professional, to which we belong, during the course of our lives. As individuals (the habitus), we both contribute to the field(s) and the field(s) affect us and the way in which we think. So, depending on our background, we will see ourselves in different ways. From some backgrounds, we form the view that we can achieve whatever we desire; from others, we may feel that certain paths in life are not open to us, so much so that these opportunities do not form part of our conscious thoughts (Hodkinson and Sparkes, 1997). Great scientists and inventors look at the same objects and events that others have viewed countless times and see them differently, making the previously unrecognized obvious to all. Our backgrounds mean that, as learners, we find some concepts and tests easy and others much harder, in completely different ways from others regarded as at the same stage of learning. All this has implications for widening participation and aspiration to access various educational tracks, as well as for teaching of more diverse groups of learners. It must be recognized that if the learning sequences we create do not work for some learners, they may never progress beyond the stage where the break occurred in that particular aspect of their thinking.

In contrast to behaviorism, where the animal gives relatively little thought to its response, social constructivism acknowledges the cognitive part that the learner plays. The social and collaborative aspects have been explored as "communities of practice" (Lave and Wenger, 1991) and iterative individual development conceptualized as a cyclical process, as in the case of Kolb's learning cycle. When new situations are encountered, the effective learner not only observes but also reflects on the experience, including the part they played and their feelings about what happened (Mann, Gordon, and MacLeod, 2009). This allows new ideas to be generated and lessons to be learned, so that when required to act in similar (or even different) situations in the future, such actions can be that much better informed.

Learning Theories and Their Relationships

Learning Theories Related to Learner Maturity

Our consideration of Bourdieu has introduced us to the idea of learner maturity, both in terms of a learner's integrated knowledge base and also the way in which their mind works around what they consider possible and not possible. Jean Piaget (1896–1980) demonstrated that at an early point in life, our physical stage of development has a marked effect on our ability to recognize volume as opposed to linear measurements, and this applies to us all. However, when we start to be able to cope with hypothetical and counterfactual thinking at the age of 11, our learning experiences themselves become increasingly important in our educational maturity and how we view our abilities (Dweck, 2003) (see Box 4.2). In early adolescence, based on the nature of the feedback that parents and teachers deliver, the learner is likely to have formed a view either that they are clever or

Box 4.2: Focus on mindset

Carol Dweck's (2006) major contribution to our understanding of learners has been the concept of "mindset." It is now clear that mindset has a profound effect on individual attitudes to learning, learning behaviors, and learner wellbeing. Parents and teachers play a crucial role in the development of a child's mindset through the type of praise they deliver. Praise focused on intelligence drives a fixed mindset; praise focused on effort to achieve a successful outcome drives a growth mindset.

A fixed mindset means that learners will:

- Fear being exposed as "not clever."
- Take the view that "nothing ventured is nothing lost."
- Tend to believe that if they do not know the answer immediately, they will not be able to solve a problem (unless they are taught).

- Choose easy "puzzles" that they are sure they can complete.
- Focus on grades, rather than the reasons for achieving a specific grade.
- Have difficulties judging their own abilities.

A growth mindset means that learners will:

- Enjoy new challenges.
- Take the view that "nothing ventured is nothing gained."
- Believe that if at first they do not succeed, they should try, and try again.
- Choose difficult puzzles that can help them to develop.
- Focus on feedback and the reason for the award of a particular grade so that they know how to improve for the future.
- Seek to develop their skills in judging their own abilities.

that they are not: either that they are capable of accomplishing certain tasks or that they are not (fixed mindset), or that they are capable of a lot provided that they work hard (growth mindset). This view of our abilities, which is fundamental to all our learning and will profoundly affect our motivation and engagement with learning opportunities, is dramatically related to the nature of the praise that we receive throughout our childhood. If, on successful completion of a task, the learner is told that their achievement is because they are a clever person, they will quickly develop a fixed mindset. If on successful completion they are told that their achievement is because they have worked hard, they will increasingly believe that with hard work and practice they can complete whatever tasks they are set: the growth mindset. For those with a fixed mindset, undertaking tests is all about performance and avoidance of being exposed as incompetent in any area. In contrast, those with a growth mindset are much more interested in

mastery. They know that this will allow them to understand advanced concepts and undertake more complicated tasks. Avoidance of exposure and mere performance in a test will not help them to develop, so they will frequently seek challenges in areas in which they know they might fail (safely) in order to learn.

A significant development in learner maturity comes with the acknowledgment that they themselves have a significant part to play in their own understanding. In the 1970s, William Perry recognized several distinct phases through which learners go in their journey from "basic dualism," with the teacher having the right answers that just need to be learned, through more relativistic positions, leading to an understanding of good and less good explanations of phenomena, to a stage of "evolving commitments," where the responsibility for recognizing and establishing current best evidence lies with the individual. This is where early educational preparation is important. Those who are well advanced in this kind of thinking at high school may progress to Perry's more advanced positions by the end of their formal education. Others may still cling to dualist perspectives, or have progressed to the position of multiplicity but no further, believing that "everyone has a right to his own opinion" and one person's is just as valid as that of another (Thoma, 1993; Dale, Sullivan, and May, 2008).

This maturity of thinking about the nature of knowledge is likely to be paralleled by a change in preference for the way it is delivered. In our youth, we accept pedagogical approaches where the teacher is the authority figure transmitting their knowledge to us, and this is appropriate both to our needs and to our educational maturity. However, as adults we are much more likely to embrace an andragogical approach, where we have a hand in directing our own learning, based on our learning preferences and our analysis of our current learning needs (Dale, Sullivan, and May, 2008). Rather than being subject oriented, the problems we are currently tackling motivate us to seek knowledge and, where necessary, individual expert support to help us solve these new challenges.

Learning Theories Related to Learner Capacity

So far, I have explored cognitive development in a social context, with only learner maturity as the limiting factor once we have progressed beyond the stages where physical development plays a significant role. However, it is clear that our brain is a limiting factor in the amount of information that we can process and integrate at any one time, and this relates to our working memory capacity. Our working memory allows us simultaneously to process new information and solve problems, by retrieving from our long-term memory prior knowledge and solutions to aid with this processing. Subsequently, it supports the transfer of new knowledge and solutions to long-term memory for future use. Working memory has two components: a phonological loop that processes sound and a visuospatial sketchpad that deals with images (Baddeley, 2003). These can work in tandem to increase our processing capacity – hence the learning advantage of well-used audiovisual aids (Mayer, 2010) – but it is well established that our working memory can only handle a small number of units of information simultaneously. Classically, the number of units available has been regarded as 7 ± 2, with some individuals having a more extensive working memory and others being more restricted in terms of working memory capacity. One key to understanding working memory is that these units can either be single pieces of information or "chunks" of related information at various levels of aggregation. So in memory games, such as remembering telephone numbers, an average individual can remember a number containing seven digits with relative ease. However, to remember longer numbers individuals have to engage in various associative strategies, involving groups of digits, so the units of working memory contain several digits as a chunk.

So far we have viewed knowledge as developing into sophisticated concepts in our long-term memory through the sequential integration of new knowledge. The recognition that working memory can handle increasing aggregates of information, retrieved from long-term memory for the purposes of problem-solving, helps us to understand how, with rehearsal and chunking, the learner is capable of solving more and more complex and sophisticated problems (van Merriënboer and Sluijsmans, 2009).

The size of working memory means that it can be easily overloaded if we are presented with too much new knowledge, too quickly, or problems that are too complex for the stage we have reached in any particular subject area. This is the basis of cognitive load theory (Van Merriënboer and Sweller, 2010), which recognizes that for any problem there will be information relevant to solving that problem (intrinsic load), information that is irrelevant to the solution (extraneous load), and learning that takes place as a result of encountering the problem (germane load). An expert will be able quickly to discard irrelevances and focus on the key information, which they will be able to handle in chunks for the solution. A novice will find it much more difficult to discriminate between the relevant and the irrelevant, and may be completely overwhelmed by the extraneous load generated. Once more, we can see the need for the sequential development of problem-solving, where, in the early stages, problems may be stripped of all their task-irrelevant features (Mayer and Moreno 2003) to ensure that the learner has the capacity for supporting both intrinsic (problem-solving)

and germane (learning) tasks (see Box 4.3). Occasionally, intrinsic load alone or intrinsic and extraneous loads together may completely absorb working memory capacity. In such situations, we may be able to solve problems at the limits of our ability, but be perplexed subsequently to find that we cannot recall their solution. The learner might then need to revise the task by simplifying one or more aspects in order to free up the necessary working memory

---

 Box 4.3: Where's the evidence? Managing cognitive load

In consideration of cognitive capacity and separate working memory processes for handling visual and verbal material (the dual channel assumption), Mayer and Moreno (2003) have proposed nine ways of managing cognitive load in multimedia teaching.

Strategies to consider are:

- *"Offloading" of one channel*. In a series of six studies, they demonstrated superior learning through scientific explanations in the form of animation and narration rather than combined on-screen animation and text.
- *Segmenting and/or pre-training in components of a class*. In a series of studies tackling the problem of complete overload of both channels, it was demonstrated that segmenting material, with students being able to pause between sections, or pre-training in various functions of individual components, led to superior learning in the subsequent class.
- *"Weeding" out extraneous material and "signaling" key information*. A rush to authenticity can lead to the inclusion of content not directly related to problem-solving and completion of a task. In a series of experiments, it was shown that both highlighting key words relevant to problem-solving and removing embellishments from narratives improved learners' subsequent problem-solving.
- *Ensuring coherence of pictorial material and on-screen text*. Temporal spacing of related

material being processed by a single channel can be challenging for learners. Animations with integrated on-screen text led to superior learning compared to animations followed by segmented on-screen text.
- *Synchronization of visual and verbal material and elimination of redundancy*. A similar lack of alignment between visual and verbal material can lead to inferior learning. In a series of studies, students performed better in subsequent problem-solving when animations and narration were synchronized rather than presented serially, and also when text on-screen that was identical to the narration was removed.
- *Individualization of learning resources*. It is important to remember that achieving an optimal cognitive load for one individual will not necessarily suit others. In some of their studies, Mayer and Moreno (2003) demonstrated that while synchronization led to improved results for those with high spatial ability, no benefits could be demonstrated for those with less capacity to hold mental images. This means that so-called high-quality multimedia design may work well as an individualized strategy for learners with high spatial ability, but more attention to pre-training and familiarization with individual components separately is likely to be required by those with more limited working memory capacity.

capacity to support learning, before revisiting the complexity of the task in its original format.

An understanding of the limitations of working memory capacity and the variations in its size between individuals is important in working with learners with special learning needs. In the United Kingdom, the lower performance that is most often encountered in the testing of those in veterinary schools in need of learning support relates to working memory. These individuals have often developed learning strategies that optimally use their long-term memory for extensive memorization of material, including solutions to problems that can be replicated under assessment conditions. Such strategies are successful as long as those affected are only tested in contexts where the retrieval of memorized material is all that is required. However, they will fail where individuals are tested on genuinely novel problems, particularly where "real-time" processing is vital, such as on the clinic floor.

Our two types of processing – novel problem-solving, dependent on the extensive use of working memory; and the retrieval of past solutions from long-term memory – have been called Type I and Type II processing (Evans, 2012). Each is best regarded as a collection of processes, Type I related to pattern recognition and behaviors based on past experiences, and Type II related to various analytic approaches that we may be able to adapt to a challenge that we face. Type II processing is slow and demands effort of us all, so where possible our brain will attempt to recognize patterns and retrieve memorized solutions to be examined for their appropriateness. This is more rapid and imposes little cognitive load, ensuring that we are able to negotiate busy lives and careers without having to work through every small challenge as though it were new.

Learning Theories Relating to Styles/Preferences/Approaches

Relatively highly functional learners with special needs related to limited working memory capacity have a clear reason for preferring an approach to learning based on memorizing as much material as possible. However, many individuals have distinct preferences that can lead to different approaches to learning, and recognition of these preferences has been very influential in various areas of education (see Box 4.4). Some writers have emphasized constitutional differences, such as visual, auditory, kinesthetic, and tactile strengths and preferences; some stable learning preferences, such as activists, reflectors, pragmatists, and theorists;

 Box 4.4: Where's the evidence? Learning styles and approaches

In a comprehensive review, Coffield *et al.* (2004) looked at over 800 references from which they identified 71 learning style models. They then examined in detail the 13 most influential models. They concluded the following as far as learning styles are concerned:

- There is little theoretical coherence and an absence of well-replicated findings.
- Claims for particular models are overblown, perhaps as a result of vested interests in a considerable industry associated with the sale of copyrighted models.

- Researchers and students have a tendency to apply labels to individuals as particular types of learner, despite the inappropriateness of this, and the potential negative consequences of students assuming that learning framed in certain ways is inappropriate for them.
- Even after more than 30 years of research, there is no consensus on the best approach to measuring learning styles or the most effective educational interventions.

and still others preferences more related to conceptions of learning and learning strategies, such as deep and surface approaches (Coffield *et al.*, 2004). Supporters of learning styles suggest that learning materials and teaching approaches that play to individual strengths will lead to superior learning. However, while this idea is superficially attractive, there is little empirical evidence that supports this hypothesis. If anything, the evidence shows that pursuing learning preferences that do not support learning outcomes (for instance, theorizing about a practical task) leads to inferior learning. Learners need to adopt appropriate approaches for the types of knowledge that they need to acquire and the particular challenges that they face.

The one exception to the earlier generalization about learning styles, preferences, and approaches is related to concepts of learning and deep and surface approaches. Learners can be identified adopting deep and surface approaches on a strategic basis, according to the tests they are set (Entwistle and Ramsden, 1983). Teaching methods based on information transmission and objective written tests of factual knowledge will tend to drive surface learning aimed at memorization for the test. In contrast, more student-centered approaches and assignments focused on solving problems will tend to drive deeper approaches where the learner is focused on understanding the material (Trigwell, Prosser, and Waterhouse, 1999).

Emotion and Learning

At the outset I distinguished motivation from learning, but any account of learning and reasoning would be incomplete without a consideration of the effects of motivation and emotion on learning (see Box 4.5). In our early years, we are largely extrinsically motivated by our parents and teachers with rewards or, in some cases, punishments of various types, motivating our behavior. This may continue into later life, as social motivation combines with a performance goal orientation to make achievement of examination certificates an end in itself. However, an important transition for those who are to go on to become effective, lifelong, self-directed learners in any area is the development of intrinsic motivation for their discipline (Dale, Pierce, and May, 2010).

 ## Box 4.5: Focus on emotion in learning

In a report that Reinhard Pekrun (2014) produced for the International Academy of Education in Brussels, he identified four different types of "academic emotions" that affect learning. These are:

- *Achievement emotions* that relate to success, including enjoyment of learning, and failure, including anxiety and shame. These emotions are particularly prominent when the importance of success is emphasized to students.
- *Epistemic emotions* that are evoked by new tasks, such as surprise, confusion, and curiosity, or frustration when efforts to solve problems

reveal obstacles. These emotions are important in learning new, non-routine tasks.
- *Topic emotions* that are triggered by the topics of classes. These can be both positive, such as empathy for an animal or person that is suffering, and negative, such as disgust over rotting vegetation, but both can stimulate interest in the topic.
- *Social emotions* that are associated with others in a learning group, such as admiration, sympathy, anger, or social anxiety. These are particularly important in teacher–student interaction and collaborative learning.

Learners need to develop a positive attitude to subjects and for this they have to understand the relevance of learning materials and have self-belief that they can master the associated learning challenge. Subsequent mastery gives pleasure and feeds back into further interest (Gläser-Zikuda *et al.*, 2005).

Positive emotion and a feeling of safety in the learning environment allow the learner's mind to focus on learning as opposed to survival (Rogers, 1969). Feeling socially challenged can lead to an individual's entire focus being on saving face and excluding themselves in as dignified a way as possible from the unsafe environment. Ultimately, this leads to avoidance behavior to prevent a recurrence of negative emotions related to perceived failure. Intriguingly, work with those who have brain lesions that reduce their ability to respond emotionally suggests that despite being able to reason, they struggle with decision-making and the ability to transfer past experience to new challenges (Immordino-Yang and Damasio, 2007). It is as though the inability to process emotional tags for their accumulated knowledge and experience prevents them from making progress in problem-solving and learning.

Positive emotions such as pleasure in success or an interesting task tend to support learning. Negative emotions, such as fear of failure, frustration at lack of progress, and social anxiety, are likely to interfere with or prevent student learning.

Emotions can be manipulated/regulated to benefit learning in four main ways:

- *Developing one's competencies* (deliberate practice) in order to promote the positive emotions associated with success.
- *Reappraisal of the factors that induce the emotions* by developing self-confidence (appraisal of ability) and identifying the relevance of learning opportunities (appraisal of task value).
- *Changing the learning environment* by choosing a particular university, degree program, or teacher that meets the student's needs.
- *Direct targeting* by relaxation techniques and even therapeutic agents to reduce anxiety.

Emotion also affects our ability to delay closure. It can be uncomfortable to deal with uncertainty and not be able to identify answers immediately (DeBacker and Crowson, 2009). Some learners will either race to a superficial and often imperfect solution or give up. However, to be effective in reaching complex decisions and learning complex concepts, the learner must be able to explore all aspects fully before coming to a conclusion. This will be supported by a preference for complexity and a growth mindset, and will also feed into a desire for lifelong learning (Dale, Pierce, and May, 2010).

Implications of Learning Theories for Teaching

All these different perspectives on the complex process of learning in the classroom, laboratory, and clinic have profound implications for curricular design and delivery, and yet frequently they seem to be ignored in veterinary programs, which at times seem to be more based on what individuals and departments are prepared to deliver, rather than the learners' needs related to a coherent set of program-level learning outcomes.

Curricular Design

Sequential Knowledge and Skills Development
The need for knowledge and skills to progress from a basic to an advanced level, in order for learning to be really effective, emphasizes the value of designs based on vertical integration of individual courses/modules, rather than having these as freestanding elements that differ only in relation to their content. Certain transitions, such as that from basic science to clinical theory and that from classroom to clinic, can be particularly difficult to navigate because of the tendency for sudden changes in the way in which knowledge is used and acquired (May, 2015). All this points to the need for specific attention to "bridging" for these stages, such as the use of clinical skills laboratories to develop simple practical skills, before learners

are confronted with live patients in busy clinics (May and Silva-Fletcher, 2015). Confronted with a disease focused on a single organ system, the learner will need simultaneously to understand the anatomy, physiology, and pathologies of that organ and, as they consider treatment, the pharmacology of the different therapeutic agents that they might choose. Our disciplinary structures relate more to the way in which we have organized propositional knowledge in these disciplines in the past, rather than considerations of clinical practice, so aids to this horizontal synthesis by the learner, even including horizontal integration of disciplines in teaching, can all be helpful in the support of high-quality learning (Brynhildsen *et al.*, 2002).

Recognition of Developing Learner Maturity

Although we want our learners to be emerging with the maturity of those who see knowledge and its application as a process of "evolving commitments," many will arrive from a first degree or high school with dualist perspectives, believing that knowledge is black and white (Knight and Mattick, 2006) and that they need to be taught the correct answers. Therefore, the curriculum design needs to follow the expected growth of learning maturity over the four to six years of the clinical veterinary program, with learning materials and teachers at the start acting as authority figures and experts, giving way to teachers acting more as facilitators and delegators in later years. In the same way that learners will not be able to cope with advanced concepts before acquiring a foundation of basic knowledge, they will not be able to cope with more andragogical, delegator-type learning formats until they have matured from dependent to more involved and self-directed learners (Grow, 1991).

Clarity over Relevance of Courses/Modules

Given that interest is stimulated by the perceived relevance of courses, it is sometimes surprising that course directors and teachers do not do more to sell the relevance of the subjects and experiences that they are offering. Many students (and teachers) will take on

trust the relevance of anatomy for surgery and physiology for medicine, but at times struggle to distinguish the most relevant aspects from material of lesser relevance. Designing the curriculum backward in terms of overall learning outcomes, together with relevant assessment methods for those outcomes and intermediate year-by-year and course-by-course learning outcomes and assessments, concentrates all minds on the appropriate learning to pass these assessments and achieve the outcomes (May and Silva-Fletcher, 2015). Although the goal of professional learning is successful entry and employability within the profession, the intermediate assessment stages can loom larger in the learner's mind and drive learning specifically for the assessment (Rust, 2002). This is particularly true of those with a fixed mindset and a high fear of failure. This powerful driver to learning can, if assessments are not well aligned to desired outcomes, lead to inappropriate learning for tests that crowds out the appropriate learning for the professional role. A clear trajectory of learning, signposted by curricular integration and alignment, emphasizes the coherence of the whole learning experience and its continued relevance to Day One knowledge and skills development.

Avoidance of Content Overload

Deep learning for the understanding and application of knowledge requires time for students to reflect on how new knowledge relates to prior learning, how current conceptualizations need to be revised, and the implications of this for further study. If this time is not available, the learner will give up on understanding and, in panic, embrace surface approaches to try to meet test requirements (Ramsden, 1992). Research indicates that a certain level of teacher–student contact is required to provide the frameworks and motivation for directed and self-directed learning activity. However, beyond an optimal level, increased contact reduces independent student effort, risking insufficient reflection to integrate new knowledge effectively (Schmidt *et al.*, 2010). Different concepts and skills will require different amounts of reflection and rehearsal for them to be mastered and integrated. However, it is known in the United Kingdom that the average medical and veterinary student studies in total for about 45 hours per week (Soilemetzidis *et al.*, 2014). If the ratio of contact to independent study is, say, 1:2, this would indicate a maximum of 15 hours or so contact time. However, depending on the ratio of lectures to more participative contact periods, such as practicals and seminars/discussions, we might justify the actual weekly contact hours for clinical courses as about 22–23 hours, with seminars playing their role, alongside independent study and reflection, in the integrative process associated with conceptual development and assimilation on the part of the individual student.

Curriculum Delivery

Key to effective learning is the activity of the learner themselves (Shuell, 1986). Reliance on information transmission approaches that require relatively passive involvement on the part of the learner is a poor strategy for fostering both understanding and long-term recall. Therefore, it is crucial that the teacher does not do all the work for the student in terms of the organization of content and identification of key points. The ability to undertake both these tasks for themselves is an essential professional skill set for learners.

Learning materials can highlight different ways of framing different arguments, helping students start to move away from dualist perspectives on knowledge and develop their own commitments to ways of organizing their knowledge (Thoma, 1993). Materials can also be designed with gaps that students complete during classes or through independent study. It is known, for instance, that where our brains have to make connections in narratives, where certain actions are implied rather than explicit, these stories are better remembered than those in which all the details are complete (Chabris and Simons, 2010). Optimal learning will occur in classes that allow students to recall prior knowledge as their starting point, and place them at their "learning edge" (in their zones of proximal development), with appropriate teacher support available to help them advance to the next stage (Fryer-Edwards *et al.*, 2006; Nelson Laird *et al.*, 2008).

Teachers' Knowledge and Skills

For a program to be maximally effective, in addition to knowledge of their respective area, all teachers should know the place that their class has in the curriculum and the learning maturity that their students have achieved. This will ensure that they know the students' prior learning, in terms of knowledge and skills, and the stage they have reached in terms of self-direction and independent learning. This allows the teacher to calibrate the content to the knowledge base and conceptual development stage of the student, and to organize the class according to students' ability to define their own goals and lead their own discussions.

For students to engage and participate fully, it is vital that they regard the learning environment as safe (Rogers, 1969). This means that the teacher must foster a culture that supports a growth mindset, with experimentation and failure not seen as something to be criticized (Dweck, 2006). Indeed, the major concern should be for those who do not participate and open themselves up to the prospect of being wrong.

Scaffolding

Some 2500 years ago, Chinese philosophy Lao Tzu is credited with saying that a good leader is a person who talks little and "when his work is done, his aims fulfilled, they (the people) will all say 'we did this ourselves.'" The target for all teachers is much the same: the development of motivated and increasingly independent learners who gain pleasure from their own achievements. A key metaphor for the way in which the teacher supports active learning is the provision of "scaffolding" that can be adjusted to learner needs and removed as the learner becomes more capable and confident (Wood, Bruner, and Ross, 1976).

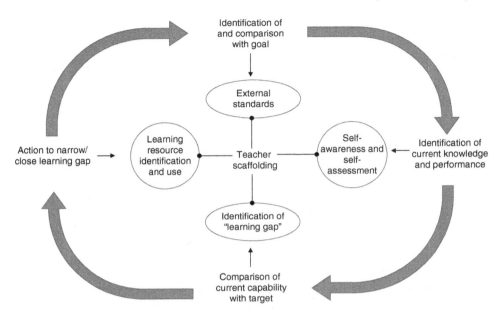

Figure 4.1 For novice learners, the teacher has a major role in setting standards, identifying and creating learning resources, and matching these to learner stage and ability. As learners become more self-directed, the teacher can increasingly signpost where standards descriptions and learning materials can be found, while still helping the learner in identifying their learning needs. As learners become more independent, they grow increasingly capable of assessing their own learning needs, and of completing the cycle for themselves. Source: Inspired by Sadler (1989).

A useful model for considering how the teacher "scaffolds" learning and weans the learner off dependence is to consider a cycle (Figure 4.1) that identifies the learning gap (Sadler, 1989). For organized learning to occur, the teacher, and increasingly the learner, must be aware of a standard that is to be targeted and the learner's current level of performance. The difference between the two is the learning gap that must be closed. For areas that appear complex or unfamiliar to the learner, the teacher has an important role in signaling the nature of the gap and the sources of knowledge and/or experience that will help the learner close that gap. In the early stages, teachers themselves will be the knowledge resource. However, as learners become more self-directed, they get better at setting learning goals around externally derived standards, self-assessment, and recognizing the learning gap for themselves. At various times, teachers and professional colleagues may help calibrate these personal judgments and aid in the identification of appropriate resources for learning. Eventually, the independent learner becomes extremely good at using databases to access primary and secondary sources of knowledge and plan their professional development programs. However, even then, peer calibration remains a vital input (Eva and Regehr, 2008). The effective independent learner can often be recognized by their ability to "train themselves" in new career avenues, hobbies, and other pursuits. These individuals have been described as "intelligent novices." They know how to learn, through being able to identify what they need to know and how to gain the desired knowledge and skills. In particular, they are very good at identifying when they can learn for themselves and when they need to seek expert help to guide them through a current zone of proximal development (Brown *et al.*, 1983).

Questioning Techniques

Teachers and learners are involved in a serious professional game (Furtak, 2006). The students suspect that the teacher has the answers, but is concealing them in the interests of the students' learning. The teacher can scaffold the students' exploration of their own knowledge and experience and the development of new knowledge through various approaches based on asking questions. Techniques such as Socratic questioning can stimulate reflection on the part of learners to explain different concepts and skills, who in so doing clarify and confirm their own knowledge and abilities. Where learners' current concepts are basic, or even wrong, teachers can engage in "discrepant questioning" to highlight how basic models that provide starting points may not stand more detailed scrutiny, and encourage learners to think individually and collectively about refinement of their thinking (Rea-Ramirez, Nunez-Oviedo, and Clement, 2009). The teacher needs to recognize that when students ask questions, it is not always appropriate to tell them the answer. This might be an opportunity for them to try out their skills at sourcing information independently and comparing notes on their findings, particularly where there are currently multiple views on the results of scientific experiments or the most appropriate methods for treating a diseased patient. In forcing delay in closure, the teacher can help the learner to better define the problem and elaborate on it in their exploration of the relevant literature. Particularly in situations where "all is not as it seems" – for instance, an unusual diagnosis for a common clinical presentation – the teacher can discourage "cognitive miserliness" (Stanovich, 2009) and encourage students in their independent study to consider all the possibilities analytically.

Important areas that learners take from teachers are their enthusiasm for their subject (Bolt, Witte, and Lygo-Baker, 2010) and their attitude to the interests of the student. Teachers who are emotionally engaged with the subject of their teaching will both inspire students and also stimulate their interest. This means that the material being taught should be fresh; where it is repeated, it is better to vary the content so that teachers still feel the anxiety associated with novelty, which boosts their performance (McAlpine *et al.*, 1999). This is easy to achieve in seminars where students affect the course of discussions and different groups may take the class in different directions. It is harder to achieve in respect of practical classes, where the class may be much more prescribed and similar each time it is repeated.

Learner-Derived Signs of Problems

A knowledge of learning theories can aid teachers in the early detection of learner problems or immaturity. Statements such as "tell me the answer" or "tell me what I need to know for the examination" (Jones, 2009; Waldrop, 2015) could be pointing to learners who still view the teacher as the authority figure, or tend to be rather superficial in their approach to knowledge and are uncomfortable with delayed closure. They may also be students prone to cognitive miserliness who either dislike the effort of analytic reasoning or, as a result of limited working memory capacity, struggle with working out problems for themselves.

Clinical teachers in particular often complain that the students "do not know anything" and want to cram revision sessions or their own classes into the period immediately preceding clinical rotations or during rotations. This can relate to at least three different issues in design and delivery. If students did not recognize material as relevant, through lack of interest or mistaken priorities, they may not have paid it much attention. If students were feeling overloaded, they may have crammed the material for a test and not integrated it into their longer-term knowledge base, leading to its being forgotten. Additionally, if the knowledge has not been integrated in a way appropriate to its application, through problem-solving and rehearsal, it may be capable of recall in response to certain triggers such as an artificial test, but not available for application as intended in relevant professional contexts (Perkins, 1995). Although teachers frequently blame students for "not knowing their stuff," if the finding applies to whole classes or large subgroups within cohorts, this points to issues with curricular design and delivery.

Similar considerations apply to students who "cannot problem-solve" and "cannot undertake practical classes." They may not have received staged instruction and opportunities to practice these skills in an appropriate manner, or the curricular design and culture of the institution may not have encouraged a growth mindset that supports trial and potential failure with feedback on how to improve and ultimately succeed. Such students are likely to have both underdeveloped reasoning and practical skills and an inclination to adopt avoidance behaviors, both of which will confirm the impression that they "cannot…"

Learner Preparation

An account of the implications of learning theories for teaching would not be complete without consideration of learner preparation. At times we confuse wants and needs, and this is particularly the case where students provide feedback in the form of student satisfaction surveys (so-called happy sheets) rather than measures of their engagement and the benefits that they derive from learning. Even with relatively simple tests, such as knot-tying, it can be demonstrated that students who receive feedback in the form of compliments, as opposed to advice on how to improve, score the teacher more highly, despite demonstrating inferior abilities compared to the advice group in subsequent tests. Learners like the process to be easy for them and they like to be told that they are clever, despite the adverse effects that each of these has on the quality of their learning and their concept of their ability (Boehler *et al.*, 2006). Every effort should be made to avoid feedback to students that has any tendency to reinforce a fixed mindset. Learners must associate their own effort with success, and be intrinsically motivated to seek out challenges that support their intellectual growth and development.

Rhetoric around "students as consumers" has dominated political discussions in English-speaking countries, as student fees and student debt have achieved greater prominence. This has served to aggravate the misunderstanding that a university degree program has

many similarities to, say, a camera or a washing machine. A better analogy for learners to consider is that of gym membership (Morgan and Brown, 2010). The gym owner is responsible for the quality and relevance of the equipment and the expertise of the trainers. However, the purchase of gym membership does not, in itself, lead to fitness. The gym member must make full use of the opportunities for all types of exercise, in a developmental way, proportionate to their physiological and mental fitness, in order progressively to achieve their training goals. Similarly, the university is responsible for the excellence and appropriateness of its curriculum and the expertise of its faculty and staff, both in their professional areas and as teachers. However, students must then fully engage with all these learning opportunities to achieve their own professional goals.

In the course of a veterinary program, we are not educating students to be teachers and educational researchers. However, a basic knowledge of how our curricula are designed, why students will face a variety of types of assessment, some of which they will not have encountered previously, and the importance of taking responsibility for and actively engaging in their own learning, will help them understand the value of what the university has designed for them, and maximally benefit from the rich variety of learning opportunities on offer. Evaluations that target informed and thoughtful feedback, based on student engagement as well as satisfaction, can then support high-quality program and teacher development, rather than undermine it, as may happen with relatively non-reflective satisfaction surveys.

Conclusion

A consideration of learning theories, each providing its own perspective on the complex process of learning, can help us understand and avoid the dysfunctional approaches to learning and teaching that we can encounter during the course of our professional lives (Ertmer and Newby, 2013). Learning theories offer insight at all levels of the educational process, including curriculum design and delivery, and individual teacher and learner practices. Ultimately, to be successful, educational leaders need to address all aspects of education – curriculum design, assessment, and teaching delivery, including the skills of individual teachers. All these features must work in parallel in order to stimulate individuals to become intrinsically motivated, self-directed, and active learners. It cannot be denied that many exceptionally gifted teachers develop tacit knowledge with empiricism and experience that supports high-quality learning. However, learning theories make effective

pedagogical approaches explicit in a way that can guide novice teachers, and also clarify for experienced teachers the larger principles related to program design, as well as ways in which, at an individual level, they can develop themselves further. Society expects all professionals, whether their roles are clinical or scientific, to work from a sound evidence base to the best of their ability. The educational role is no different (DiCarlo, 2006). Our classes should be well designed and well delivered. Learning theories provide the evidence base for sound educational practice.

References

Alexander, P.A., Schallert, D.L., and Reynolds, R.E. (2009) What is learning anyway? A topographical perspective considered. *Educational Psychologist*, **44** (**3**), 176–192. doi:10.1080/00461520903029006

Amirault, R.J., and Branson, R.K. (2006) Educators and expertise: A brief history of theories and models, in *The Cambridge Handbook of Expertise and Expert Performance* (eds. K.A. Ericsson, N. Charness, P.J. Feltovich, and R.R. Hoffman), Cambridge University Press, Cambridge, pp. 69–86.

Baddeley, A. (2003) Working memory: Looking back and looking forward. *Nature Reviews. Neuroscience*, **4** (**10**), 829–839. doi:10.1038/nrn1201

Boehler, M.L., Rogers, D.A, Schwind, C.J., et al. (2006) An investigation of medical student reactions to feedback: A randomised controlled trial. *Medical Education*, **40** (**8**), 746–749. doi:10.1111/j.1365-2929.2006.02503.x

Bolt, D.M., Witte, T.H., & Lygo-Baker, S. (2010) The complex role of veterinary clinical teachers: How is their role perceived and what is expected of them? *Journal of Veterinary Medical Education*, **37** (**4**), 388–394.

Bordage, G. (2009) Conceptual frameworks to illuminate and magnify. *Medical Education*, **43** (**4**), 312–319. doi:10.1111/j.1365-2923.2009. 03295.x

Bower, G.H., and Hilgard, E.R. (1981) *Theories of Learning*, Prentice-Hall, London.

Brown, A.L., Bransford, J.D., Ferrara, R.A., and Campione, J.C. (1983) Learning, remembering and understanding, in *Handbook of Child Psychology: Cognitive Development*, Vol. **3** (eds. P. Mussen, J.H. Flavell, and E.M. Markman), John Wiley & Sons Ltd, Chichester.

Brynhildsen, J., Dahle, L.O., Behrbohm Fallsberg, M., et al. (2002) Attitudes among students and teachers on vertical integration between clinical medicine and basic science within a problem-based undergraduate medical curriculum. *Medical Teacher*, **24** (**3**), 286–288. doi:10.1080/01421590220134105

Chabris, C., and Simons, D. (2010) *The Invisible Gorilla and Other Ways Our Intuition Deceives Us*, HarperCollins, London.

Coffield, F., Moseley, D., Hall, E., and Ecclestone, K. (2004) *Learning Styles and Pedagogy in Post-16 Learning: A Systematic and Critical Review*, Learning and Skills Research Centre, London.

Dale, V.H.M., Pierce, S.E., and May, S.A. (2010) The importance of cultivating a preference for complexity in veterinarians for effective lifelong learning. *Journal of Veterinary Medical Education*, **37** (**2**), 165–171. doi:10.3138/ jvme.37.2.165

Dale, V.H.M., Sullivan, M., and May, S.A. (2008) Adult learning in veterinary education: Theory to practice. *Journal of Veterinary Medical Education*, 35 (4), 581–588. doi:10.3138/jvme.35.4.581

DeBacker, T., and Crowson, H. (2009) The influence of need for closure on learning and teaching. *Educational Psychology Review*, 21 (4), 303–323. doi:10.1007/s10648-009-9111-1

DiCarlo, S.E. (2006) Cell biology should be taught as science is practised. *Nature Reviews. Molecular Cell Biology*, 7 (**April**), 290–296. doi:10.1038/nrm1894

Dweck, C.S. (2003) Ability conceptions, motivation and development, in *BJEP Monograph Series II, 2: Development and Motivation* (eds. P. Tomlinson, J. Dockrell, and P. Winne), British Psychological Society, Leicester, pp. 13–27.

Dweck, C.S. (2006) *Mindset: How You Can Fulfill Your Potential*, Random House, New York.

Entwistle, N., and Entwistle, A. (1992) Experiences of understanding in revising for degree examinations. *Learning and Instruction*, 2, 1–22.

Entwistle, N.J., and Ramsden, P. (1983) *Understanding Student Learning*, Croom Helm, London.

Ertmer, P.A., and Newby, T.J. (2013) Behaviourism, cognitivism, constructivism: Comparing critical features from an instructional design perspective. *Performance Improvement Quarterly*, 26 (2), 43–71.

Eva, K., and Regehr, G. (2008) "I'll never play professional football" and other fallacies of self-assessment. *Journal of Continuing Education in the Health Professions*, 28 (1), 14–19. doi:10.1002/chp

Evans, J.S.B.T. (2006) The heuristic-analytic theory of reasoning: Extension and evaluation. *Psychonomic Bulletin and Review*, 13, 378–395.

Evans, J.S.B.T. (2012) Spot the difference: Distinguishing between two kinds of processing. *Mind and Society*, 11 (1), 121–131. doi:10.1007/s11299-012-0104-2

Fryer-Edwards, K., Arnold, R.M., Baile, W., *et al.* (2006) Reflective teaching practices: An approach to teaching communication skills in a small-group setting. *Academic Medicine*, 81 (7), 638–644. doi:10.1097/01.ACM. 0000232414.43142.45

Furtak, E.M. (2006) The problem with answers: An exploration of guided scientific inquiry teaching. *Science Education*, 90 (3), 453–467. doi:10.1002/sce.20130

Gladwell, M. (2006) *Blink*, Penguin, London.

Gläser-Zikuda, M., Fuß, S., Laukenmann, M., *et al.* (2005) Promoting students' emotions and achievement: Instructional design and evaluation of the ECOLE-approach. *Learning and Instruction*, 15 (5), 481–495. doi:10.1016/j.learninstruc.2005.07.013

Grow, G.O. (1991) Teaching learners to be self-directed. *Adult Education Quarterly*, 41 (3), 125–149. doi:10.1177/0001848191041003001

Hodkinson, P., and Sparkes, A.C. (1997) Careership: A sociological theory of career decision making. *British Journal of Sociology of Education*, 18 (1), 29–44.

Immordino-Yang, M.H., and Damasio, A. (2007) We feel, therefore we learn: The relevance of affective and social neuroscience to education. *Mind, Brain, and Education*, 1 (1), 3–10. doi:10.1111/j.1751-228X.2007.00004.x

Jones, A. (2009) Redisciplining generic attributes: The disciplinary context in focus. *Studies in Higher Education*, 34 (1), 85–100. doi:10.1080/03075070802602018

Knight, L.V., and Mattick, K. (2006) "When I first came here, I thought medicine was black and white": Making sense of medical students' ways of knowing. *Social Science and Medicine*, 63 (4), 1084–1096. doi:10.1016/j.socscimed. 2006.01.017

Lave, J., and Wenger, E. (1991) *Situated Learning: Legitimate Peripheral Participation*, Cambridge University Press, Cambridge.

Mann, K., Gordon, J., and MacLeod, A. (2009) Reflection and reflective practice in health professions education: A systematic review. *Advances in Health Sciences Education: Theory and Practice*, 14 (4), 595–621. doi:10.1007/s10459-007-9090-2

May, S.A. (2008) Modern veterinary graduates are outstanding, but can they get better? *Journal of Veterinary Medical Education*, 35 (4), 573–580.

May, S.A. (2015) Creating the consummate professional: Historical and contemporary perspectives (based on the BEVA John Hickman Memorial Lecture 2014). *Equine Veterinary Education*, **27** (**9**), 489–495. doi:10.1111/eve.12319

May, S.A., and Silva-Fletcher, A. (2015) Scaffolded active learning: Nine pedagogical principles for building a modern veterinary curriculum. *Journal of Veterinary Medical Education*, **42** (**4**), 332–339. doi:10.3138/jvme.0415-063R

Mayer, R.E. (2010) Applying the science of learning to medical education. *Medical Education*, **44** (**6**), 543–549. doi:10.1111/j.1365-2923.2010.03624.x

Mayer, R.E., and Moreno, R. (2003) Nine ways to reduce cognitive load multimedia learning. *Educational Psychologist*, **38** (**1**), 43–52. doi:10.1207/S15326985EP3801_6

McAlpine, L., Weston, C., Beauchamp, J., *et al.* (1999) Building a metacognitive model of reflection. *Higher Education*, **37**, 105–131.

Morgan, M., and Brown, S. (2010) Commencement of the academic year: Welcoming, inducting and developing students, in *A Practical Guide to University and College Management: Beyond Bureaucracy* (eds. S. Denton and S. Brown), Routledge, Abingdon, pp. 47–68.

Nelson Laird, T.F., Shoup, R., Kuh, G.D., and Schwarz, M.J. (2008) The effects of discipline on deep approaches to student learning and college outcomes. *Research in Higher Education*, **49** (**6**), 469–494. doi:10.1007/s11162-008-9088-5

Pekrun, R. (2014). *Educational Practices Series 24: Emotion and Learning*, International Academy of Education, Brussels.

Perkins, D. (1995) The alarm bells, in *Smart Schools: Better Thinking and Learning for Every Child* (ed. D. Perkins), Free Press, New York, pp. 19–42.

Ramsden, P. (1992) *Learning to Teach in Higher Education*, Routledge, London.

Rea-Ramirez, M.A., Nunez-Oviedo, M.C., and Clement, J. (2009) Role of discrepant questioning leading to model element modification. *Journal of Science Teacher Education*, **20** (**2**), 95–111. doi:10.1007/s10972-009-9128-9

Reeve, J. (2010) Interpretive medicine: Supporting generalism in a changing primary care world. *Occasional Paper (Royal College of General Practitioners)*, **88**, 1–20. http://www.pubmedcentral.nih.gov/articlerender.fcgi?artid=3259801&tool=pmcentrez&rendertype=abstract (accessed October 23, 2016).

Rogers, C.R. (1969) *Freedom to Learn*, Charles E. Merrill, Columbus, OH.

Rowe, K.J. (2002) Issue analysis: The importance of teacher quality. *Issue Analysis*, **22**, 1–12. https://www.cis.org.au/publications/issue-analysis/the-importance-of-teacher-quality (accessed October 23, 2016).

Rust, C. (2002) The impact of assessment on student learning: How can the research literature practically help to inform the development of departmental assessment strategies and learner-centred assessment practices? *Active Learning in Higher Education*, **3** (**2**), 145–158. doi:10.1177/1469787402003002004

Sadler, D.R. (1989) Formative assessment and the design of instructional systems. *Instructional Science*, **18** (**2**), 119–144. doi:10.1007/BF00117714

Säljö, R. (2009) Learning, theories of learning, and units of analysis in research. *Educational Psychologist*, **44** (**3**), 202–208. doi:10.1080/00461520903029030

Schmidt, H.G., Cohen-Schotanus, J., Molen, H.T., *et al.* (2010) Learning more by being taught less: A "time-for-self-study" theory explaining curricular effects on graduation rate and study duration. *Higher Education*, **60** (**3**), 287–300. doi:10.1007/s10734-009-9300-3

Schwartz, D.G. (2006) Aristotelian view of knowledge management, in *Encyclopedia of Knowledge Management* (ed. D.G. Schwartz), Idea Group Reference, London, pp. 10–16. http://api.ning.com/files/bbXaWNVZL*AQDIRSKAnext1LmbrvepP0mstpALe2bSls CoyrPjFaRYzE5yhHDjMkrbUmNhn9GOiifl5ey U02oZfWR8jiTBIA/AristotelianViewof

KnowledgeManagement.pdf (accessed October 23, 2016).

Shuell, T.J. (1986) Cognitive conceptions of learning. *Review of Educational Research*, **56** (**4**), 411–436. doi:10.3102/00346543056004411

Soilemetzidis, I., Bennett, P., Buckley, A., *et al.* (2014) *The HEPI–HEA Student Academic Experience Survey 2014*. Higher Education Policy Institute. http://www.hepi.ac.uk/2014/05/21/hepi-hea-2014-student-academic-experience-survey/ (accessed October 24, 2016).

Stanovich, K.E. (2009) The thinking that IQ tests miss. *Scientific American Mind*, **20** (**6**), 34–39.

Thoma, G.A. (1993) The Perry Framework and tactics for teaching critical thinking in economics. *Journal of Economic Education*, **24** (**2**), 128–136.

Tosey, P. (2002) Teaching on the edge of chaos: Complexity theory, learning systems and enhancement. Working paper. Faculty of Arts and Social Sciences, Surrey Business School. http://epubs.surrey.ac.uk/1195/ (accessed October 24, 2016).

Trigwell, K., Prosser, M., and Waterhouse, F. (1999) Relations between teachers' approaches to teaching and students' approaches to learning. *Higher Education*, **37** (**1**), 57–70. doi:10.1023/A:1003548313194

van Merriënboer, J.J.G., and Sluijsmans, D.M.A. (2009) Toward a synthesis of cognitive load theory, four-component instructional design, and self-directed learning. *Educational Psychology Review*, **21**, 55–66. http://www.springerlink.com/content/m2623w025u3wn627/ (accessed October 24, 2016).

van Merriënboer, J.J.G., and Sweller, J. (2010) Cognitive load theory in health professional education: Design principles and strategies. *Medical Education*, **44** (**1**), 85–93. doi:10.1111/j.1365-2923.2009.03498.x

Waldrop, M.M. (2015) The science of teaching. *Nature*, **523**, 272–274. doi:10.1177/019263655704122614

Wood, D., Bruner, J.S., and Ross, G. (1976) The role of tutoring in problem solving. *Journal of Child Psychology and Psychiatry*, **17** (**2**), 89–100. doi:10.1111/j.1469-7610.1976.tb00381.x

5

Integrated Learning

Jan E. Ilkiw

School of Veterinary Medicine, University of California, Davis, USA

 Box 5.1: Key messages

- Integration in medical education is important because medical practice itself requires a great deal of integration.
- Integration promotes the blending of the basic sciences with each other as well as with the clinical sciences.
- For integration to be effective it must focus on the learner. It should be looked at as a cognitive function that occurs within the learner as the learner links clinical concepts with basic science.
- The benefits of integration are attributed to presenting information and problems in a way that mimics how they are encountered in the real world, and presenting facts in relevant, meaningful, and connected ways.
- There are two main types of integration: integration through dedicated approaches and

integration through specific contexts. In the first, integration is facilitated by organizing content around themes or problems; in the latter, integration occurs through the rich environment associated with authentic learning in the workplace.
- Integration should be viewed as a strategy of curricular design and development and therefore should be considered at the program, course, and session levels.
- Learning outcomes and assessment methods must be aligned and therefore integrated learning must be assessed in an integrated manner.
- While there are a number of identified advantages of integration, there are also challenges that should be considered prior to implementation.

Introduction

While much has been written about integration and education, little in the literature is specific to veterinary medicine. However, the fundamentals of how students learn and how curricula are designed and implemented are similar regardless of the situation. This chapter will discuss integration in the context of medical education and conclude with a short section on integration and veterinary medicine. Most veterinary school curricula today follow a traditional medical school design, in which two years of basic and paraclinical (foundational)

Veterinary Medical Education: A Practical Guide, First Edition. Edited by Jennifer L. Hodgson and Jacquelyn M. Pelzer.
© 2017 John Wiley & Sons, Inc. Published 2017 by John Wiley & Sons, Inc.

sciences are followed by two years of clinical (applied) sciences. Courses in the first two years are usually discipline based, delivered independently, and include subjects such as anatomy, embryology, neuroscience, histology, physiology, biochemistry, microbiology, pharmacology, and pathology. The effectiveness of this traditional approach in medical education has been questioned in recent years, resulting in a call for integration of the basic sciences with each other as well as with the clinical sciences (Cooke *et al.*, 2010). This chapter defines integration, provides support for why integration is a good strategy for a learner, describes approaches to integration and how a session, course, or curriculum could be integrated, and discusses how integration affects assessment. It concludes with the reported benefits and challenges of integration and a short section on integration and veterinary medicine.

Definitions

While there are a number of definitions in the literature, most start with the dictionary and define integration as combining two or more things to make something more effective, more harmonious, or more coordinated, often by the addition or rearrangement of elements (Achike, 2016; Schmidt, 1998).

When applied to teaching, Harden defined integration as "the organization of teaching matter to interrelate or unify subjects frequently taught in separate academic courses or departments" (Harden, Sowden, and Dunn, 1984).

When applied to medical education, integration refers to situations in which knowledge from different sources (basic science, clinical, factual, experiential) connects and interrelates (Regehr and Norman, 1996) in a way that fosters understanding and performance of the professional activities of medicine (Kulasegaram *et al.*, 2013).

Some writers believe that a very precise definition is necessary to aid in designing, implementing, and reviewing integrated curricula and integrated curricular units (Brauer and Ferguson, 2015). Utilizing the spiral model as

the ideal goal, they propose that an "integrated curriculum" be defined as "fully synchronous, trans-disciplinary delivery of information between the foundational sciences and the applied sciences throughout all years of a medical school curriculum."

Others refer to an integrated curriculum as interdisciplinary teaching, thematic teaching, and synergistic teaching (Malik and Malik, 2011).

In this chapter, integration is discussed in its broadest context: within learning sessions, within courses, and within programs.

Why Integrated Learning?

Many aspects of veterinary education are modeled after medical education. The traditional curricular design of two by two harks back to the first call for reform in medical education (Flexner, Carnegie Foundation for the Advancement of Teaching, and Pritchett, 1910). Flexner had observed that most medical schools relied on lectures to transmit information to students and he contended that this passive form of learning was ineffective if it was not connected to practice. He argued that a better model was to apply knowledge through more active forms of laboratory and clinical experience, providing opportunities for integrated learning (Irby, Cooke, and O'Brien, 2010). Flexner naively assumed that students would be able to apply what they learned in the class and the laboratory to the bedside. This fundamental model of education continues today in many medical schools and most veterinary schools and recently, 100 years after the first call for reform, a second call by the Carnegie Foundation was issued. The key findings (Cooke *et al.*, 2010) recommended four goals for medical education for the future: standardization and individualization; integration; insistence on excellence; and formation of professional identity. The specific recommendations for integration included:

- Connect formal knowledge to clinical experience, including early clinical immersion and adequate opportunities for more advanced learners to reflect and study.

Box 5.2: Reflections on integration within the curriculum

"There is a fundamental difference between a curriculum in which many disciplines are represented simultaneously, reflecting many interconnections among them but not requiring the student to achieve any transfer, and a curriculum in which the student is required to generalize, to identify commonalities and to draw conclusions applicable to other disciplines .... The former type of curriculum demonstrates integration on the part of the planner, at the macro-level; the latter, on the learner's at the micro-level." (Benor, 1982, p. 357)

- Integrate basic, clinical, and social sciences.
- Engage learners at all levels with a more comprehensive perspective on patients' experience of illness and care, including more longitudinal connections with patients.
- Provide opportunities for learners to experience the broader professional roles of physicians, including educator, advocate, and investigator.
- Incorporate interprofessional education and teamwork into the curriculum (Cooke *et al.*, 2010).

Rather than leaving integration to chance, the report called for medical schools to implement integration actively throughout all levels of the curriculum. Such integration would allow medical students to appreciate the relevance and clinical context of information encountered in the classroom, to build experiential knowledge to complement formal knowledge, to transfer and apply formal knowledge to the clinical setting, and, ultimately, to be better prepared for the complex tasks involved in patient care (Dyrbye *et al.*, 2011).

Integration, as a fundamental requirement of medical school curricula, has also been advocated by those who oversee education in Canada (Bandiera *et al.*, 2013) and the United Kingdom (GMC, 2015).

Integration and the Learner

If integration is to be used as an effective learning strategy, then integration must focus on the learner (see Box 5.2). It should be looked at as a cognitive function that occurs within the learner as the learner links clinical concepts with basic science.

Students in a classroom generally organize medical knowledge according to the structure of the curriculum. For example, if pathophysiology is taught according to organ systems, then the student's knowledge will be similarly organized, and the retrieval of information will be triggered by questions related to a specific organ system or to the context in which the material was taught. However, in the clinical setting, wellness and disease are the focus. Clinical problems cross organ systems and disciplines and so the transition for the student from preclinical to clinical is awkward and difficult (Bowen, 2006). Only after learners make new connections between their knowledge and specific clinical encounters can they also make strong connections between clinical signs and the knowledge stored in their memory. Integrating information in teaching sessions, courses, or across the curriculum and helping students make the connections between prior knowledge and new knowledge, especially in the context in which they will use this information, will provide students with opportunities for meaningful and relevant storage and retrieval of information.

The earlier that students begin to accumulate a mental database of cases, the sooner they will develop a firm foundation on which to allow nonanalytic processes to contribute to the development of clinical reasoning. Context specificity and the need to build an adequate database from which to reason by way of analogy demand that many examples be seen, that students actively engage in the problem-solving process, and that the examples provide an accurate representation of different ways in which specific diseases present (Eva, 2005). Using comparisons of clinical examples can help students identify deep features of basic science concepts that will assist them in elaborating on that knowledge as they progress into clinical education (Woods, Brooks, and Norman, 2005).

The benefits of integration are attributed to presenting information and problems in a way that mimics how they are encountered in the real world, and presenting facts in relevant, meaningful, and connected ways. The responsibility for learning resides with the learners, who must construct their own meaning, and hence integrate, from available learning opportunities. Cognitive psychology has demonstrated that facts and concepts are best recalled and put into service when they are taught, practiced, and assessed in the context in which they will be used (Bransford *et al.*, 1999). Since the ability to perform thinking tasks is related to success in retrieving relevant knowledge from memory, educational strategies should be directed at enhancing meaning, reducing dependence on context, and providing repeated, relevant practice in retrieving information (Regehr and Norman, 1996).

For new information to have meaning, it must be integrated into the semantic network, an elaborate set of connections between abstract concepts and/or specific experiences. These linkages between concepts and experiences are based on meaning. By linking basic science material to clinical problems, often through patient- or case-based learning, students are able to integrate the material into their existing networks for better retrieval. Likewise, clinical reasoning skills should be taught with clinical content, as the two must be integrated in the development of expertise (Regehr and Norman, 1996). The context in which we teach information also affects the ability to retrieve that content later. Retrieval depends on the similarity between the context or condition of

retrieval, and the context or condition in which the item was originally learned. Thus, teaching students about basic science in the context of clinical examples and explicitly making connections are ways in which integration can enhance long-term retention and deeper understanding. Finally, practice is vital to the development of expertise. The work on the specialization of routines suggests that individuals must practice the same problem-solving routines repeatedly. In addition, the novice must have extensive practice in identifying the situations in which a particular problem-solving routine is likely to be useful.

The use of authentic learning, connecting knowledge to real-world issues, problems, and applications, is a powerful learning strategy. Adult learners prefer meaningful learning: they learn best when they understand the topic's relevance and how it can be immediately applied to current relevant problems. Thus, students are more likely to be interested in what they are learning, more motivated to learn new concepts and skills, and better prepared to succeed in careers, if what they learn mirrors real-life contexts. This then equips them with practical and useful skills and addresses topics that are relevant and applicable to their lives outside of school. Another principle of authentic learning is that it mirrors the complexities and ambiguities of real life.

Therefore, when examining integrated learning from the learners' perspective, the following are important considerations (Prideaux, Ash, and Cottrell, 2013):

- Learners can achieve integration from constructing learning in real work settings.
- Learning will be facilitated when there is integration of content beyond the single context into multiple contexts, and when the learning contexts are similar to those in which information must be retrieved.
- Integrated learning should be holistic rather than atomistic.

While there is ample indirect evidence that integration enhances memory and retrieval and therefore facilitates thinking tasks, there is little direct evidence. One example involves the use of progress testing in a contextual medical curriculum with integration of the basic and clinical sciences. The change to this type of curriculum was reported to lead to a more gradual, steadier, and finally higher level of mastery of clinical knowledge. At the same time, the study showed that a stronger emphasis on the basic sciences in the early years of a curriculum led to a steeper learning curve in the mastery of clinically relevant basic knowledge. This type of knowledge continued to develop, even without formal teaching in this domain, during the later years of the curriculum (van der Veken *et al.*, 2009).

Integration and the Curriculum

Within a curriculum, there are a number of ways to approach integration. The two main types of integration are integration through dedicated approaches and integration through specific contexts (see Box 5.3). In the first of these, the program is deliberately structured to organize or facilitate learning across the disciplines through the use of key concepts, themes, or problems. Within this, integration is referred to as horizontal or vertical or both.

Integrated learning through context is commonly found in clinical settings. Community, ambulatory, primary care, and general practice settings offer excellent opportunities for integrated learning in current veterinary school curricula, providing students with chances to gain entry-level knowledge, skills, and behaviors.

While educators can provide integrative opportunities within the curriculum through either dedicated approaches or specific contexts, this will not necessarily translate into integrative learning. Integration should always emphasize the cognitive activity that occurs within the learner.

In an integrated curricular model, the underlying principle is synthesis or blending. Instead of individual subjects or disciplines dominating a curriculum, there tends to be themes that draw on different subjects or disciplines, and these run longitudinally throughout the year or the entire curriculum. In this way, students are encouraged to see the links between subjects or disciplines and to understand how subject- or discipline-based knowledge is applied to real-world cases. With the shift to more integrated curricula, there are also other shifts such as weak framing (Loftus, 2015). This is because there are many ways of implementing pedagogy; for example, problem-based learning sessions can be dovetailed with traditional lectures and laboratories.

Horizontal Integration

In horizontally integrated courses, the disciplines are combined and organized around concepts or ideas in each year or level of the course (see Box 5.4). The focus then moves from subjects such as anatomy or physiology to blocks or units corresponding to body systems, such as cardiovascular or gastrointestinal. In some cases body systems are integrated within the block or unit, for example cardiovascular with respiratory or endocrine with reproduction. Within these blocks, normal structure and

---

 Box 5.3: Focus on types of integration

- Dedicated approaches:
  - Horizontal
  - Vertical
- Specific contexts

 Box 5.4: What's the meaning of horizontal integration?

Horizontal integration is defined as integration across disciplines, but within a finite period of time (Brauer and Ferguson, 2015).

function are taught in Year 1 and abnormal structure and function are taught in Year 2. More recently, some medical schools have organized and integrated their content around stages in the life cycle (Prideaux and Ash, 2013).

Horizontal integration can be achieved with a division between normal and abnormal or preclinical and clinical, or these can be combined – normal and abnormal or preclinical and clinical – supporting both horizontal and vertical integration.

Vertical Integration

Vertical integration implies that clinical science is taught at the same time as basic science (see Box 5.5). This may be organized on the basis of body systems or as a number of "vertical themes" that run through all years of the curriculum. A common form of vertical integration involves the early introduction of clinical contact in a course. As time goes on, the amount of clinical contact increases and the amount of basic science content decreases (Leinster, 2013). Many medical courses are now organized around four main themes, which, while given different names, generally contain the following: clinical and communication skills; basic and clinical sciences; social, community, and population health; and law, ethics, and professionalism (Prideaux and Ash, 2013).

A common way of organizing a vertically integrated curriculum is to use a spiral approach. In a spiral curriculum, there is iterative revisiting of topics throughout the curriculum with increasing levels of difficulty. New knowledge builds on

---

Box 5.5: What's the meaning of vertical integration?

Vertical integration represents integration across time, usually attempting to improve education by disrupting the traditional barrier between the basic and clinical sciences (Brauer and Ferguson, 2015).

---

prior knowledge and the students' competence increases with each visit to the top of the spiral (Harden, 1999). In one such curriculum, basic science knowledge was reported to improve as students moved through the curriculum compared with traditional curricula, where basic science knowledge usually declines after the early years (Davis and Harden, 2003). This approach was reported to allow purposeful repetition over time, such that detail and complexity increased, allowing progression toward independent, professional clinical practice (Finnerty *et al.*, 2010).

Integration around Problems or Cases

Problem-based learning (PBL) and case-based learning (CBL) provide opportunities for both horizontal and vertical integration. When used to provide opportunities for horizontal integration, specifically constructed cases become the focus for learning over a week or two. The cases or problems may be organized by body system or life cycle; however, they are structured around the context of patients. They are designed so that students must draw on knowledge, ideas, and concepts from across the disciplines in order to generate and pursue learning goals.

Problem-based learning, as an instructional method, relies on patient problems as the major learning methodology, and these provide the context for students to acquire knowledge about basic and clinical sciences. Problem-based learning is a very useful way of integrating learning, since the information acquired comes from many disciplines and is structured around the context of patient problems (Barrows, 1985). In these curricula, the PBL design facilitates both horizontal and vertical integration, and it is often implemented to achieve integration between the basic and clinical sciences. This integration has been found to stimulate deep rather than superficial learning, a better understanding of important biological principles, and better retention of knowledge (Dahle *et al.*, 2002).

However, it is not necessary to adopt a problem-based approach to learning in order to use PBL as a learning strategy. May and Silva-Fletcher discuss "scaffolded active learning," where core knowledge was provided through framework lectures, and context-related problem-solving was supported through various group exercises, such as case-, problem-, or team-based learning (May and Silva-Fletcher, 2015). In this case, the interest stimulated by context-related problem-solving, and the associated active learning, will build on the framework knowledge to allow personal and integrated knowledge construction in a way that is similar to but more efficient than PBL (May and Silva-Fletcher, 2015).

Integration and Outcome-Based Education

Outcome-based approaches to curricular design and development are advocated for medical courses (Harden, Crosby, and Davis, 1999). In an outcome-based approach, those responsible for the course define broad and significant outcomes that students must attain on graduation. There is then a process of "designing down" so that learning and assessment systems match the outcomes. Courses are therefore defined by outcomes that cross disciplinary boundaries.

Integration and Clinical Teaching

The clinical years provide many opportunities for integrated learning and are a rich environment for authentic learning and authentic integration. Here clinicians apply an integrated body of knowledge to patient care, and so students' knowledge becomes integrated as they actively reason to solve clinical cases. Evidence supports the idea that this integration is best achieved early, such that students learn basic sciences in the context of clinical sciences (Irby, 2011). This then provides contextual relevance to foundational knowledge and allows students to maintain the connection throughout the program, so that they concurrently link clinical cases to evidence-based knowledge.

Veterinary clinical education is similarly challenged: educators question how to provide students with an integrated and generalist clinical learning experience within specialized tertiary-level hospitals associated with university-based veterinary teaching hospitals (see Box 5.6). While there are reports of some innovative approaches (Coe, 2012; Stone *et al.*, 2012), strategies reported in medical curricula might also provide answers for veterinary medicine. Those strategies include task-based learning, longitudinal clerkships, and community-based longitudinal placements.

Task-based learning has been recommended as a strategy to integrate clinical teaching (Harden *et al.*, 2000). In task-based learning, the focus for learning is a set of tasks addressed by a doctor in clinical practice. The learning is built around the tasks and takes place as the student tries to understand not only the tasks themselves, but also the concepts and mechanisms underlying the tasks. These tasks are designed to provide an appropriate focus on clinical rotations for learning clinical medicine,

---

 Box 5.6: Reflections on the clinical year

When specifically considering the clinical year, the literature supports the notion that there are important challenges in medical schools that may negate the benefits of integration. Continuity of learning is considered very important, and is complicated by the traditional division of the core clinical clerkship experience into a "disconnected series of independently governed, discipline-specific, randomly ordered, sequential blocks each characterized by largely ad hoc patient assignments and poorly coordinated learning objectives" (Hirsh *et al.*, 2007).

allowing review of the basic foundational sciences as well as the development of generic competencies.

Longitudinal integrated clerkships (LICs) involve learners spending an extended time in a clinical setting (or a variety of interlinked clinical settings). Here, their clinical learning opportunities are interwoven through continuities of patient contact and care, continuities of assessment and supervision, and continuities of clinical and cultural learning. Some of the reported advantages of LICs include improvement in student learning and professional development, as well as greater satisfaction (Hirsh *et al.*, 2012).

Community-based longitudinal placements are similar to the distributed model of veterinary education, except that in medicine, compared with veterinary medicine, placements are longer. This allows students greater access to patients and clinical learning opportunities, and the ability to learn clinical decision-making in the context of the whole patient, their family, and the available community resources (Worley *et al.*, 2000).

Integration and Interprofessional Education

Interprofessional education is also a form of integration, in which learning is integrated across health and social care professional programs. Interprofessional education occurs when two or more different professions learn with, from, and about each other. Mostly, students from different professions come together in the early part of the curriculum and work in small groups around cases or problems. The literature documents a few examples of fully integrated interprofessional student training wards, where five to seven students work in teams. Together, the students plan and deliver care to inpatients, while learning about teamwork, handover, and communication across professions (Thistlethwaite, 2013).

Integration as an Educational Strategy

Educational strategies are an important consideration when planning a curriculum or reviewing an existing curriculum. The SPICES model reports six strategies that are often viewed at different ends of the spectrum as either traditional or innovative (Harden, Sowden, and Dunn, 1984). One of these strategies represents integrated at one end and subject or discipline based at the other. Another way to consider educational strategies is on a continuum and this is facilitated by the 11 steps on the integration ladder, as outlined in Figure 5.1 (Harden, 2000).

When the continuum is viewed as steps on the ladder, educationalists are provided with

Figure 5.1 Educational strategy.

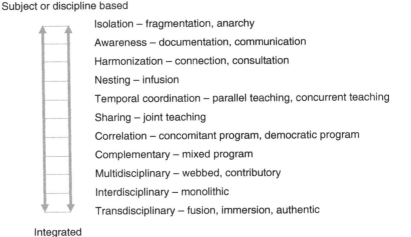

Subject or discipline based

Isolation – fragmentation, anarchy

Awareness – documentation, communication

Harmonization – connection, consultation

Nesting – infusion

Temporal coordination – parallel teaching, concurrent teaching

Sharing – joint teaching

Correlation – concomitant program, democratic program

Complementary – mixed program

Multidisciplinary – webbed, contributory

Interdisciplinary – monolithic

Transdisciplinary – fusion, immersion, authentic

Integrated

Box 5.7: Reflections on the integration continuum

"The question that should be asked of teachers and curriculum designers is not whether they are for or against integration, but rather where on the continuum between the two extremes they should place their teaching." (Harden, Sowden, and Dunn, 1984)

opportunities to explore and to decide at the program level, the course level, and the individual session level where on the ladder they would like to be (Harden, 2000) (see Box 5.7).

Implementing Integration

Integration should be considered as a strategy of curricular design and development and not a goal in itself (Goldman and Schroth, 2012). It should not be carried out in isolation, but rather decisions should be made at program, course, and session levels and should be in line with curricular design and development decisions. If an organized and logical approach is followed, integration as a learning strategy is more likely to be successful. A three-level framework has been suggested as one way to accomplish this (Goldman and Schroth, 2012):

- At the program level, the educational mission of the institution will inform the program goals, and these in turn will determine the specific educational requirements. As part of this, a decision is made as to whether integration will be a strategy to achieve these goals. Once this decision is made, a number of program-level integration decisions follow and a framework is designed. Goldman and Schroth (2012) provide a synopsis of five crucial considerations and decisions, with associated examples.
- At the course level, decisions relate to course learning outcomes, content, and sequencing,

as well as assessment. Goldman and Schroth (2012) view the integration ladder (Harden, 2000) as a useful way to determine where on the continuum of integration the course should lie.

- Session-level course development decisions relate to session learning outcomes, content, sequencing, and strategies. An important concept is that the individual learner's cognitive processing dimensions related to integration occur at the final two levels of Bloom's taxonomy, "synthesis" and "evaluation" (Bloom, 1956). Teaching methods should target these two levels and include problems, cases, simulations, projects, exercises, and critiques.

An alternative step-wise approach to total curricular integration, with 12 suggestions, has been reported as being successful (Malik and Malik, 2011). These authors discuss how integration can be achieved by avoiding commonly committed mistakes. They include subjects such as staff development, establishing working groups, organizing the teaching/learning materials under themes, and developing some innovative teaching/learning and assessment strategies.

Although students, faculty, and curricular leaders share similar perspectives on many aspects of curricular integration, they also have differing perceptions of what integration means, how it succeeds, and where it faces important challenges. As schools embark on curricular revision and integration, it is important to listen to different perspectives (Muller *et al.*, 2008).

Integrated Learning and Assessment

Learning outcomes and assessment methods must always be aligned (see Box 5.8). Therefore, if integrated learning is to be promoted by curricular design, it must be assessed in an integrated manner. Integrated learning assessment methods must be chosen that will promote and encourage students to think in an integrated

Box 5.8: Focus on integration and assessment

Learning outcomes and assessment methods must always be aligned, and this is especially so in an integrated curriculum.

way (Prideaux, Ash, and Cottrell, 2013). Assessments should focus on the application of basic science knowledge, often to clinical problems, and on the integration of knowledge across topics and courses. This requires test materials that are very different from those produced on a lecture-by-lecture and course-by-course basis (Swanson and Case, 1997). These authors provide examples of how to construct assessments that test for integration of knowledge within and across courses or blocks.

An important step is to ensure that integrated learning is represented in assessment blueprints. This requires a central process of test and examination construction, with responsibility for assessment residing within the school rather than within individual departments (Prideaux and Ash, 2013).

Designing integrated learning assessments is reported to be quite challenging and requires sufficient time and resources. Some of the reported challenges include developing questions that cross subject disciplines and yet retain validity and reliability. Often multidisciplinary input is needed, requiring faculty with different expertise from both basic and clinical sciences to work together (Achike, 2016). In some schools, integrated assessment has been referred to as "stapled integration," where discipline-based faculty write discipline-based questions and just staple them together (Schmidt, 1998). Generally, schools that designed student assessment to be congruent with the integrated curricula reported fewer problems (Schmidt, 1998).

Advantages of Integration

There are a number of articles that discuss the advantages of integrated learning (Harden,

Sowden, and Dunn, 1984; Cavalieri, 2009; Harden and Laidlaw, 2012). These advantages include the following (also see Box 5.9):

- Integrated learning reflects how medicine is practiced. As highlighted at the beginning of this chapter, integration in medical education is important because medical practice itself requires a great deal of integration.
- A well-planned, integrated curriculum has been reported to significantly streamline the foundational sciences curriculum, resulting in a reduction in classroom hours (Schmidt, 1998). It highlights what it is important for the student to know and can be seen as a solution to the problem of information overload.
- For the many reasons discussed under the heading of integration and learning, integration should provide students with opportunities that allow better retention and retrieval of information. It allows students to see connections between disciplines and topics, thus reinforcing their relevance and helping students to apply their knowledge. Authentic learning connects knowledge to application in the world beyond the classroom, improving not only the retention and retrieval of information, but students' participation, engagement, excitement, and satisfaction. It allows students to see why foundational knowledge is important for their careers and how they will use that knowledge.
- Building connections and establishing relevance may promote greater student interest and motivation. Rigorous training in foundational sciences without a connection to application can result in decreased enthusiasm and motivation early in a course, together with concerns about relevance.
- Teaching together as part of an integrated curriculum promotes collaboration and communication between faculty. It enables faculty to share teaching methodologies and learn from one another, and faculty find teaching a richer and more rewarding experience. Sometimes teaching together provides faculty with opportunities to find common areas for research collaboration.

Box 5.9: Focus on advantages to integration

- It reflects how medicine is practiced
- It streamlines the basic science curriculum
- It offers opportunities for storage and retrieval of knowledge, authentic learning, and development of clinical reasoning skills

- It provides relevance, interest, and motivation
- It leads to a richer teaching environment for faculty

 Box 5.10: Focus on challenges to integration

- Integration is a curricular strategy, not a goal
- It is time consuming and resource intensive
- It raises challenges about who owns the curriculum
- It requires central curricular management
- It demands that multidisciplinary teams work together for the greater good

- It can marginalize and devalue faculty
- It requires a curricular map to determine where disciplines are taught
- It requires the realignment of resources and expectations

Challenges Associated with Integration

Integration also involves a number of challenges (also see Box 5.10):

- While there is much literature in support of curricular integration, there is also literature that contains criticisms of the practices associated with its implementation. Goldman and Schroth contend that these criticisms most often arise from a failure to understand that integration is a strategy of curricular development and not a goal. The basis for using this strategy – that is, the goal that it is designed to achieve – should be clear, and the application of the strategy at all three levels should be carefully executed (Goldman and Schroth, 2012).
- Creating an integrated curriculum can be time consuming and resource intensive. Many references discuss the time and work commitment in terms of planning,

organization, and execution (Prideaux, Ash, and Cottrell, 2013; Malik and Malik, 2011; Brauer and Ferguson, 2015). Delivering an integrated curriculum requires faculty to collaborate and work closely together to design and deliver course content and assessment tasks. Faculty need to be collegial and creative as they strategically select the topics that are most relevant and decide how they can be integrated. Delivering learning sessions and assessing integrated content may also require faculty from a variety of disciplines to meet and work together, which can make scheduling difficult and place more demands on faculty time. A high level of cooperation and time to plan and deliver the integrated content are required (Cavalieri, 2009).

- Any form of integration within the curriculum raises challenges as to who owns that curriculum. Traditionally, each discipline or department is responsible for the selection of material and the delivery of teaching within its own domain. With integration, curricula are no longer managed within departments but across the school, resulting in a loss of departmental control of course content and management. In most cases, the administration of the curriculum is centrally managed, with curriculum content and organization overseen by a central committee.

- Unlike the traditional curriculum, the integrated curriculum requires multidisciplinary basic and clinical sciences teams to develop course content. This includes the biases that faculty bring to the table regarding their perception of integration and the tendency to push or not push their discipline. Unless a group or holistic view is taken, discipline content can be over- or underrepresented in the new design (Achike, 2016).
- Centralized curriculum planning can lead to disengagement of teachers, who may feel that they can no longer cover their disciplinary content in the allotted time. It is important that the teachers who are to deliver the curriculum feel that they have a stake in it (Leinster, 2013).
- Academic faculty tend to identify themselves by their specialty, which tends to be discipline based. In moving to an integrated curriculum, faculty may perceive that their discipline is no longer important, and therefore by inference that the content they teach is devalued.
- Academic faculty tend to teach within their disciplines, so there is a need to map curricular content to be able to determine the amount of time allocated to disciplines, and also to help faculty identify where their specific discipline is now taught throughout the curriculum.
- Transitions from one curricular model to the other often require the realignment of resources and expectations. In traditional curricula, nonphysicians usually teach basic science content, whereas physicians teach clinical sciences content. Integration of basic and clinical sciences content can result in debates between basic scientists and clinicians as to who is better able to teach the content (Bandiera *et al.*, 2013).

Integration and Veterinary Medicine

While much has been written about integration and education within human medicine, there are only a few reports addressing the topic in veterinary education. Curriculum integration in veterinary education was reported to represent one approach to delivering a learning experience that aims to mimic more closely the way in which information and problems are encountered in the workplace (Cavalieri, 2009). Cavalieri explores examples of steps on the integration ladder and reports that these examples are included in many undergraduate veterinary degree programs. In attempting to contextualize a definition for the teaching of veterinary science, Cavalieri suggested that integration of a veterinary science curriculum should involve the following:

- Organizing student learning in an authentic way that is linked to what veterinarians do.
- Designing the curriculum to reflect how problems are encountered in real life.
- Promoting linkages between disciplines and topics, allowing students to connect and construct their learning across fields and thereby promoting deeper learning and reinforcing greater relevance.
- Encouraging the development of skills to assist students to be able to locate, assess, and use a variety of sources of information. This may help equip students to be lifelong learners.
- Enhancing communication, self-management, and interpersonal skills, recognizing their critical importance in professional life and the application of knowledge and skills.
- Acknowledging and embracing the contribution of academic disciplines, but limiting their contribution to what is needed in the application of knowledge and seeing their place in the context of a more holistic view of knowledge.
- Interrelating different subjects and topics, both horizontally between parallel disciplines such as anatomy, physiology, and biochemistry, and vertically between different

disciplines that are traditionally taught in the early or later years of the curriculum, such as physiology and medicine.

Specific Examples of Integration in Veterinary Medicine

Curriculum Integration for a Veterinary Program (James Cook University)

James Cook University implemented a five-year veterinary science degree built on an integrated learning program (Cavalieri, 2009). Integration within the curriculum started toward the end of Year 1 and continued in Years 2 and 3, with full integration around the following themes: structure and function; disease, defense, and chemical agents; animal production, management, and behavior; veterinary services; veterinary practice; and professional life. Years 4 and 5 were still to be implemented at the time of writing, with integration accomplished by designing problems based on clinical signs within each species.

Problem-Based Learning as a Strategy for Integration of Basic and Clinical Sciences in a Traditional Veterinary Curriculum (University of Tennessee)

As part of an overall curricular modification, PBL experiences were introduced into a professional curriculum at the University of Tennessee (Howell *et al.*, 2002). PBL was introduced into the traditional curricular format in dedicated week-long experiences (application-based learning exercises) at specific points during the first six semesters. These experiences were implemented to encourage students to take

more responsibility for their education, to reinforce students' curiosity and enthusiasm for learning, to integrate basic and applied information across disciplines, to promote professional behavior and attitudes, and to enhance written and verbal communication skills. The inclusion of "thin slices" of PBL in a modified traditional curriculum was reported as a successful method of introducing problem-solving, self-directed learning, and small-group work into the veterinary curriculum.

Curriculum Integration for a Veterinary Program (University of California, Davis)

In 2011, the School of Veterinary Medicine at the University of California, Davis introduced a curriculum in which content in Years 1 and 2 was integrated horizontally and vertically, mostly around body systems but also themes. As a result, these blocks formed the majority of the coursework. Where appropriate, topics are integrated within blocks: musculoskeletal; neuroscience, senses, and behavior; gastrointestinal and metabolism; cardiovascular and respiratory; urinary and renal; and endocrine and reproduction. Other topics include basic and clinical foundations; pharmacology, nutrition, and toxicology; immunology, hematology, and coagulation; skin; oncology; population health; and immunology and infectious diseases. A professional and clinical skills course threads through all three years, in some cases introducing new content, such as ethics, regulatory medicine, and law, and in other cases revisiting the same content, such as communication and business but at a more advanced level. In Year 3, students select either a small animal or large animal stream, and again content is horizontally integrated around body systems or themes.

References

Achike, F.I. (2016) The challenges of integration in an innovative modern medical curriculum. *Medical Science Educator*, **26** (**1**), 153–158.

Bandiera, G., Boucher, A., Neville, A., *et al.* (2013) Integration and timing of basic and clinical sciences education. *Medical Teacher*, **35**, 381–387.

Barrows, H.S. (1985) *How to Design a Problem-Based Curriculum for the Preclinical Years*, Springer, New York.

Benor, D.E. (1982) Interdisciplinary integration in medical education: Theory and method. *Medical Educator*, **16**, 355–361.

Bloom, B.S. (1956) *Taxonomy of Educational Objectives: The Classification of Educational Goals*, Longmans, Green, New York.

Bowen, J.L. (2006) Educational strategies to promote clinical diagnostic reasoning. *New England Journal of Medicine*, **355**, 2217–2225.

Bransford, J., Brown, A.L., Cocking, R.R., and National Research Council (US) Committee on Developments in the Science of Learning (1999) *How People Learn: Brain, Mind, Experience, and School*, National Academy Press, Washington, DC.

Brauer, D.G., and Ferguson, K.J. (2015) The integrated curriculum in medical education: AMEE Guide no. 96. *Medical Teacher*, **37**, 312–322.

Cavalieri, J. (2009) Curriculum integration within the context of veterinary education. *Journal of Veterinary Medical Education*, **36**, 388–396.

Coe, J.B. (2012) Primary care: An important role in the future of veterinary education. *Journal of Veterinary Medical Education*, **39**, 209.

Cooke, M., Irby, D.M., O'Brien, B.C., and Carnegie Foundation for the Advancement of Teaching (2010) *Educating Physicians: A Call for Reform of Medical School and Residency*, Jossey-Bass, San Francisco, CA.

Dahle, L.O., Brynhildsen, J., Behrbohm Fallsberg, M., *et al.* (2002) Pros and cons of vertical integration between clinical medicine and basic science within a problem-based undergraduate medical curriculum: Examples and experiences from Linkoping, Sweden. *Medical Teacher*, **24**, 280–285.

Davis, M.H., and Harden, R.M. (2003) Planning and implementing an undergraduate medical curriculum: The lessons learned. *Medical Teacher*, **25**, 596–608.

Dyrbye, L.N., Starr, S.R., Thompson, G.B., and Lindor, K.D. (2011) A model for integration of formal knowledge and clinical experience: The advanced doctoring course at Mayo Medical School. *Academic Medicine*, **86**, 1130–1136.

Eva, K.W. (2005) What every teacher needs to know about clinical reasoning. *Medical Educator*, **39**, 98–106.

Finnerty, E.P., Chauvin, S., Bonaminio, G., *et al.* (2010) Flexner revisited: The role and value of the basic sciences in medical education. *Academic Medicine*, **85**, 349–355.

Flexner, A., Carnegie Foundation for the Advancement of Teaching, and Pritchett, H.S. (1910) *Medical Education in the United States and Canada: A Report to the Carnegie Foundation for the Advancement of Teaching*, Carnegie Foundation, New York.

GMC (2015) *Promoting Excellence: Standards for Medical Education and Training*. General Medical Council. http://www.gmc-uk.org/education/26828.asp (accessed 4 January 2016).

Goldman, E., and Schroth, W.S. (2012) Perspective: Deconstructing integration: A framework for the rational application of integration as a guiding curricular strategy. *Academic Medicine*, **87**, 729–734.

Harden, R.M. (1999) What is a spiral curriculum? *Medical Teacher*, **21**, 141–143.

Harden, R.M. (2000) The integration ladder: A tool for curriculum planning and evaluation. *Medical Educator*, **34**, 551–557.

Harden, R.M., Crosby, J.R., and Davis, M.H. (1999) AMEE guide no. 14: Outcome-based education: Part 1 – An introduction to outcome-based education. *Medical Teacher*, **21**, 7–14.

Harden, R., Crosby, J., Davis, M.H., *et al.* (2000) Task-based learning: The answer to integration and problem-based learning in the clinical years. *Medical Educator*, **34**, 391–397.

Harden, R.M., and Laidlaw, J.M. (2012) *Essential Skills for a Medical Teacher: An Introduction to Teaching and Learning in Medicine*, Churchill Livingstone, Edinburgh.

Harden, R.M., Sowden, S., and Dunn, W.R. (1984) Educational strategies in curriculum development: The SPICES model. *Medical Educator*, **18**, 284–297.

Hirsh, D., Gaufberg, E., Ogur, B., *et al.* (2012) Educational outcomes of the Harvard Medical School-Cambridge integrated clerkship: A way forward for medical education. *Academic Medicine*, **87**, 643–650.

Hirsh, D.A., Ogur, B., Thibault, G.E., and Cox, M. (2007) "Continuity" as an organizing principle for clinical education reform. *New England Journal of Medicine*, **356**, 858–866.

Howell, N.E., Lane, I.F., Brace, J.J., and Shull, R.M. (2002) Integration of problem-based learning in a veterinary medical curriculum: First-year experiences with application-based learning exercises at the University of Tennessee College of Veterinary Medicine. *Journal of Veterinary Medical Education*, **29**, 169–175.

Irby, D. (2011) Educating physicians for the future: Carnegie's calls for reform. *Medical Teacher*, **33**, 547–550.

Irby, D.M., Cooke, M., and O'Brien, B.C. (2010) Calls for reform of medical education by the Carnegie Foundation for the Advancement of Teaching: 1910 and 2010. *Academic Medicine*, **85**, 220–227.

Kulasegaram, K.M., Martimianakis, M.A., Mylopoulos, M., *et al.* (2013) Cognition before curriculum: Rethinking the integration of basic science and clinical learning. *Academic Medicine*, **88**, 1578–1585.

Leinster, S. (2013) The undergraduate curriculum and clinical teaching in the early years, in *A Practical Guide for Medical Teachers*, 4th edn (eds. J.A. Dent and R.M. Harden), Churchill Livingstone/Elsevier, London, pp. 16–22.

Loftus, S. (2015) Understanding integration in medical education. *Medical Science Educator*, **25**, 357–360.

Malik, A.S., and Malik, R.H. (2011) Twelve tips for developing an integrated curriculum. *Medical Teacher*, **33**, 99–104.

May, S.A., and Silva-Fletcher, A. (2015) Scaffolded active learning: Nine pedagogical principles for building a modern veterinary curriculum. *Journal of Veterinary Medical Education*, **42**, 332–339.

Muller, J.H., Jain, S., Loeser, H., and Irby, D.M. (2008) Lessons learned about integrating a medical school curriculum: Perceptions of students, faculty and curriculum leaders. *Medical Educator*, **42**, 778–785.

Prideaux, D., and Ash, J.K. (2013) Integrated learning, in *A Practical Guide for Medical Teachers*, 4th edn (eds. J.A. Dent and R.M. Harden), Churchill Livingstone/Elsevier, London (pp. 183–189).

Prideaux, D., Ash, J., and Cottrell, A. (2013) Integrated learning, in *Oxford Textbook of Medical Education* (ed. K. Walsh), Oxford University Press, Oxford.

Regehr, G., and Norman, G.R. (1996) Issues in cognitive psychology: Implications for professional education. *Academic Medicine*, **71**, 988–1001.

Schmidt, H. (1998) Integrating the teaching of basic sciences, clinical sciences, and biopsychosocial issues. *Academic Medicine*, **73**, S24–S31.

Stone, E.A., Conlon, P., Cox, S., and Coe, J.B. (2012) A new model for companion-animal primary health care education. *Journal of Veterinary Medical Education*, **39**, 210–216.

Swanson, D.B., and Case, S.M. (1997) Assessment in basic science instruction: Directions for practice and research. *Advances in Health Sciences Education, Theory and Practice*, **2**, 71–84.

Thistlethwaite, J.E. (2013) Interprofessional education, in *A Practical Guide for Medical Teachers*, 4th edn (eds J.A. Dent and R.M. Harden), Churchill Livingstone/Elsevier, London, pp. 190–198.

van der Veken, J., Valcke, M., de Maeseneer, J., *et al.* (2009) Impact on knowledge acquisition of the transition from a conventional to an integrated contextual medical curriculum. *Medical Educator*, **43**, 704–713.

Woods, N.N., Brooks, L.R., and Norman, G.R. (2005) The value of basic science in clinical diagnosis: Creating coherence among signs and symptoms. *Medical Educator*, **39**, 107–112.

Worley, P., Silagy, C., Prideaux, D., *et al.* (2000) The parallel rural community curriculum: An integrated clinical curriculum based in rural general practice. *Medical Educator*, **34**, 558–565.

6

Collaborative Learning

Elizabeth Tudor, Laura Dooley and Elise Boller

Faculty of Veterinary and Agricultural Sciences, University of Melbourne, Australia

---

 Box 6.1: Key messages

- Learning is a social construct.
- Collaborative learning can contribute to the development of higher-order thinking skills and professional abilities.
- Collaborative learning can enhance the development of professional socialization and enculturation, and is an essential attribute of the graduate veterinarian.
- Teamwork skills employed in collaborative learning situations model those used in professional life.
- Fostering development of "soft skill" attributes such as teamwork and communication are core responsibilities of veterinary colleges.
- Collaborative learning approaches are consistent with adult learning styles and can leverage the potential of the self-regulating adult learner.

- The notion that collaborative learning is a skill that must be learned must be overtly communicated and developed in both the teacher and the student.
- In veterinary medical colleges, the student characteristics of elite performance and a propensity for individual and competitive learning must be managed for effective use of collaborative learning.
- Building a culture of collaborative learning requires strong leadership and buy-in from the whole of the faculty.
- Collaborative learning strategies can be applied across all disciplinary areas and levels of a veterinary learning program.
- Resource limitations need not restrict opportunities and outcomes in collaborative learning.

Introduction

This chapter will examine the role of collaborative learning activities within the veterinary curriculum. Although numerous studies have demonstrated the value of collaborative activities in achieving learning outcomes of great relevance to veterinary education, collaborative learning activities are commonly perceived to be difficult to implement. Many students and educators are largely accustomed to individualistic forms of learning, assessment, and achievement, and this has led to some reluctance to implement collaborative learning tasks in curricula.

Veterinary Medical Education: A Practical Guide, First Edition. Edited by Jennifer L. Hodgson and Jacquelyn M. Pelzer.
© 2017 John Wiley & Sons, Inc. Published 2017 by John Wiley & Sons, Inc.

Here, we will discuss the nature of collaborative learning, why its inclusion is of benefit in veterinary curricula, and, most importantly, *how* collaborative activities can be integrated into each level of veterinary education.

Defining Collaborative Learning

Defining collaborative learning has proven challenging, with authors from wide-ranging disciplines providing varied perspectives, as described by Dillenbourg (1999). Most broadly, a collaborative task can be viewed as any task that involves the contributions of more than one person. Many authors have utilized the following definition of collaborative learning, as noted by Roschelle and Teasley (1995):

> a coordinated, synchronous activity that is the result of a continued attempt to construct and maintain a shared conception of a problem.

In a veterinary context, collaborative learning has been described as something that occurs "when small groups of students help each other to learn" (Klemm, 1994). Klemm goes on to describe collaborative learning in the veterinary context as "the process whereby each member contributes personal experience, information, perspective, insight, skills, and attitudes with the intent of improving learning accomplishments of the others." Other authors argue that students working in groups may work independently on individual aspects of a group task that are then collated, and that this represents *cooperative* learning rather than true *collaborative* learning (Dillenbourg, 1999). By this definition, when groups work together but learning tasks are divided and then compiled, students may well produce the assessed outcome of group work, without any engagement in collaborative processes. A review of the literature reveals that these terms are variably defined. Davidson and Major (2014) provide an excellent review of the origins of the terms collaborative, cooperative, and problem-based learning, explaining that differences appear to lie along disciplinary lines, and that, to some degree, the distinction between them is semantic.

For the purposes of this chapter, we will examine collaborative learning in the broadest sense and within the veterinary context, drawing on illustrative examples of collaborative learning approaches from different countries. We will focus on activities that involve learning through the co-construction of knowledge and understanding that are developed together via social interactions between and among groups of peers and educators, and carefully designed, collaborative learning activities that can transpire through both face-to-face and virtual interactions. In this process, each individual student contributes their perspective to create new knowledge that the group as a whole then possesses.

Collaborative Learning: Why Do It?

Collaborative Learning Aids in the Development of General Professional Attributes

Becoming a veterinarian demands not only the acquisition of a large body of knowledge and practical skills, but also the process of gaining entry to a professional community of practice. Professional learning is often collaborative in nature, therefore students must be equipped with the skills to participate effectively in, and learn from, collaborative opportunities that may present themselves within and outside of the workplace (Eraut, 2007). The recent NAVMEC *Roadmap for Veterinary Medicine Education in the 21st Century* lists collaboration as a core professional competency for graduate veterinarians (Shung and Osburn, 2011). Indeed, many veterinary colleges reference the ability to engage in lifelong learning as a key graduate attribute. We must therefore give explicit consideration to how students will acquire these skills through the course of their veterinary program. It has been argued that the learning and teaching of professionalism in veterinary medicine should be reframed as a sociocultural construct (Scholz, Trede, and Raidal, 2013). Early learning in the form of collaborative preclinical activities and clinical and extramural rotations may strongly support enculturation into the profession. Thoughtfully crafted collaborative learning activities may back up this process of professional socialization, the evolution from knowing how to "do" veterinary medicine to "being" a veterinarian. This is addressed in more detail in Part Two, Chapter 7: Teaching Interprofessionalism.

Working with peers also provides an opportunity for students to develop and exercise professional skills in the early preclinical years, when they may have limited access to clinical contexts. For example, communication (verbal, non-verbal, and written), listening, and reflection skills are required to interact effectively with peers. Through collaboration, students also have the opportunity to develop cultural awareness and build friendships across ethnic and sociocultural boundaries. This understanding is directly applicable to the work environment of many veterinarians who service ethnically diverse communities. Collaborative work can result in conflict and disagreements associated with differences in expectations between peers. These experiences mirror the types of disputes that may arise in the workplace between colleagues, or between a veterinarian and a client. The challenges associated with collaborative work therefore also provide an opportunity for students to develop and try out strategies to manage conflict, and the leadership and management skills required to move the group forward.

Collaborative Learning Is Consistent with Adult Learning Styles

A growing body of research indicates that adults learn differently than children, and are differently motivated to learn. Kolb's experiential learning model has shaped our understanding of how adults learn (Kolb, 1984). According to Kolb, adults learn through a series of cycles of experience, reflection, and planning (see Figure 6.1). In this model, it is the dissonance between the concrete experience and the prior knowledge/experience of the learner that provides the stimulus for new learning. In this way, the prior knowledge of an individual shapes their perception of an experiential task. Collaborative learning tasks provide an opportunity for students to expose and discuss their pre-existing knowledge or assumptions of relevant content, and to experiment actively with applying concepts in new situations. Collaborative activities

Figure 6.1 Experiential learning model. Source: Kolb, 1984. Reproduced with permission of Prentice Hall.

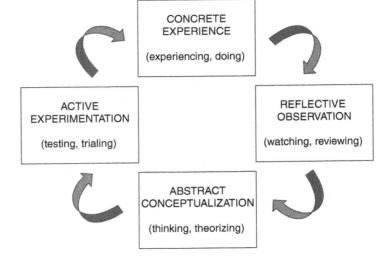

therefore create a new experience on which to reflect. Within a single collaborative task, students can undertake multiple iterative cycles of experience, planning, and reflection.

Collaborative Learning Allows Students to Leverage the Knowledge and Experience of Peers

Collaborative learning activities provide an opportunity for students to uncover new knowledge by leveraging the varied experiences of their peers. Luft and Ingram (1955) designed the Johari window through a study of personality traits and interpersonal skills (see Figure 6.2). This construct highlights that for any individual there are characteristics that exist that are not known to them, but are known to others. It emphasizes that interactions with others can enable the uncovering of knowledge beyond that which is known to individuals. Through peer interactions, students can discover new approaches and expose gaps in their understanding. Perry (1999) observed that college students progress from a learning approach of "duality" (clear right and wrong, with direction from teachers) toward "multiplicity" (recognition that solutions may be uncertain, context is important, and peers can be a relevant source of experience). At each stage of their veterinary

education, students will be variably progressed along this spectrum. Collaboration with peers provides an opportunity for them to reveal and discuss their individual approach to a task, and come to a collective understanding that builds on the individual knowledge base. This is particularly relevant in graduate-level veterinary education, where students begin the program with varied undergraduate experience and knowledge. There is a clear opportunity for veterinary students to learn from each other, and one method for harnessing this opportunity is through the delivery of well-designed collaborative learning tasks.

Collaborative Learning Is Central to the Development of Self-Regulation of Learning

Collaborative learning shifts considerable responsibility for learning onto the learners themselves. This models the reality for qualified veterinarians seeking continuing professional development, whereby they are required to identify their individual development needs, and to identify strategies by which to achieve their stated learning goals. Self-regulation of learning involves planning, performance, and reflection, thus the "self-regulated" learner is able to regulate their thinking, their motivation, and their behavior during the learning process (Pintrich and Zusho, 2002). A study by Sungur and Tekkaya (2006) demonstrated that students undertaking a problem-based program of study in small collaborative groups showed higher self-reported levels of self-regulated learning than those exposed to a traditional teacher-centered mode of delivery. However, a study by Raidal and Volet (2009) demonstrated that veterinary students show a strong preference for teacher-driven learning experiences. Therefore, the integration of student-centered collaborative learning tasks within a veterinary curriculum can be challenging. The importance of developing the skills of self-regulated learning for future career progression must be clearly articulated to both faculty and veterinary students.

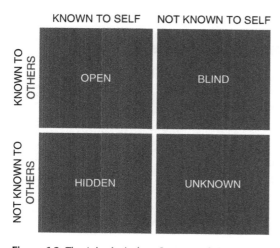

Figure 6.2 The Johari window. Source: Luft & Ingram, 1955. Reproduced with permission of UCLA.

How Can Collaborative Learning Be Integrated into Veterinary Curricula?

The evidence and argument are there: there is an imperative to create a curriculum and employ a pedagogy that foster collaborative learning practices in our students, that enhance their interpersonal skills of teamwork and communication, and that discourage competitive behavior. At its core, collaborative learning involves a shift in focus from instructor-centered learning to student-driven and student-shared learning. As such, collaborative learning is not an "add-on," provided as a supplement to an existing course, but rather an approach to be embraced and owned at the highest levels of the faculty leadership and teaching teams and to be applied throughout a program. The adoption of this approach should be fostered through the professional development of educators and in the design of learning spaces, and should be encouraged and made visible to students.

Student-Centered and Collaborative Learning Practices Must Be Embraced at a Whole-Faculty Level

When in 2008 the University of Melbourne (UoM) embarked on a major curriculum renewal project and development of the graduate Doctor of Veterinary Medicine (DVM), a first step was a process of faculty consultation that led to redefinition of graduate attributes. From these, the *goals* of curriculum renewal emerged. Foremost among these were:

- To develop a curriculum that enhanced opportunities for developing transferable skills in problem-solving.
- To develop a more integrated and systems-based approach to the curriculum.
- To create more time within the teaching program for students to cogitate and to develop intellectual curiosity.

Collaborative learning approaches were identified as central to the attainment of these goals.

At the UoM, our approach to collaborative learning is grounded on several premises:

- Graduate learners come to the classroom with valuable prior knowledge, and students can learn from the prior knowledge and experience of others.
- Deep understanding requires mastery of the language of veterinary science; opportunities to use the language in conversation will aid in that mastery.
- Veterinary students are inherently vocationally focused, and they will learn best when learning is placed in the context of the vocation to which they aspire.
- The learning context must embrace the elements of Kolb's experiential model of adult learning, with opportunities for:
  - experiencing and doing → clinical problem-solving
  - watching and reviewing → listening to and observing the thought patterns of others (peers and instructors)
  - thinking and theorizing → applying current knowledge to a new situation or context
  - active experimentation → testing understanding against peers' knowledge and understanding, and against formative feedback tasks.

Throughout the development of the new curriculum, an increased focus was maintained on the progressive acquisition of the attributes of a graduate veterinary scientist. This focus was formalized through the definition of student learning domains, strands of learning (and assessment) that traverse every subject area of the DVM program, and that are used to describe the student's progressive acquisition of the graduate attributes of a veterinary scientist: the *technical*, the *academic*, the *professional*, the *ethical*, and those relating to *population health and biosecurity*. Collaborative learning practice is woven as a vertical, integrative pedagogical element through each of these domains, throughout the curriculum (see Part Two, Chapter 5: Integrative Learning).

Progressive Attainment of Graduate Outcomes, Including Attainment of Professional Collaborative Skills, Must Be Explicit and Visible to Students

Consistent with our commitment to student-centered learning, we needed to find ways to make these learning domains visible to students, so that they could see that each learning activity in their program was a further step toward acquisition of the skills, knowledge, and aptitudes relevant to them as a graduate veterinarian.

Icons were developed for each of the five learning domains (see Figure 6.3): clinical skills; scientific basis of clinical practice; personal and professional development; ethics and animal welfare; and population health and biosecurity.

Students "see" these icons in study guides and notes for didactic, collaborative, and practical learning activities, and there is visible and constructive alignment of learning outcomes, teaching and learning activities, and feedback and assessment that relate back to one or more of these domains. Teamwork and collaboration are fundamental elements of the personal and professional development learning domain.

Professional Development in Teaching and Curriculum Design should be Encouraged and Supported

In their studies of the factors influencing seminar learning for veterinary students, Spruijt *et al.* (2012, 2013, 2015) identified teacher factors (see Box 6.2) as a key to successful learning outcomes. The ability of the teacher to facilitate group discussion with an appropriate questioning style, to encourage students to participate actively, to stimulate deep thinking, and to guide students toward a case outcome

will have a substantial impact on what students learn. This requires appropriate preparation by the teacher for each learning activity, but also professional development in the form of formal training in small-group teaching. One approach to the provision of preparation is the "tutor briefing session" and "tutor study guide" often provided in problem-based learning programs. Many veterinary colleges now recognize the need for more extensive and formal training of faculty.

Physical Spaces for Collaborative Learning Must Accommodate and Encourage Small-Group Interaction

In recent years we have seen a progressive shift in curriculum design away from more traditional delivery modes like the lecture to more active modes of learning, and in addition the inclusion of a range of information technologies in learning and teaching. Nordquist and Laing (2015) argue that the curriculum must be aligned with learning spaces and that learning spaces must be designed so that collaboration can be achieved. They illustrate this in the cognitive map that they refer to as the "hybridization of learning spaces" in their networked learning landscape model (see Figure 6.4). On the X axis is the direction of change in provision of learning spaces, from single-purpose didactic teaching spaces such as lecture theaters to increasingly flexible-use spaces with multiple applications for both formal and informal learning.

At the UoM our goals for the degree, the premises regarding collaborative learning, and key elements of activity design helped to determine the requirements for the learning spaces where collaborative learning takes place and for

Figure 6.3 University of Melbourne student learning domains: clinical skills; scientific basis of clinical practice; personal and professional development; ethics and animal welfare; and population health and biosecurity.

Box 6.2: Where's the evidence?

One of the most comprehensive studies of factors that influence learning in small-group settings was conducted at Utrecht University (Spruijt *et al.*, 2012, 2013, 2015). Specifically, these researchers looked at factors influencing the learning of veterinary students in a seminar setting (up to 25 students working with a content expert tutor for a two-hour class). While this class is somewhat larger than a typical small-group class, the objectives were entirely consistent with those of small-group teaching: "promotion of active and deep learning in interactive student-centred sessions in which students discuss questions and issues relating to subjects of practical relevance" (Spruijt *et al.*, 2012).

Spruijt *et al.* considered factors affecting learning from the perspectives of both students and teachers, and also analyzed whether these factors accounted for differences in student achievement scores. Factors consistently identified by both students and teachers were the following:

- *The teacher*: the didactic approach, the teacher's facilitating approach, and the teacher's role in preparation of the case and hence "ownership" of it.
- *The students*: their motivation, their preparedness or prior knowledge, their level of active participation, and the continuity of group composition.

- *Preparation for the session*: availability and quality of self-study materials.
- *Group functioning*: "safety" of the group and its inclusivity.
- *Content of the seminar* and its suitability to small-group learning.
- *Course coherence*: the course schedule, and the alignment of small-group learning activities with other elements of the learning program, such as lectures and practical classes.
- *The learning space* and its appropriateness for interaction.
- *Assessment*: alignment of assessment with the goals of small-group learning, such as problem-solving, deep learning, and reflective practice.

However, when these seminar factors were compared to student achievement (examination results), there did not appear to be a strong correlation between positive seminar factors and student achievement scores; instead, student achievement scores correlated more strongly with prior achievement scores (Spruijt *et al.*, 2015). A possible explanation for this finding is that the intended learning outcomes of the seminar (active learning and the adoption of a deep learning approach) were not reflected in the nature of the exam questions.

the size of student learning groups. Effective collaboration requires the following:

- *Dialogue*, a space for which will be facilitated by proximity, visibility, face-to-face contact, and appropriate acoustics.
- *Visualization* of prior knowledge and of new theories and concepts, which can be facilitated in many different ways that are not necessarily technologically advanced or expensive, such as chalkboards, whiteboards, smart whiteboards, shared computer monitors, and so on.

- *"Hybridization"* (Nordquist and Laing, 2015) of the physical and digital learning space, with access to information technology for presentation, simulation, data, and virtual forms of collaboration, such as wikis and blogs.

The efficacy of a learning space is not necessarily directly related to its sophistication. Many examples are now available of more sophisticated interpretations of collaborative learning spaces that bridge the formal and informal learning landscapes, but spaces do not have to be sophisticated or technologically advanced as

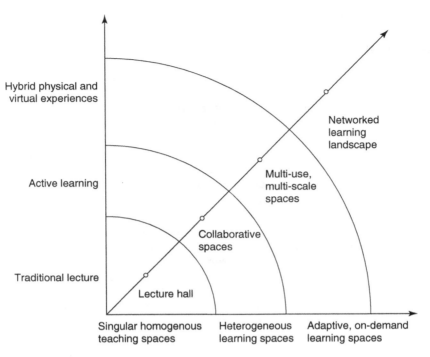

Figure 6.4 Hybridization of learning spaces. Source: Nordquist & Laing, 2015. Reproduced with permission of Taylor and Francis Ltd. http://www .informaworld.com.

long as the key elements required for effective dialog and collaboration in a digital world are provided. At the UoM our small-group work in the pre-clinical years takes place in open pods and small meeting rooms in the library; learning materials for case studies are delivered electronically through the Blackboard Learning Management® system, and large wall-mounted computer screens and white boards are used to facilitate group wiki work. In the Chemistry Learning Laboratory at UoM, a traditional tiered lecture theater has been transformed into a collaborative learning space, where sharing of knowledge within and between groups and with

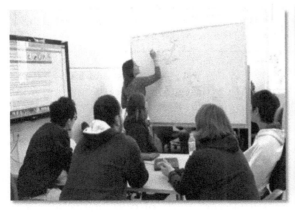 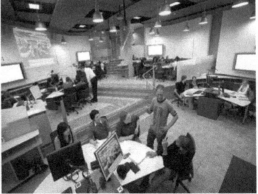

Figure 6.5 Small-group work with a whiteboard and shared flat-screen monitor for group wiki work in case studies at the University of Melbourne (left); a technologically advanced classroom for small-group work in the Department of Chemistry at the University of Melbourne (right).

instructors is facilitated by a range of digital technologies (see Figure 6.5).

Visualization Is a Key Element of Collaborative Learning

The whiteboard, and its predecessor the blackboard, plays a critical role in promoting teamwork and shared thinking. The role of shared visualization has been formalized in recent years by the Lean Enterprise Institute. In lean practice, the visual management board (VMB) is designed to enable all members of a team to see work in progress, recognize impediments to progress, create common information for shared understanding, improve communication between team members, and enhance collaboration. More simply, in our collaborative learning setting at UoM, whiteboards help students to visualize one another's thinking: exposing different points of view, clarifying points of confusion, or summarizing shared progress and understanding. In Figure 6.6 you can see a group of first-year students using a hybridized environment for learning. There is electronic delivery of content on a virtual case with the use of physical tools (e.g., the whiteboard and collaborative discussion) to reinterpret what they have viewed on the radiograph; in doing so, they are sharing their knowledge of urinary tract anatomy in the dog

as it relates to their understanding of a case of urolithiasis.

The Effectiveness of Small-Group Learning Will Depend on Core Discussion Skills

Irrespective of the small-group collaborative methodology (problem-based learning, PBL; team-based learning, TBL; or case-based learning, CBL), learning materials, or physical space, the effectiveness of small-group learning will depend on core discussion skills. This is a truism of collaborative learning: the best-quality learning materials, the most stimulating of cases, and the best alignment of learning outcomes with learning activities will not result in effective and collaborative learning if the students in the group lack the skills required to interact. Effective dialog should involve all members of the group, and the productive participation of group members will depend on their feeling "safe." Is the group the right size? Can they make eye contact with all group members? Is the group a culturally safe place for all students? A very useful guide to the essential elements of effective small-group teaching and learning is provided by Edmunds and Brown (2010). As previously discussed, faculty professional development is very important in this regard: teachers should be skilled at asking questions, listening, reflecting, summarizing, and reinforcing.

Figure 6.6 Students use a hybridized classroom (digital delivery of content of a virtual case with physical tools such as the whiteboard) to reinterpret what they have viewed on the radiograph.

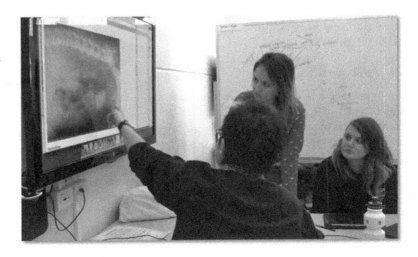

On Effective Questioning

In all group work, the questions that instructors pose are the stimulus for thinking, discussing, refining understanding, and problem-solving. Questions should be carefully crafted to achieve specific learning outcomes (see Box 6.3). When CBL activities are conducted in student-led groups, provision of appropriately framed questions becomes vital to achieving successful learning outcomes. As we developed case-based workshops at UoM, our authors repeatedly asked themselves these key questions:

- What learning outcomes are we trying to achieve?
- What style of thinking or what shared understanding are we looking for at this point?
- What misunderstandings might arise?
- What question should I be posing next?

 Box 6.3: Focus on questioning

Getting started: Prompts to thinking and discussion

Our workshops often start with questions of a fairly standard format, following presentation of a "trigger" scenario. For example, at the start of a case study that investigates hypovolemic shock in a dog, students watch a video that records an initial triage conversation between a veterinarian and the owner of a collapsed dog. Initial trigger questions – Can you list the key information about Murphy? How would you describe Murphy's presenting problem or problems? Does the veterinarian use open or closed questions for this initial triage? – encourage broad thinking about the situation while starting simply and then gradually increasing the complexity of the tasks and thinking required.

Are we all "on the same page"?

An important role of the tutor is to ensure that all students in the group have a shared foundational understanding, so that the group can move forward together in analyzing the problem. This is a fundamental requirement for building a trusting and collaborative learning group. Is everyone clear about the meaning of a clinical term, or the explanation of a clinical acronym? In a student-driven learning environment, the same form of questioning can be achieved with simple formative online testing. At the UoM we use the Blackboard Learning Management® system to introduce low-risk formative assessments that student groups undertake together. These tests provide opportunities for clarification and review in a safe, non-threatening context. We introduce multiple-choice test items, tasks that require matching of definitions with their meanings, or ranking/ordering questions that explore cause and effect. In addition, these tests enhance students' perception of mastery and provide valuable feedback on learning. Some questions confirm background knowledge, some check that students share a common understanding of mechanisms as the case unfolds, and others expand student thinking, perhaps to test hypotheses that have not previously been considered.

Asking probing questions: Is that all there is to know?

One of the great benefits of small-group and collaborative learning is the opportunity it provides for students to test their understanding against the unknown and to apply their knowledge to new situations. When appropriately supported, questions asking "why", "how", or "what if" can provide opportunities for deep learning that students find both empowering and exhilarating.

Is Effective Listening Practised and Valued?

Listening is a critical component of all communication, particularly of small-group work. In the PBL methodology it is common practice for group members to take turns reading aloud the case content, in order to encourage good listening techniques. Respectful listening enhances a positive group dynamic, and creates a space where it is safe for all to contribute. Given the centrality of communication and teamwork skills as attributes of graduate veterinarians, explicit instruction of students on these elements of group functioning should be part of the small-group learning curriculum.

Discussion Embodies All Elements of Communication

Discussion involves questioning and responding, reviewing and reflecting, and sharing understanding. This is where deep learning occurs. As described earlier, it is greatly enhanced by visualization – by sharing of ideas, summaries, and processes on whiteboards, and by collective rephrasing and reframing of ideas. Here, the content of the task at hand becomes very important: the task must be difficult enough that students benefit from working in groups, so that they can help one another through the zone of proximal development. Consider the following questions relating to a DVM first-year, Week 2 case study about "choke" in a horse. Students come to this learning activity with little knowledge of the topic other than classes in anatomy of the upper digestive tract and the physiology of swallowing. The disparate prior knowledge and experience of group members will benefit the group significantly as they find responses to these questions.

- How is it possible that oesophageal content can pass out the nasal passages?
- Does this happen in all animal species?
- Why is the stomach tube not passed down through the mouth?
- What evidence could be used to establish that the tube is in the stomach?

Discussion time also provides valuable opportunities for students to practice both the language of veterinary science and the vernacular of animal management and to hear them spoken – an important step in mastery and the building of professional confidence.

Where students are testing and taking risks with language in this way, "group safety" is paramount. Group composition should be determined by the teacher, ensuring diversity and inclusivity within groups, and group composition should be consistent over time. In PBL formats, equitable assignment of roles is achieved through rostered role allocation: whiteboard scribe, note taker, and so on. In other settings, groups develop social contracts with agreed behaviors and grievance procedures (see Box 6.4).

Reflection Is a Critical Activity for the Self-Regulating Learner

Opportunities for internal and group reflection can be built into collaborative learning activities by providing appropriate structure and questioning. Questions such as "How would you refine your hypotheses, in the light of the findings of your physical examination and the new problems that you have identified?" or "Which of your earlier hypotheses now seem less likely, and which are more likely?" signpost the need to reflect, to discuss, and to refine understanding in the light of new knowledge. Further opportunities for reflection are provided when the co-constructed knowledge of individual groups is brought to the bigger group in a concluding plenary. The role of the teacher is important here. In these sessions, groups can raise questions and seek explanation from other groups, and the teacher can challenge students with questions of "How?," "Why?," and "What if?" that test their understanding and interpretation of clinical signs, of physiological process, or of disease progression. This activity often provides moments of "cognitive dissonance" for students, as they recognize the need to go further and seek deeper clarity and understanding in their learning.

Box 6.4: Example of use of group contracts to foster effective communication skills in small group work

The Regional Anatomy of the Dog (RAD) course at the UoM is taught by Helen Davies (who devised the course with Christopher Philip) and Christina Murray. The RAD course is intended to provide knowledge of the integrated anatomy of the whole animal, as well as to promote skills in identifying and manipulating structures, as a foundation for the surgical and other clinical skills that will be taught in the later years of the DVM program. Further objectives of this course are the development of generic skills (graduate attributes), including communication, conflict negotiation, self-directed learning, facilitating the learning of others, and collaborative problem solving.

Students work in small groups to develop collaborative learning skills and so that each member can facilitate the learning of the others. The group contract strategy was devised to reduce conflict within groups and give individual students a means of communicating their needs in a non-confrontational and effective way. The contract is an agreement by the group on how the group dissection sessions will be conducted and how problems will be dealt with if they arise. The group devises its own rules, except for one rule that it must include, which is that each student must complete at least one session as team leader and one session as chief dissector.

We wish to thank Dr. Christina Murray in the Faculty of Veterinary and Agricultural Sciences for her contribution to this case example.

Feedback Is One of the Most Powerful Influences on Learning and Achievement

Feedback is information provided by a peer (group member) or an instructor regarding the student's performance or understanding. In settings where students co-construct knowledge (group work), feedback is particularly important, as there may otherwise be no guarantees of whether the knowledge constructed is right or wrong. Feedback provides the "intellectual safety net" that checks for and detects inaccuracies. Hattie and Timperley (2007) identify three major feedback questions: "Where am I going?," "How am I going?," and "Where to next?" The answers to these questions, they assert, "enhance learning, when there is a discrepancy between what is understood and what is aimed to be understood. Feedback can increase effort, motivation, or engagement to reduce this discrepancy, and/or it can increase cue searching and task processes that lead to understanding." Feedback, they further claim, is among the most critical influences on student learning.

In the context of collaborative learning, feedback can be provided in a range of ways; again, the nature of the question is critical. In their model of feedback to enhance learning, Hattie and Timperley (2007) describe four levels of feedback questioning:

- The *task level*: which we could interpret in the context of collaborative veterinary learning as "Your answers to those questions are correct."
- The *process level*: "Your hypotheses are sound, but I think you may have confused cause and effect here."
- The *self-regulation level*: "Yes, I agree with your diagnosis, but how can you explain this clinical sign?"
- The *self (or affective) level*: "We've all worked really well together today. I was so impressed when…"

Each of these levels of questioning can be built into the teacher's repertoire of questions, used during the collaborative activity, as a part of the text in a student-led activity, or in a concluding plenary.

Collaborative Learning May Take a Range of Different Forms

A number of specific pedagogies broadly incorporating collaborative learning principles have been reported in the medical education literature, and it is beyond the scope of this chapter to describe each of these in detail. It is also certain that in the future new, modified approaches will gain in popularity. These pedagogies do share many similarities, and the terms are sometimes used interchangeably in the literature, leading to some difficulties in the interpretation and comparison of reported outcomes. We advocate that no matter the precise format of specific types of learning activities, it is the collaborative processes in which students engage that most contribute to the effectiveness of these learning activities. Moreover, specific activities should be designed to align tightly with the intended learning outcomes relevant to the individual contexts of veterinary school curricula. To aid the reader in navigating the terminology presented in the literature, we have summarized the key features of more commonly described small-group learning formats in Table 6.1 and the four case examples that follow.

Case Example 6.1: Seminar Teaching at Utrecht University, The Netherlands

What Is It?

Annemarie Spruijt and her colleagues use seminar teaching extensively at Utrecht University in The Netherlands for veterinary students at all levels. A seminar is a collaborative group learning method that is characterized by interaction between student peers and a teacher, typically with group sizes around 25 students, focusing on more advanced content. Content expert(s) guide discussion regarding issues arising from preparatory readings and in-seminar assignments. The underlying premise of seminar learning is that by discussing and explaining concepts, specifically those with clinical and practical relevance, to their peers, students get to build on former knowledge, make connections, and experience their own gaps in knowledge and abstraction (Dennick and Spencer, 2011; Jaarsma *et al.*, 2008).

Table 6.1 Key features of commonly described small-group learning formats.

	Problem-based learning (PBL)	Team-based learning (TBL)	Case-based learning (CBL)
Underlying principles	The problem provides context and focus to the activity and drives a self-directed problem-solving approach.	Instructor-directed activities that require learners to be accountable for their learning before and during class.	Learning activities contextualized within a decision-making or case scenario, provided in a structured, sequential manner.
Distinguishing design elements	Students are presented with the problem before they have all the information required to solve it. Students must define the problem and acquire the relevant resources to create a recommendation.	Students are provided with detailed preparatory material in advance. Readiness testing of individuals and groups provides for learning accountability. Immediate feedback is provided by peers and instructor.	Guided enquiry approach in which students are directed to key issues and relevant concepts within the scenario. Students link this to previously presented material and create solutions to open-ended questions.
Relevant references	Hyams and Raidal (2013) Lane (2008) Newman (2005)	Hazel *et al.* (2013) Koles *et al.* (2010) Malone and Spieth (2012) Michaelsen, Knight, and Fink (2002)	Grauer *et al.* (2008) Monahan and Yew (2002) Patterson (2006)

What Resources Are Required and How Does It Work?

Students prepare for seminars by completing assigned readings with stimulating guiding questions. Except for length (typically 105 minutes maximum), there is no prescribed facilitating format for seminars. In practice, instructors either ask students to discuss the seminar questions in small "buzz" groups of two to six students, followed by plenary discussion, or they may ask students to address questions and concepts individually first; students often favor the former approach (Kurtz, Silverman, and Draper, 2005; Spruijt *et al.*, 2015).

Seminar learning requires a classroom with flexible seating arrangements and suitable audiovisual equipment, and a seminar teacher for each student group.

Feedback from Instructors

"It is easier to provide a safe learning environment and go into depth with the students. Besides veterinary expertise, they also develop their communication, collaboration, and even negotiating skills. Because students have permanent groups during a course they get an idea of each other's strengths and weaknesses as well."

Feedback from Students

"I really learn more in a seminar when I participate actively and know what I'm talking about as a result of good preparation for the seminar."

We wish to thank Annemarie Spruijt, DVM, PhD, Assistant Professor, School of Health Professions Education, Maastricht University, for her contribution to this case example.

Case Example 6.2: Team-Based Learning at Iowa State University

What Is It?

Team-based learning, as introduced by Michaelsen, Knight, and Fink (2002), is a collaborative learning format used by several instructors in core courses at the Iowa State University (ISU) College of Veterinary Medicine. One example is the core clinical pathology course in the second year of the DVM curriculum, which is coordinated by Sharon Hostetter and Jared Danielson.

What Resources Are Required and How Does It Work?

The TBL approach as used at ISU involves instructors forming teams of five to seven students that remain set throughout the course. The students prepare for class with either outside reading or previously delivered lectures. Class time begins with an individual readiness assurance test (RAT) followed by a team RAT (tRAT) prior to commencing the group work. The RATs and tRATs must be completed and scored in class in real time, requiring electronic testing or a Scan Tron®–based testing solution. There are then a number of group application exercises that engage students in solving diagnostic problems together, using what they have learned through their reading and practice. In this way, the majority of class time is spent on group learning activities rather than a one-way delivery of content from instructor to student.

One essential characteristic of TBL as it is used at ISU is that groups simultaneously respond to a question regarding a significant problem that is the same for all groups. This is usually accomplished by having students participate in real-time quizzing using Blackboard Learn® and either an audience response system, or simple laminated placards that are color and letter coded. All students are equipped with a laptop computer in class, which facilitates the real-time response system and electronic testing.

One unique aspect of ISU's implementation of TBL is that approximately 25 students (5 TBL groups) participate fully in the TBL activities from a distance using real-time conferencing. The remote students use the exact same tools for real-time testing and audience response; they are also connected via two-way video, so that they can participate with the rest of the class in justifying their group responses and hearing explanations from the instructor and other groups. TBL can be done with an entirely paper-based approach; however, working with a remote group does require two-way video.

Assessment

Part of the assessment involves each student evaluating each member of the group regarding how well they contributed to the group's learning. Students who prepare more thoroughly for class and participate in group discussions typically receive a higher peer score than students who do not prepare well or who do not participate in group discussions. Students do an initial peer evaluation midway through the course, which does not contribute to the grade, and a final peer evaluation at the end, which does. Other forms of assessment include RATs, tRATs, and in-class individual and group quizzes.

Feedback from Instructors

"Team-based learning is designed to engage students in solving problems together as a team… students spend much of their class time discussing the merits and/or flaws in various explanations to content-related problems. When students come prepared with a strong grasp of the material, they are able to help the group to succeed and earn a better grade. Much of the discussion entails students explaining concepts to each other, either to justify a response that has not yet been scored, or to explain one that has been scored. There is a very strong motivation to understand the material, help the team succeed, and to explain concepts to and/or learn concepts from teammates."

Feedback from Students

"I really liked how interactive this course was – it really helped me learn the material… I was skeptical of the group format because I am an introvert, but I think it worked out well."

"As much as I hate to admit this, working in groups was actually a great experience in this course. I like the way the class is set up in terms of evaluations. The weekly quizzes keep you on top of the material and the individual and group quizzes really do give you a chance to keep a good grade, but also learn from your group members."

We wish to thank Associate Professor Jared Danielson, DVM, PhD, and Assistant Professor Sharon Hostetter, DVM, PhD, Iowa State University College of Veterinary Medicine, for their contributions to this case example.

Case Example 6.3: The Clinical Integrative Puzzle in the Large Lecture at the University of Melbourne

What Is It?

Elise Boller, Natalie Courtman, and Cathy Beck use the clinical integrative puzzle (CIP) as an in-class collaborative teaching and learning activity (TLA) in large lecture settings (125 students). The CIP is a paper-and-pencil or computer-based activity that combines disciplinary knowledge (e.g., physical assessment, diagnostic imaging, clinical pathology, microbiology) with diagnostic reasoning and clinical problem-solving. The puzzle is presented as a table (see Table 6.2) with some cells filled in and some empty; the students must work together in small groups of two to four students to complete the empty cells. The rows contain a series of cases, but only signalment, history, and physical exam data are given. The columns are filled in by choosing from sets of data that are grouped by domain area (e.g., lab work, imaging, cytology, diagnoses, treatment). The properly completed puzzle will show coherent "illness scripts" for each case in the rows. As such, the CIP is structurally similar to the extended multiple-choice question format. However, it may help students to practice clinical reasoning, and they may find it a more fun and engaging way to test their knowledge and identify gaps.

Assessment

The CIP may be used as a formative teaching and learning activity in a collaborative context, or as a group or individual assessment task (e.g., as continuous assessment tasks over the course of a subject, or in the context of an examination).

In a large lecture theater at the UoM, completion of a CIP is used as a formative TLA.

Table 6.2 Clinical integrative puzzle grid.

Case number	Signalment	History	Physical Examination Findings	SECTION 1 Clinical Pathology	SECTION 2 Imaging	SECTION 3 Peritoneal fluid analysis and cytology	SECTION 4 Diagnosis
1	8 yo female entire Maltese Terrier	• Vomited this morning • Bloody discharge on bed last night	• Temp 39.2, HR 180, RR 36 • Mild hypoperfusion • Pink mucus membranes • CRT 2 s • Abd – moderate diffuse abdominal pain • Bloody diarrhoea on perineum	Question 1	Question 2	Question 3	Question 4
2	8 yo female entire Maltese Terrier	• Vomited this morning • Bloody discharge on bed last night • Distended abdomen • PU/PD for 10 days	• Temp 39.9, HR 180, RR 36 • Moderate hypoperfusion • Hyperaemic mucous membranes • CRT 0.5 sec • Abd – moderate abdominal pain, caudal abdominal mass effect • Blood tinged vulvar discharge	Question 5	Question 6	Question 7	Question 8
3	8 yo female entire Maltese Terrier	• Vomiting (3 times) and anorexic for 48 hours • History of abdominal trauma 2 weeks (hit by car)	• T 39.2, P 150, RR 48 • Moderate hypoperfusion • Pale MMs • CRT 2s • Markedly icteric • Abd - moderate abdominal pain and mild distension	Question 9	Question 10	Question 11	Question 12
4	8 yo female entire Maltese Terrier	• Vomiting intermittently for 4 weeks • PU PD for 3 months • Weight loss	• T 38.0, P 100, RR 24 • Normal hydration and perfusion • Diffusely thickened, firm intestines • BCS 2/5	Question 13	Question 14	Question 15	Question 16

Students work collaboratively, but have their own computers for viewing the content and entering their own answers into a "test" in the electronic learning management system (LMS). After all the students have entered their answers, data analysis is performed in real time and cases are discussed. Data analysis allows the instructors immediately to see the discrimination of each question and what the most commonly entered incorrect answers are. Discussion ensues that involves reviewing the salient points for each case, perhaps with additional trigger questions, and unpacking why students chose the answers they did.

Feedback from Instructors

"The CIP had some unexpected benefits, such as the pleasure and fun associated with collaborating with colleagues in different specialty areas as we developed the puzzles. Also, our interactions with students during delivery really stoked positive feelings about the student–teacher relationship."

"The immediate feedback from the LMS analytics enables us to immediately identify the most common incorrect answers and to have a discussion about why students chose that answer, for example the incorrect answer may have been plausible in some way or the associated teaching needed to be reviewed."

Feedback from Students

"I really liked the way that we had to actively think for ourselves in the lecture theatre rather than just being presented with another lecture. It really drew together different aspects of the diagnostic process."

"I very much enjoyed that we were able to interact with peers and work together in the process of reviewing broad concepts and approaches to working up a case."

We wish to thank Senior Lecturer Cathy Beck, BVSc, and Lecturer Natalie Courtman, BVSc, University of Melbourne Faculty of Veterinary and Agricultural Sciences, for their contributions to this case example.

Case Example 6.4: Wiki-Based Collaborative Poetry Writing Project for Learning Pathology at the University of Minnesota College of Veterinary Medicine

What Is It?

Rob Porter, Erik Olson, and Deb Wingert created a wiki-based interactive cooperative learning poetry project, in an attempt to enhance engagement in and understanding of selected pathology topics in second-year veterinary students. Veterinary students were randomly placed in one of 23 wiki groups, each corresponding to a specific pathology topic. Students used their wiki sites and followed a rubric to research and build a list of key words and phrases. From this list they created an online poem about the specific topic, with the understanding that this poem would be used to educate their peers. For instance:

Clostridial Enterotoxemia type D

C. perfringens is nothing strange
In the guts of animals that live on the range.
But sheep and goats that eat far too much
Will have GI tracts full of mush.
Normal flora will multiply
Releasing toxins that cause small ruminants to die.
What will you find on necropsy?
Hemorrhaged GI and pulpy kidney!
Bloody diarrhea and animals that can't stand,
You know that Clostridial enterotoxemia type D played a hand.
On histology you'll find rods that are gram positive.
If it wasn't for that bacteria on culture that sheep might have lived.
How do I keep my animals movin'?
Prevention is the magic solution.
Vaccination and stopping gluttons
Will keep sheep from becoming mutton.

What Resources Are Required?

Students need computers with an online connection. The wiki format is particularly suited to collaborative work, in that it is open and allows for students to build on each other's input and share resources. Work on the project can theoretically take place at any time and anywhere, with students having the choice of working together in person, online, or a combination of both.

Why Is This TLA Better as a Collaborative Activity Than as an Individual Effort?

The poetry project capitalizes on the idea that collaboration (in person or online) on a challenging and enjoyable activity engenders engagement, co-construction of knowledge, and possibly improved retention of that knowledge. With a guiding framework or rubric to follow, the poetry project gives students clear direction regarding the intended learning outcomes and a structure that all participants can see and understand. An online survey of student opinions indicated that the cooperative learning poetry project engaged most students and enhanced learning through the required research to satisfy the construction rubric.

We wish to thank Professor Rob Porter, DVM, PhD, Associate Professor Erik Olson, DVM, PhD, and Associate Dean for Academic and Student Affairs Laura Molgaard, DVM, from the University of Minnesota College of Veterinary Medicine, and Deb Wingert, MS, PhD, Center for Educational Innovation, University of Minnesota for their contributions to this case example.

Box 6.5: How to implement a collaborative case-based learning approach

- *Constructive alignment*: the curriculum at UoM is tightly integrated and systems based. Learning outcomes of the weekly case study are closely aligned to those of the whole week of study, and small-group, case-based workshops take place at the end of the week. Learning outcomes are provided in study guides at the level of each week of the study program, and at the level of the workshop activity.
- *Workshops are student driven*: students work in groups of six to eight. Learning materials are released at the start of each two-hour session. One or two faculty members concurrently act as facilitators for to up to nine student groups (60 students), and lead a 20-minute "wrap-up"/plenary at the end.
- *Electronic delivery of all learning materials enhances media richness*: typically a case study includes up to 2000 words of text, as well as images, video, and audio, including consultations with "mock" clients, radiographs, histomicrographs, and the like.
- *Case study approach employs a hypothetico-deductive approach to clinical reasoning*:

information is released sequentially to students as they work through the case, from the "trigger" to formulation of a question list and then history taking, physical examination, clinical investigation, and so on.
- *Guidance is provided through carefully structured questions and sequential release of information*: see earlier for tips on questioning techniques.
- *Outcomes of collaborative activities are recorded electronically using a group wiki*: each student group is enrolled in their own wiki, enabling them to build on one another's knowledge, capture discussion points for future revision, as well as allowing academic staff to review the results and provide feedback.
- *Feedback is provided through collaborative online quizzes and faculty-led plenary discussion ("wrap-up")*: simple online feedback tests ensure that students share a common understanding, before they move on to the next step in the workshop.

Implementing Integrated Case-Based Collaborative Learning at the University of Melbourne

In order to reach our major "degree-level" curriculum goal of promoting teamwork and problem-solving skills at the UoM, we established collaborative CBL activities as a core component of the first two years of the DVM program, with a commitment to engaging students in student-driven group work in every week of their academic program. As a means to achieve this, against a backdrop of limited resources, the authors developed an approach that employed the key elements described in Box 6.5.

In course evaluation questionnaires, students frequently cite their CBL as "the most valuable and enjoyable learning activity of the week." This successful outcome depends on the alignment of CBL learning outcomes with other elements of their learning program, the safety of the student group, the quality and richness of the supporting case materials that are provided online (text, video, audio, and image files), the crafting of probing open-ended questions that promote lively discussion and sharing of prior knowledge, the feedback and guidance provided through formative online assessments (true/false, matching, and multiple-choice questions), and the leadership and facilitating skills of the teacher in concluding plenaries.

How Should Collaborative Learning Activities Be Assessed?

Collaborative learning necessarily requires a group effort, but assessment in higher education is traditionally individualistic and competitive (Boud, Cohen, and Sampson, 1999). In a constructively aligned curriculum, assessment tasks must be aligned with both the intended learning outcomes and the specific nature of the learning activity (Biggs and Tang, 2011). Herein lies the key challenge in designing appropriate assessment strategies for collaborative learning activities. For this reason, there has been a tendency not to assess group activities, or to assign them very little weight within a grading strategy. However, assessment serves as an indicator to students of the relative importance of a particular activity, and therefore of the amount of attention that should be devoted to it (Boud, Cohen, and Sampson, 1999). There is no doubt that working collaboratively with others requires considerable effort and commitment. Therefore, it is important that veterinary educators design assessment strategies that provide crucial feedback, and recognize and reward students' efforts.

Assessing collaborative tasks completed by groups of students fairly and validly is challenging. Many of the learning outcomes that we aim to achieve through collaborative learning activities are traditionally difficult to assess, such as communication, listening, enquiry, and team processes. If collaborative effort is to be truly evaluated, it may be argued that assessment of the collective effort of a group of students is necessary. Group assessment of collaborative work should therefore include a detailed instructional briefing to enhance collaborative group processing, as is done at Murdoch University (Australia) (Khosa, Volet, and Bolton, 2010). However, group assessment can be challenging for both students and educators who are accustomed to individualistic performance assessment. Students may perceive that others are receiving credit for their work, or that the submitted work does not meet the standards of their individual effort. In these instances, a mix of both individual and group assessment may alleviate some of this anxiety while maintaining an emphasis and focus on the importance of group processing.

Assessment should address group processes in addition to the outcomes of learning activities (Boud, Cohen, and Sampton, 1999; Falchikov, 2013). Peers are arguably best placed to assess collaborative group processes, with educators well situated to assess the quality of the outcome. A good compromise can be to assign a group mark to the outcome of the group work, and an individual mark for student contribution to the group processes involved in producing this outcome. A component of peer assessment on the processes of the group can assist in the development of critical reflection skills, and enable students to voice concerns related to the inequality of efforts within the group. Such an approach has been reported by Hazel *et al.* (2013) within a veterinary TBL context. Students provide formative and summative peer feedback on team processing based on a set of clearly structured criteria. Additionally, the outcome of the team application exercise is assessed by an instructor. Peer assessments can also be utilized to inform self-assessment in the form of reflective writing activities. For example, students could be tasked with providing qualitative feedback on the collaborative activities of their peers. They are then asked to think about their own performance and the feedback of their peers in a reflective writing task that is individually assessed. Excellent practical advice on assessment design for group work is provided in Falchikov (2013).

Conclusion

The benefits of collaborative learning extend far beyond the simple attainment of knowledge. As described in this chapter, adult learning is experiential and fundamentally social. It is therefore imperative for veterinary educators to create learning activities that both enable social interplay and facilitate experiential learning by veterinary students. Collaborative learning activities align with our understanding of how adults learn and model the environment in which most veterinary graduates will go on to work. These tasks also provide an opportunity to foster the development of professionalism and professional skill development in veterinary students from the very early stages of their education.

Taken from Spruijt *et al.* (2015), crucial elements for the design of small-group collaborative curricula that promote active learning and the adoption of a deep learning approach include the following:

- Clearly define the rationale behind active learning methods.
- Engage and train faculty and students with this rationale, to create a "community of learners."
- Create seminar teacher teams and outline their responsibilities.
- Train faculty for their roles as facilitators.
- Facilitate interaction between students by seating arrangements and group activities.
- Provide learning materials of high quality and suitability.
- Ensure perfect alignment and coherence between different instructional methods and assessments.
- Involve students to help improve active learning formats.

Some of the complex and intangible learning outcomes that can be achieved through the delivery of well-structured collaborative learning activities include:

- Asking thought-provoking questions.
- Challenging the assumptions underlying the comments of others.
- Providing explanations and teaching peers.
- Providing justification for assertions.
- Using reasoning and influencing tactics.
- Exploring and elaborating ideas.
- Relating evidence to conclusions.
- Relating concepts to previous knowledge.
- Two-way exchange of ideas (both communication and listening).
- Completing tasks that are either too onerous or too difficult to achieve on one's own.

No matter the precise format of specific types of learning activities or the physical spaces in which they occur, the collaborative processes in which students engage contribute most to the effectiveness of these learning activities. The adoption of the approach at the highest levels of the faculty, robust faculty development programs in teaching, and careful construction of collaborative learning activities will aid in ensuring optimal outcomes for students, veterinary colleges, and the profession.

References

Biggs, J., and Tang, C. (2011) *Teaching for Quality Learning at University*, Open University Press/McGraw-Hill Education, New York.

Boud, D., Cohen, R., and Sampson, J. (1999) Peer learning and assessment. *Assessment and Evaluation in Higher Education*, **24**, 413–426.

Davidson, N., and Major, C.H. (2014) Boundary crossings: Cooperative learning, collaborative learning, and problem-based learning. *Journal on Excellence in College Teaching*, **25**, 7–55.

Dennick, R.G., and Spencer, J. (2011) Teaching and learning in small groups. *Medical Education: Theory and Practice*, **2011**, 131–156.

Dillenbourg, P. (1999) What do you mean by collaborative learning?, in *Collaborative-Learning: Cognitive and Computational Approaches* (ed. P. Dillenbourg), Elsevier, Oxford, pp. 1–19.

Edmunds, S., and Brown, G. (2010) Effective small group learning: AMEE guide no. 48. *Medical Teacher*, **32**, 715–726.

Eraut, M. (2007) Learning from other people in the workplace. *Oxford Review of Education*, **33**, 403–422.

Falchikov, N. (2013) *Improving Assessment through Student Involvement: Practical Solutions for Aiding Learning in Higher and Further Education*, Taylor and Francis, London.

Grauer, G.F., Forrester, S.D., Shuman, C., and Sanderson, M.W. (2008) Comparison of student performance after lecture-based and case-based/problem-based teaching in a large group. *Journal of Veterinary Medical Education*, **35**, 310–317.

Hattie, J., and Timperley, H. (2007) The power of feedback. *Review of Educational Research*, **77**, 81–112.

Hazel, S.J., Heberle, N., McEwen, M.M., and Adams, K. (2013) Team-based learning increases active engagement and enhances development of teamwork and communication skills in a first-year course for veterinary and animal science undergraduates. *Journal of Veterinary Medical Education*, **40**, 333–341.

Hyams, J.H., and Raidal, S.L. (2013) Problem-based learning: Facilitating multiple small teams in a large group setting. *Journal of Veterinary Medical Education*, **40**, 282–287.

Jaarsma, A.D.C., de Grave, W.S., Muijtjens, A.M.M., *et al.* (2008) Perceptions of learning as a function of seminar group factors. *Medical Education*, **42**, 1178–1184.

Khosa, D.K., Volet, S.E., and Bolton, J.R. (2010) An instructional intervention to encourage effective deep collaborative learning in undergraduate veterinary students. *Journal of Veterinary Medical Education*, **37**, 369–376.

Klemm, W.R. (1994) Using a formal collaborative learning paradigm for veterinary medical education. *Journal of Veterinary Medical Education*, **21**, 2–6.

Kolb, D.A. (1984) *Experiential Learning: Experience as the Source of Learning and Development*, Prentice Hall, Englewood Cliffs, NJ.

Koles, P.G., Stolfi, A., Borges, N.J., *et al.* (2010) The impact of team-based learning on medical students' academic performance. *Academic Medicine*, **85**, 1739–1745.

Kurtz, S., Silverman, J., and Draper, J. (2005) *Teaching and Learning Communication Skills in Medicine*, 2nd edn, Radcliffe Medical, Manchester.

Lane, E.A. (2008) Problem-based learning in veterinary education. *Journal of Veterinary Medical Education*, **35**, 631–636.

Luft, J., and Ingham, H. (1955) The Johari Window, a graphic model of interpersonal awareness. *Proceedings of the Western Training Laboratory in Group Development*, UCLA Extension Office, Los Angeles, CA.

Malone, E., and Spieth, A. (2012) Team-based learning in a subsection of a veterinary course as compared to standard lectures. *Journal of the Scholarship of Teaching and Learning*, **12**, 88–107.

Michaelsen, L.K., Knight, A.B., and Fink, L.D. (2002) *Team-Based Learning: A Transformative Use of Small Groups*, Greenwood, Santa Barbara, CA.

Monahan, C.M., and Yew, A.C. (2002) Adapting a case-based, cooperative learning strategy to a veterinary parasitology laboratory. *Journal of Veterinary Medical Education*, **29**, 186–192.

Newman, M.J. (2005) Problem based learning: An introduction and overview of the key features of the approach. *Journal of Veterinary Medical Education*, **32**, 12–20.

Nordquist, J., and Laing, A. (2015) Designing spaces for the networked learning landscape. *Medical Teacher*, **37** (**4**), 337–343. Figure reprinted by permission of the publisher (Taylor & Francis Ltd, http://www.informaworld.com)

Patterson, J.S. (2006) Increased student self confidence in clinical reasoning skills associated with case-based learning (CBL). *Journal of Veterinary Medical Education*, **33**, 426–431.

Perry, W.G. (1999) *Forms of Intellectual and Ethical Development in the College Years: A Scheme*, Holt, Rinehart, and Winston, New York.

Pintrich, P.R., and Zusho, A. (2002) The development of academic self-regulation: The role of cognitive and motivational factors, in *Development of Achievement Motivation* (ed. A.W.S. Eccles), Academic Press, San Diego, CA, ch. 10.

Raidal, S.L., and Volet, S.E. (2009) Preclinical students' predispositions towards social forms of instruction and self-directed learning: A challenge for the development of autonomous and collaborative learners. *Higher Education*, **57**, 577–596.

Roschelle, J., and Teasley, S. (1995) The construction of shared knowledge in collaborative problem solving, in *Computer Supported Collaborative Learning* (ed. C. O'Malley), Springer, Berlin, pp. 69–97.

Scholz, E., Trede, F., and Raidal, S.L. (2013) Workplace learning in veterinary education: A sociocultural perspective. *Journal of Veterinary Medical Education*, **40**, 355–362.

Shung, G., and Osburn, B.I. (2011) The North American Veterinary Medical Education Consortium (NAVMEC) looks to veterinary medical education for the future: "Roadmap for Veterinary Medical Education in the 21st Century: Responsive, Collaborative, Flexible." *Journal of Veterinary Medical Education*, **38**, 320–327.

Spruijt, A., Jaarsma, A.D.C., Wolfhagen, H.A.P., *et al.* (2012) Students' perceptions of aspects affecting seminar learning. *Medical Teacher*, **34**, E129–E135.

Spruijt, A., Leppink, J., Wolfhagen, I., *et al.* (2015) Factors influencing seminar learning and academic achievement. *Journal of Veterinary Medical Education*, **42**, 259–270.

Spruijt, A., Wolfhagen, I., Bok, H., *et al.* (2013) Teachers' perceptions of aspects affecting seminar learning: A qualitative study. *BMC Medical Education*, **13**, n.p.

Sungur, S., and Tekkaya, C. (2006) Effects of problem-based learning and traditional instruction on self-regulated learning. *Journal of Educational Research*, **99**, 307–317.

7

Teaching Interprofessionalism

John H. Tegzes

College of Veterinary Medicine, Western University of Health Sciences, USA

Box 7.1: Key messages

- Interprofessional practice and education (IPE) is an effective way to operationalize One Health across health professions education.
- Collaboration is a core skill for all practicing veterinarians, both the ability to collaborate with other health professions as well as within the veterinary healthcare team.
- Interprofessional competencies emphasize communication and collaboration skills and behaviors.

- IPE curriculum development itself brings health professions together in a collaborative manner.
- IPE curriculum implementation requires both university administrative support and grass-roots faculty involvement.
- Various teaching methods such as team-based learning and problem-based learning are useful in providing information and providing opportunities for skills acquisition.

Introduction: Why it is Time for Interprofessional Practice and Education in Veterinary Education

Dr. Jones, a small-animal general practice veterinarian, sees an 8-year-old golden retriever for a 3-month follow-up examination after the dog has been diagnosed with hypothyroidism and initiated on synthetic thyroxine replacement therapy. However, the dog does not seem to have improved since the start of the drug therapy; in fact, it seems quite a bit worse. The client was provided with a written prescription for the drug after diagnosis and had the prescription filled at a neighborhood retail pharmacy. She has brought the medication with her to the veterinary visit, and when Dr. Jones reads the label she realizes that the prescription was filled at one-tenth the dose that was prescribed. She quickly blames the pharmacist for making a mistake, unaware that the pharmacist's scope of practice allows for alterations in dosage if they suspect an error on the part of the prescriber. Both professions believe that the other is to blame.

Dr. Smith is in the exam room with a mom, her 5-year-old daughter, and their pet rat. The rat is freely climbing over the girl's shoulders and the child repeatedly kisses the rat every

Veterinary Medical Education: A Practical Guide, First Edition. Edited by Jennifer L. Hodgson and Jacquelyn M. Pelzer.
© 2017 John Wiley & Sons, Inc. Published 2017 by John Wiley & Sons, Inc.

time it crosses in front of her face. Dr. Smith notices a sizable pustule on the girl's upper lip. She asks the mom if she has seen her pediatrician for it. The mom replies yes, and that the pediatrician referred the child to her dentist, since she thought it was an oral health issue. The dentist has since prescribed two different antimicrobials, but neither has made any difference. Dr. Smith asks the mom if she mentioned to the dentist that her daughter has a pet rat that she regularly kisses. The mom responds that she hasn't. "Is that important?" she asks. Dr. Smith calls the dentist to talk about the normal flora of the rat, and to suggest perhaps selecting a different antimicrobial that might be more efficacious.

As is apparent from these scenarios, veterinarians are important members of the healthcare team. While the One Health concept reminds us of that, it is important to work collaboratively in everyday practice. Interprofessional practice and education (IPE) prepares veterinary students to work collaboratively (see Figure 7.1).

The everyday practice of veterinary medicine is changing, and has been for the past few decades. Such change is evident everywhere there are animals. There are increasing numbers of veterinary specialty organizations with

record numbers of clinicians achieving Diplomate status. There are many new internship and residency programs within academia and in private practice and industry. The availability of veterinary specialists is spreading far and wide, and the public demand for high-tech and high-quality care by competent veterinarians is increasing every year. Corporate veterinary practices are getting to be the norm in the United States, and the day of the solo veterinary practitioner is becoming a distant memory.

At the same time, the growth of the scientific body of knowledge and advances in the practice of medicine have challenged the veterinary curriculum. It has become extraordinarily difficult to prepare veterinary graduates with all the knowledge, skills, attitudes, and behaviors necessary to be successful veterinarians and meet the needs of a rapidly changing profession and demanding society within a four-year curriculum. Collaboration is the key to success, yet today's veterinary curricula have not necessarily taken on the challenge of preparing veterinary graduates to be successful collaborators. IPE is one way for the veterinary curriculum to prepare veterinary graduates for the necessities of collaborative practice.

A One Health approach to healthcare was first formally introduced in Calvin Schwabe's textbook *Veterinary Medicine and Human Health* in 1964. Today, virtually every veterinarian is familiar with the term One Health and the concepts that it promotes. Put simply, it calls for collaboration between human and veterinary medicine to effectively cure, prevent, and control illnesses that affect both humans and animals. Yet if we were to take a quick poll of the general public or even any of the other health professions, there would be very few who would recognize the term, or understand its focus.

The veterinary profession is somewhat insular, yet we often become defensive when other health professions seem to misunderstand our roles and responsibilities in improving the health of animals, humans, the environment, and society. It is time to share our wisdom! Again, IPE is an excellent way to begin educating health professionals during their early

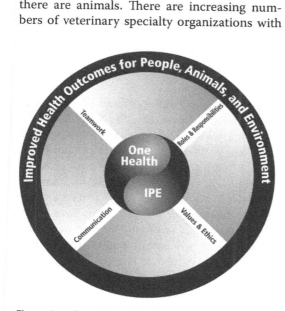

Figure 7.1 The relationships between interprofessional practice and education (IPE) and One Health.

professional education so that collaboration and wisdom-sharing become a natural part of their practice. Many of those involved in the One Health initiative focus their efforts, research, and conferences on the science and treatment of zoonotic diseases. There is less emphasis on developing collaboration skills. IPE emphasizes collaboration and develops effective communication habits and professionalism. It is less focused on disease pathogenesis, diagnosis, and treatment protocols and therefore pairs well with One Health. This is the primary reason why it is important for veterinary curricula to embrace and participate in IPE.

History of Interprofessional Practice and Education in Human Health

Just as the One Health initiative can trace its roots back to the 1960s, IPE had its early beginnings in 1972 after an Institutes of Medicine (IOM) report entitled "Educating for the Health Team" called on academic institutions to begin educating students in the health professions to practice collaboratively. The IOM called on healthcare teams to share common goals and incorporate the patient, family, and communities as members of the team. Moreover, the report noted that the existing educational system was not adequately preparing health professionals for such teamwork. Initially, not much changed in how health professions students were educated; the same educational silos remained common throughout the 1970s, 1980s, and 1990s. Universities and health professions colleges remained rather insular, establishing their own cultures and educational practices without conferring much with other health professions. It was not until students entered the clinical environment that they even encountered other health professions, and then contact was brief and focused on specific functions. Even healthcare records were kept separate, with rarely a chance for sharing patient goals and treatment plans across professions.

The IOM (2000, 2001, 2003) published further reports identifying the need for healthcare delivered by interprofessional teams. These new reports largely cited preventable errors as the impetus for better collaboration, noting that communication failures are major obstacles in delivering quality care across the professions, and calling for systematic changes in order to create cultures of cooperation and coordination.

In 2003 the IOM sponsored a summit on health professions education where five competencies central to the education of all health professions were identified. The IOM competencies recommend that students should be able to provide patient-centered care; apply quality improvement; employ evidence-based practice; utilize informatics; and work in interdisciplinary teams. Every one of these competencies is just as relevant to the practice of veterinary medicine. In veterinary medicine, patient-centered care not only includes a focus on the individual animal patient, but also incorporates a client-centered focus, where the specific goals of the client/animal owner are addressed and the client is embraced as a member of the veterinary healthcare team.

The World Health Organization (WHO) has also noted the need for collaborative practice in mitigating the global health workforce crisis by publishing the "Framework for Action on Interprofessional Education and Collaborative Practice" in 2010. The WHO defines IPE as occurring when students from two or more professions learn about, from, and with each other to enable effective collaboration and improve health outcomes. From a global health perspective, this describes the One Health initiative to a tee.

Setting the One Health perspective aside, veterinary medicine still needs interprofessional practice and education to meet the ongoing needs and demands of society. In the developed world, increased veterinary specialization and vast improvements in diagnostic capabilities and treatment strategies are de rigueur. Just step into any general or specialty veterinary clinic in the United States to see the array of diagnostic equipment and therapeutic tools that are commonly used. Computed tomography (CT) scans, magnetic resonance imaging (MRI), digital radiography, endoscopy, arthroscopic and laparoscopic surgeries, chemotherapy regimens, ventilators, portable complete blood cell (CBC) and serum chemistry machines – the list goes on and on. All of these technologies and advances require special knowledge, skills, and behaviors. As a result, more veterinarians are pursuing advanced training, certifications, and specialty boards. With these advances comes an increased need for veterinary care delivered by teams. Often, educators will suggest that because veterinary students do not deliver human care, they need not participate in IPE. Yet this is the wrong assumption. IPE is not about human healthcare; rather, it is about team-based healthcare, regardless of the species of focus. As the WHO has defined it, IPE occurs when students learn about, from, and with one another to enable effective collaboration and improve health outcomes. Such students need not be treating the same patients, or even practicing in the same settings. Collaboration skills are universal, and can be learned and practiced across settings. When students are challenged to learn and practice such skills together, they will gain the added benefits of learning about all the health professions, and be better prepared to coordinate care when their professions do in fact intersect.

Veterinary medicine has continued to change in ways very similar to how human healthcare has evolved over the past three or four decades, with increased specialization and, unfortunately, fragmented healthcare delivery as a consequence. Let us face the challenge of providing coordinated, collaborative care by learning from the other health professions, examining their systems, and proactively shaping the future of veterinary practice so as not to repeat those professions' past errors. IPE can help with this too, by providing veterinary students and faculty with insights into the systems that have driven and shaped the human healthcare system.

Collaborative care saves lives. Plainly and simply, creating healthcare that is coordinated

and collaborative can prevent suffering and premature deaths. Based on 1984 data, the IOM estimated that up to 98 000 Americans die each year from medical errors, with most of those errors a result of communication failures. An updated analysis published in 2013 estimated that more than 400 000 human patients experience premature deaths annually associated with preventable harm in healthcare (Interprofessional Education Collaborative Expert Panel, 2011; James 2013). While such a high number of incidents does not occur in veterinary practice, increased specialization and the challenges that it poses to care coordination and communication mean that it is not unreasonable to assume that veterinary patients may also experience preventable harm. While most veterinary curricula incorporate communications skills, these are largely focused on doctor–client communication, with less time devoted to building communication skills within the veterinary or interprofessional healthcare team. Even the veterinary primary literature notes the incidence of patient harm due to communication failures between veterinarians and pharmacists (Cima, 2014; Wells *et al.*, 2014). Such examples of preventable errors in veterinary practice are the reason that IPE is needed universally across veterinary education today.

Interprofessional Competencies and Curriculum Development

In 2011 a multidisciplinary health professions panel (IPEC) convened to define and establish educational competencies to be used across health professions and IPE programs throughout the United States. Four competency domains and specific competencies within each domain were established. IPEC published its report, findings, and recommendations that same year (Interprofessional Education Collaborative Expert Panel, 2011). A similar effort in Canada had already published a national interprofessional competency framework the year before (Canadian Interprofessional Health Collaborative, 2010). A similar report was published in the United Kingdom even earlier (UK Centre for the Advancement of Interprofessional Education, 2007). All of these reference similar core competencies across the health professions, yet individual national reports are necessary considering the differences in how both health professions education and healthcare delivery are regulated, accredited, funded, and delivered in each nation. This section will refer primarily to the US publication.

In the United States, the four core competency domains for IPE that have been established are (Interprofessional Education Collaborative Expert Panel, 2011):

- Values and ethics for interprofessional practice.
- Professional roles and responsibilities.
- Interprofessional communication and collaboration.
- Teams and teamwork.

The competency domains and the specific competencies that follow are purposely general in nature and are meant to function as guidelines, allowing flexibility within the professions and at the institutional level. The desired principles of the interprofessional competencies are (Interprofessional Education Collaborative Expert Panel, 2011):

- Patient/client/family centered.
- Community/population oriented.
- Relationship focused.
- Process oriented.
- Linked to learning activities, educational strategies, and behavioral assessments that are developmentally appropriate for the learner.
- Able to be integrated across the learning continuum.
- Sensitive to the systems context/applicable across practice settings.
- Stated in language common and meaningful across the professions.
- Outcome driven.

As is evident in Box 7.2, the overarching goals of the IPE competencies reach beyond educational methods and professional behaviors. The general nature of these competencies therefore poses significant challenges in assessment, since

 Box 7.2: Focus on the overarching goals of the core competencies

- Create a coordinated effort across the health professions to embed essential content in all health professions education curricula.
- Guide professional and institutional curricular development of learning approaches and assessment strategies to achieve productive outcomes.
- Provide the foundation for a learning continuum in interprofessional competency development across the professions and the lifelong learning trajectory.
- Acknowledge that evaluation and research work will strengthen the scholarship in this area.
- Prompt dialogue to evaluate the "fit" between educationally identified core competencies for interprofessional collaborative practice and practice needs/demands.

- Find opportunities to integrate essential interprofessional education content consistent with current accreditation expectations for each health professions education program.
- Offer information to accreditors of educational programs across the health professions that they can use to set common accreditation standards for interprofessional education, and to know where to look in institutional settings for examples of implementation of those standards.
- Inform professional licensing and credentialing bodies in defining potential testing content for interprofessional collaborative practice (Interprofessional Education Collaborative Expert Panel, 2011).

the specific competencies describe skills more than they do knowledge. Likewise, specific curriculum components tend to focus on skills development, such as communication, rather than on knowledge acquisition, which requires more complex assessment strategies. Other competencies are more knowledge based and can be assessed with traditional multiple-choice format exams, for instance professional roles and responsibilities.

As this is an educational endeavor that crosses professions and universities, it is important to note that the stated goals aim for changes in systems and policy as well as in the education of health professions students. While this is very useful in the formative years of interprofessional education globally, it makes it particularly difficult to design and evaluate curricula. Suddenly, designing curricula around the basic sciences seems easy! Specific strategies for designing curricula around these competencies will be described later in this chapter.

Table 7.1 lists the specific competencies under each competency domain. Additionally, it details specific types of educational assessment that can be used to assess students' proficiency and mastery of the competency.

It is clear from this table that a variety of teaching methods need to be developed and implemented to achieve these competencies. Likewise, a variety of assessment strategies are also necessary and may include traditional written exams, objective structured clinical exams (OSCEs), portfolio evaluations that include reflective practice exercises, and evaluations by clinical preceptors using rubrics developed for interprofessional practice, such as the ICAR (Curran *et al.*, 2011).

Curriculum Development and Implementation

As it is a relatively new educational endeavor, there is no one single formula for creating and implementing an IPE curriculum. Although many of the health professions accrediting bodies now require IPE as an accreditation

standard, they do not specify during which years of the curriculum or even how much IPE is required. There are many logistical challenges that must be met and each individual academic institution has unique needs and cultures to be considered. The approach used at Western University of Health Sciences (WesternU) to overcome these challenges is highlighted in Box 7.3. This is just one example of the work that is sometimes necessary to create an educational program that spans multiple professions in various colleges and programs.

Some academic institutions introduce learners to IPE during the clinical years of instruction, while others begin during the preclinical stages of the curriculum. There are advantages and disadvantages to both approaches. Beginning early in the preclinical years allows learners to begin thinking differently and critically about their own roles and responsibilities as well as those of the other health professions. Students will then enter their clinical years with new ideas about how their profession fits into the healthcare team. On the other hand, if IPE is offered during the clinical years, learners can apply new concepts and collaboration strategies right away while they rotate in the clinics; such an approach may cement the learning more deeply.

Each university must consider its unique needs when developing an IPE curriculum. There are many very successful IPE programs that only begin when students are in the later stages of the clinical years of instruction. Such programs tend to occur at academic health centers, where having students and faculty from multiple programs come together for learning sessions is logistically possible. In these situations, students collaborate where they are already assembled on clinical rotations. On the other hand, such an approach may exclude professions that are not normally onsite, but are important members of a patient's healthcare team. Such is the case for veterinary medicine, since it is not usual or common for veterinary students to be on clinical rotation in academic health centers. It is possible that veterinary students may be on rotation in a laboratory medicine setting there, but these

Table 7.1 Core competencies for interprofessional practice.

Specific competencies	Assessment strategies (knowledge, skills, attitudes, behaviors)
Values/ethics	
Place the interests of patients and populations at the center of interprofessional healthcare delivery	Attitudes, behaviors
Respect the dignity and privacy of patients while maintaining confidentiality in the delivery of team-based care	Attitudes, behaviors
Embrace the cultural diversity and individual differences that characterize patients, populations, and the healthcare team	Knowledge, skills, attitudes, behaviors
Respect the unique cultures, values, roles/responsibilities, and expertise of other health professions	Knowledge, attitudes, behaviors
Work in cooperation with those who receive care, those who provide care, and others who contribute to, or support the delivery of, prevention and health services	Attitudes, behaviors
Develop a trusting relationship with patients, families, and other team members	Skills, attitudes, behaviors
Demonstrate high standards of ethical conduct and quality of care in one's contributions to team-based care	Attitudes, behaviors
Manage ethical dilemmas specific to interprofessional patient/population-centered care situations	Knowledge, skills, attitudes, behaviors
Act with honesty and integrity in relationships with patients, families, and other team members	Attitudes, behaviors
Maintain competence in one's own profession appropriate to scope of practice	Knowledge, skills
Roles/responsibilities	
Communicate one's roles and responsibilities clearly to patients, families, and other professionals	Knowledge, skills, behaviors
Recognize one's limitations in skills, knowledge, and abilities	Attitudes, behaviors
Engage diverse healthcare professionals who complement one's own professional expertise, as well as associated resources, to develop strategies to meet specific patient care needs	Knowledge, skills, behaviors
Explain the roles and responsibilities of other care providers and how the team works together to provide care	Knowledge
Use the full scope of knowledge, skills, and abilities of available health professionals and healthcare workers to provide care that is safe, timely, efficient, effective, and equitable	Knowledge, attitudes, behaviors
Communicate with team members to clarify each member's responsibility in executing components of a treatment plan or public health intervention	Knowledge, skills, behaviors
Forge interdependent relationships with other professions to improve care and advance learning	Attitudes, behaviors
Engage in continuous professional and interprofessional development to enhance team performance	Knowledge, skills, behaviors
Use unique and complementary abilities of all members of the team to optimize patient care	Attitudes, behaviors

(Continued)

Table 7.1 (Continued)

Specific competencies	Assessment strategies (knowledge, skills, attitudes, behaviors)
Interprofessional communication	
Choose effective communication tools and techniques, including information systems and communication technologies, to facilitate discussions and interactions that enhance team function	Knowledge, skills, behaviors
Organize and communicate information to patients, families, and healthcare team members in a form that is understandable, avoiding discipline-specific terminology when possible	Knowledge, skills
Express one's knowledge and opinions to team members involved in patient care with confidence, clarity, and respect, working to ensure common understanding of information and treatment and care decisions	Attitudes, behaviors
Listen actively, and encourage ideas and opinions of other team members	Skills, behaviors
Give timely, sensitive, instructive feedback to others about their performance on the team, responding respectfully as a team member to feedback from others	Attitudes, skills, behaviors
Use respectful language appropriate for a given difficult situation, crucial conversation, or interprofessional conflict	Attitudes, behaviors
Recognize how one's own uniqueness, including experience level, expertise, culture, power, and hierarchy within the healthcare team, contributes to effective communication, conflict resolution, and positive interprofessional working relationships	Knowledge, skills, attitudes, behaviors
Communicate consistently the importance of teamwork in patient-centered and community-focused care	Attitudes, behaviors
Teams and teamwork	
Describe the process of team development and the roles and practices of effective teams	Knowledge
Develop consensus on the ethical principles to guide all aspects of patient care and teamwork	Knowledge, attitudes, behaviors
Engage other health professionals – appropriate to the specific care situation – in shared patient-centered problem-solving	Attitudes, behaviors
Integrate the knowledge and experience of other professions – appropriate to the specific care situation – to inform care decisions, while respecting patient and community values and priorities/preferences for care	Knowledge, attitudes, behaviors
Apply leadership practices that support collaborative practice and team effectiveness	Knowledge, skills, attitudes, behaviors
Engage self and others to constructively manage disagreements about values, roles, goals, and actions that arise among healthcare professionals and with patients and families	Skills, attitudes, behaviors
Share accountability with other professions, patients, and communities for outcomes relevant to prevention and healthcare	Skills, attitudes, behaviors
Reflect on individual and team performance for individual, as well as team, performance improvement	Skills, attitudes, behaviors
Use process improvement strategies to increase the effectiveness of interprofessional teamwork and team-based care	Knowledge, skills, attitudes, behaviors
Use available evidence to inform effective teamwork and team-based practices	Knowledge, attitudes, behaviors
Perform effectively in teams and in different team roles in a variety of settings	Knowledge, skills, attitudes, behaviors

Source: Adapted from Interprofessional Education Collaborative Expert Panel (2011).

Box 7.3: Example of a model of interprofessional practice, educational development, and implementation at Western U

Began with "top-down" direction from president, provost, and college deans:

- Common time dedicated for IPE class sessions across all programs (dental medicine, nursing, optometry, osteopathic medicine, pharmacy, physical therapy, physician assistant, podiatric medicine, and veterinary medicine).
- Sufficient classroom space for small-group sessions.
- Faculty time committed for curriculum development and implementation.
- Required for graduation for all students from all nine professions, including veterinary medicine.

Continued with "grassroots" efforts by faculty:

- Interprofessional curriculum committee formed to oversee curriculum development.

- Interprofessional committees formed to implement curriculum over the preclinical years of all programs.
- Various curricular models piloted to assess and evaluate effectiveness and outcomes.

Current curriculum:

- Utilizes problem-based learning (PBL) to deliver content in first year analyzing case studies.
- Utilizes an online platform to practice asynchronous communication skills among multiple professions in second year.
- Conducts clinical simulations with standardized patients and standardized clinicians in clinical years.
- Organizes student-led case conferences, focusing on complicated clinical cases benefiting from interprofessional collaborative care.

students would not normally cross paths with students from other health professions on clinical rotations in the same institution.

A term that is embedded in most IPE programs is "patient-centered" care. This refers to a basic tenet of collaborative care that places the patient in the center of the healthcare team, and gives patients a voice in their own care. The corollary to this in veterinary medicine would be "client-centered" care, where the animal owner is a member of the veterinary healthcare team, and their goals, wishes, and opinions are taken into account in treatment plans in a very active and proactive manner. In veterinary medicine we already have a long history of doing this well, so in IPE sessions it is important to share our insights and techniques for including clients as members of the healthcare team.

It is vital to emphasize that a core component of an IPE curriculum is students learning from, with, and about one another in order to improve health outcomes and the care that is provided to patients. It is not necessary for students to be treating the same patient in order to benefit from this approach; it is more about sharing the gems from each program, and how each profession cares for patients with similar conditions. By sharing this information with one another, students will learn about the roles and responsibilities of each profession. Perhaps even more importantly, they will begin to see where overlaps and gaps in care exist. This is how health outcomes will begin to improve.

Consider obesity rates and the prevalence of diabetes mellitus across developed and developing nations. In the United States, more than one-third of adults are obese (Ogden *et al.*, 2014). As for diabetes, a report by the CDC estimated that 9.3% of the US population was affected (Centers for Disease Control and Prevention, 2014). A national pet obesity survey (Association for Pet Obesity Prevention, 2012) found that 55% of US dogs and cats were overweight or obese. Regardless of the health profession or clinical specialty, all students will encounter patients with either obesity or diabetes during their clinical rotations and in their careers. This can then be the central focus of IPE class discussions. Opening with a broad, population-based health issue enables students to begin to reflect on their own profession's roles and responsibilities. Then in interprofessional discussions, they can be challenged to find solutions to the problems. All students, including veterinary students, have an equal voice, and this levels the discussions so that no professions are excluded. Even if a student represents a profession that does not directly diagnose or treat obesity and diabetes, they can still have an impact on the quality of life of those affected, and educate patients and family members about preventive strategies. By including veterinary medicine in such discussions, the One Health approach may then be addressed with all the health professions, bringing awareness of the connectedness of human, animal, and environmental health.

While there is much variability regarding when IPE is delivered, how often it is delivered, and which professions to include, some common practices are emerging. First, most IPE programs include small-group work and can incorporate PBL or case-based learning (CBL) in both preclinical and clinical years of the curriculum. These can also occur in seminar-type sessions where cases are reviewed in an interprofessional, rounds-like format. PBL works very well with IPE because there are no clear solutions to some of the problems that are discussed. While some of the communication techniques could be delivered in a large-group lecture format, practicing the communication skills will still require small-group work.

The key to successful and engaging small-group interprofessional sessions is creating relevance for all participants. For example, focusing a session on hospital-based care may alienate students who normally will not work in an inpatient setting. This is particularly true for veterinary students. While a PBL case could be developed that includes hospital-based care,

it should do so as a component of the case and not as the primary focus. Since IPE class discussions often focus on communication between healthcare providers, hospital-based discussions should focus on interprofessional core competencies rather than the mechanics of hospital-based care. This re-engages those professions who would not be present in that particular care setting. As an example, students could be asked to focus on how new diagnostic findings discovered during an inpatient hospitalization could be shared with professions outside of primary care. If the patient of focus has suffered serious sequelae from a chronic disease that potentially affects multiple body systems, how could those professions who are likely to see the patient in the near future in ambulatory care settings be informed about these changes? Is it only the patient's responsibility to share this information with their dentist, their physical therapist, or their optometrist? By discussing the logistical, legal, and ethical challenges of communicating important patient information across professions, students will begin to seek solutions to these real and common problems in healthcare, and might be more likely to overcome them and improve health outcomes when they are in clinical practice. They may also recognize the shared responsibility in caring for the whole person, the whole animal, or the whole community, as opposed to the kind of specialized parts care that is more of the norm in healthcare today, and is becoming ever more common in veterinary medicine as well.

Specific Teaching Methods in Interprofessional Education

Large-Group Teaching and Learning

Large-group lectures can be used to deliver information, theories, data, and specific communication and collaboration techniques and strategies. Team Strategies and Tools to Enhance Performance and Patient Safety (TeamSTEPPS™) is one such program designed to deliver core content in large groups, with time also devoted to small-group break-out sessions to practice specific skills and techniques. Team-STEPPS is a systematic approach developed by the US Department of Defense and the Agency for Healthcare Research and Quality that is designed to integrate teamwork into clinical practice (Agency for Healthcare Research and Quality, 2014a). It is evidence based and is available online and via DVD. There are frequent meetings and conferences throughout the United States, including master trainer courses to help faculty and healthcare providers disseminate and teach the techniques. In addition, many of the communication skills presented in the TeamSTEPPS curriculum are becoming policy and standard operating procedures in healthcare facilities across the United States (Kaiser Permanente, 2007). Specific communication techniques can be introduced in large-group lectures and demonstrations. However, it is important that learners have opportunities to practice the techniques in small groups so that every learner can try them out and receive feedback.

Small-Group Teaching and Learning

Small-group sessions are an excellent way to forge relationships among students from multiple professions while allowing them to engage in active learning and discussion about interprofessional core competencies. Specific teaching techniques that can be implemented in small groups include PBL, team-based learning (TBL), or other modified case-based discussions. Teaching materials used during these sessions should be designed to emphasize interprofessional core competencies. While including some clinical science in the cases helps to illustrate roles and responsibilities and highlight One Health issues, teamwork skills and communication strategies should be significant parts of the case discussions. One such open-source example can be found on MedEdPortal (Tegzes *et al.*, 2013). Specific TeamSTEPPS communication tools like SBAR (Situation, Background, Assessment, Recommendation) can be used to illustrate communication strategies (Agency for Healthcare Research and Quality, 2014b). Likewise, it is important to include values

and ethical considerations in the design of teaching cases (Interprofessional Education Collaborative Expert Panel, 2011).

Clinical Simulations

Using standardized patients and standardized clinicians to focus on interprofessional core competencies is an excellent way to give learners opportunities to learn new techniques and skills, and to receive feedback and debriefing on their proficiencies and areas for improvement and future work. Clinical simulations can be developed for ambulatory settings, with individual students working alone with the patient/client. They can also be developed to deliver care as a team in a hospital-based setting, where students' direct interactions can be analyzed and debriefed. Both types offer enormous opportunities for learning and improvement. Along with students from multiple professions working together in the simulations, standardized (actor) clinicians can also be included to emphasize interprofessional core competencies by challenging students with poor communication or collaboration techniques. Video recording of these encounters allows faculty to evaluate and offer debriefing on these sessions with learners, greatly improving their educational impact. As is obvious from the description, such sessions tend to be resource intensive for the university, and this may limit their utility. However, there are some validated tools and rubrics that can help to guide and implement clinical simulations (Curran *et al.*, 2011; Dickter, Stielstra, and Lineberry, 2015).

Clinical Rotations

An interprofessional clinical rotation with actual patients and clients, students from multiple professions, and clinicians from more than one profession is the ultimate utilization of IPE. Veterinary students could benefit from rotating alongside pharmacy students in either an inpatient or outpatient human pharmacy, observing and discussing therapeutic interventions, and hearing pharmacy students explain how drug therapies and prescriptions are evaluated according to the pharmacy scope of practice. In addition, pharmacy students would benefit from hearing unique animal considerations from veterinary students. Ultimately, both professions would benefit from learning with, from, and about one another in an actual practice setting. Such rotations would also forge relationships that can foster ongoing collaborations throughout individuals' careers. Pharmacists may gain awareness of unique veterinary considerations and may be more likely to call a veterinarian in the future to discuss unique species considerations. Veterinarians would gain insight into the responsibilities of pharmacists and their scope of practice in altering written prescriptions when they encounter a therapeutic issue, and may be more proactive in speaking with and collaborating with them to ensure that there is understanding between the two professions when caring for specific patients. Medication errors are still one of the most common types of medical error that effective collaboration can prevent. Since these are two professions that will work with one another, but not directly side by side, such a rotation could bridge current gaps in understanding and build relationships that potentially will improve collaboration and patient care.

Case Conferences and Rounds

Student-run case conferences give opportunities to discuss challenging clinical cases among various health professions in order to gain insight and perspectives on possible solutions to improving care and health outcomes. These are sessions that can engage veterinary students in presenting One Health considerations for human patients. Likewise, veterinary students can present challenging animal cases and seek One Health input from the human health professions in a collaborative environment.

Assessment

One of the major challenges to IPE throughout academia today is measuring outcomes. Because the core competencies have been defined largely in relation to skills, attitudes, and behaviors, this makes them very difficult to assess in learners, particularly in programs with large numbers of students. Similarly, some of the core competencies refer to improved patient health outcomes, which are extremely difficult to tease out and measure with attribution to IPE alone. Still, assessment is critical in credit-bearing academic courses, and is essential for measuring academic program outcomes. Since IPE is a relatively new and evolving academic focus, there currently are no definitive resources or methods for assessment. Many efforts are underway to assess interprofessional learning, and the literature will likely see many new publications in the coming years.

Written (Multiple Choice, Short Answer, Essay)

Written examinations remain a key method of veterinary student assessment. They tend to be easier to create, easier to grade, and analyzing outcomes is easier. Since the veterinary licensing boards still rely heavily on multiple-choice-type questions, many academicians also utilize them as primary assessment tools, often commenting that it helps students prepare for success on the boards. Interprofessional core competencies are difficult to assess with only multiple-choice-type questions. Communication often requires subtle interpretations of cues, both verbal and nonverbal, in order to decide which specific techniques to use. Context is also very important, making a written question challenging to write and challenging to answer when one is only faced with the question itself. Still, specific communication techniques such as SBAR could be assessed to some extent with a multiple-choice-type question. The bigger challenge, however, is that a student's correct response to the written question does not necessarily indicate that the student will be able to utilize SBAR successfully in a future clinical encounter.

Multiple-choice questions can be designed to assess knowledge of the roles and responsibilities of various healthcare professions, which tend to be easier to assess in objective question formats.

Objective Structured Clinical Examinations

The OSCE is an excellent tool to assess students in simulated clinical encounters. It has been modified to assess teamwork and collaboration skills in healthcare. The University of Toronto has developed the iOSCE (interprofessional Objective Structured Clinical Exam), and WesternU has developed the ATOSCE (Ambulatory Team Objective Structured Clinical Exam) (Simmons *et al.*, 2011). Both of these assessment techniques include the use of standardized patients, and the WesternU model also includes standardized clinicians. In both models, professional actors are used to play the roles of patients and family members. In the WesternU model, professional actors play the roles of healthcare professionals. These actors are directed to challenge the students vigorously to allow them to implement and practice various communication and collaboration techniques. Both universities have validated rubrics to assess students during the encounters. The WesternU rubric was also validated for inter-rater reliability, since the encounters are video recorded and viewed subsequently by faculty from various professions (Dickter, Stielstra, and Lineberry, 2015). Additionally, faculty and actors involved in the exercises provide feedback and debriefing on the encounters with participating students immediately after the exercises. The video recordings can also be used to provide directed feedback to learners.

Such assessments have been very useful in assessing skills, behaviors, and even attitudes, and they are ideal for assessing interprofessional core competencies. Nevertheless, their widespread utility is limited by the availability of resources. Each encounter requires the use of a clinical skills simulation space, professional actors, video-recording equipment and operators, faculty and staff.

Portfolios and Reflections

Since interprofessional competencies require opportunities to practice various communication and collaboration skills, portfolios and self-reflections can be very useful. They allow learners to track the opportunities they have had to observe and practice interprofessionalism, and to receive feedback from faculty on their observations and reflections. Learning interprofessionalism requires some reflecting on one's experiences in clinical settings, and portfolios provide a method to record and reflect on these experiences. At the same time, they require faculty commitment to read and provide useful feedback if they are to have the greatest impact. Therefore, faculty engaged in portfolio reviews need to be versed in the interprofessional core competencies. Veterinary students in particular should be encouraged to record their experiences within the veterinary healthcare team, as well as with any other health profession. There are opportunities to learn and practice interprofessional skills with veterinary technicians, animal assistants, and general and specialist referral veterinarians.

Clinical Preceptor Evaluations and Rubrics

Regardless of clinical rotation, clinical preceptor rubrics can be used to assess collaboration and teamwork skills and behaviors. There are several validated rubrics available and others currently in the validation process are expected to be available on an open-source basis in the near future (Curran *et al.*, 2011). While clinical preceptors and faculty are assessing veterinary students in clinical medicine, they can also assess communication and collaboration skills in the clinical work environment, regardless of area of practice. The practice of veterinary medicine requires interaction with people both within the veterinary profession and increasingly outside of the profession. Effective patient care and patient outcomes rely on effective collaboration with the entire veterinary healthcare team. Assessing learners and providing effective feedback are critical to developing these skills and behaviors. Adequate faculty and preceptor development is also necessary so that the feedback is effective and formative for the learner.

Conclusion

We live in a collaborative society. With the increasing use of technology, effective communication and teamwork skills and behaviors are coming to be as important as hands-on clinical skills in arriving at optimal patient outcomes. Interprofessional practice and education are becoming essential components of veterinary practice. Including core competencies in the veterinary curriculum is also essential.

Acknowledgments

With kind appreciation and gratitude to Sheri Kling for her editing and feedback skills; to Katy Avila for her writing guidance; and to Edith Jennison for her graphics expertise.

References

Agency for Healthcare Research and Quality (2014a) *TeamSTEPPS®: Strategies and Tools to Enhance Performance and Patient Safety.* http://www.ahrq.gov/professionals/education/curriculum-tools/teamstepps/index.html (accessed December 28, 2015).

Agency for Healthcare Research and Quality (2014b) *TeamSTEPPS® 2.0: SBAR Provides...* http://www.ahrq.gov/professionals/education/curriculum-tools/teamstepps/instructor/fundamentals/module3/igcommunication.html#sbarprov (accessed November 4, 2016).

Association for Pet Obesity Prevention (2012) *National Pet Obesity Survey Results.* http://www.petobesityprevention.org/2012-national-pet-obesity-survey-results/ (accessed December 27, 2015).

Canadian Interprofessional Health Collaborative (2010) *A National Interprofessional Competency Framework*, Canadian Interprofessional Health Collaborative, Vancouver.

Centers for Disease Control and Prevention (2014) *National Diabetes Statistics Report: Estimates of Diabetes and Its Burden in the United States, 2014.* US Department of Health and Human Services, Atlanta, GA. http://www.cdc.gov/diabetes/pubs/statsreport14/national-diabetes-report-web.pdf (accessed December 27, 2015).

Cima, G. (2014) Substitution errors: Surveys describe harm from differences between prescriptions and drugs dispensed. *JAVMAnews*, **September 1**. https://www.avma.org/News/JAVMANews/Pages/140901a.aspx (accessed December 26, 2015).

Curran, V., Casimiro, L., Banfield, V., et al. (2011) *Interprofessional Collaborator Assessment Rubric*, Academic Health Council. https://www.med.mun.ca/getdoc/b78eb859-6c13-4f2f-9712-f50f1c67c863/ICAR.aspx (accessed December 28, 2015).

Dickter, D.N., Stielstra, S., and Lineberry, M. (2015) Interrater reliability of standardized actors versus nonactors in a simulation based assessment of interprofessional collaboration. *Simulation in Healthcare*, **10** (**4**), 249–255.

Institutes of Medicine (1972) *Educating for the Health Team*, National Academy of Sciences, Washington, DC.

Institutes of Medicine (2000) *To Err Is Human: Building a Safer Health System*, National Academy Press, Washington, DC.

Institutes of Medicine (2001) *Crossing the Quality Chasm*, National Academy Press, Washington, DC.

Institutes of Medicine (2003) *Health Professions Education: A Bridge to Quality*, National Academy Press, Washington, DC.

Interprofessional Education Collaborative Expert Panel (2011) *Core Competencies for Interprofessional Collaborative Practice: Report of an Expert Panel*, Interprofessional Education Collaborative, Washington, DC.

James, J.T. (2013) A new, evidence-based estimate of patient harms associated with hospital care. *Journal of Patient Safety*, **9** (**3**), 122–128.

Kaiser Permanente (2007) *Shifting Perspectives.* http://share.kaiserpermanente.org/article/shifting-perspectives/ (accessed November 4, 2016).

Ogden, C.L., Carroll, M.D., Kit, B.K., and Flegal, K.M. (2014) Prevalence of childhood and adult obesity in the United States, 2011–2012. *Journal of the American Medical Association,* **311** (**8**), 806–814.

Schwabe, C.W. (1964) *Veterinary Medicine and Human Health,* Williams & Wilkins, Baltimore, MD.

Simmons, B., Egan-Lee, E., Wagner. S.J., et al. (2011) Assessment of interprofessional learning: The design of an interprofessional objective structured clinical examination (iOSCE) approach. *Journal of Interprofessional Care,* **25** (**1**), 73–74.

Tegzes, J.H., Mackintosh, S., Meyer, T.M., et al. (2013) *To Be or Not To Be: An Interprofessional Problem-Based Learning Case Introducing the One Health Initiative,* MedEdPORTAL Publications, Washington, DC. https://www.mededportal.org/publication/9623 (accessed November 4, 2016).

UK Centre for the Advancement of Interprofessional Education (2007) *Creating an Interprofessional Workforce: An Education and Training Framework for Health and Social Care in England,* Department of Health, London.

Wells, J.E., Sabatino, B.R., Whittemore, J.C., et al. (2014).Cyclophosphamide intoxication because of pharmacy error in two dogs. *Journal of the American Veterinary Medical Association,* **245** (**2**), 222–226.

World Health Organization (2010) *Framework for Action on Interprofessional Education and Collaborative Practice,* World Health Organization, Geneva. http://www.who.int/hrh/resources/framework_action/en/ (accessed December 26, 2015).

8

Peer-Assisted Learning

Laura K. Molgaard[1] and Emma K. Read[2]

[1] College of Veterinary Medicine, University of Minnesota, USA
[2] Faculty of Veterinary Medicine, University of Calgary, Canada

---

 Box 8.1: Key messages

- Peer-assisted learning (PAL) is used extensively in health sciences education to provide academic (remedial) support, develop clinical and professional skills (including teaching skills), and provide additional resources for assessment.
- Peer learners generally report comfort and satisfaction in working with peer tutors.
- There are limited published works describing PAL in veterinary education, but an unpublished survey indicates that many schools are using PAL for one-to-one or small-group support of struggling students.
- Best practices in PAL include training of tutors and evaluation of outcomes for tutees, but are not uniformly implemented in existing PAL programs.
- In human medical education, PAL has evolved from a focus on remedial academic support to an emphasis on skill development and assessment through objective structured clinical examinations and in clinical settings.

Introduction

Peer-assisted learning (PAL) has been shown to be a valuable strategy in health sciences education, and while it is not yet widely adopted or described in veterinary medical education, there are many possible benefits that could be explored. PAL has been defined as "people from similar social groupings who are not professional teachers helping each other to learn and learning themselves by teaching" (Topping, 1996, p. 322). This chapter will focus on uses of PAL identified to date and attempt to define relevant terminology for the veterinary education context. It will also outline the potential benefits of implementing PAL, explore considerations for both tutors and tutees, and describe several applications of PAL that may be particularly relevant to veterinary medical education.

Terminology

Group work and cooperative learning differ from PAL. Group work and cooperative learning are about peers working together on faculty-designed interactions. With PAL, the emphasis is on peer teaching and peer direction (Ross and Cameron, 2007). For the purposes of this chapter, group and cooperative learning will not be considered under the working definition of PAL.

Peer tutors are often tasked with "helping others to learn," but this does not fully encompass the role they may play. Peers can play a role in teaching new material, helping to revise previously acquired knowledge, producing learning resources, mentoring study or life skills, and assessing progress related to learning (Ross and Cameron, 2007).

Confusion exists regarding terminology commonly employed in the literature, with many authors using the same term to describe a variety of activities or roles. In peer-assisted learning the peer teacher may be from the same year of study as the learners (peer) or from a more advanced year (near-peer), although this distinction is not clearly articulated in many references. The peer teacher is often referred to as the tutor and is responsible for assisting in the teaching of, mentoring of, or assessment of the tutee. The tutor has less content knowledge, less formal teacher training, and less authority than the formal course instructors (Damon, 1989). The tutee is the one being assisted. The term "learner" is sometimes used to describe the tutee, but because all students are learners, and in fact some PAL programs are designed with the primary goal of the tutor learning to teach, this term might best be avoided in the context of PAL.

Definitions relating to PAL are summarized in Box 8.2.

Framework for Planning and Implementation of Peer-Assisted Learning

In a 2007 Association for Medical Education in Europe (AMEE) guide, Ross and Cameron (2007) articulated a planning and implementation framework for PAL with 23 questions organized into 7 categories to help guide an institution through the process of creating and implementing a PAL program. We have consolidated and adapted this framework to include background and objectives, a discussion of roles and responsibilities of participants, and a description of published outcomes and best practices.

Background to and Objectives of PAL

Programs may have a variety of reasons for considering the implementation of PAL. Educational institutions ranging from primary schools to those offering undergraduate, graduate, and professional programs have created PAL programs to serve a variety of needs, many of which are relevant to veterinary education. Objectives of these programs include support of individual students through social support, remedial support, or additional opportunities to practice new technical skills. While PAL cannot replace the role or expertise of the faculty instructor, it can provide another mechanism for students to have basic or common questions answered in a setting that may be considered more comfortable and less intimidating (Micari, 2006). Peer tutors and peer learners have "cognitive congruence" with the peer tutee, meaning that in many cases they are better able to understand and answer the questions that a tutee poses. This often relates to their use of simpler language for explanation and to their ability to more readily identify problem areas that are making learning challenging for the tutee (Lockspeiser *et al.*, 2008).

In addition to benefit to the individual student, peer support can provide benefit to the institution through decreased attrition (Higgins, 2004). An institution may also choose to offer PAL to alleviate the teaching burden or address limited resources (Ten and Durning, 2007). This can be critical when the cohort is large and the institutional resources, particularly the budget, are limited. It has been especially useful in the area of clinical skills teaching and learning when demand for repeated practice exceeds the staff resources available. It should be noted that programs using PAL to alleviate resource limitations have been criticized by some commentators for ethical concerns regarding possibly disadvantaging students

Box 8.2: What's the meaning – PAL definitions

Tutor = student as leader, mentor, trainer, teacher Tutee = student as participant, mentee, trainee, student Dyad = a tutor–tutee pairing Reciprocal PAL = students take successive turns in being the tutor and the tutee, playing both roles in a single exercise	Peer = from the same cohort Horizontal peer = from the same cohort Near peer = from cohorts that are similar but not equal in training or education Vertical peer = from cohorts further into their training Source: Black and MacKenzie, 2008.

with what might be perceived as lower-quality education (Ross and Cameron, 2007).

The resources needed to create and manage a PAL program must be considered, including recruitment and training of tutors, design of interactions, development of materials, scheduling of sessions, oversight of peer tutors, and assessment of outcomes (Topping, 1996). Stakeholders, including faculty, need to be involved early in order to obtain buy-in and minimize political resistance (Ross and Cameron, 2007). Faculty may worry that students who require additional support through PAL are not capable of meeting the requirements of a rigorous program or that PAL encourages grade inflation (Widmar, 1994). If peer tutors are perceived as a replacement for instructors, students may be skeptical about the knowledge and skill of the peer tutors, and faculty may be suspicious of administrative motives in using students to replace faculty effort (Smith, 2013). The quality and variability of the tutoring may also be a concern that needs to be mitigated by training and evaluation (Topping, 1996). Clear guidelines must be created to delineate when peers will be used to support instruction. In the case of peer tutoring for academic support, faculty and students alike need to understand the role of the peer tutor as a facilitator, not as replacement for the instructor. Students who look to the peer tutor for quick-fix learning or as a mechanism simply to increase grades will not benefit from

the potential benefits of deeper learning and social support (Smith, 2013).

In a review of the literature, there are four main purposes for which one may wish to consider PAL in a veterinary institution: academic support, skill development, development of teaching skills, and assessment. The following sections will include some uses of PAL at veterinary schools that have not been described in the published literature previously, although most have been discussed at educational meetings. These interactions have come to light following an informal survey of Association of American Veterinary Medical Colleges (AAVMC) veterinary colleges, and are presented here as some examples of how peer programs may be useful in meeting current educational challenges.

PAL to Provide Academic Support

A common objective for PAL programs in undergraduate and health science programs is to provide additional study support to learners or mentoring in case of remediation or gaps in preparation for high-stakes assessments. Additionally, support may be required for specific courses in a curriculum with a high volume of difficult-to-master material, and relatively high failure rates (Hurley *et al.*, 2003). The structure of a PAL academic support tutor program may be one-to-one, in which a student, typically a near-peer from a more senior class, acts in a fixed role (Topping, 1996). An alternative structure is small-group tutoring, where a tutor works with a small group or multiple small groups to provide remedial content support as well as more effective approaches to studying or understanding the content. The rigors of a veterinary curriculum invariably put demands on learners and stretch their ability to cope with the tremendous volume and complexity of content they are expected to learn. While little has been published in veterinary medical education about PAL as it is defined in this chapter, with the peer tutor acting in a fixed role to support the learning of another student or students, in an informal survey of veterinary colleges (unpublished) the most commonly reported use of PAL was for near-peer tutor programs to support struggling learners. Most colleges did not provide training to tutors beyond a brief

orientation. Supervision was also similarly variable. An example of a near-peer tutor program is provided in Box 8.3.

PAL to Support Skills Development

Using peers to support anatomical, professional, and clinical skills training and assessment is intuitively beneficial because this sort of teaching does not always lend itself well to the efficiency of one teacher working with a large classroom filled with students. The dominant mode of learning in anatomy is student-led dissection with accompanying lectures, and living anatomy demonstrations using imaging and animals (Evans and Cuffe, 2009). The University of Glasgow medical school was one of the first institutions to use near-peers to

---

Box 8.3: Example of remedial tutoring program at the University of Minnesota

Veterinary peer-assisted coaching (VetPAC) was implemented in 2008 to provide struggling students with additional support and to lessen the burden on faculty for providing that support through office hours.

Tutors

- Selected based on past performance in a particular course and overall academic excellence.
- Typically near-peers, but in some cases high-ability students coach within the same year.
- Training involves five online modules followed by one face-to-face session covering topics such as expectations, learning theory, Bloom's taxonomy, facilitation, feedback, study skills, and troubleshooting difficulties.
- Paid a nominal hourly wage.
- Benefit from training and experience as a coach.

Tutees

- Students who receive a mid-term deficiency letter are referred to the VetPAC program for one-to-one coaching.

- Students can also self-identify as struggling because of current or past academic difficulty.
- May be in any year of the program.

Oversight

- By faculty member who provides training and ongoing support.
- Details managed by a staff member, including matching tutee and tutor.

Process

- Tutor and tutee arrange meeting times directly.
- May occur on campus or off.
- Walk-in coaching also available to all students during advertised hours in the library.

Source: Unpublished example provided by Margaret Root Kustritz.

teach clinical examination to junior veterinary students (Field *et al.*, 2007). Clinical skills training courses have recently seen an increased emphasis in many curricula as part of the focus on outcomes-based programming. Many of these programs incorporate peer tutors to help with teaching, learning, and assessing clinical skills, including a novel use of peers to teach rectal palpation skills with the Haptic Cow simulator at the Royal Veterinary College in London, UK (Kinnison *et al.*, 2009). PAL was combined with an automated self-teaching version of this computerized simulator and role-playing exercises were used to improve tutee communication skills. There was an emphasis on the preparation and support of tutors.

Examples of using PAL to enhance anatomical training exist in both the medical and veterinary medical literature. Near-peer programs have been employed in medical schools to allow upperclassmen to gain teaching experience and a deeper understanding of the material, while enhancing the student–teacher ratio in labs and providing educational materials aimed at highlighting some of the challenges in retaining large volumes of material (Evans and Cuffe, 2009). With the advent of outcomes-based programs in medical and veterinary schools, some educators have highlighted concerns about the reduction in contact hours for teaching anatomical principles (Hall *et al.*, 2013). This shift in ideology was partly instituted to create more time to develop non-technical competencies (also referred to as SKAs or Skills Knowledge Aptitudes and Attitudes; Brown and Silverman, 1999; Lloyd *et al.*, 2004) that provide essential social and professional skills that will benefit students in becoming well-rounded professionals on graduation (Hall *et al.*, 2013), but some educators insist that this additional training has compromised time spent on core content knowledge. Educators at the Royal Veterinary College in London developed a novel anatomy training system with four defined roles for students in a reciprocal PAL exercise, and reported enhancements in learning, pre-class preparation efforts, and use of available resources (Hall *et al.*, 2013).

Examples of PAL in veterinary skills training are provided in Box 8.4.

Communication skills, history taking, and physical examination skills are the most common discipline areas for PAL implementation via peer teaching in medical and nursing schools (Burgess, McGregor, and Mellis, 2014). Medical schools also use peers for assessment and feedback in these same areas using formative objective structured clinical examinations (OSCEs) with near-peers (Burgess, McGregor and Mellis, 2014). In a novel interprofessional peer-assisted skill development project, final-year medical students were recruited and trained to provide small-group near-peer training to nursing students (Gill *et al.*, 2006). Skills laboratory facilities allow training of students in simulated and sheltered learning environments prior to entering the workplace. Use of task trainers, models, and simulated clients/patients enables repetitive practice in a safe environment with expert feedback (Weyrich, 2008). It is the feedback during development of the skills that is critical. As American football coach Vince Lombardi is reported to have said, "Practice does not make perfect. Only perfect practice is perfect," which highlights the challenge of self-directed learning. It can be obvious during an OSCE that a student shows efficiency and confidence in performing the skill, indicating time spent practicing, but the skill can be poorly performed because obvious components are missing or conducted incorrectly (Marteau, 1990). In addition, self-assessment has been shown to be notoriously unreliable as a measure of performance outcome in skills training (Davis, 2006). Peer tutors in the skills lab can be useful to help offset high student–teacher ratios and allow more dedicated teaching and feedback (Weyrich, 2008). It has been shown that use of peer teachers for surgical skills training with novices can worsen the learning outcome; the same authors reported that efforts must be made to provide thorough structured training of tutors and continual oversight (Ketele *et al.*, 2010). In properly structured PAL events, learning has been shown in some cases to be equally successful using peer

Box 8.4: Example of clinical skills peer tutoring at the University of Calgary Faculty of Veterinary Medicine (UCVM) and Royal (Dick) School of Veterinary Studies (RDSVS), University of Edinburgh

The Royal (Dick) School of Veterinary Studies and the University of Calgary Faculty of Veterinary Medicine incorporated peer learning into the teaching of physical examination skills.

Tutors

- Third-year students at UCVM and fourth-year students at RDSVS.
- At both schools, required to complete a PAL teaching and learning exercise as part of their clinical skills training program, and assessment of the program provides a portion of the students' final grade for the course (UCVM), and is a required summative element (tutors' lesson plan) of the fourth-year portfolio (RDSVS).
- Plan an hour-long session reviewing physical examination of a domestic animal species (dog, cow, or horse); encouraged to develop teaching materials and to use models or live animals in teaching.
- Encouraged to remember the challenges they had in learning the skills and in their skills assessments when developing informative sessions for tutees.

Tutees

- First-year students at UCVM and at RDSVS.
- Voluntarily participate and sign up for sessions that are conducted in lunch hours and after school (UCVM).
- Participate on a compulsory basis during scheduled class time (RDSVS).

Process

- A faculty member provides a three-hour session for tutors in class time to explain the benefits of PAL, teach them some learning theory, provide assistance with lesson planning, and explain the logistics of the PAL activity.

Evaluation

- Tutors asked to evaluate one another and required to submit a lesson plan and reflective blog for grading.
- Tutees asked to evaluate tutors.
- Feedback about the utility of the program collected from all participants.

Source: Unpublished example provided by Emma Read, Neil Hudson, and Catriona Bell.

---

tutors and experienced faculty (Weyrich *et al.*, 2009).

PAL to Develop Teaching Skills in Tutors

Joseph Joubert reportedly stated that "to teach is to learn twice" (Durling and Schick, 1976). Evidence in the literature suggests that it is the act of teaching, especially the vocalizing of content and addressing learners' questions, that reinforces learning in the "teacher" (Durling and Schick, 1976). Development of professional competence and confidence through serving in the role of a PAL tutor is identified as a frequent driver for PAL initiatives, especially in human medical education (Burgess, Black, Chapman *et al.*, 2012a; Burgess, McGregor,

and Mellis, 2014). PAL has been widely used in health professional education and its perceived importance can be partially attributed to the UK General Medical Council's document stating that graduates "must be able to demonstrate appropriate teaching skills" (Education Committee of the General Medical Council, 2003). Leadership skills development, enhanced confidence, and improved intrinsic motivation are all cited as reasons for incorporating peer learning for medical students (Burgess, Black, Chapman *et al.*, 2012a; Burgess, McGregor, and Mellis, 2014). It is an expectation that throughout graduate medical education the next generation of doctors will be educators of their future trainees, and will also be patient educators throughout their careers (Dandavino, Snell, and Wiseman, 2007). Other health professional education programs have also incorporated PAL to serve similar purposes. For example, in one report advanced paramedic students were recruited to teach first-year students, with the primary goal of developing teaching skills and confidence in the more advanced learners (Williams, Olausson, and Peterson, 2015). An example of a veterinary student teaching rotation is provided in Box 8.5.

PAL for Use in Assessment

There is a renewed call for specific outcome measures in veterinary education. Examples are emerging whereby peers are trained in the critical evaluation of one another after faculty, not peer, instruction. Many PAL or team-based projects have incorporated student assessment, usually in a formative capacity, as part of the grading schema (Danielson *et al.*, 2008; Iblher *et al.*, 2015). Recently student assessors have been used to integrate assessment practices into existing class time as a learning exercise for all involved, and to minimize the time and expense required for expert raters across the program. An example of the use of peers for assessment via OSCEs is provided in Box 8.6.

Box 8.5: Example of PAL for development of teaching and leaderships skills: UC Davis Educational Leadership Rotation

Tutors

- Fourth-year students can elect to take a two-week teaching rotation and act as teaching assistants in preparation of teaching materials, and in presentation and facilitation of case- and team-based learning.
- Program created to provide an opportunity to develop leadership and teaching skills.
- Can select content area of choice in a discipline of interest (e.g., ophthalmology) or through mentorship of new students enrolled in a graded course.

Tutees

- All incoming students work with the tutors (students enrolled in the rotation) during the professional and clinical skills unit.
- Students enrolled in selected "blocks" (integrated body system units) where tutors provide a session in a particular content area (variable).

Process

- Rotation is tailored to the tutors' interests and professional development goals. Training includes assigned readings on learning theory, educational methodology, facilitation, analysis of personality type, and opportunities for self-reflection.
- Students enrolled in the rotation develop learning outcomes, sessions (lecture, laboratory, etc.) and assessments for their tutees in a specific content area, under the supervision of the educational specialist and relevant faculty content expert.

Evaluation

- Tutors submit an evaluative portfolio consisting of an analysis of learning outcomes, development of assessment items aligned to learning outcomes, presentation or summary of methodology used to convey content to achieve the learning outcomes, and a metacognitive self-reflection on the processes over the two weeks.
- The tutor's portfolio is evaluated with an educational rubric by the educational specialist. Content-related items and performance are evaluated by the content area faculty, although the emphasis of this rotation is on the educational processes.

Source: Unpublished example provided by Karen Boudreaux.

Box 8.6: Example of using peers for formative assessment in OSCEs at the University of Veterinary Medicine Hannover

Near-peer tutors augment teaching staff for formative procedural skill OSCEs that are offered in preparation for high-stakes assessments for students tracking in selected species.

Tutors

- Selected based on clinical experience and references.
- Most have been veterinary technicians (nurses) prior to veterinary school.
- Compensation is provided but is not a primary motivator.
- Participate in two-day training on preparing a session, content, set-up, assessment, and giving feedback.
- Must pass a skills assessment.

Tutees

- All students tracking in small animals, small ruminants, and swine.

Process

- Tutors and staff alike use a detailed description of procedural skills.
- A binary checklist with 15–30 items is used for each skills station.
- There is no interaction during the OSCE, but tutees receive a completed checklist.
- Feedback is standardized and provided as a group debrief.

Evaluation

- Tutees show no preference for near-peer tutors versus staff as evaluators.

Source: Unpublished example provided by Marc Dilly.

Role and Responsibilities of Participants

In addition to determining the broader institutional needs that a PAL program is intended to address, it is also important to consider the specific objectives of the tutors and tutees involved, including selection, training, and rewards.

Tutors

There are numerous potential benefits to the tutor that have been documented. Most commonly cited is the development of professional attributes such as the ability to admit uncertainty, an increase in confidence, a willingness to contribute to educating others, and autonomy in learning (Burgess, McGregor, and Mellis, 2014). Tutors gain the opportunity to develop skills that can extend to client education as a future practitioner (Ross, 2012). They must formulate and deliver constructive feedback to others as part of these exercises, and this is a

critical skill for their future interactions in a professional organization (Burgess, McGregor, and Mellis, 2014). Volunteer medical students' participation in an OSCE tutor program showed positive influences in their perception of their teaching skills and interest in further education in teaching (Buckley and Zamora, 2007). However, less than half of medical schools surveyed indicated that they provided formal training in teaching, although all indicated that students "made significant teaching contributions" in their programs (Soriano *et al.*, 2010, p. 1726). Development of tutor training should begin by defining outcomes and objectives such as general knowledge about adult learning and education, teaching skills and strategies, and attitudes toward teaching (Dandavino, Snell, and Wiseman, 2007).

Tutors are often first motivated to work with their peers to further their own content knowledge through review (Ross and Cameron, 2007). The teaching experience typically provides an opportunity to reflect on their knowledge gaps and to develop a deeper understanding of the subject matter (Ross and Cameron, 2007). The medical literature has not always been able to demonstrate a clear advantage for the tutor in skills development. Some studies show that peer tutors have higher OSCE and multiple-choice question scores compared to controls (Knobe *et al.*, 2010), while others show minimal changes in skill level when assessed (Nestel and Ridd, 2005).

The time required for participation as a tutor may be a concern to the tutors and to the faculty, because it has been reported to distract tutors from their own studies (Capstick, 2004). The reward system for tutors is another important consideration and care must be taken that they are not exploited. While many programs provide hourly compensation for tutors, it has been suggested that creation of a credit-bearing course is one way to provide ongoing support and training, as well as appropriate recognition of the tutor's efforts (Smith, 2013).

Tutees

The benefits to the tutee are often more obvious and sometimes perceived to be greater (Ross and Cameron, 2007). Tutors can impart a large amount of knowledge to learners, who are often motivated to learn in the less intimidating environment (Burgess, McGregor, and Mellis, 2014). Tutees may develop close relationships with tutors that allow for much-needed social support and help in developing study skills (Yu *et al.*, 2011). Tutors frequently create a cognitively congruent environment whereby they only demonstrate a small step up in knowledge, which in turn motivates tutees to learn and develop (Lockspeiser *et al.*, 2008). Tutors tend to be better able to express themselves at the learner's level than are experts (Ross and Cameron, 2007).

While some studies have shown that tutees may use PAL to improve grades through strategies that focus on understanding assessment demands rather than deeper understanding of

the material (Ashwin, 2003), others assert that PAL contributes to deeper understanding, not just higher scores (Capstick, 2004).

In the case of one-to-one or small-group coaching, consideration must be given to resource limitations in order to ensure that students who need this support most have access to it. Students in need of peer support may be identified by the instructor and referred to the PAL program, or may be identified centrally based on class rank or grade point average (GPA). However, there is the risk of stigmatization or a perception of elitism if only certain students have access to PAL programs (Smith, 2013). The Supplemental Instruction (SI) model is a particular manifestation of group peer tutoring that has been adopted across multiple medical schools (Bridgham and Scarborough, 1992; Blanc and Martin, 1994; Sawyer *et al.*, 1996; Hurley *et al.*, 2003) and avoids this pitfall. David Arendale defines SI as "a student academic assistance program that increases academic performance and retention through its use of collaborative learning strategies" (Arendale, 1994, p. 11). Rather than matching struggling students with tutors, SI focuses on high-risk courses, not high-risk students, and begins in the first week of the class as a voluntary form of support that aims to prevent academic difficulty. Like other manifestations of PAL, SI provides not only content support but also peer modeling of learning strategies, such as development of test questions, creating charts to show relationships between information, and construction and analysis of diagrams (Bridgham and Scarborough, 1992). SI "leaders" (the designation for the near-peer tutor) are trained and the SI sessions are designed to be interactive, rather than a passive transfer of information (Arendale, 1994). There are no published reports of the use of SI in veterinary schools, but there are at least two examples of SI-like programs that have been developed in recent years. The VetPALs program at the Royal (Dick) School of Veterinary Studies, University of Edinburgh has been in place since 2012 and is described in Box 8.7.

 Box 8.7: Example of group academic support at the Royal (Dick) School of Veterinary Studies (RDSVS)

VetPALs was created to provide support for students during their first year of this difficult program, with a focus on study skills and the intentional development of the teaching and facilitation skills of tutors ("leaders").

Tutors

- Apply by explaining interest, what skills they will bring, and what skills they hope to develop; academic performance does not influence selection.
- A two-day training course is provided, including facilitation techniques and simulated Vet-PALs sessions.

Tutees

- Open to all first-year students and attendance varies, but up to one-third of the cohort attends some sessions.

Process

- Tutors ("VetPAL leaders") design the interactions, which focus on study skills, time management, and exam-taking skills, sometimes using illustrative content (e.g., on anatomy).
- Tutees rotate among various stations aimed at helping them consider how a particular technique may work for them.

Evaluation

- No identifying information is collected from students in order to prevent stigmatization; only the numbers of students attending are tracked. Attendance has increased over the first three years of the program.
- Tutors report perceived benefits of better communication skills and increased engagement. Organizers state that the unintended benefit has been the development of a community between students in different years of the program.

Source: Unpublished example provided by Jessie Paterson.

Evaluation

The variability of schemas for PAL complicates the evaluation of outcomes, but in some formats educational achievement has been shown to be equal to or better than faculty-led tutoring (Topping, 1996).

Evaluation of Students' Ability to Assess

When peers are used for assessment, controversy exists in the literature as to whether tutors are stricter in their assessment of their peers when compared to faculty (Bucknall *et al.*, 2008) or more lenient (Burgess *et al.*, 2012b; Iblher *et al.*, 2015). In a study evaluating the feasibility of using near-peers to assess a written assignment, peers were able to provide valid, reliable ratings without specific training, demonstrating a cost-effective use of PAL in assessment in veterinary education. Third-year students evaluated final-year students' performance on a case analysis assignment in pathology. Final-year student performance was used as a benchmark of the veterinary pathology program's success. There was good agreement between experts and peer evaluators, and it allowed a cost-effective multirater accounting of pathology knowledge and skills within the program (Danielson *et al.*, 2008). In another project, peers authored and rated multiple-choice questions for use in assessment of veterinary courses. The degree of student engagement with the development and rating of the questions was correlated to student performance overall (Rhind and Graham, 2012).

Evaluation of Students' Ability to Teach

There are studies in favor of peer tutors compared to more highly trained faculty. A 2010 study with medical students demonstrated that students who learned from their peers had comparable outcomes to those who learned from experienced doctors. Students in that study received a short (30-minute) training session and underwent one week of self-teaching prior to teaching a complicated technical skill (ultrasound of the shoulder joint) to peers with the same level of experience (Knobe *et al.*, 2010). Interestingly, the learners still placed more confidence in the competence of the experts, even though no difference was identified in the performance outcomes (Knobe *et al.*, 2010). Near-peer medical students recruited to teach basic clinical skills (e.g., injection techniques, setting up an infusion) to third-year medical students were found to be better teachers, as demonstrated by a superior performance rating of their tutees compared to those taught by faculty members (Weyrich *et al.*, 2009). Peer teachers have also been praised when recruited and trained to provide near-peer teaching in an anatomy laboratory (Evans and Cuffe, 2009). A study looking at the effectiveness of and first-year medical student perceptions of tutorials led by new ("junior") doctors showed that 95% of learners had a strong preference for learning from near-peers versus from faculty, citing the near-peers as more approachable (Gibson *et al.*, 2014). Boylan *et al.* found that tutor training was one of the most important determinants of success and that tutor programs with untrained tutors had no effect on grades or retention (Boylan, 1997).

Evaluation of Students' Ability to Learn

Published literature reviews show widely varied implementations of dyadic and small-group tutoring, with inconsistent and often incomplete methods of evaluation making it very difficult to judge the outcomes of the various iterations (Topping, 1992, 1996). A 2014 review reported that "all studies showed that student learners were not disadvantaged by ... PAL initiatives"

(Burgess, McGregor, and Mellis, 2014). Determining where there has been greater tutor content knowledge or an improved ability to teach is often based on self-reporting and is rarely if ever assessed objectively (Burgess, McGregor, and Mellis, 2014). In some studies, the only outcome evaluated for tutees' learning was their perception regarding peer feedback being better than faculty feedback (Reiter *et al.*, 2004). More recent studies have tried to demonstrate a change in content knowledge or skills performance for tutees (Weyrich *et al.*, 2009; Knobe *et al.*, 2010; Yu *et al.*, 2011). In an example of SI to retain disadvantaged students at a medical school, SI participants who took part in 80% of sessions performed at about half a standard deviation higher than comparable students who did not, and achieved comparably to students who had better Medical College Admission Test (MCAT) scores and undergraduate science GPAs (Bridgham and Scarborough, 1992).

Evaluation of Students' Ability to Feel Supported

Much has been published on tutees' perceptions of academic PAL programs as being supportive of their learning (Topping, 1996; Micari, Streitwieser, and Light, 2006; Lockspeiser *et al.*, 2008; Smith, 2013). PAL must meet certain requirements in order to create a safe and supportive learning experience, and it has been asserted that the peer tutor cannot be perceived as having an evaluative role that creates a power differential (Ladyshewsky, 2010). In a study of veterinary students used as simulated clients in communications training, learners reported a comfort level that indicated emotional safety in this program involving non-evaluative feedback by near-peers, with the majority indicating a preference for a trained peer over a non-familiar paid actor (Strand, Johnson, and Thompson, 2013). One veterinary program has created a peer program specifically aimed at providing non-academic support (Spielman, Hughes, and Rhind, 2015). In a school-wide survey, 74% of respondents indicated that peer support is important, but only 26% responded that they would be likely to use this system, with stated reasons for avoiding such support being greater comfort with others (friends, family, or staff) and a small community perceived as competitive (Spielman, Hughes, and Rhind, 2015).

Conclusion

Peer-assisted learning in medical schools in the 1980s and 1990s focused on dyadic or small-group remedial tutor programs, with little detail published about the purpose of those programs, which appeared to be based more on tradition and practical drivers than on evidence (Schaffer, Wile, and Griggs, 1990; Trevino and Eiland, 1980; Moore-West and Hennessy, 1990;

Ten and Durning, 2007, p. 546). In a recent literature review, the majority of PAL programs in medical schools focused on teaching clinical skills and assessment using OSCEs rather than on remedial tutoring (Burgess, McGregor, and Mellis, 2014). While there is much less published in the veterinary literature, it is likely that the profession will follow suit and that in the future PAL in veterinary education will focus less on one-to-one remedial support and more on building on the evidence of the value of SI for academic support and on the use of peers to teach and assess skills. Regardless of the use of peers to support teaching and learning, it will be important to follow best practices in training tutors, and to evaluate and publish the outcomes of PAL programs in veterinary education.

References

Arendale, D.R. (1994) Understanding the supplemental instruction model. *New Directions for Teaching and Learning*, **60**, 11–21.

Ashwin, P. (2003) Peer support: Relations between the context, process and outcomes for the students who are supported. *Instructional Science*, **31** (**3**), 159–173.

Black, F.M., and McKenzie, J. (2008) Quality enhancement themes: The first year experience: Peer support in the first year. *Enhancement Themes*, Quality Assurance Agency for Higher Education, Mansfield. http://dera.ioe.ac.uk/11603/1/peer-support-in-the-first-year-1.pdf (accessed November 5, 2016).

Blanc, R., and Martin, D.C. (1994) Supplemental instruction: Increasing student performance and persistence in difficult academic courses. *Academic Medicine*, **69** (**6**), 452–454.

Boylan, H.R., Bliss, L.B., and Bonham, B.S. (1997) Program components and their relationship to student performance. *Journal of Developmental Education*, **20** (**3**), 2–8.

Bridgham, R.G., and Scarborough, S. (1992) Effects of supplemental instruction in selected

medical school science courses. *Academic Medicine*, **67** (**10**), 69–71.

Brown, J.P., and Silverman, J.D. (1999) The current and future market for veterinarians and veterinary medical services in the United States. *Journal of the American Veterinary Medical Association*, **215**, 161–183.

Buckley, S., and Zamora, J. (2007) Effects of participation in a cross year peer tutoring programme in clinical examination skills on volunteer tutors' skills and attitudes towards teachers and teaching. *BMC Medical Education*, **7** (**1**), 20.

Bucknall, V., Sobic, E.M., Wood, H.L., *et al.* (2008) Peer assessment of resuscitation skills. *Resuscitation*, **77** (**2**), 211–215.

Burgess, A., Black, K., Chapman, R., *et al.* (2012a) Teaching skills for students: Our future educators. *Clinical Teacher*, **9** (**5**), 312–316.

Burgess, A., Clark, T., Chapter, R., and Mellis, C. (2012b) Senior medical students as peer examiners in an OSCE. *Medical Teacher*, **35** (**1**), 58–62.

Burgess, A., McGregor, D., and Mellis, C. (2014) Medical students as peer tutors: A systematic review. *BMC Medical Education*, **14** (**1**), 115–122.

Capstick, S. (2004) Benefits and shortcomings of peer assisted learning (PAL) in higher education: An appraisal by students. *Peer Assisted Learning Conference*, January, Bournemouth. https://www1.bournemouth.ac .uk/sites/default/files/asset/document/stuart-capstick.pdf (accessed November 5, 2016).

Damon, W., and Phelps, E. (1989) Critical distinctions among three approaches to peer education. *International Journal of Educational Research*, **13** (**1**), 9–19.

Dandavino, M., Snell, L., and Wiseman, J. (2007) Why medical students should learn how to teach. *Medical Teacher*, **29** (**6**), 558–565.

Danielson, J.A., Fales-Williams, A.J., Sorden, S.D., *et al.* (2008) Peer assessment of a final-year capstone experience for formative evaluation of a pathology curriculum. *Journal of Veterinary Medical Education*, **35** (**3**), 466–474.

Durling, R., and Schick, C. (1976) Concept attachment by pairs and individuals as a function of vocalization. *Journal of Educational Psychology*, **68** (**1**), 83–91.

Davis, M., Ponnamperuna, G.G., McAleer, S., and Dale, V.H.M. (2006) The objective structured clinical examination (OSCE) as determinant of veterinary clinical skills. *Journal of Veterinary Medical Education*, **33** (**4**), 578–587.

General Medical Council – Education Committee (2003) *Tomorrow's Doctors: Recommendations on Undergraduate Medical Education*. General Medical Council, London.

Evans, D.J., and Cuffe, T. (2009) Near-peer teaching in anatomy: An approach for deeper learning. *Anatomical Sciences Education*, **2** (**5**), 227.

Field, M., Burke, J.M., McAllister, D., and Lloyd, D.M. (2007) Peer-assisted learning: A novel approach to clinical skills learning for medical students. *Medical Education*, **41** (**4**), 411–418.

Gibson, K.R., Qureshi, Z.U., Ross, M.T., and Maxwell, S.R. (2014) Junior doctor-led 'near-peer' prescribing education for medical students. *British Journal of Clinical Pharmacology*, **77** (**1**), 122–129.

Gill, D., Parker, C., Spooner, M., *et al.* (2006) Tomorrow's doctors and nurses: Peer assisted learning. *Clinical Teacher*, **3** (**1**), 13–18.

Hall, E.R., Davis, R.C., Weller, R., Powney, S. and Williams, S.B. (2013) Doing dissections differently: A structured, peer-assisted learning approach to maximizing learning in dissections. *Anatomical Sciences Education*, **6** (**1**), 56–66.

Higgins, B. (2004) Relationship between retention and peer tutoring for at-risk students. *Journal of Nursing Education*, **43** (**7**), 319–321.

Hurley, K.F., Mckay, D.W., Scott, T.M., and James, B.M. (2003) The supplemental instruction project: Peer-devised and delivered tutorials. *Medical Teacher*, **25** (**4**), 404–407.

Iblher, P., Zupanic, M., Karsten, J., and Brauer, K. (2015) May student examiners be reasonable substitute examiners for faculty in an undergraduate OSCE on medical emergencies? *Medical Teacher*, **37** (**4**), 374–378.

Ketele, P., Jacobs, A., Boruett, N., and Derese, A. (2010) PerSIST: A PAL system for clinical skills training: A planning and implementation framework: Guide supplement 30.8 – Practical application. *Medical Teacher*, **32**, 782–784.

Kinnison, T., Forrest, N.D., Frean, S.P., and Baillie, S. (2009) Teaching bovine abdominal anatomy: Use of a haptic simulator. *Anatomical Sciences Education*, **2** (**6**), 280–285.

Knobe, M., Münker, R., Sellei, R.M., *et al.* (2010) Peer teaching: A randomised controlled trial using student-teachers to teach musculoskeletal ultrasound. *Medical Education*, **44** (**2**), 148–155.

Ladyshewsky, R.K. (2010) Building competency in the novice allied health professional through peer coaching. *Journal of Allied Health*, **39** (**2**), 77E–82E.

Lloyd, J.W., King, L.J., Maccabe, A.T., and Heider, L.E. (2004) Skills, knowledge, aptitude, and attitude colloquium. *Journal of Veterinary Medical Education*, **31**, 435–440.

Lockspeiser, T.M., O'Sullivan, P., Teherani, A., and Muller, J. (2008) Understanding the experience of being taught by peers: The value of social and cognitive congruence. *Advances in Health Sciences Education*, **13** (**3**), 361–372.

Marteau, T.M., Wynne, G., Kaye, W., and Evans, T.R. (1990) Resuscitation: experience without feedback increases confidence but not skill. *British Medical Journal*, **300** (**31**), 849–850.

Micari, M., Streitwieser, B., and Light, G. (2006) Undergraduates leading undergraduates: Peer facilitation in a science workshop program. *Innovative Higher Education*, **30** (**4**), 269–288.

Moore-West, M., and Hennessy, S.A. (1990) The presence of student-based peer advising, peer tutoring and performance evaluation programs among U.S. medical schools. *Academic Medicine*, **65** (**10**), 660–661.

Nestel, D., and Kidd, J. (2005) Peer assisted learning in patient-centred interviewing: The impact on student tutors. *Medical Teacher*, **27**, 439–444.

Reiter, H.I., Rosenfeld, J., Nandagopal, K., and Eva, K.W. (2004) Do clinical clerks provide candidates with adequate formative assessment during objective structured clinical examinations? *Advances in Health Sciences Education*, **9** (**3**), 189–199.

Rhind, S.M., and Graham, W.P. (2012) Peer generation of multiple-choice questions: Student engagement and experiences. *Journal of Veterinary Medical Education*, **39** (**4**), 375–379.

Ross, M.T. (2012) Teachers who study and students who teach: Are we really so different? *Medical Teacher*, **34** (**5**), 351–353.

Ross, M.T., and Cameron, H.S. (2007) Peer assisted learning: A planning and implementation framework: AMEE guide no. 30. *Medical Teacher*, **29**, 527–545.

Sawyer, S.J., Sylvestre, P.B., Girard, R.A., and Snow, M.H. (1996) Effects of supplemental instruction on mean test scores and failure rates in medical school courses. *Academic Medicine*, **71** (**12**), 1357–1359.

Schaffer, J.L., Wile, M.Z., and Griggs, R.C. (1990) Students teaching students: A medical school peer tutorial programme. *Medical Education*, **24** (**4**), 336–343.

Smith, T.S. (ed.) (2013) *Undergraduate Curricular Peer Mentoring Programs: Perspectives on Innovations by Faculty, Staff, and Students*, Lexington Books, Lanham, MD.

Soriano, R.P., Blatt, B., Coplit, L., *et al.* (2010) Teaching medical students how to teach: A national survey of students-as-teachers programs in US medical schools. *Academic Medicine*, **85** (**11**), 1725–1731.

Spielman, S., Hughes, K., and Rhind, S. (2015) Development, evaluation, and evolution of a peer support program in veterinary medical education. *Journal of Veterinary Medical Education*, **42** (**3**), 176–183.

Strand, E.B., Johnson, B., and Thompson, J. (2013) Peer-assisted communication training: Veterinary students as simulated clients and communication skills trainers. *Journal of Veterinary Medical Education*, **40** (**3**), 233–241.

Ten, C.O., and Durning, S. (2007) Dimensions and psychology of peer teaching in medical education. *Medical Teacher*, **29** (**6**), 546–552.

Topping, K.J. (1992) Cooperative learning and peer tutoring: An overview. *The Psychologist*, **5** (**4**), 51–57.

Topping, K.J. (1996) The effectiveness of peer tutoring in further and higher education: A typology and review of the literature. *Higher Education*, **32**, 321–345.

Trevino, F.M., Eiland, D.C., Jr., (1980) Evaluation of a basic science, peer tutorial program for first-and second-year medical students. *Academic Medicine*, **55** (**11**), 952–953.

Weyrich, P., Schrauth, M., Kraus, B., *et al.* (2008) Undergraduate technical skills training guided by student tutors -analysis of tutors' attitudes, tutees' acceptance and learning progress in an innovative teaching model. *BMC Medical Education*, **8** (**1**), 18.

Weyrich, P., Celebi, N., Schrauth, M., *et al.* (2009) Peer-assisted versus faculty staff-led skills laboratory training: A randomised controlled trial. *Medical Education*, **43** (**2**), 113–120.

Widmar, G.E. (1994) Supplemental instruction: From small beginnings to a national program. *New Directions for Teaching and Learning*, **60**, 3019.

Williams, B., Olaussen, A., and Peterson, E.L. (2015) Peer-assisted teaching: An interventional study. *Nurse Education in Practice*, **15** (**4**), 293–298.

Yu, T.C., Wilson, N.C., Singh, P.P., *et al.* (2011) Medical students-as-teachers: A systematic review of peer-assisted teaching during medical school. *Advances in Medical Education and Practice*, **2011** (**2**), 157–172.

Part III

Learning Opportunities

9

Learning in Classrooms and Laboratories

Susan M. Matthew[1], Jacqueline M. Norris[2] and Mark B. Krockenberger[2]

[1] *College of Veterinary Medicine, Washington State University, USA*
[2] *Sydney School of Veterinary Science, University of Sydney, Australia*

 Box 9.1: Key messages

- Seven interrelated core principles guide effective teaching in classrooms and laboratories: authenticity, constructive alignment, integration, synergy, culture, relationships, and sustainability.
- Veterinary educators should use these principles in designing and evaluating learning outcomes, activities, and assessments by critically reflecting on how strongly these teaching practices are aligned with the key characteristics of each principle.

- Critical reflection on teaching encompasses reviewing published literature and examples of best practice; seeking 360° feedback on performance from peers, students, supervisors, and experienced colleagues; and undertaking critical self-reflection on performance.
- By considering the alignment of teaching practices with each of the key principles and using the reflective process with the examples provided, educators can continuously evolve their teaching to achieve high-quality learning outcomes.

Introduction

Seven interrelated core principles guide effective teaching in classrooms and laboratories: authenticity, constructive alignment, integration, synergy, culture, relationships, and sustainability. Table 9.1 outlines the educationally significant variation in each of these core principles. This is followed by an explanation and case study illustrating each principle. A star rating indicates the extent to which the case study aligns with each of the seven core principles. Guidelines are provided on how educators may use these principles in deliberate, reflective practice to evaluate and improve the quality of their teaching.

Core Principles Guiding Effective Teaching

Authenticity

Authenticity is fundamental to effective teaching in veterinary degree programs. Authentic

Veterinary Medical Education: A Practical Guide, First Edition. Edited by Jennifer L. Hodgson and Jacquelyn M. Pelzer.
© 2017 John Wiley & Sons, Inc. Published 2017 by John Wiley & Sons, Inc.

Table 9.1 Criteria for reflective practice when designing and evaluating teaching practices – a system for utilizing the core principles in reflective practice to improve your teaching.

Principle	* Minimally addressed	** Developing	*** Strongly Aligned
Authenticity	The learning activity and/or assessment task has minimal connection to, or obvious relationship with, the tasks required of a graduate veterinarian		The learning activity and/or assessment task draws realistically on knowledge and skills relevant to those performed by a graduate veterinarian
Constructive alignment	The learning activity and/or assessment task minimally informs or assists the development of the intended learning outcome		The learning outcome is an accurate reflection of the competency required and is practiced and demonstrated through the learning activity and assessment
Integration	The learning activity utilizes interpretation of data from only one discipline in the investigative process		The learning activity overtly requires analysis of data generated by multiple disciplines in the overall learning activity, to arrive at a unified investigative approach
Synergy	Teachers and/or students have little awareness of what and how students are learning, or do not work together in teams to enhance learning outcomes		Teachers are focused on how students are learning and adjust their approach accordingly; students are focused on what and how they are learning; and groups of teachers and students work together to enhance learning outcomes, including incorporating student contributions in learning activities
Culture	The learning activity offers limited opportunities for learners to develop lifelong learning and reflective practice skills, or minimally demonstrates the principles of student-centered learning, constructive alignment, innovation, and sustainability		The learning activity helps to create and sustain a mutual commitment to lifelong learning, critical reflection, and evidence-based outcomes assessment for both learners and teachers, as well as demonstrating a focus on student-centered learning, constructive alignment, innovation, and sustainability
Relationships	The teaching and learning activity shows limited regard to the importance and skills of effective relationships among learners and teachers		The teaching and learning activity and assessment task explicitly develop emotional intelligence competencies and demonstrate effective teacher–learner and peer relationships founded on mutual trust, respect, enjoyment, and commitment
Sustainability	The learning activity requires a high staff-to-student ratio and is based solely in the physical classroom		The learning activity utilizes peer learning, online resources, and self-directed learning to enhance face-to-face teaching and create new learning material. Typically, this activity develops a bank of learning resources through ongoing development of these resources by successive student cohorts.

learning involves a clear connection between essential graduate attributes and the learning activities, teaching methods, and assessment of the course (Barrows and Tamblyn, 1980; Boud and Falchikov, 2006). These need to reflect the complexities and variabilities of the real world, while still providing students with a supportive scaffold to ensure effective learning (May and Silva-Fletcher, 2015). Through this, students can be progressively equipped with practical skills and knowledge that they can easily adapt to address the issues they will face after graduation.

Authenticity usually leads to greater learner motivation and engagement, as the benefit and future application of the knowledge are explicit (Hafen *et al.*, 2015). For technical skills such as suturing or venipuncture, the importance of the skills rarely needs explanation. Depending on the competence being taught, scaffolding of the learning activity may be required either to highlight the real-world relevance and importance of required skills and knowledge (e.g., detailed interpretation of clinical pathology data in diagnostic investigation), or to demonstrate the need for more extensive competence than the student currently has (e.g., clinical consultation skills and hand hygiene practices) (Hafen *et al.*, 2015).

Achieving authenticity goes beyond the simple inclusion of case material within learning activities. Authenticity encompasses teachers genuinely sharing both their limitations and their expertise, creating engagement and connection with learners that enhance learning outcomes (Kreber and Klampfleitner, 2013). Teachers striving for authenticity in their curricula need to balance the relevance of learning activities with what is practical, sustainable, and achievable given the resources available (see Box 9.2). In taking this pragmatic approach, however, it is important to ensure that the fundamental disciplinary basis is not sacrificed to expediency.

Constructive Alignment

Constructive alignment is the meaningful connection between the desired learning outcomes, learning activities, and assessment of the course (Biggs and Tang, 2007). Central to this in a veterinary degree is the understanding that all three elements need to be authentic and directly relevant to the skills and knowledge required of a graduate veterinarian.

In a constructively aligned course, the learning activities meaningfully illustrate and allow exploration and practice of the desired skills and knowledge (Kurtz, Silverman, and Draper, 2005), enabling students to construct meaning through discovery and actions rather than simply receiving information from the teacher. As Shuell (1986, p. 429) discussed over three decades ago:

"Without taking away from the important role played by the teacher, it is helpful to remember that *what the student does* is actually more important in determining what is learned than what the teacher does."

The role of the teacher in this context is to create the culture, structure, and assessment tasks that stimulate student engagement and learner success. Assessment tasks need to explicitly provide a genuine and accurate evaluation of student achievement of the intended learning outcomes (Taylor, 2009).

The easiest way to create constructive alignment is to honestly to consider and express in the form of a clearly written learning outcome what is reasonably achievable and expected of students at the completion of each course (Taylor, 2009). These course-level learning outcomes are then explicitly linked to program-level outcomes expressed as a statement of desired new graduate attributes (Taylor, 2009). The next step is to review all of the available learning activities that allow students to explore and practice their abilities through learning activities that nurture

Box 9.2: Example of authenticity: Professional skills classes

Main principle illustrated: Authenticity
Secondary principle(s) illustrated: Integration, constructive alignment

Explanation of the activity

Design and philosophy
Professional Skills classes in Year 2 of a four-year veterinary degree are designed to integrate prior learning in fundamental sciences with clinically relevant skills and knowledge. The case material is designed to balance authenticity with the pre-clinical developmental stage of the learners. The class described in this case study builds on prior learning in urogenital anatomy and physiology, and regional anatomy of the abdomen.

Intended learning outcomes
The intended learning outcomes are to apply a working knowledge of topographical and regional anatomy of the caudal abdomen (especially the urogenital tract) to perform bladder palpation, cystocentesis, and exploratory laparotomy in the cat.

Learning activities
The class is designed for small groups, with students working in pairs. It uses feline cadavers to actively engage students in catheterizing the male feline urethra and distending the bladder with saline. This facilitates caudal abdominal palpation and cystocentesis of the bladder using external topographical landmarks. A mock laparotomy is performed by the students following these procedures to allow them to practice surgical skills and revise essential regional anatomy in situ.

Assessment
The Professional Skills course requires active participation and achievement of core skills in all classes for a satisfactory grade to be achieved. The students receive individual feedback from demonstrators and are assisted during the class to ensure that a satisfactory level of competence is achieved. These skills are subsequently tested with a range of other skills in an Objective Structured Clinical Exam (OSCE) at the end of Year 2. Students must successfully complete this OSCE to progress to the third year of the degree.

Vertical and horizontal integration

This learning activity relies on the fundamental knowledge of structure and function and surgical skills classes taught in Year 1. It is horizontally integrated with a Year 2 Principles of Animal Disease course in which the importance of urinary tract diseases across species is explored and the role of urinalysis as a diagnostic test is explained.

Auth: ***　　Align: ***　　Intgr: ***　　Syn: ***　　Cult: ***　　Rel: ***　　Sust: **

the desired knowledge, skills, and attitudes in each area. Offering a range of different learning activities allows students to practice and demonstrate their knowledge in ways that best suit their needs as learners (Ramsden, 2003). Finally, to focus the students on achieving the learning outcome in a way that is meaningful for their future practice, the design and nature of assessment

tasks need to reflect the expectations of a new graduate veterinarian. In contrast to common assessment methods that evaluate lower-level knowledge and disparate skills, assessment of the higher-order learning outcomes expected of new graduates requires students to synthesize and apply their knowledge and skills in practice (Cheek and Lamb, 2010) (see Box 9.3). The consequences of misaligning learning outcomes, learning activities, and assessment tasks are that students may be unable to apply disciplinary

knowledge to practical problem-solving in the workplace, despite potentially attaining good grades throughout the course.

 Box 9.3: Focus on constructive alignment: Learning activities that support modified essay questions

Main principle illustrated: Constructive alignment
Secondary principle(s) illustrated: Integration, synergy

Explanation of the activity

Design and philosophy
This assessment task is designed for a course in Principles of Animal Disease in Year 2 of a four-year program. The course builds on prior learning in the disciplines of microbiology, parasitology, clinical and anatomical pathology, and pharmacology, and integrates these as common clinical syndromes, for example hematuria in dogs, fever in cats, dyspnea in horses, sudden death in cattle. Each syndrome is addressed over eight hours of learning activities spread throughout the week. The intention is to develop students' skills in an investigative approach to case scenarios that allow for effective therapeutic intervention, and to bring each case to a rational resolution that embeds an understanding of ongoing disease management for individuals and populations.

Intended learning outcomes
The intended learning outcomes are to:

- Apply a problem-based approach to investigating disease.
- Demonstrate appropriate knowledge of disease-causing agents and factors to select appropriate diagnostic techniques for the investigation of each case, and be able to interpret the results accurately.
- Recommend suitable strategies for treatment and control of diseases in animals and be able to convey these to a client.

- Demonstrate skills in researching information from a range of sources and presentation of material in a clear and efficient manner using both oral and written communication.
- Work in a team to investigate disease issues.

Learning activities
Each syndrome uses a similar format, illustrated here by the "hot cat" (fever of unknown origin in cats). An interactive "trigger" session probes students to assess the case presentation, pose questions for the owner, make an assessment of likely body systems affected, and discuss approaches to diagnosis that ensure students are mindful of the owner's wishes and limitations. Following this, students are divided into small tutorial groups and assigned new cases of "hot cats" with different presentations. In teams, the students use a custom-made online program (ResourceBuilder©) to "purchase" diagnostic tests sequentially within an enforced budget, knowing that they will be asked both to justify their choices based on evidence and to interpret all findings (normal and abnormal). The program permits the purchase of over 100 tests, from diagnostic imaging to polymerase chain reaction (PCR) to hematology. The learning activities are supported by roving tutors, whose role is not to instruct but to help teams overcome an impasse in their rationalization of the case scenario. Cases are easily changed and updated through a user-friendly interface.

Assessment
Summative assessment involves a modified essay exam based on a clinical scenario. In these exams, the signalment and presentation of the case scenario are provided on the front cover, which

students may read during reading time. The exam booklet is divided into sections through which the student must progress sequentially without turning back. The sections are designed to progressively test the student's capacity to "approach" a case, consider potential diagnoses, and develop a diagnostic plan; "interpret" new information from diagnostic investigation of this case; and "rationalize and communicate" the implications of a specific disease entity and/or its control or treatment. The sequential format of the exam tests a range of skills that would not be possible in an open-framework exam, and it is suitable for paper-based or online formats.

Vertical and horizontal integration

This course is preceded by all anatomy and physiology units, general and anatomical pathology, microbiology, parasitology, pharmacology, and behavior. It is taught concurrently with small animal medicine, therapeutics, and clinical pathology.

Auth: ***	Align: ***	Intgr: ***	Syn: ***	Cult: ***	Rel: ***	Sust: ***

Integration

Being an effective veterinarian requires integration of knowledge, skills, and professional attributes. Therefore, effective teaching of veterinarians requires the integration of theoretical and practical material, and development of professional attributes, to achieve the intended learning outcomes (Baillie, Pierce, and May, 2010). This requires thoughtful sequencing of teaching materials, learning activities, and assessment tasks to ensure that preclinical and paraclinical disciplines are learned in a manner that facilitates their use in clinical decision-making (May and Silva-Fletcher, 2015). This contextualization or integration of preclinical, paraclinical, and clinical learning activities creates authenticity in learning, and is effective in engaging learners in the underlying basis of disease (Krockenberger, Bosward, and Canfield, 2007).

The key to integration that is often overlooked in clinical teaching is the fundamental discipline-specific detail that underpins a deep understanding of diagnostic processes and clinical case management. The analogy of the iceberg is relevant here. While it may be true that the analytical use of the preclinical and paraclinical disciplines in diagnostic reasoning utilizes a relatively small knowledge base, it is increasingly understood that this relies greatly on intuitive thinking that utilizes a much larger body of knowledge (Canfield *et al.*, 2016). Therefore, the exposed tip of the iceberg of clinical knowledge requires the submerged bulk of detailed preclinical and paraclinical knowledge to position and contextualize the clinical knowledge into a useful relevant resource. Integration therefore has two overt levels that potentially require two approaches: the acquisition of contextualized fundamental knowledge; and the advanced integration of specific discipline-based knowledge in authentic problems. The success of the second, more advanced integration relies heavily on the fundamental groundwork of the first approach. Encouraging students to consider overtly how they interact with clinical problems and the investigative approach will allow them to utilize the tools at their discretion to arrive at appropriate conclusions (Canfield and Malik, 2016; Canfield *et al.*, 2016). This applies as much to learning in the laboratory as it does to clinical learning (see Box 9.4).

Box 9.4: How to integrate theoretical and practical material

Main principle illustrated: Integration
Secondary principle(s) illustrated: Constructive alignment, authenticity, sustainability, culture

Explanation of the activity

Design and philosophy
An investigative approach to the diagnosis of disease is built on a conceptual framework that overtly identifies analytical components. This begins with defining the problem through the detection and description of abnormalities; continues with interpretation of the detected abnormalities at the level of the test, organ function, and whole animal; and then uses that interpretation to design further investigative pathways. These approaches are made authentic by utilizing real case scenarios.

Intended learning outcomes

The intended learning outcomes include detection and interpretation of diagnostic data, and integration of knowledge of normal structure and function with pathophysiology and pathology and agents of disease, in order to make a diagnosis and formulate a plan for further investigation, control, or treatment if required.

Learning activities and assessment

The activity is a group-based exercise with online access to real case data. A key feature is the presentation of raw data from diagnostic laboratory tests, mainly hematology, serum biochemistry, gross pathology, cytopathology, and histopathology. Interpreted findings of other diagnostic tests such as imaging are included to provide additional contextual data and support the students in disciplines for which they have not yet had extensive training.

Access to all information is open so the learner may access material in any sequence. A pattern of access to data is suggested through the nature of the assessable outcome, but is not mandated through the presentation of material online. This does not provide workflow authenticity, but allows the learner an exploratory approach to learning, thereby building independent discovery into the process, while influencing them to form a framework that achieves the assessment outcome. The raw data presented requires the student to understand the basic principles of reference intervals and categorization requirements for various data types. This introduces the student to the management of clinical and diagnostic information as data, and managing the interpretation and certainty associated with different data types.

The assignment template provides the framework for learning using a sequential approach to diagnostic interpretation, with increasing levels of certainty as interpreted data is added to the framework. The first step is the translation of clinical data into a clinical problem list and an initial interpretation of body system involvement. This level of interpretation asks the learner to consider the sensitivity and specificity of clinical data in the diagnosis of disease. The next step involves the learner making a prediction as to the likely pathological process that would result in the dysfunction manifested in the clinical abnormality, followed by interpreting diagnostic data to establish evidence that builds a diagnosis. The assignment template builds toward a morphological diagnosis, suggests a list of likely specific diseases, and then offers an investigative pathway to achieve a specific disease diagnosis.

Learners are asked to engage in independent research into the diagnostic differentials and to present information about those diseases. Part of this research asks the learner to critically examine the strength of the clinical and diagnostic data in the case scenario against the published literature. This introduces the learner to concepts of certainty and the reliance on interpretation of the type of data on which it is built. The learner is asked to outline an investigative approach that would increase the certainty of diagnosis. The final step is to prognosticate and formulate simple conceptual therapeutic or preventive interventions, based on the published literature.

The process is designed to build clinical decision-making skills, with an emphasis on the interpretation of descriptive and numerical pathology data.

Vertical and horizontal integration

This activity concentrates on pathology and pathophysiology, requiring a detailed understanding of normal structure and function. These are the disciplines of morphology (gross anatomy, microscopic anatomy), function (physiology), and general pathology (pathological processes). The approach builds toward designing therapeutic interventions in clinical medicine and surgery, which are elucidated later in the degree.

Auth: ***	Align: ***	Intgr: ***	Syn: ***	Cult: ***	Rel: ***	Sust: ***

Source: Krockenberger, Bosward, and Canfield, 2007.

Synergy

Synergy in teaching is a multifaceted concept. Synergy is broadly defined as the interaction between elements or contributions that when combined produce a total effect that is greater than the sum of the individual parts, and therefore enhance the result. Synergy in teaching can be created in many ways if both teachers and students adopt an open-minded framework for their own learning and for the format and focus of learning activities. Weimer (2014) aptly describes the essential element of part of this synergy occurring when teachers are "thinking, observing and focusing" on how learning is occurring for the student and constantly considering what approaches are best, given the content and desired learning outcomes. This encourages flexibility, dynamism, and reflective practice in teaching (Kurtz, Silverman, and Draper, 2005; Brookfield, 1995). Synergies can be enhanced by the use of various learning resources and activities appropriate to the content, which complement and improve students' capture of key elements. This allows for variation in students' learning preferences (Ramsden, 2003).

A second element of synergy that Weimer (2014) describes is that which occurs when students become focused on "what they are learning" and "how they are learning it." Synergies can occur when students recognize and embrace the learning that they gain from the explanations of classmates as well as the experience of teachers (Khosa, Volet, and Bolton, 2010). The learning environment is enriched when teachers are also open to contributions and comments from students whose past experiences or novice interpretations can provide valuable insights that add to the learning of teachers and students. These synergies allow for the development of a learning culture that is open and builds respect and positive relationships among teachers and students. Synergies in learning can also be created through the integration of disciplines and team teaching that model for the student collegial discourse and appreciating the perspectives and knowledge of others.

In the case study in Box 9.5, and as proposed by Canfield and colleagues (2016, p. 40–41), a blend of "intuitive reasoning" as well as the "analytical, problem-oriented, forward reasoning approach" permits synergies between the knowledge and understanding of the "novice" and the "expert." It gives credence to the value of each and supports a clinical approach that does not rely entirely on either "gut instinct" or "objective data."

Box 9.5: Where's the evidence that synergy enhances learning outcomes: "Flipped" classrooms and student designed leaning tool

Main principle illustrated: Synergy
Secondary principle(s) illustrated: Integration, constructive alignment, relationships, culture

Explanation of the activity

Design and philosophy
An investigative approach to veterinary microbiology is taught in Year 2 of a four-year degree program using a flipped classroom technique. This creates synergies between the online learning activities used in class preparation and the active discussion of case studies that occurs during face-to-face teaching. Examples of previous students' assignments in the form of visual learning tools are incorporated into the discussion. Through the eyes of their peers, the use of the visual learning tool assignment can provide a synergistic learning activity to enhance the case discussion. It also builds the culture of respect in the classroom by illustrating the inherent value that the learners themselves can bring. Equally, synergy is created by blending different disciplines, learning resource formats, and reflection on how graduates best use information regarding pathogens in their day-to-day practice, without minimizing the importance of paraclinical knowledge.

Intended learning outcomes
The overarching intended learning outcomes are to use clinical cases and research studies to explore the unique features of highlighted infectious agents and their role in the development of animal disease; critically analyze the strategies used for their diagnosis, treatment, and control; and encourage an approach to investigating problems that acknowledges an evidence-based approach and intuitive reasoning.

Learning activities
The key principles and background information regarding the agent of disease (e.g., canine parvovirus, CPV) are introduced through a seven-minute interactive PowerPoint™ presentation with audio commentary available online. In the classroom, case studies are presented and students are asked in an interactive discussion to consider how the clinical signs have developed. Integration of information relevant to the case from the online background video is sequentially embedded through these discussions. As the case progresses with more information presented, students are asked to explain how their understanding of the pathogenesis of disease, diagnosis, and control fits the case information, and the advice they would give to owners. This

illustrates the application of knowledge and the value of intuitive reasoning as well as an analytical problem-oriented approach. To complement the activity, during class discussions an assignment video produced by students in current or previous years is shown, which illustrates and brings to life the virus or the disease it causes.

Assessment
Examinations in this course are entirely case based, where the student's intellectual engagement in learning activities and independent learning is rewarded by their ability to interpret case data using their knowledge of the organism. An assignment in this course in which students develop a visual learning tool

for their peers that brings to life the organism and/or the disease it creates is embedded back into the learning activities of their cohort and subsequent ones.

Vertical and horizontal integration

This subject is preceded by all anatomy and physiology units, and is taught concurrently with other pathobiology disciplines such as general and anatomical pathology, parasitology, pharmacology, and clinical pathology. It precedes but aligns vertically with the practice units (e.g., small animal practice, equine practice, etc.).

Auth: ***   Align: ***   Intgr: ***   Syn: ***   Cult: ***   Rel: ***   Sust: ***

Culture

It is challenging to create and sustain a ubiquitous culture of high-quality teaching and learning. Creation of this culture rests on the principles of lifelong learning for staff and students, together with critical reflection and evidence-based outcomes assessment. For effective lifelong learning and reflective practice, individuals need to analyze the strengths and gaps in their current performance; set Specific, Measurable, Action-oriented, Realistic, and Time-oriented (SMART) goals for improvement; and seek feedback from a range of perspectives on whether these goals have been achieved (Goleman, Boyatzis, and McKee, 2002). These perspectives are gained from reviewing published literature and examples of best practice; seeking 360° feedback on performance from peers, students, supervisors, and experienced colleagues; and undertaking critical self-reflection on performance (Brookfield, 1995).

A culture of student-centered learning and constructive alignment is vital to guide the

effective selection and implementation of teaching methods appropriate for particular content (Prosser and Trigwell, 1999; Biggs and Tang, 2007). This includes a culture of physical and emotional safety for experiential learning activities, coupled with gradual challenge and extension of individuals' confidence and competence (Kurtz, Silverman, and Draper, 2005). A culture of innovation and a willingness to embrace change enable individuals and institutions to make rapid progress. To support this, learning spaces and technology must be consistently reviewed and upgraded to support a positive and effective student learning experience (Ellis and Goodyear, 2010). Implementation of the proposed changes must be tempered by evaluation of their costs and benefits to the full range of stakeholders. In most instances compromises are needed to ensure that changes are sustainable, creating situations of "practical" best practice, or best practice tempered by context (see Box 9.6).

Box 9.6: Reflections on building a positive culture for student learning: simulated clinical consultations

Main principle illustrated: Culture
Secondary principle(s) illustrated: Relationships, constructive alignment, integration

Explanation of the activity

Design and philosophy
Simulated clinical consulation skills classes are built on the philosophies that effective communication consists of learnable skills, and that lifelong improvement is possible through focused, self-reflective practice. This is aided by critical review of video-recorded performances based on ongoing, constructive feedback from self, peers, and teachers (Kurtz, Silverman, and Draper, 2005). The theoretical framework used for development and analysis of students' consultation skills is the Calgary Cambridge Model (Kurtz, Silverman, and Draper, 2005) modified for the veterinary context (Radford *et al.*, 2006). This case study describes simulated Clinical Consultation Skills classes in Year 1 of a four-year degree program.

Intended learning outcomes
The intended learning outcomes are focused on the skills required to conduct an effective consultation, receive constructive feedback on performance, and effectively critique others' consultations.

Learning activities
Students are allocated to small groups with stable membership throughout the six-week clinical consultation skills course. This helps to create an environment of trust and emotional safety for the experiential learning activities involved. Each group has a trained staff facilitator who guides the group in attempting the cases and providing feedback on each other's performance. Supporting resources are provided for the consultation skills being taught and the basic veterinary information for the case, with an expectation that

students will use these independently to prepare for each case. Consultation topics chosen are relatively simple so that the students can address them early in their degree.

Students set SMART goals for their performance in each simulated consultation they undertake. This enables individuals to create an independent, personalized learning program within the overall requirements of the course. The student receives verbal and written constructive feedback from their peers and the facilitator on their performance after each consultation. Each consultation is also video-recorded, and the video uploaded to the university's online learning system for central storage and access. The students review their video after class and provide a brief critique of the strengths and gaps in their performance at the start of the following class. This process of constructive feedback, critical review, and reflection forms the foundation for the SMART goals that they set for their next consultation.

In the first four classes students develop their consultation skills by working with their peers as simulated clients. In the fifth class actors are used to extend and enhance the students' learning experience. The final class involves a detailed critique by each student of their performance with the actor. Each student shows their small group short vignettes from their consultation to highlight strengths and gaps in their performance based on the feedback they received, together with any differences in the perspective on their consultation given by the client. Finally, they are asked to list strategies for how they can use their strengths to improve their clinical communication in future, and to give a brief demonstration of one of these strategies to the group.

Assessment
Formative assessment is provided throughout the classes by the constructive feedback from the student, peers, actor, and facilitator, together

with review of the video-recorded consultation. After each class the facilitator evaluates whether the student achieved each of the key consultation and constructive feedback skills allocated for the classes, grading each as satisfactory/unsatisfactory. Grades are uploaded to the university's online system for the students to reflect on and review before the next class. Grades received in Classes 1–4 are formative, while grades received in Class 5 (consultation skills) and Class 6 (constructive feedback skills) are summative. Students are given the opportunity to perform further consultations if their skills are judged inadequate in summative assessment.

Vertical and horizontal integration

The small-group practical classes are preceded by an introductory large-group workshop scheduled in a veterinary professional practice foundational unit at the start of the degree program. Clinical consultation skills classes in Year 2 build on those in Year 1 by incorporating a greater range of scenarios and more challenging contexts, as well as integrating medical veterinary content taught previously or contemporaneously in other parts of the Year 2 curriculum. In Years 3 and 4 the skills will be applied to the various clinical and workplace contexts that students will face after graduation.

| Auth: ** | Align: *** | Intgr: *** | Syn: ** | Cult: *** | Rel: *** | Sust: ** |

Relationships

Teaching is a relational activity. The quality of the relationships between teachers and learners, and among groups of teachers and learners, is instrumental to the success of learning. Effective relationships are based on trust, respect, enjoyment, and mutual commitment to desired outcomes. For teachers this encompasses being authentic, creating an enjoyable learning environment, and providing constructive feedback that respectfully challenges learners to help them grow as junior colleagues in the profession (Kreber and Klampfleitner, 2013). It also involves ensuring that learners are held accountable for their progress and performance in a way that reflects the expectations of the workplace. Teachers need to create a context for learning where learners care for others, feel supported in respectfully challenging others' perspectives, and hold each other accountable for the achievement of desired learning outcomes. In a strong and constructive learner–teacher relationship, learners feel empowered to provide feedback to

teachers on their performance in an environment of mutual empathy and commitment to shared learning goals.

Ultimately, the characteristics of effective relationships in teaching are based on the competencies of emotional intelligence (Goleman, Boyatzis, and McKee, 2002):

- *Self-awareness*: knowing the aspects of your character likely to influence your interactions with others; understanding your values, strengths, limitations, emotions, and common responses to situations that you encounter; and having both confidence in and a sense of humor about your capabilities.
- *Self-management*: the ability to manage your emotions and impulses in ways that foster successful interpersonal interactions, together with setting effective and motivational goals for self-improvement and adapting to changing circumstances.
- *Social awareness*: the ability to empathize with and respond to others' needs and emotions in the context of social networks and

the policies of the organization in which you work.

- *Relationship management*: the ability to inspire, influence, work with, and develop other people while managing conflict. It incorporates the skills of inspirational leadership, influence, developing others,

communication, catalyzing change, conflict management, building bonds, and teamwork.

Encouraging learners and teachers to develop these capabilities improves the quality of relationships not only in the classroom, but also throughout professional life (see Box 9.7).

 Box 9.7: Quick tips for group assessment - case study in veterinary professional practice

Main principle illustrated: Relationships
Secondary principle(s) illustrated: Culture, sustainability, constructive alignment, synergy

Explanation of the activity

Design and philosophy
This assessment task is built on the philosophies that student learning outcomes are enhanced when students are given choice in what they learn, that emotional intelligence competencies need to be put into action to be developed, and that peer and self-assessment of performance is valued as well as faculty assessment in evaluating and providing feedback on outcomes.

Intended learning outcomes
The intended learning outcomes are in-depth knowledge of professional practice principles in an area of choice, the development of emotional intelligence competencies required for effective relationships and teamwork, and the capacity to provide feedback accurately and constructively on other people's performance.

Learning activities
Students form self-chosen groups of five to six members and create a case study that critically analyzes a veterinary workplace situation using theoretical principles of professional practice. Each group is free to decide which area of professional practice they wish to focus on in their presentation. Students are provided with

the marking criteria for the task and given an opportunity to apply these in evaluating a prior presentation by the teacher. This provides an opportunity to give the class feedback on their understanding of the grading standards, the marking criteria, and their application prior to use in peer assessment. It also has the dual benefit of gathering feedback on the teacher's presentation that can be used in reflective practice by the teacher, modeling a joint commitment to learning, trust, vulnerability, mutual respect, and how to effectively receive constructive feedback.

Students are asked to provide feedback to each group member on the extent of emotional intelligence competencies demonstrated during completion of the assessment task, as well as the effectiveness of the team. Self-assessment spans all core competencies of emotional intelligence, while peer assessment focuses on those of relationship management only.

Assessment
The case study is a 10-minute presentation involving all group members, followed by 2 minutes for questions. Formative assessment and feedback on each group's presentation idea are provided halfway through the course. Of each group's final mark for the presentation, 50% is determined by the peer assessments they received from the other groups in the audience, while the remaining 50% is by staff assessment. One student group is tasked with providing detailed constructive feedback on the presenting team's performance.

The final mark and detailed feedback are shared with each presenting team immediately after assessment.

To encourage honest, accurate, and helpful feedback on the development of emotional intelligence competencies, students are not graded on the extent to which they and their peers evaluated whether they demonstrated emotional intelligence competencies during completion of the task. Instead, a small percentage of the final grade for the course is attributed to simple completion of this task.

Vertical and horizontal integration

The emotional intelligence competencies and presentation skills evaluated in this assessment are applicable to other courses taught in the same semester. Future plans include incorporation of peer and self-feedback on emotional intelligence competencies using the same rubric halfway through preparation for the assessment task, and in a subsequent year of the course. This will provide further feedback to individuals on their progress in emotional intelligence, effective relationships, and teamwork.

Auth: ***   Align: ***   Intgr: **   Syn: **   Cult: ***   Rel: ***   Sust: ***

Sustainability

Sustainability refers to the likely longevity of a learning activity after it has been implemented in the curriculum. This is influenced by a number of teacher and learner factors. The most limiting resource in most veterinary schools is staffing, with the addition of the school's teaching and learning culture and other potential local limitations. Building curricula and learning activities with a focus on constructive alignment and integration represents a high workload at first, initially implemented in an intensive teaching effort requiring increased resourcing. The ultimate success of such tools depends on both staff and institutional commitment to continuing to support the initiative (Lam, 2005).

Because staffing is often the most limiting factor, the challenge with sustainability is maintaining learner engagement while minimizing workload impact on faculty staff and budget. A range of strategies can be employed to achieve this, including group and peer learning environments, technological solutions, and suitably

supported problem-based learning, resulting in a blended learning approach (Krockenberger, Bosward, and Canfield, 2007; Powell and Steel, 2003) (see Box 9.8). In most modern veterinary schools, sustainability will include at least some aspect of web-based delivery. When skillfully done, this is usually the easiest way to promote the sustainability of a teaching tool, but the capacity to support this at both a school and institution level, including culturally, needs to be carefully considered (Ellis and Goodyear, 2010).

Sustainability is often primarily considered from a teaching and resourcing perspective, but the learner perspective cannot be ignored. To achieve sustainability from a learner perspective, engagement is key (Ramsden, 2003). The critical drivers of learner engagement – constructive alignment, authenticity, and integration – will be the biggest determinants of overall sustainability. The result of encouraging learners to consider how they learn will also be, if not enhanced engagement, then at least the learner's consciousness of the framework of the knowledge they are creating and how they can access it (Canfield and Malik, 2016).

Box 9.8: Example of creating sustainable web-delivered learning resources -Virtual Microscopy and Resource Builder

Main principle illustrated: Sustainability
Secondary principle(s) illustrated: Constructive alignment, authenticity, integration, culture

Explanation of the activity

Design and philosophy
Microscopic structural changes are important in the pathogenesis of disease. Recognizing microscopic change and relating it to gross structural abnormalities and dysfunction is a difficult process for novices, requiring time and extensive support from experts. Contextualization into real case scenarios is aimed at enhancing relevance and therefore engagement by the learner.

The Sydney School of Veterinary Science has developed a web delivery platform called ResourceBuilder that allows teachers easily to enter case data to create multiple different types of learning tools. Text, images, and laboratory data are readily integrated into the system. This includes integration of digital whole-slide scans (virtual microscopy) based on case histopathological and cytological slides. Students can obtain all case data at any time they are able to access the Internet with a standard bandwidth. No specialized programs are required beyond an Internet browser. The development of web-based resources involves a combination of the development of task-specific platforms and collaboration with or purchase of "off-the-shelf" solutions. In this case, our veterinary school developed ResourceBuilder and purchased a virtual microscopy software solution to integrate and extend its capability.

For graduates, the tasks described in this case study are performed utilizing microscopes in clinics as well as via understanding reports from specialist pathologists. The balance between sustainability and constructive alignment requires a blending of technologies.

Underpinning this approach are parallel laboratory classes including the use of microscopes for examination of material to be compared with that available for review on virtual microscopy afterward.

Intended learning outcomes
The intended learning outcomes from these activities are the development of a framework for the detection and interpretation of structural and functional abnormalities from case diagnostic data; and the description, detection, and interpretation of gross pathology, histopathology, clinical pathology, microbiology, and parasitology data in clinical case scenarios.

Learning activities and assessment
There are four major groups that build cases for learners from real case material:

- *Learners* engaging with the paraclinical disciplines for the first time (Years 2 and 3 of a five-year curriculum). Case material presented for examination through the university's Veterinary Pathology Diagnostic Service is presented to small groups of students (three students per group) for examination. As students compile a report on the case they enter the data into ResourceBuilder, including their completed case report. This forms a sizable proportion of their summative assessment. During the marking process, the teacher moderates the resource, allowing potential use for further cohorts in ResourceBuilder. The case can be utilized in learning activities for further cohorts, either supported by the initial student case report or without it.
- *Final-year veterinary students*. Case material gathered by final-year students on their paraclinical rotations is entered into ResourceBuilder with supporting case reports and referencing. This forms part of their case report and communication assessment tasks

in the final year. The expert supports the development of the resource by regular feedback during the diagnostic process and then moderates its content, approach, and interpretation before adding it to the learning resource bank.

- *Discipline residents.* Case material gathered by residents is entered into ResourceBuilder with the supporting case report and referencing. This cohort requires less formal feedback in the development of case material.
- *Faculty.* All faculty teaching the paraclinical disciplines are involved in diagnostic services and utilize case material to create learning resources. This allows for specific targeting of curricular deficiencies with case material. This cohort is able to provide the most strategic

development of learning resources within the overall curriculum.

Vertical and horizontal integration

The activity facilitates peer learning between cohorts to provide vertical integration (final-year interns creating resources for Year 2 and Year 3 students and cohorts to create learning resources for subsequent cohorts at the same stage of development). Vertical integration is also encouraged by the interpretation of paraclinical data activities, building on preclinical knowledge in the context of clinical cases. Horizontal integration is encouraged through the inclusion of data from multiple paraclinical disciplines in the clinical scenario assessment.

| Auth: *** | Align: *** | Intgr: *** | Syn: *** | Cult: ** | Rel: ** | Sust: *** |

Applying the Principles

In this chapter we have presented seven interrelated, core principles for effective teaching in classrooms and laboratories. These principles form a useful framework for encouraging reflective practice by educators seeking to improve their teaching. Explicitly considering each of these principles in turn when designing and evaluating the success of individual learning activities and course curricula overall can be used to create high-quality learning and teaching experiences.

We have provided an explanation of each core principle, followed by an example of how the principle has been implemented in our hands. We have explicitly linked each case study to one or more secondary principles that it also clearly illustrates. A star rating indicates the extent to which the case study aligns with each of the seven core principles. This system links to the criteria for reflective practice when designing learning activities that were

outlined in Table 9.1. It is intended to make explicit the process of reflective practice that we have undertaken in designing these learning activities and assessments. The evaluation system has been designed to illustrate that no learning activity or curriculum is perfect, that high-quality learning outcomes can be achieved by emphasizing and integrating particular principles in curricula implementation while broadly upholding others, and that structured reflective practice is essential in the evolution of effective learning activities and curricula.

While a particular activity or assessment is likely to be rated highly (three stars) in one or more core principles presented in this chapter, it may not rank highly on all, but it should be strongly aligned with at least three of the principles presented. If the learning activity or assessment demonstrates strong alignment with only one or two principles and the rest are ranked as developing (two stars) or below, alignment with these remaining principles should be critically considered. After the activity or assessment has been completed, the same principles can be used to evaluate its effectiveness and identify ongoing areas for improvement in the cycle of lifelong learning and reflective practice. A consistent focus on critical reflective practice to create an upward spiral of teaching and learning quality will benefit not only individual learners and teachers, but ultimately the overall veterinary profession.

References

Baillie, S., Pierce, S.E., and May, S.A. (2010) Fostering integrated learning and clinical professionalism using contextualised simulation in a small-group role-play. *Journal of Veterinary Medical Education*, **37** (**3**), 248–253.

Barrows, H., and Tamblyn, R. (1980) *Problem-Based Learning: An Approach to Medical Education*, Springer, New York.

Biggs, J., and Tang, C. (2007) *Teaching for Quality Learning at University*, 3rd edn, McGraw-Hill/Society for Research into Higher Education/Open University Press, Maidenhead.

Boud, D., and Falchikov, N. (2006) Aligning assessment with long-term learning. *Assessment and Evaluation in Higher Education*, **31** (**4**), 399–413.

Brookfield, S. (1995) *Becoming a Critically Reflective Teacher*, Jossey-Bass, San Francisco, CA.

Canfield, P.J., and Malik, R. (2016) Think about how you think about cases. *Journal of Feline Medicine and Surgery*, **18** (**1**), 4–6.

Canfield, P.J., Whitehead, M.L., Johnson, R., et al. (2016) Case-based clinical reasoning in feline medicine: 1: Intuitive and analytical systems. *Journal of Feline Medicine and Surgery*, **18** (**1**), 35–45.

Cheek, B., and Lamb, E. (2010) *The Miller Pyramid and Prism*. http://www.gp-training.net/training/educational_theory/adult_learning/miller.htm (accessed January 27, 2016).

Ellis, R.A., and Goodyear, P. (2010) *Students' Experiences of e-Learning in Higher Education: The Ecology of Sustainable Innovation*, Routledge, New York.

Goleman, D., Boyatzis, R., and McKee, A. (2002) *Primal Leadership: Realizing the Power of Emotional Intelligence*, Harvard Business School Press, Boston, MA.

Hafen, M., Jr.,, Drake, A.A., Rush, B.R., and Sibley, D.S. (2015) Engaging students: Using video clips of authentic client interactions in pre-clinical veterinary medical education. *Journal of Veterinary Medical Education*, **42** (**3**), 252–258.

Khosa, D.K., Volet, S.E., and Bolton, J.R. (2010) An instructional intervention to encourage effective deep collaborative learning in undergraduate veterinary students. *Journal of Veterinary Medical Education*, **37** (**4**), 369–376.

Kreber, C., and Klampfleitner, M. (2013) 'Lecturers' and students 'conceptions of authenticity in teaching and actual teacher actions and attributes students perceive as helpful.' *Higher Education*, **66** (**4**), 463–487.

Krockenberger, M., Bosward, K., and Canfield, P. (2007) Integrated Case-based Applied Pathology (ICAP): A diagnostic-approach model for the learning and teaching of veterinary pathology. *Journal of Veterinary Medical Education*, **34** (**4**), 396–408.

Kurtz, S.M., Silverman, J., and Draper, J. (2005) *Teaching and Learning Communication Skills in Medicine*, 2nd edn, Radcliffe Medical Press, Abingdon.

Lam, A. (2005) Organizational innovation, in *The Oxford Handbook of Innovation* (eds J. Fagerberg, D.C. Mowery, and R.R. Nelson), Oxford University Press, Oxford, pp. 115–147.

May, S.A., and Silva-Fletcher, A. (2015) Scaffolded active learning: Nine pedagogical principles for building a modern veterinary curriculum. *Journal of Veterinary Medical Education*, **42** (**4**), 332–339.

Powell, V., and Steel, C. (2003) Search for the woolly mammoth: A case study in inquiry-based learning. *Journal of Veterinary Medical Education*, **30** (**3**), 227–230.

Prosser, M., and Trigwell, K. (1999) *Understanding Learning and Teaching: The Experience in Higher Education*, SRHE/Open University Press, Buckingham.

Radford, A., Stockley, P., Silverman, J., *et al.* (2006) Development, teaching and evaluation of a consultation structure model for use in veterinary education. *Journal of Veterinary Medical Education*, **33** (**1**), 38–44.

Ramsden, P. (2003) *Learning to Teach in Higher Education*, 2nd edn, Routledge Falmer, London.

Shuell, T.J. (1986) Cognitive conception of learning. *Review of Educational Research*, **56** (**4**), 411–436.

Taylor, R. (2009) Defining, constructing and assessing learning outcomes. *Revue Scientifique et Technique (International Office of Epizootics)*, **28** (**2**), 779–788.

Weimer, M. (2014) The teaching-learning synergy. Faculty Focus. http://www.facultyfocus.com/articles/teaching-professor-blog/teaching-learning-synergy/ (accessed January 27, 2016).

10

Learning and Teaching in Clinical Skills Laboratories

Marc Dilly[1] and Sarah Baillie[2]

[1] *scil Animal Care Company, Germany*
[2] *School of Veterinary Medicine, University of Bristol, UK*

 ### Box 10.1: Key messages

- Clinical skills laboratories provide a dedicated area where students can practice using a range of models and simulators.
- Having an academic lead for clinical skills and a laboratory manager is highly recommended.
- The clinical skills program should be embedded in the curriculum.
- Feedback on learning should be an integral part of teaching in a clinical skills laboratory.
- Supporting learning resources (instruction manuals, videos, etc.) should be provided for students to use during taught classes and for self-directed learning.
- Instructor training ("train the trainer") is helpful for all involved in delivering teaching (faculty, practitioners, technicians, and students).
- Clinical skills laboratories are an ideal venue in which to run assessments such as objective structured clinical examinations (OSCEs).

Introduction

There has been rapid growth in the use of clinical skills laboratories in medicine since the 1970s, with their role now well established in undergraduate and postgraduate training. Other names for such a facility include clinical skills center, simulation center, clinical simulation laboratory, and skills lab. Clinical skills laboratories are used to train students in specific practical, clinical, and procedural skills (sometimes referred to as psychomotor skills), using models and simulators with the aims of increasing competence and confidence, improving patient safety, reducing technical errors, and complementing bedside teaching. The facility provides a safe, relatively stress-free environment in which learners can practice repeatedly. Compared to the sometimes variable opportunities in the hospital setting, it provides greater standardization and more structured feedback. There is an increasing body of evidence supporting the effectiveness of models used in clinical skills laboratories and the benefits for trainees' skill development (Akaike *et al.*, 2012). Ongoing initiatives in simulation-based training (McGaghie *et al.*, 2010) draw from advances in other areas, such as aviation, and increasingly

Veterinary Medical Education: A Practical Guide, First Edition. Edited by Jennifer L. Hodgson and Jacquelyn M. Pelzer.
© 2017 John Wiley & Sons, Inc. Published 2017 by John Wiley & Sons, Inc.

incorporate additional skills such as teamwork, decision-making, leadership, and situational awareness.

Veterinary education is following medicine's lead and clinical skills laboratories are becoming more commonplace in recognition of the potential benefits in preparing students for the modern workplace (Jaarsma *et al.*, 2008). The acquisition of clinical skills is a key aim of veterinary education in order to achieve the competencies defined by accrediting bodies and required of new graduates. However, there is a risk that some students will complete their studies armed with the prerequisite knowledge, but lacking in some essential practical and clinical skills (Remmen, 1998). The reasons relate to a number of challenges encountered when learning and teaching clinical skills. For instance, the clinical environment (during clinical rotations or extramural studies) can be variable for the student and challenging for the teacher (Remmen *et al.*, 1999). It is important for students to gain experience in real-life situations and have access to clinical cases, but at times the clinician has to prioritize the animal's safety and the needs of the client. Additionally, when students are learning on a live animal some feel nervous and anxious, especially the first time, and are mindful that mistakes may have serious consequences. Other factors that may limit opportunities for practice include larger cohorts, competing demands on faculty budgets, difficulties sourcing cadavers, and the need to consider the welfare and ethical implications around the use of live animals in education (de Boo and Knight, 2005). Clinical skills laboratories can address many of these challenges and provide training in simple practical skills, more complex clinical and procedural skills, and communication skills, as well as being a suitable venue for assessments such as objective structured clinical examinations (OSCEs). Unlike workplace-based education (e.g., clinical rotations), students can practice without pressure, stress, or anxiety about harming animals, while learning new skills or consolidating and refining existing skills (Langebaek *et al.*, 2012).

Clinical skills laboratories house a variety of models, part-task trainers, and simulators, which promote the development of competencies while supporting the principles of reduction, replacement, and refinement (the 3Rs) of the use of animals in education. Teaching in the clinical skills laboratory provides useful preparation for clinical training, but it is important to note that learning on models is meant to be a supplement, not a complete replacement for animals. However, there seems little doubt that the amount of veterinary training using models in such laboratories will continue to grow, with associated benefits for student learning and animal welfare.

Students have opportunities to learn a range of skills as well as being able to target their practice of specific techniques in a timely manner. Staffing is crucial and should include enough instructors, who may be faculty, practitioners, technicians, and/or students (peer-assisted learning). A manager for the laboratory, and its associated equipment and facilities, will ensure efficient organization and administration and oversight of the budget. Having an academic lead is highly recommended, and they should have responsibility for the design, promotion, and coordination of the clinical skills program and quality assurance of teaching and assessment.

At veterinary colleges with existing laboratories, the clinical skills program is usually closely linked to the curriculum and preferably has specific practical classes embedded in the formal timetable. Teaching and learning of practical and clinical skills should run throughout the period of study (a longitudinal design), with competencies building year on year and with the aim that graduates are able to provide safe and effective entry-level care. Additionally, using the clinical skills laboratory as an assessment center not only extends its utilization, but also provides outcomes assessment data. It is worthwhile considering having an open access policy, with a "drop-in" area where students can repeat skills in their own time and at their individual pace (Dilly *et al.*, 2014). Another benefit of having a clinical skills laboratory and providing as much access as possible is to decrease students' anxiety prior to their first "hands-on" experience with live animals or before practical assessments and exams.

There are recognized challenges in teaching and learning clinical skills. As a result, an increasing number of veterinary colleges are opening clinical skills laboratories and developing clinical skills programs. In the following sections, further points will be discussed relating to developing clinical competencies, designing and equipping the laboratory, and considerations for the teaching, learning, and assessment of clinical skills.

Developing Clinical Competencies: From Basic Skills to Complex Procedures

The types of skills that can be taught, learned, and assessed range from simple basic skills (e.g., knot tying) to more "complex" procedures (e.g., surgeries). The facility is sometimes also used for teaching communication skills (e.g., history taking) in mock consulting rooms with role players (see Part Six, Chapter 23: Communication).

Early and repeated opportunities to practice a variety of skills in the laboratory will support and enhance the development of competencies (Lynagh, Burton, and Sanson-Fisher, 2007). Most competencies are defined by accrediting bodies and organizations and encompass the spectrum of skills, knowledge, and attitudes expected of a newly graduated veterinarian. These lists tend to be overarching rather than providing details of all skills or exact levels of competence to be achieved. Nevertheless, a list of competencies (from the relevant regulatory body) can be used to define learning outcomes for the clinical skills program, and to identify and map skills that can be taught and assessed in the clinical skills laboratory. It is also important to align teaching in the clinical skills laboratory with other learning opportunities within the curriculum, ensuring that these complement each other while building

progressively year on year, thereby enabling students to develop a skill set that ultimately prepares them for the needs and demands of veterinary practice. The approach to teaching clinical skills should include opportunities for feedback, to enable students to reflect on their performance and identify areas needing further improvement. The clinical skills laboratory provides an environment where students can practice repeatedly and develop proficiency while applying knowledge, but it is not somewhere just to gain knowledge or study facts – it is crucially about hands-on "doing" skills, not only "knowing how."

In medical education the term clinical skill is used to embrace three aspects of teaching, learning, and assessment: knowledge, procedural steps, and clinical reasoning (Michels, Evans, and Blok, 2012). In the context of a clinical skills laboratory, the focus is primarily on the psychomotor (procedural) component. A skill can be defined as the learned or possessed ability to perform a task, and represents a set of coordinated movements required to perform part or all of a clinical, practical, or procedural task. Clinical skills training can be seen as a continuum from learning basic tasks or steps to performing complex procedures; it is also helpful to classify the different skills in relation to their difficulty and stage of learning with reference to the clinical skills program and overall curriculum. There are often logical ways to divide complex procedural skills into simple steps performed on basic models, for instance part-task trainers (Low-Beer *et al.*, 2011), before learning the more complete or complex procedure using for example high-fidelity simulators or cadavers. The more complex the skill or procedure, the more likely students are to be overwhelmed with the situation, and therefore there are benefits if the component skills or "building blocks" are the initial focus of training. With the acquisition, maintenance, and refinement of skills the student becomes an advanced learner, thus teaching and learning (as well as assessment) may place the skill into a clinical context. In addition, the specific skill and skill acquisition depend increasingly on more advanced underlying

Table 10.1 Examples of skills that can be taught, learned, and assessed in a clinical skills laboratory.

Animal handling and husbandry	Basic clinical skills	Clinical, procedural, and other skills
Apply a halter or head collar	Surgical preparation, e.g., gloving	Perform basic surgeries
Apply a muzzle	Basic surgical skills, e.g., knot tying	Anesthesia techniques
Collect a milk sample	Clinical examination	Fluid therapy
Bandaging	Venipuncture	Diagnostic imaging
Hand wash	Injection techniques	Emergency procedures
Basic nursing techniques	Laboratory techniques, e.g., PCV (packed cell volume)	Communication skills

knowledge and other professional skills such as communication and teamwork (Kinnison, May, and Guile, 2014). Therefore, it is helpful to consider the learner's stage and what skill should be taught in the clinical skills laboratory and/or during work-based learning opportunities, such as extramural studies or rotations and in the teaching hospital, and how these complement each other. Examples of the types of skills that may be taught, learned, and assessed in a clinical skills laboratory are given in Table 10.1.

Designing a Clinical Skills Laboratory

When building a clinical skills laboratory, local physical constraints and financial resources are major factors, but the decisions should still focus on optimizing teaching and learning. The clinical skills laboratory should be designed to support the types of teaching required – that is, hands on, small group – and be easily adaptable for different classes and for use in assessments, such as an OSCE circuit. In addition, the provision of a drop-in area, which may be open access or bookable (sign-in), is beneficial for self-directed learning and provides students with opportunities for repeated practice and to revisit the laboratory when needing to refresh or perfect skills in preparation for a clinical rotation, work placement, or assessment. Suggestions for setting up a clinical skills laboratory are summarized in Box 10.2.

Veterinary clinical skills laboratories have been set up in a variety of ways, sometimes as a bespoke new center or by refurbishing existing buildings, for example an old operating

Box 10.2: Quick tip – useful areas and rooms in a clinical skills laboratory

- Reception and sign-in area
- Large teaching (and assessment) area (with room dividers/screens)
- Designated drop-in/open-access area
- Mock operating theater (including prep area with sinks)
- Multiple single rooms (small-group teaching)
- Consulting rooms
- Locker rooms
- Storage rooms (often overlooked!) with shelves and enough space for boxes of equipment, replacements, models, and simulators
- Prep room (to prepare for practical classes, make and repair models)
- Office (staff, manager)

theater, laboratory, or practice, and they may be included within a learning complex, the clinic, or a surgical teaching area. The laboratory may be in one building or more spread out and may or may not be linked to other teaching areas. There are several good reasons for having one center known as the clinical skills laboratory, as it helps signpost the facility to students and faculty, and there are efficiencies in staffing and managing the space. Ideally, when deciding on the location it should be in close proximity to other areas used by students. For example, students on clinical rotations are more likely to drop in and practice if the facility is adjacent to the teaching hospital, although that may not be the best location for students in lower years for learning more basic animal handling skills. In some instances there is more than one facility, with each tailored to the needs of students and staff at different stages in the curriculum and at the most appropriate venues.

The size and number of rooms can range from one single space (preferably large) to a multi-room layout or a complete building complex. The room layout should ideally facilitate multiple training sessions at the same time, and the rooms should be flexible for use in teaching and assessment. One of the benefits of large rooms is being able to run several groups or classes in parallel, or an OSCE circuit when screens can be used to divide the space into multiple smaller areas or OSCE stations. Although the space may appear busy and noisy, students are still able to learn, as the primary focus is on hands-on practice and "doing." Other rooms may be specific to certain types of teaching, such as consulting and communication skills training. If the facility is based in an existing building, some rooms may already be equipped and are therefore more suitable for specific skills (e.g., surgical preparation, including sinks and flooring with drainage) and often existing equipment can be repurposed. Careful consideration should be given when selecting or purchasing equipment (tables, benches, etc.) to ensure that it will fit within the room(s) and can be moved as required (e.g., to set up an OSCE circuit). Each skill station should have sufficient

space for teaching and for students to practice, while there also needs to be enough surfaces for the model(s), equipment, and any supporting learning resources (e.g., instruction sheets).

Ideally, the clinical skills center should include a reception and sign-in area, plenty of storage space (for equipment, spares, and consumables), a prep room (e.g., to prepare for practical classes, to make and repair models), somewhere for students' belongings, and an office for the laboratory manager and staff. Another important consideration is to provide an area set aside for drop-in and self-directed learning in addition to the formal teaching spaces. The facility should be equipped with technology such as large screens and tablets. Some rooms may be set up for the use of video cameras and links to videos are helpful, for example via QR (quick response) codes. The area will need computer network infrastructure and wi-fi so that e-learning resources, including video recordings, can be used to support student learning, teaching, and assessment. It is worth noting that most technology, as well as other equipment, will require regular updating, ongoing maintenance, and modernization.

Equipping the Clinical Skills Laboratory

As the main focus of a clinical skills laboratory is to provide an environment where students can learn practical and clinical skills in a hands-on way, the most important resources are the models, part-task trainers, simulators, and associated equipment. Some models and part-task trainers from medical education are suitable for use in veterinary clinical skills laboratories, and there are some specific veterinary models available commercially. However, there are significant gaps, and as a result a growing array of home-made models and simulators has been developed by veterinary educators. The veterinary community is proactive in sharing ideas, tips, and "recipe" sheets for home-made simulators via online forums and web pages, for example the Veterinary Clinical Skills &

Simulation group on NOVICE (Baillie *et al.*, 2011), and face to face during workshops at conferences (Baillie, Crowther, and Dilly, 2015). When buying commercial models or constructing, adapting, and using home-made ones, it is useful to consider the following aspects:

- Cost (initial, parts, and repair).
- Reusability (single or multiple use: how many times a model or component can be used before needing replacement).
- Alignment with (usefulness in relation to) the aims of the clinical skills program.
- Appropriateness for the stage and needs of the learner.
- Limitations compared to performing the task on the real animal.
- Transferability of skills to the real task.
- Storage requirements.

Even though the focus of most clinical skills laboratories is on teaching with models, there are times when the use of live animals and cadavers is appropriate. However, sourcing of cadavers and policies around the use of live animals in teaching will be dependent on the regulations and ethical guidelines of each country and university. The clinical skills laboratory will also need to include the appropriate biosecurity measures. In order to promote animal welfare and the principles of humane veterinary education, the following questions should be considered:

- Which skills can be taught or assessed with simulators and models or using nonharmful teaching methods?
- What types of models and simulators are available to train and prepare students for their practical handling and clinical experiences?
- What types of supporting learning resources (e.g., videos) are accessible and available to demonstrate a specific skill and/or complex procedure (e.g., spaying or neutering)?
- Is there a need to use cadavers (if yes, are these cadavers ethically sourced)?

- What type of noninvasive self-examination could be undertaken (e.g., ultrasound)?
- What is the maximum acceptable use of a live animal for teaching purpose (e.g., number of students, time period)?

Simulation aims to complement teaching and learning by replacing live animals with reasonably realistic but nonetheless artificial substitutes. There is a wide range of models and types of simulator, which are broadly classified as follows:

- *Low fidelity*: simple, usually cheap models and part-task trainers designed for a specific skill, task, or part of a procedure (Scalese and Issenberg, 2005). Examples include suture pads, toy dogs for bandaging, home-made venipuncture models, and a range of injection models (different species and sites).
- *Intermediate fidelity*: typically simulating several skills or steps of a technique, incorporating more aspects of the real task. Examples include a home-made heart sounds simulator, canine intubation (home-made or commercial; Aulmann *et al.*, 2015), and an ophthalmology model.
- *High fidelity*: often simulating complete procedures or techniques, closer to representing the real task or animal, and usually more expensive than simpler models. Examples include physical or virtual-reality simulators for rectal palpation of the cow and the horse, and surgical models, such as a bitch spay.
- *Simulated clients (SCs)*: if communication skills training is run in the clinical skills laboratory, then SCs are usually recruited and are individuals (actors or role players) trained to portray a client in a scripted and standardized encounter (Adams and Kurtz, 2006) during teaching and OSCE-type assessments.
- *Contextualized simulation*: a hybrid form of simulation that supports training combining technical with other skills, including communication, application of knowledge,

and decision-making (Kneebone and Baillie, 2008; Baillie, Pierce, and May, 2010).

Teaching and Learning in the Clinical Skills Laboratory

The clinical skills laboratory provides an active learning environment and supports teaching of psychomotor skills in ways that lectures do not. There is an increasing body of evidence that learning on models and simulators positively influences the learning experience and skill acquisition; and evidence-based protocols have emerged that provide guidance for effective simulation-based training (Akaike *et al.*, 2012; McGaghie *et al.*, 2010). As well as practicing skills on the models, students will be able to receive feedback on performance from teachers and peers and, in some cases, the simulator. Videotaping can also be used to review performance and as part of a debriefing exercise.

When considering how to support the learner, a distinction should be made between two types of delivery: participating in taught practical classes and self-directed learning. Whatever the approach, the skill station must be well designed, with clear, step-by-step instructions provided. This is particularly important for an open-access or drop-in area, for when students return after the formal teaching to revise, improve, and further develop their skills. Without clear instructions there is a risk that students will be reluctant to return and practice on their own, or that they may develop inappropriate skills or approaches. The supporting learning resources can be provided in various formats, such as instruction booklets (see Box 10.3) or sheets (the text illustrated with good-quality photographs and diagrams), videos, posters, information cards, and slide shows. The resources should be easily accessible to students, not just in the clinical skills laboratory but at other times and places – that is, for private study and when undertaking extramural rotations and off-site work placements.

Box 10.3: Example of the structure of a learning booklet

- Title of station or skill
- Learning outcome
- Scenario/contextualization
- What is needed when practicing the skill (e.g., equipment, an assistant)
- What needs to be considered (e.g., safety, biosecurity)
- How to perform the skill: step-by-step written instructions with photos and/or illustrations
- Limitations of the model
- Resetting the station (tidying up and leaving it ready for the next learner)
- Top tips/useful to know or "I wish I'd known…"
- Frequently asked questions (FAQs)
- References and further reading or resources, e.g., QR code to access a video

One of the advantages of teaching in a clinical skills laboratory is that the delivery and learning outcomes can be standardized and consistent for each student. It is also important to provide training for instructors, whether faculty, practitioners, technicians, or students (peer tutors). The most frequently adopted approaches to teaching students psychomotor skills are the five-step method by George and Doto (2001) and Peyton's approach (Walker and Peyton, 1998). A teaching session involves initially ensuring that the learner understands the objectives and can conceptualize the relevance. It may be obvious to students why they need to learn surgical skills, but check that they are as clear about the importance of good bandaging technique; that is, that a bandage falls off if applied too loosely or causes discomfort and damage if too tight. The instructor demonstrates the skill silently, allowing students to visualize the steps (the demonstration may be "live" or using a video), and then repeats the demonstration while also describing the steps. Students should outline the steps to the instructor or a peer before finally performing the skill. It is important that the instructor provides feedback and that the student appreciates that mastery only develops over time and with repeated, deliberate practice. It is also helpful to consider how best to support the learner on their journey from novice toward the required level of expertise. This will vary depending on the stage in the curriculum and type of skill; the rate of acquisition will depend on the individual student, but can be enhanced by good instructions, from both teachers and supporting resources. Typically training takes place in small groups, which allows all students the opportunity for hands-on practice, enables the instructor to provide feedback, and tends to generate a relaxed atmosphere conducive to learning.

Peer-assisted learning (Topping, 2008) is commonplace in clinical skills laboratories, either as a formal part of the clinical skills program or informally during practical classes and drop-in sessions. There are a number of benefits, including that peers are supportive, accessible, and less intimidating than faculty, which help to promote learning. However, the limited experience and skills of the peer tutor may present potential risks and issues. In more formal peer-assisted learning programs, tutors will undergo training for the skill(s) being taught and in how to structure a session, support learning, and give feedback (see Part Two, Chapter 8: Peer-Assisted Learning).

Whether teaching in the clinical skills laboratory is delivered by faculty, practitioners, technicians, or students, the importance of training the teacher cannot be overemphasized; that is, having a specifically designed staff development program, preferably delivered on an annual basis.

Using a Clinical Skills Laboratory for Assessments

The main purpose of a clinical skills facility is to support the acquisition, maintenance, and enhancement of clinical skills. However, assessment of clinical skills is essential to demonstrate that the required outcomes, skills, and competencies have been achieved, and inevitably student learning will, in part, be driven by assessment. An assessment method widely used in medical education is the OSCE (see also Part Four, Chapter 16: Performance and Workplace-Based Assessment), where students demonstrate to an examiner their ability to perform a skill, typically on a model rather than a real patient (Harden and Gleeson, 1979). The OSCE is usually organized as a circuit consisting of multiple stations, each lasting the same amount of time, and is often set up in the clinical skills laboratory, for instance in a large space divided using screens to create multiple examination "rooms." The exam is frequently controlled by an automated announcement system. At each station the student reads a scenario, then performs a specific task in front of an examiner, then moves on to the next station. The examiner has a brief script, for example to confirm the student's identity, and marks the parts of the skills performed (done, not just described, by the student) using a checklist and/or a global rating scale. OSCEs are employed as formative and summative assessments and at different stages in the curriculum. Formative OSCEs aim to provide feedback that students can use to improve and focus their learning. The goal of summative OSCEs is to measure the level of performance/proficiency that has been achieved at the end of a stage of the clinical skills program or the entire curriculum. The pass mark is determined using a standard setting method (Dwyer *et al.*, 2016), of which borderline regression is one of the most widely adopted (although borderline group and modified Angoff are alternatives, particularly for small cohorts). The selection of stations should be blueprinted against the learning outcomes and competencies, and can range from basic skills (e.g., handling and restraint, injection techniques) to surgical skills (e.g., a type of suture), or performing part or all of a physical examination. In some instances the circuit includes communication skills (e.g., history taking). It is sometimes commented that OSCEs, which are run in the laboratory using models, are too artificial and assess skills "in vitro." However, there is a growing body of evidence that OSCEs are a valid and reliable way of testing at the "shows" level of Miller's pyramid, for instance when the student demonstrates their ability to place a simple interrupted suture on a skin pad. OSCEs are useful in ensuring that students prepare and are ready for clinical placements and rotations, where a workplace-based assessment, such as direct observation of procedural skills (DOPS), is more typically used to assess clinical skills performed on patients (at the "does" level of Miller's pyramid).

The resourcing of OSCEs is not trivial, especially with an increasing number of stations (skills to be assessed per year of the program) and larger cohort sizes. The resources include space – for instance to set up 15 stations in one circuit, equipment and consumables, manpower to prepare and reset the stations during the OSCE, as well as the examiners (one per station, and the OSCE will run over several days in order to assess the whole cohort) – and expertise – for example a psychometrician to process and evaluate the results. The use of OSCEs for assessing clinical skills is summarized in Box 10.4.

What are the Limitations of Simulation and Clinical Skills Laboratories?

Simulation mimics reality to a greater or lesser extent, and as a result there can be limitations, including the potential lack of transferability of skills to the real task (Norman, Dore, and Grierson, 2012). Ways of mitigating the risks include establishing face validity: do experts consider that the model or simulation is realistic enough for students to learn? However, in some instances a lack of reality is helpful, as a student can focus on acquiring the technical or psychomotor competence without having to deal with aspects of a situation that could be distracting, or worrying about hurting the animal. It is important that any limitations related to learning on a particular model are identified and made clear to students prior to performing the skill on a live animal, in order to manage expectations and avoid students being unprepared.

The stage of a learner's development should also be considered and could possibly be a limitation for a particular simulation or model. For example, novices may learn better with low fidelity, whereas more experienced students may need greater realism and higher fidelity to support the level of skills to be learned and for them to become sufficiently immersed

---

Box 10.4: Focus on the use of objective structured clinical examinations (OSCEs) in assessing clinical skills

- A valid and reliable method for assessing practical and clinical skills
- Scenario- or task-driven assessment
- At the "shows" level of Miller's pyramid (demonstrate a skill on a model)
- Multiple stations (usually 10–20 tasks or scenarios) in a circuit
- The same scenarios and tasks for every student; that is, at each station

- Standardized time per station (simple skills 5 minutes, more complex tasks 15–20 minutes)
- Examiners typically mark using a checklist, often with a rating scale
- Formative or summative assessment
- The time and resources required to run OSCEs should not be underestimated

in the learning experience. Sometimes using low-fidelity or task-specific models is more effective in promoting learning, but it may not be realistic enough to provide competence in the more challenging real situation (e.g., hemostasis during surgery).

Although teaching and learning in clinical skills laboratories make intuitive sense, it is important to consider whether there is a beneficial effect on students' performance in the clinical setting. Therefore, the use of models and simulators should be carefully planned, using the most appropriate teaching method and context at each stage in the curriculum. Additionally, where possible it is best to use simulators or models that have already been evaluated; that is, where there is evidence that students develop the required skills as a result of training on the model.

Another consideration is whether the buy-in for the clinical skills initiative is as widespread as was anticipated. It is important to raise awareness of the clinical skills laboratory and the supporting learning resources among faculty as well as students. Clear academic leadership and committed staff are crucial to the success of a clinical skills program and laboratory, as is having a sufficient budget for the purchase, maintenance, and replacement of models and other consumables. The overall resourcing (equipment and staff) for a clinical skills program should not be underestimated when establishing a new clinical skills laboratory, as well as for annual maintenance and to accommodate increasing demands on its use.

What is Next for Clinical Skills Laboratories?

The clinical skills initiative has been partly driven by a greater emphasis in competency frameworks on hands-on practice and ensuring that new graduates are able to deliver entry-level care. Other factors include societal expectations for humane veterinary education and finding opportunities to further promote animal welfare. As a result, clinical skills laboratories are becoming increasingly important in veterinary education and are having a positive impact on the student learning experience. All these factors are only likely to boost the need for, and demands placed on, clinical skills laboratories in the future.

One factor that has contributed to the recent and rapid growth in veterinary clinical skills has been the veterinary community's willingness to share, whether in online forums, via publicly available media sites (e.g., YouTube), at conferences, or by hosting site visits. In the future it will be important to continue to build the community, encouraging others to join and identifying additional areas for sharing, for instance staff development, as well as making new models.

Another exciting opportunity afforded by having a clinical skills laboratory and a greater emphasis on clinical skills within the curriculum is to undertake educational research. Until recently there has been a paucity of evidence to support simulation-based training in medicine, and even less in veterinary medicine. However, as more veterinary educators engage in research, there is the potential to generate a growing evidence base that will further underpin clinical skills training. Areas include stakeholder consultation to define clinical competencies, validating (evaluating) models, deconstructing procedures and expert performance, monitoring outcomes assessment, and investigating the impact of staff development programs.

Capitalizing on the progress in supporting and improving teaching and learning, willingness to share expertise, and opportunities to undertake educational research will all contribute to the ongoing development and growth of the veterinary clinical skills initiative worldwide.

References

Adams, C.L., and Kurtz, S.M. (2006) Building on existing models from human medical education to develop a communication curriculum in veterinary medicine. *Journal of Veterinary Medical Education*, **33**, 28–37.

Akaike, M., Fukutomi, M., Nagamune, M., *et al.* (2012) Simulation-based medical education in clinical skills laboratory. *Journal of Medical Investigation*, **59**, 28–35.

Aulmann, M., Marz, M., Burgener, I.A., *et al.* (2015) Development and evaluation of two canine low-fidelity simulation models. *Journal of Veterinary Medical Education*, **42**, 151–160.

Baillie, S., Crowther, E., and Dilly, M. (2015) The veterinary clinical skills laboratory initiative. *REDU Revista de Docencia Universitaria*, **13**, 73–81.

Baillie, S., Kinnison, T., Forrest, N., *et al.* (2011) Developing an online professional network for veterinary education: The NOVICE project. *Journal of Veterinary Medical Education*, **38**, 395–403.

Baillie, S., Pierce, S.E., and May, S.A. (2010) Fostering integrated learning and clinical professionalism using contextualized simulation in a small-group role-play. *Journal of Veterinary Medical Education*, **37**, 248–253.

de Boo, J., and Knight, A. (2005) "Concepts in animal welfare": A syllabus in animal welfare science and ethics for veterinary schools. *Journal of Veterinary Medical Education*, **32**, 451–453.

Dilly, M., Tipold, A., Schaper, E., and Ehlers, J.P. (2014) Setting up a veterinary medicine skills lab in Germany. *GMS Zeitschrift für Medizinische Ausbildung*, **31**, Doc20.

Dwyer, T., Wright, S., Kulasegaram, K.M., *et al.* (2016) How to set the bar in competency-based medical education: Standard setting after an Objective Structured Clinical Examination (OSCE). *BMC Medical Education*, **16**, 1.

George, J.H., and Doto, F.X. (2001) A simple five-step method for teaching clinical skills. *Family Medicine*, **33**, 577–578.

Harden, R.M., and Gleeson, F.A. (1979) Assessment of clinical competence using an objective structured clinical examination (OSCE). *Medical Education*, **13**, 41–54.

Jaarsma, D.A., Dolmans, D.H., Scherpbier, A.J., and van Beukelen, P. (2008) Preparation for practice by veterinary school: A comparison of the perceptions of alumni from a traditional and an innovative veterinary curriculum. *Journal of Veterinary Medical Education*, **35**, 431–438.

Kinnison, T., May, S.A., and Guile, D. (2014) Inter-professional practice: From veterinarian to the veterinary team. *Journal of Veterinary Medical Education*, **41**, 172–178.

Kneebone, R., and Baillie, S. (2008) Contextualized simulation and procedural skills: A view from medical education. *Journal of Veterinary Medical Education*, **35**, 595–598.

Langebaek, R., Eika, B., Jensen, A.L., *et al.* (2012) Anxiety in veterinary surgical students: A quantitative study. *Journal of Veterinary Medical Education*, **39**, 331–340.

Low-Beer, N., Kinnison, T., Baillie, S., *et al.* (2011) Hidden practice revealed: Using cognitive task analysis and novel simulator design to evaluate the teaching of digital rectal examination. *American Journal of Surgery*, **201**, 46–53.

Lynagh, M., Burton, R., and Sanson-Fisher, R. (2007) A systematic review of medical skills laboratory training: Where to from here? *Medical Education*, **41**, 879–887.

McGaghie, W.C., Issenberg, S.B., Petrusa, E.R., and Scalese, R.J. (2010) A critical review of simulation-based medical education research: 2003–2009. *Medical Education*, **44**, 50–63.

Michels, M.E., Evans, D.E., and Blok, G.A. (2012) What is a clinical skill? Searching for order in chaos through a modified Delphi process. *Medical Teacher*, **34**, e573–e81.

Norman, G., Dore, K., and Grierson, L. (2012) The minimal relationship between simulation fidelity and transfer of learning. *Medical Education*, **46**, 636–647.

Remmen, R. (1998) Unsatisfactory basic skills performance by students in traditional medical curricula. *Medical Teacher*, **20**, 579–582.

Remmen, R., Derese, A., Scherpbier, A., *et al.* (1999) Can medical schools rely on clerkships to train students in basic clinical skills? *Medical Education*, **33**, 600–605.

Scalese, R.J., and Issenberg, S.B. (2005) Effective use of simulations for the teaching and acquisition of veterinary professional and clinical skills. *Journal of Veterinary Medical Education*, **32**, 461–467.

Topping, K. (2008) Peer-assisted learning: A planning and implementation framework. Guide supplement 30.1– Viewpoint. *Medical Teacher*, **30**, 440.

Walker, M., and Peyton, J. (1998) Teaching in theatre. In *Teaching and Learning in Medical Practice* (ed. J.W.R. Peyton), Manticore Europe, Rickmansworth, pp. 171–180.

Further Reading

Baillie, S., Booth, N., Catterall, A., *et al.* (n.d.) *A Guide to Veterinary Clinical Skills Laboratories.* http://www.bris.ac.uk/vetscience/media/docs/csl-guide.pdf (accessed November 7, 2016).

NOVICE (n.d.) *Network Of Veterinarians In Continuing Education (NOVICE).* http://www.noviceproject.eu/ (accessed November 7, 2016).

University of Veterinary Medicine Hannover, *Foundation. TiHo YouTube Channel*: www.youtube.com/tihovideos

University of Bristol, School of Veterinary Sciences (2016) *Clinical Skills Booklets.* http://www.bristol.ac.uk/vetscience/research/comparative-clinical/veterinary-education/clinical-skills-booklets/ (accessed November 30, 2016).

11

Learning in the Electronic Age

Jodi A. Korich[1] *and Lisa M. Keefe*[2]

[1] College of Veterinary Medicine, Cornell University, USA
[2] College of Veterinary Medicine & Biomedical Sciences, Texas A&M, USA

Box 11.1: Key messages

- Technology does not replace teaching. However, when used as a tool, technology has the capacity to expand an instructor's capabilities and deepen students' understanding of the learning material.
- When designing technology-enhanced learning activities, it is essential to consider content, pedagogy, and technology simultaneously and in equal measure.

- When incorporating technology into a course, the best learning outcomes will be achieved when the instructor adheres to the philosophy of learner-centered teaching and utilizes the backward course design method.
- Two of the most common mistakes made when using technology in teaching are failing to consider pedagogy during the design and incomplete project planning.

Introduction

Despite the integration of technology into many aspects of our modern lives, the use of technologies to augment veterinary teaching remains surprisingly minimal. Why do so many veterinary teaching faculty avoid using technology? There are no doubt many reasons. However, after a decade of working in veterinary academia, we have noticed that many faculty who eschew technology do so out of fear and misconceptions about the role of educational technologies in teaching. The goal of educational technologies is *not* to replace faculty, but rather to augment their capacity to teach.

Like any successful teaching effort, teaching with technology requires an understanding of and adherence to pedagogical principles. Nevertheless, all too often educational technologies are applied to courses indiscriminately. Such approaches typically lead to disappointing results, causing many faculty to give up on technology altogether.

Can Technology Enhance Teaching?

Dr. Turner is a veterinary oncologist who teaches small animal oncology to third-year veterinary

Veterinary Medical Education: A Practical Guide, First Edition. Edited by Jennifer L. Hodgson and Jacquelyn M. Pelzer.
© 2017 John Wiley & Sons, Inc. Published 2017 by John Wiley & Sons, Inc.

students. Originally he was allotted seven hours for his oncology lectures in a team-taught small animal medicine course. Over the past decade, the knowledge base for oncology has expanded significantly and, after numerous requests to the curriculum committee, Dr. Turner was eventually granted an additional six hours to teach oncology. At first he was delighted, since he thought he would finally have time to cover everything that students needed to know about oncology. However, he quickly realized that despite the expanded contact time, the students continued to struggle to recall the material on clinical rotation.

After reviewing the third-year student evaluations, Dr. Turner noticed that many students complained that he went through his lectures too quickly. He had to admit that he did talk fast; after all, there was so much important material to cover. Determined to help his students be successful, he decided to turn to technology to fix the problem. He had recently heard about a new lecture-capture system installed at the college. He decided that he would videotape his lectures and post them online for students to watch after class. This solution seemed ideal, because he would not have to eliminate any material from his lectures. Meanwhile, the students could watch his lectures as many times as necessary to master the concepts.

The lecture-capture solution was implemented; however, much to Dr. Turner's surprise, students continued to struggle in applying the oncology lecture material to patients on clinical rotation. Based on this experience, he concluded that using technology in his class did not enhance student learning. What was really needed, he decided, was simply more lecture time to prepare the students adequately for clinical rotation. He resolved to go back to the curriculum committee yet again and argue for an increase to 20 hours of lecture time. He knew that it would not be easy to convince the committee to allot him more time. These days, it seemed that everyone wanted more time to teach their subject matter.

Do you identify with any aspects of Dr. Turner's story? Most veterinary faculty have grappled with the problem of how to present a growing body of material in the same amount of time. After all, new medical discoveries add more knowledge, but unfortunately not more hours in the day. Likewise, the struggle to help students bridge the gap between theory and practice is a universal challenge across many professional schools, including veterinary medicine. Maybe you serve on a curriculum committee and bear witness to the never-ending pleas from faculty for more time to cover their material. Perhaps, like Dr. Turner, you have attempted to use technology to solve an educational problem in your class, only to be disappointed with the results. In this chapter, we will show you how to design, build, and deliver technology-enhanced learning activities successfully to enhance your courses.

Common Reasons Why Technology-Enhanced Teaching Fails

As you begin your journey learning how to utilize technology to teach more effectively, let us examine some common mistakes. In our experience working with many groups to develop technology-enhanced educational programs, we have observed eight common stumbling blocks resulting in suboptimal student learning outcomes (see Box 11.2). As you review this list, recall the story of Dr. Turner and see how many mistakes you can recognize.

Now that we have introduced some common mistakes to avoid when using technology in teaching, let us analyze Dr. Turner's story more closely. You will recall Dr. Turner's observation that students on his clinical rotation had difficulty remembering the lecture material that he had taught them the previous year. In our experience, short-term retention of material from one class to the next is a problem that engenders more frustration among teaching faculty than any other. Often, we hear instructors make comments such as: "If only students would believe me when I tell them that this material is important and they need to remember it after the test." Unfortunately, many instructors,

Box 11.2: Quick tip – common mistakes in technology-enhanced teaching

- *Technology-driven instructional design*: designing a learning activity around a particular technology versus selecting the appropriate technology to support the learning goals.
- *Ill-defined learning goals*: lack of clearly articulated learning goals leading to unfocused learning activities.
- *Clinging to teacher-centered techniques*: failure to adopt learner-centered teaching techniques when designing and delivering new learning activities.
- *Too much material*: trying to cover excessive volumes of content, leaving few opportunities for students to practice applying their knowledge.

- *Poor assessment strategies*: missing the opportunity to incorporate better assessment, including using formative assessment to support learning.
- *Taking on too much*: initiating a large-scale and/or complex project without understanding the time, budget, and expertise required.
- *Making too many changes, too quickly*: failure to take a phased approach to course updates and thereby missing the opportunity for small-scale pilot testing, feedback, reflection, and refinement of the new technique.
- *Not managing student expectations*: failure to explain adequately the learning value of the technology-enhanced activity to students.

like Dr. Turner, fail to recognize the underlying cause of students' apparent forgetfulness. Thus, any course improvements that are implemented to correct the problem are unlikely to achieve the desired outcomes.

To acquire deep learning and achieve long-term retention, students must engage in the materials and undertake the mental effort of learning. Teacher-centric strategies, such as didactic lectures, rely on passive listening on the part of students. Material presented in this manner is prepackaged and organized according to the instructor's own expert understanding, which diminishes the students' learning experience. During the learning process, students must develop their own model (context) to understand the circumstances under which they will use the information. This includes an opportunity to practice applying the new knowledge in the appropriate context. If the goal is for students on clinical rotations to be able to utilize clinical reasoning skills to work up patients, hopefully you can appreciate that Dr. Turner would not be helping his students to reach this goal through an increase in lecture hours. If not lectures, how could Dr. Turner

teach students instead to help prepare them better? Learner-centered teaching (LCT) is a well-documented strategy that pushes students beyond short-term memorization of facts to a deeper level of mastery. LCT techniques yield significantly improved learning outcomes (see Table 11.1).

Educational technologies offer many opportunities to introduce learner-centered teaching techniques to veterinary courses. However, all too often, as in Dr. Turner's case, technologies are merely used to "digitize" the same unsuccessful, passive, teacher-centered instructional approaches. The migration of slide carousels to PowerPoint™ lectures and the introduction of lecture-capture software brought lectures into the digital age. However, these technologies on their own do little to prepare students to reason like a clinician. Too often technology is wielded with little or no regard for the underlying pedagogy of how students learn, and when technology is treated like a teaching method instead of a teaching tool, the results are typically disappointing. Sound instructional design is the underpinning of any successful application of technology to teaching. It is for this reason

Table 11.1 Learner-centered teaching.

Reference	Publication type	Synopsis
Armbruster *et al.* (2009)	Journal article	Comparison study ($n = 520$, introductory undergraduate biology course) showed that learner-centered methods increased academic performance with higher Bloom's taxonomy levels, and significant improvement of student self-reported engagement and satisfaction when compared to traditional lecture taught by same teacher.
Hake (1998)	Journal article	Comparison meta-analysis ($n = 6542$, 62 high school and undergraduate courses) of Force Concept Inventory (FCI) exam results. The score comparisons by class teaching methods strongly indicate that use of interactive engagement methods in the classroom increased student learning outcomes (higher FCI scores) well beyond traditional classroom practices.
Knight and Wood (2005)	Journal article	Comparison study ($n = 146$, upper-division lecture course in developmental biology) showed that learner-centered pedagogy resulted in significantly higher learning gains and better conceptual understanding compared to traditional lecture taught by same pair of teachers.
Prince (2004)	Research review	Active learning pedagogies play an important role in learner-centered teaching. This review finds broad support for improved learning outcomes with common active learning pedagogies.
Reh *et al.* (2014)	Journal article	Prospective longitudinal study ($n = 59$, residents over 11 years) implemented a learner-centered curriculum with otolaryngology head and neck surgery residents. The four years following implementation of an LCT curriculum showed significant improvement of otolaryngology training examination (OTE) scores.
Weimer (2013)	Book	A concise review of literature supporting LCT, combined with case studies and practical tips for developing LCT classroom experiences.

that we have chosen to discuss educational technologies within the context of pedagogy throughout the remainder of this chapter.

The TPACK Framework

Teaching is a complex activity, and successful teachers do more than simply impart information to students. Mishra and Koehler (2006, p. 1021) describe teaching as a process whereby "the teacher interprets the subject matter and finds different ways to represent it and make it accessible to learners." Constructing meaningful student learning experiences requires teachers to blend their content expertise with the art of teaching, known as pedagogy. The idea of integrating content knowledge with pedagogy was first proposed by Lee Schulman (1986). Building on this idea, Mishra and Koehler (2006) proposed the Technological Pedagogical Content Knowledge (TPACK) framework. Figure 11.1 depicts the TPACK framework, showing the intersection of content knowledge, pedagogical knowledge, and technological knowledge. In this model, each of these three elements is critical to consider when designing and developing technology-enhanced learning activities. Unfortunately, as Kinchin (2012, p. E44) points out, all too often "content

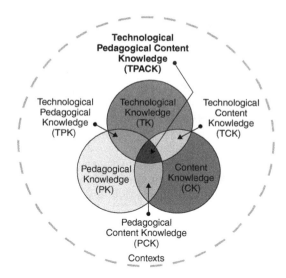

Figure 11.1 TPACK framework. Reproduced by permission of the publisher, © 2012 by tpack.org.

is the driving force and takes up most of the development energy. Technology is then added to the mix (typically by those without an academic background in the content), whilst pedagogy is often tacitly presumed to somehow 'be there.'" The lesson to be learned here is that when designing technology-enhanced learning activities, a balanced approach, one that marries content, pedagogy, and technology, offers the best possibility of optimizing student learning outcomes.

Case Studies in Technology-Enhanced Teaching

In this section we will explore a series of three case studies that demonstrate the successful integration of content, pedagogy, and technology in teaching. These cases range from simple techniques that are easily implemented in any classroom, to more complex learning activities that require extensive planning and production. In each case, you will see that all three TPACK elements were considered in equal measure from the project's inception, ensuring good results.

Case Study 11.1

Content
Small animal medicine course.

Technology
Virtual patients/web-based case studies:

- HTML5 SCORM-compliant case-study development tool.
- Learning management system.
- Student wi-fi–enabled tablet devices or laptops.

Pedagogy
- Contextualized learning.
- Formative assessment.

The Problem
The small animal medicine course is a 12-credit, team-taught course that spans the spring and fall semesters of the third-year curriculum. The large class size and rigid lecture-hall seating afforded limited flexibility to instructors. Faced with these constraints, faculty contributing to this course had a tendency to default to a lecture-style presentation as their primary mode of teaching. Students, who spent between four and eight hours per day in lectures, reported problems paying attention during class. Meanwhile, some clinical faculty who taught downstream noticed that students were struggling to apply concepts covered in this course to patients in the teaching hospital.

The Solution
To help overcome these challenges, one course instructor decided to convert six hours of passive PowerPoint lectures into active learning exercises using virtual patients. Working with an instructional designer, the course instructor defined a set of learning objectives for each exercise. Care was taken to write learning objectives that had precise, measurable learning outcomes, using terms from Bloom's taxonomy of learning. This ensured that the entire project team would have a shared understanding of the "content" goals, guiding the myriad of "pedagogy" and "technology" decisions that would be

made throughout the design and development of the virtual patients.

Storylines for a series of six virtual patients were written as a vehicle to teach each of the learning objectives. These storylines were entered into a case-study system. A number of open-source and commercial software platforms are available for developing virtual patients. The team utilized StepStone, an in-house web-based application created to support rapid, flexible development of virtual patients (go.tamucet.org/StepStone).

Media assets (e.g., photographs and videos) needed to support student learning throughout the cases were jointly identified by the clinical instructor and instructional designer. Clinical procedures (e.g., bone marrow aspiration) were marked for video production, and scripts were prepared. Patient photographs, used to support the flow of the storylines, were obtained, and a variety of illustrations, tables, and so on were created to help convey key concepts. The interplay between "content," "pedagogy," and "technology" was especially evident at this stage of the project. The course instructor worked closely with the instructional designer and educational technologists in a dynamic, collaborative manner to produce the media for the cases. The completed media files were uploaded into the case-study software, and the cases were published in a SCORM 1.2–compliant file (a file format that runs on learning management systems). The SCORM files were uploaded into a Moodle learning management system (LMS) for access during class.

Students enrolled in the course were given access to a set of course notes on the LMS to read before class. During class, they were expected to apply information found in the notes to the virtual patients. The course instructor presented each case study in a one-hour block. During the exercises, students were asked to interpret data (e.g., review diagnostic test results) and make a series of clinical decisions (e.g., formulate an appropriate therapeutic plan) as they worked through each case. Multiple-choice questions, incorporated throughout the cases, allowed the instructor to assess students' ability to apply knowledge within the context of the cases. Importantly, a free-text box was provided for students to explain how they arrived at their answers. Students submitted their answers via the LMS, which was monitored by the instructor in real time. Following each question, the instructor presented a short, 5–10-minute mini-lecture, summarizing the key points and clarifying any misconceptions revealed through the students' answer submissions. The case studies, which included answer feedback, were made available to students online after class for review.

Why Does It Enhance Learning Outcomes?

Traditional didactic lectures emphasize factual knowledge. The in-class exercises described here utilized virtual patients to give students an opportunity to contextualize their understanding of the material. Contextualized learning helps students to develop the complex mental models that are necessary to apply knowledge to patient care (Bowen, 2006). These exercises also supported a dynamic interplay between the students and the instructor, allowing her to practice the art of "pedagogy" in the classroom. By monitoring student answers on the LMS, the instructor could easily flex the mini-lectures according to the needs of the students in the class to address any misconceptions. This formative assessment served as a powerful tool to foster student learning.

Lessons Learned

- The application of factual knowledge to virtual patients is challenging for many students, who are accustomed to passive didactic lectures. To avoid excessive student frustration, we recommend taking the time to set expectations before beginning class. Explain the goal of the exercises and help students understand that they will be learning skills that will help them to think like a clinician. Once students understood that making mistakes is part of the learning process, we found that most strongly preferred the virtual patient exercises to didactic lectures.

- When converting lecture material into active learning exercises, many instructors struggle with how to include all the same information in a class. The truth is that you will likely need to reduce the volume of content you currently deliver in class to make room for student interaction and discussion. Many instructors find this difficult to accept at first. Keep in mind, however, that using virtual patients in your teaching will significantly enhance long-term retention of the material and teach valuable clinical reasoning skills that will help prepare students for clinical practice.

Acknowledgments

We wish to thank the following individuals from Texas A&M University College of Veterinary Medicine & Biomedical Sciences who contributed to this project:

- Ashley Saunders, DVM, ACVIM (cardiology).
- Audrey Cook, BVM&S, MRCVS, ACVIM, ECVIM.
- Kevin Cummings, DVM, PhD.
- The team at the Center for Educational Technologies.

For more information about collaborative case-based learning, visit go.tamucet.org/CCBL.

Case Study 11.2

Content

One-credit-hour elective course on feline internal medicine taught in the spring semester of the third-year curriculum.

Technology

Audience polling technology:

- Web-based audience polling system.
- Student wi-fi–enabled mobile devices.

Pedagogy

- Formative assessment.
- Contingent teaching.
- Peer calibration.
- Peer instruction.

The Problem

The abrupt transition from the relatively passive environment of the large classroom to the examination room, where opinions and recommendations are sought, can be very stressful for the veterinary student. To help prepare students for their transition into clinical rotations, the instructor teaches a feline elective course to approximately 80 third-year veterinary students utilizing a student-centered teaching format. The course is based on a series of case-based discussions intended to cultivate decision-making and communication skills. The challenge was finding a way to engage the students in dialog in which they were expected to express their opinion in front of peers. Student evaluations suggested that hand-raising as a method of student engagement had a detrimental impact on learning. When fellow students raised their hands, students reported that their own clinical reasoning process shut down. They were also very anxious about the prospect of answering questions incorrectly in front of the instructor and their peers, which significantly reduced overall student participation in the course.

The Solution

Audience polling technology (APT) was incorporated into the course to encourage student engagement and build confidence in clinical decision-making. The Poll Everywhere™ APT was selected due to its flexibility, allowing students to use their own wi-fi–enabled smartphones, tablets, and laptops during class. Prior to class, the instructor prepared a variety of questions designed to foster discussion of diagnostic and therapeutic strategies. Both multiple-choice and narrative questions were developed and entered into the Poll Everywhere system. A unique web page address for each question was generated (e.g., www.pollev.com/add-unique-poll-name-here) and inserted directly into the PowerPoint presentation. Students accessed the questions during the presentation via the web page addresses on the PowerPoint slides and used their mobile devices to submit their answers anonymously. The instructor monitored response submission via a laptop, waiting for the majority of students to reply to the poll before displaying the results to the class. This allowed all students to complete their clinical reasoning thought process and avoided them being influenced by other students' responses. The poll results were presented to the class and the correct answer was discussed. Multiple-choice questions that focused on comprehension of essential concepts and produced discordant student responses were particularly effective. In those cases, the instructor would clear the screen and ask the students to persuade their peers sitting close by that their original response was correct. After a peer-to-peer discussion, the students were asked to answer the original question again. Results from the first and second rounds of questions were compared, and the correct answer and clinical reasoning process were discussed in depth.

Why Does It Enhance Learning Outcomes?

Formative assessment is an essential component of student learning. Students should be provided with regular opportunities to test their understanding in a low-stakes, ungraded environment. The APT described here provides students with frequent opportunities throughout class to assess their ability to apply the material in a context-specific manner (i.e., making clinical decisions). The classroom delivery of the polls also supports peer learning and calibration, as students are able to engage with one another and gauge their mastery of the material relative to that of their peers. APT allows the instructor to gauge how well the class as a whole understood the concepts versus calling on only one or two students at a time. This approach supports the use of contingent teaching, wherein the instructor can focus the discussion on the important concepts that the majority of the class has not yet mastered.

Lessons Learned

- Students may resist the use of clickers in class because they are often linked to grades and attendance rather than learning. They appeared to view positively the use of the Poll

Everywhere web-based audience response system.

- To ensure good results, questions must be formulated carefully to align with the instructor's goals. Questions may be used to emphasize content, support contingent teaching (alter discussion based on student feedback), encourage peer instruction, and assess student knowledge at the beginning and end of a class period.

- Questions should be used sparingly, preferably no more than five or six in each one-hour presentation.

- Ideally, questions of different types should be asked during the presentation and their difficulty should increase throughout the hour, building students' confidence.

- Questions that prompt bimodal or split responses promote more productive discussion than those with clear-cut answers.

Acknowledgments

We wish to thank Dr. John August, Dean of Faculties and Associate Provost at Texas A&M University, for his contributions to this case study.

Case Study 11.3

Content

General surgical skills course.

Technology

Computer-aided tutorials:

- Mixed-media, web-based modules.
- Learning management system.
- Students' computers with internet access.

Pedagogy

- Blended learning.
- Deliberate feedback.
- Reusable learning objects.

The Problem

Traditional veterinary surgical training programs utilize a procedure-based approach. Students are taught how to perform common procedures (e.g., ovariohysterectomy) by practicing on patients under the apprenticeship of a surgeon. While this system tends to work well in surgical residency programs, where students have access to a long period of mentoring and ample patients on which to practice, it is arguably less successful for training general practitioners. In recent years, many veterinary colleges have experienced reductions in primary care caseload, as well as a movement away from terminal surgeries in teaching due to ethical concerns and budget reductions. These constraints place additional strain on the procedure-based model for teaching surgery, making it challenging for students today to master the basic surgical skills necessary for general practice. A team of educators at three veterinary colleges set out to address this pedagogical challenge. They observed that many surgery laboratories did not make efficient use of student contact time with surgeons. Instructors spent a great deal of time demonstrating how to perform basic skills, such as gripping surgical instruments, reducing the time available for students to refine their surgical skills via instructor observation and feedback.

The Solution

The instructors decided to make a shift from a procedure-based to a skills-based approach to teaching surgery. The goal was to teach students the core surgical skills necessary to perform *any* entry-level procedure. Emphasis would be placed on students building a foundation of transferable surgical skills to support lifelong learning. Next, the instructors decided to use a blend of online learning and hands-on laboratories to help students achieve the learning objectives. To some observers, computers and surgical training seem like an unnatural combination. However, the team believed that online learning modules reviewed by students prior to attending the laboratories would free up time in the laboratory, allowing students to derive maximum benefit from their limited time with live animals and surgical instructors. To accomplish their goal, the team developed a seven-contact-hour, web-based auto-tutorial covering basic instrument handling. The

modules are media rich, featuring narrated "how to" videos and interactive practice exercises with feedback. A competency checklist was also included to aid instructors in assessing and documenting student proficiency during the hands-on laboratories. The tutorial, mounted on an LMS, was designed in a modular format to facilitate implementation in a variety of pre-existing surgery courses at various colleges. At present, nine veterinary colleges have successfully utilized the training modules to augment their surgery courses. Student and instructor feedback is very positive, with instructors reporting significant improvement in student competence and confidence.

Why Does It Enhance Learning Outcomes?

This project exemplifies the blended learning approach, wherein online learning is combined with traditional hands-on laboratories to optimize the students' learning experience. The online modules provide an opportunity for students to acquire baseline knowledge and skills prior to the laboratories. During the surgery labs, instructors circulate among the students, providing one-on-one coaching. This pedagogical approach aligns with that of deliberate feedback (Ericsson, 2008), a powerful technique that allows novices to correct errors and progress toward mastery. Lastly, this project highlights the benefits of creating reusable learning objects that can be easily adopted by other academic institutions. The flexible, modular nature of these resources allows them to be incorporated into pre-existing surgery courses at other veterinary colleges. Media-rich, web-based resources are often expensive and time-consuming to produce. The sharing of reusable learning objects among veterinary colleges is a model that should receive greater attention, as it promotes leveraging of strengths for the collective benefit of our students.

Lessons Learned
- Developing media-rich, web-based modules requires extensive upfront planning. The team wrote detailed scripts for all of the videos prior to video production. These

scripts were used to generate shot lists to ensure that all media would be properly captured. This was particularly important in this project, as the team could not easily reshoot surgical scenes.

- Student feedback on the modules was very positive. Extensive survey feedback showed that students especially liked the use of instructional videos to teach procedural material. Moreover, students appreciated the interactive practice exercises that allowed them to apply knowledge and receive feedback in a low-stakes, ungraded environment.

- Pilot testing is an important aspect of developing any technology-enhanced learning activity. After the first year of running this course, student feedback indicated problems with the final examination. A new test was implemented the following year, correcting the problem. This experience underscores the importance of pilot testing new activities and gathering feedback from users to make subsequent improvements.

Acknowledgments

We wish to thank the following individuals who contributed to this project:

- Daniel Smeak, DVM, ACVS, Colorado State University College of Veterinary Medicine and Biomedical Sciences.
- Lawrence Hill, DVM, ABVP, The Ohio State University College of Veterinary Medicine.
- The team at the Center for Educational Technologies, Texas A&M University College of Veterinary Medicine & Biomedical Sciences.

For more information about the core surgical skills initiative, visit go.tamucet.org/CSS.

Future Trends in Technology-Enhanced Teaching

The adaptation of technologies to teaching is a constantly evolving landscape, and a chapter focused entirely on the educational technologies in vogue today would soon be obsolete. Nevertheless, there is value in taking a forward-thinking approach to how we educate the veterinary students of tomorrow. Here are four emerging trends in technology to which veterinary educators should look in the future.

Digital Social Networking

Facebook, Twitter, YouTube – these are just a few of the popular digital social networking (DSN) technologies currently available. Some veterinary educators have balked at the idea of using DSN to teach. After all, we frequently admonish students to exercise caution about posting inappropriate information on social media sites. However, the adoption of DSN for teaching is accelerating as educators begin to grasp the power of e-communities to augment student learning. This should not be surprising, as DSN can so easily harness the power of peer instruction.

E-Portfolios

The e-portfolio is a web-based application that facilitates the accrual, organization, and management of digital files. Students can gather learning resources, track academic achievement, exchange ideas, and receive feedback using these systems. One could imagine that in the future, veterinary students would use e-portfolios as a communication tool with potential employers, allowing them to highlight their skills and professional goals, perhaps utilizing social networking websites such as LinkedIn to share their portfolios.

Web 3.0

The term Web 3.0 is sometimes used to describe platforms that combine aspects of both the digital and the physical worlds. Combined hardware and software platforms such as zSpace and echopixel offer the potential to transform education through virtual reality. Imagine students being able to manipulate a realistic three-dimensional model of an animal as they review the regional anatomy in preparation for performing an unfamiliar surgery.

Adaptive Testing and Customized Teaching

The typical veterinary program is a largely homogeneous experience. A student enrolled within a course has virtually the same experience as every other student within that course. In the future, veterinary education will likely offer a much more customized learning experience, one that immediately flexes to a student's specific needs. Using computer-based assessments, administered at regular intervals throughout a course, students will be assigned customized learning pathways. Imagine a technology platform that allows students to hone their clinical reasoning skills by feeding them the appropriate cases at the right time to help them progress toward mastery.

Putting It All Together

In this final section, we present a project-planning exercise to demonstrate how to design and incorporate effective technology-enhanced learning activities. Recall from the TPACK model that successful implementation of technology requires a consideration of content, pedagogy, and technology in order to achieve your goals. Although all three elements are critical, pedagogy is often the most challenging to plan. This is reflected in the following thought exercise, in which thinking through the pedagogical needs takes up the majority of the planning time.

Simply put, pedagogy is a word for principles and methods of instruction, and these can be infinitely varied. However, there is a fundamental process to framing and planning your methods for instructing students. Backward design is a process of designing pedagogy in educational programs, whether it is a one-hour class period, a semester-long course, or an entire curriculum. This process is a foundational component of the philosophy of learner-centered teaching, because it helps instructors align their courses with the learning outcomes that students must achieve, rather than falling back to what information the teacher wants to cover. Wiggins and

McTighe (2005) called this backward design; Fink (2013) named it integrated design. No matter the name, the process is the same. In this chapter we will stick with the name backward design because it is the easiest way to remember where the process begins – with the end, of course! As you see in Figure 11.2, there are four steps to creating educational encounters when using backward design. In the previous case studies, you saw three examples where instructors successfully implemented technology in the classroom. These cases were successful in large part due to the planning done using the backward design process.

Now let us work through a simplified planning process for utilizing technology to address an educational need common to many veterinary schools – antibiotic use. As you review this thought exercise, keep in mind that it does not represent a finished product, but rather a dip into the pool of backward design, so that you can begin to appreciate the thought process necessary for including pedagogy in your technology-enhanced learning activities.

The Educational Need

Antimicrobial drug resistance is increasing at an alarming rate, with major implications for both human and animal health. The ability to formulate antibiotic treatment plans that support the appropriate and judicious use of antibiotics is critical for veterinary practice. Although most veterinary school curricula provide 16–20 hours of general antibiotic-related instruction, the average contact time dedicated to the topic of "antibiotic stewardship" is as little as 3 hours (Fajt *et al.*, 2013). Furthermore, the most common strategy for instruction on antibiotics is lecture with PowerPoint or slides (Fajt *et al.*, 2013). Therefore, students are rarely given the opportunity to practice antibiotic use decision-making. The goals in this thought exercise are to give students opportunities to practice antibiotic prescription decision-making in a risk-free environment to build competence and confidence; and to better coordinate and deliver antibiotic-related

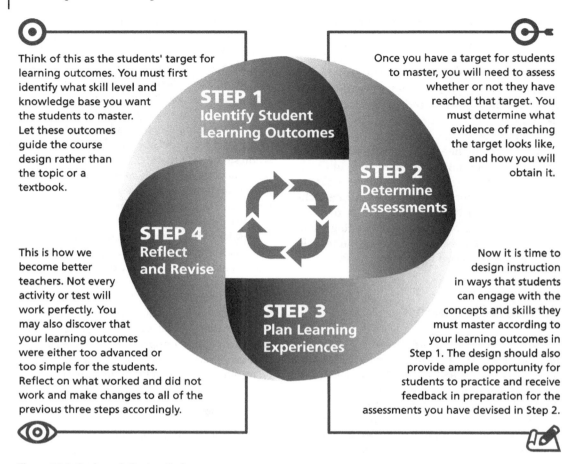

Think of this as the students' target for learning outcomes. You must first identify what skill level and knowledge base you want the students to master. Let these outcomes guide the course design rather than the topic or a textbook.

Once you have a target for students to master, you will need to assess whether or not they have reached that target. You must determine what evidence of reaching the target looks like, and how you will obtain it.

STEP 1 Identify Student Learning Outcomes

STEP 2 Determine Assessments

STEP 4 Reflect and Revise

STEP 3 Plan Learning Experiences

This is how we become better teachers. Not every activity or test will work perfectly. You may also discover that your learning outcomes were either too advanced or too simple for the students. Reflect on what worked and did not work and make changes to all of the previous three steps accordingly.

Now it is time to design instruction in ways that students can engage with the concepts and skills they must master according to your learning outcomes in Step 1. The design should also provide ample opportunity for students to practice and receive feedback in preparation for the assessments you have devised in Step 2.

Figure 11.2 Backwards Design Cycle.

instruction across multiple courses in the four-year curriculum.

Step 1: Identify the Student Learning Outcomes

Ask yourself:

> What should the students be able to do by the time this class or course is completed?

To answer this question, we consider what knowledge and skills the students are missing from their understanding of antibiotics, in order to be responsible veterinary practitioners. We conclude that students lack the ability to apply knowledge about antibiotics to real-life practice situations, including when to prescribe antibiotics and which antibiotics to prescribe under what circumstances. Next, we write a set of learning objectives to document what we will expect of students who complete the new learning activity.

Here are some potential appropriate learning outcomes:

- Students will choose antibiotics appropriate for the bacterial infection, patient conditions, and client circumstances.
- Students will execute appropriate judgment when prescribing antibiotics based on the principles of judicious antimicrobial use.

Notice that these statements begin with the phrase "students will" and are followed by a demonstrable and measurable outcome. It is essential that you are clear in your wording about what skills and knowledge you expect the student to possess at the end of this experience. Do not fall into the trap of using the term "understand." Understanding is difficult to observe and assess, whereas a word like "choose" or "judge" is more precise and measurable. For assistance in selecting appropriate words that define what the student is expected to do, consult Bloom's taxonomy chart. A good resource on Bloom can be found at Heer (2009). Writing good-quality learning outcomes is essential to the design process, yet many instructors skip this step. The necessity for clarity in writing learning outcomes will become more obvious in Step 2 of the backward design method.

As you write learning outcomes, you will need to think carefully about what knowledge and skills are *essential* for students to possess versus those that are just helpful to know. Either of the learning outcomes mentioned could be appropriate to meet our needs, depending on what students have time to master and the training you can feasibly deliver in the time allotted. For purposes of this thought exercise, let us continue with the second outcome: Students will execute appropriate judgment when prescribing antibiotics based on the principles of judicious use.

Step 2: Determine the Assessments

Ask yourself:

How will I know if the students can "execute appropriate judgment when prescribing antibiotics based on the principles of judicious use"?

Now that you have identified what outcomes the students need to achieve during your contact time, you can devise a way to assess whether or not they have achieved the learning outcomes. There are many ways to assess student mastery of learning outcomes. Most instructors immediately think of multiple-choice tests, since that method has been a very common strategy.

However, it would be nearly impossible to create a multiple-choice test that replicates the various circumstances and variables that influence a veterinarian's judgment about whether or not to prescribe an antibiotic, and, if so, selecting the appropriate drug.

A better assessment choice would be to simulate situations in which students must demonstrate good judgment throughout the simulation in order to minimize their contribution to antibiotic resistance. How could we create such a simulation? This is where technology can help. You could create a series of web-based case studies (like those in Case Study 11.1) to simulate the types of decisions that students will face in practice. As students move through the case, they would need to make decisions about what to do at key points where good judgment is required. If the student successfully finishes the case, you know that they have the basic knowledge and judgment to use antibiotics according to the principles of judicious use.

Step 3: Plan Learning Experiences

Ask yourself:

What instructional experiences do the students need that will provide opportunities both to acquire judgment in antibiotic use and to practice these skills in order to achieve the learning outcome?

We decided to use a web-based case-study assessment to measure students' mastery of judgment. It is therefore logical to provide students with similar case studies as part of our instructional design plan. This affords students the opportunity to practice and receive feedback in an authentic environment as they progress toward mastery. Here again, technology provides an advantage. Rather than us creating a static case study on paper, a computer-based case can include photos and videos to make the case as close to the real thing as possible, and branching pathways allow students to see the consequences of their decisions. Additionally, each decision point can be programmed with appropriate feedback explaining why the choice was correct, partially correct, or incorrect. This function is invaluable to the student just learning a new skill, because it provides real-time feedback so that they can immediately correct any misconceptions.

Notice in this thought exercise that the technology solution was selected *after* the learning outcomes were written and was therefore well suited to helping students achieve the learning outcomes. The importance of matching the technology to the outcomes cannot be overemphasized.

Step 4: Reflect and Revise

Ask yourself:

> Where did the students seem to excel? What could I do differently to improve student mastery of my learning outcomes? Since the course ended, have new skills or knowledge been added to veterinary medicine that it would be vital for students to learn?

After delivering the learning activity and examination, you must take time to reflect on how the instruction worked. Even though this last step in the backward instructional design cycle is often overlooked, it is essential to determining whether or not your strategies have been successful. In this example, the cases may have been a little too simple, and the students may have been capable of something more advanced. Additionally, when dealing with technology, logistical issues may occur and adjustments may significantly improve the learning experience for future students. Pilot testing, student

evaluations, and, for large installations, student focus group interviews are some of the many ways in which student feedback can be gathered to facilitate reflection and improvement. Lastly, veterinary medicine is always adding knowledge, skills, and new procedures. If you do not reflect and then revise instruction accordingly, your course may quickly become out of sync with real-world veterinary practice needs.

This thought exercise illustrates just one simplified way for integrating content, pedagogy, and technology while using backward design. There are infinite ways in which you could design instruction, but all good instruction begins with the same process of backward design.

We would like to thank Kevin Cummings, DVM, PhD, Assistant Professor of Epidemiology, Texas A&M University College of Veterinary Medicine & Biomedical Sciences, for his contributions to this exercise.

Conclusion

In this chapter we have endeavored to share with you a proven methodology to develop high-impact, technology-enhanced learning activities in your courses. Through the thoughtful application of technology to support learning goals, you can significantly improve student satisfaction and learning outcomes in your courses. The use of technology to enhance teaching and learning is still in its infancy. It will take a commitment to pedagogy and creativity by veterinary educators who are willing to experiment with new approaches to harness the true potential of educational technologies.

References

Armbruster, P., Patel, M., Johnson, E., and Weiss, M. (2009) Active learning and student-centered pedagogy improve student attitudes and performance in introductory biology. *CBE-Life Sciences Education*, **8** (3), 203–213.

Bowen, J. (2006) Education strategies to promote clinical diagnostic reasoning. *New England Journal of Medicine*, **355**, 2217–2225.

Ericsson, K. (2008) Deliberate practice and acquisition of expert performance: A general overview. *Academic Emergency Medicine*, **15** (**11**), 988–994.

Fajt, V., Scott, H., McIntosh, W., *et al.* (2013) Survey of instructors teaching about antimicrobial resistance in the veterinary professional curriculum in the United States. *Journal of Veterinary Medical Education*, **40** (**1**), 35–44.

Fink, L. (2013) *Creating Significant Learning Experiences: An Integrated Approach to Designing College Courses*, 2nd edn, Jossey-Bass, San Francisco, CA.

Hake, R. (1998) Interactive-engagement versus traditional methods: A six-thousand-student survey of mechanics test data for introductory physics courses. *American Journal of Physics*, **66** (**1**), 64–74.

Heer, R. (2009) *Revised Bloom's Taxonomy*. http://www.celt.iastate.edu/teaching-resources/effective-practice/revised-blooms-taxonomy/ (accessed March 2009).

Kinchin, I. (2012) Avoiding technology-enhanced non-learning. *British Journal of Educational Technology*, **43** (**2**), 42–48.

Knight, J., and Wood, W. (2005) Teaching more by lecturing less. *Cell Biology Education*, **4** (**4**), 298–310.

Mishra, P., and Koehler, M. (2006) Technological pedagogical content knowledge: A framework for teacher knowledge. *Teachers College Record*, **108** (**6**), 1017–1054.

Prince, M. (2004) Does active learning work? A review of the research. *Journal of Engineering Education*, **93**, 223–232.

Reh, D., Ahmed, A., Li, R., *et al.* (2014) A learner-centered educational curriculum improves resident performance on the otolaryngology training examination. *Laryngoscope*, **124** (**10**), 2262–2267.

Schulman, L. (1986) Those who understand: Knowledge growth in teaching. *Educational Researcher*, **15** (**2**), 4–14.

Weimer, M. (2013) *Learner-Centered Teaching: Five Key Changes to Practice*, 2nd edn, John Wiley & Sons, Inc., Hoboken, NJ.

Wiggins, G., and McTighe, J. (2005) What is backward design?, in *Understanding by Design* (eds G. Wiggins and J. McTighe), Association for Supervision and Curriculum Development, Alexandria, VA, pp. 7–19.

12

Learning in the Veterinary Teaching Hospital
Elizabeth M. Hardie

College of Veterinary Medicine, North Carolina State University, USA

 Box 12.1: Key messages

- Excellent clinical teachers act as "multipliers," using their entire team to solve problems.
- Clear learning outcomes for clinical rotations make learning less haphazard.
- Clinical teaching can be broken into components that are easily taught, called microskills.

- Talking through the cognitive process helps to make the expert's thought process overt for novices.
- The problem-oriented medical record allows students to develop critical thinking skills.

Characteristics of a Good Clinical Educator

Academic veterinarians balance many roles (Kochevar and Peycke, 2008; Magnier *et al.*, 2014; Smith and Lane, 2015). When asked to rank the characteristics that the best clinical teachers exhibit, both students and other clinicians ranked enthusiasm (energetic, positive attitude, enjoys their job), competence/knowledge (competent in case management, professional skills, knows literature, engaged in continuing professional development), and clarity (answers questions clearly, summarizes important points, able to explain difficult topics) as the top three characteristics (Bolt, Witte, and Lygo-Baker, 2010; Smith and Lane, 2015; Sutkin *et al.*, 2008). Other important skills were availability, positive relationship with students, being nonjudgmental, feedback skills, being a role model, professionalism, sincerity, being organized, being well prepared, demonstrating evidence-based practice, scholarly activity, and listening skills (Bolt, Witte, and Lygo-Baker, 2010; Sutkin *et al.*, 2008).

Recent attention in the medical literature has focused on defining the model of the clinical teacher as an individual who can "multiply," rather than "diminish," the intelligence of the clinical team (Wiseman, Bradwejn, and Westbroek, 2014). As medicine has become more of a team effort, the brilliant lone clinician has become less effective than the clinician who can use the skills of their entire team to produce an outcome that is better than that achieved by any one individual (Reader *et al.*, 2009). The Multiplier (Wiseman, Bradwejn, and Westbroek, 2014) makes sure that decision-making and responsibility are spread among the team,

Veterinary Medical Education: A Practical Guide, First Edition. Edited by Jennifer L. Hodgson and Jacquelyn M. Pelzer.
© 2017 John Wiley & Sons, Inc. Published 2017 by John Wiley & Sons, Inc.

with each member taking on tasks that are important. In this way, each level of the team is contributing to the overall outcome. Each time the team functions in this way, learning happens, new ideas and expertise are incorporated, and the ability of the team to work together to achieve a better outcome is enhanced. In contrast, the Diminisher (Wiseman, Bradwejn, and Westbroek, 2014) is directive, making all the important decisions, relying on their expertise. The team members are good at executing orders, but do not contribute in a meaningful way to the knowledge or the plan that is used to manage the case. Learning is stifled and the case outcome may be poorer, because the team members have little incentive to stretch their knowledge or to take responsibility for the safety and welfare of the patient.

Creation of a Good Learning Environment

The first step in making the hospital accessible and friendly to students is to develop clear policies and procedures. The functioning of the hospital may seem self-evident to the experienced clinicians who live and breathe the clinic's formal and informal rules, but having written policies clarifies the environment for the novice. Some examples would be:

- Dress code.
- Treatment responsibilities and times.
- Drug-dispensing protocols.
- Medical record navigation and policies.
- Client communication expectations.
- Interprofessional communication expectations.
- Service schedules.

The physical layout of the hospital should include spaces that allow discussion outside the main work flow. These can be "nooks" that allow the clinician to confer quickly with team members, or they can be rounds rooms with doors that can be closed (Lane and Cornell, 2013). If the work flow is constant in the service rounds room, it may be necessary to find a space

elsewhere. Since the majority of information will be recorded in electronic format, a projector and screen will also be needed. Focusing the learner's attention on one main screen will help prevent the multitasking that occurs if many small screens are open.

The service atmosphere that encourages learning is one in which each student is encouraged to speak, there are no "stupid" questions, and "I don't know" is regarded as an opportunity to learn. The information flow is multidirectional (Lane and Cornell, 2013). The team practices self-care and notices if any member is getting overwhelmed or needs help. Everyone on the team is reflecting on and working on their learning issues. When an individual masters a concept or skill that has been difficult, the team celebrates.

Developing Learning Outcomes

Learning outcomes set the teaching goals for each clinical rotation. Writing these outcomes will help determine if the rotation activities allow each student to accomplish the outcomes or if additional resources are needed. Writing outcomes that include the development of noncognitive skills helps focus students on the acquisition of key skills that they might otherwise ignore. Teachers should also encourage students to produce their own individualized rotational learning goals, recorded on an index card or a personal computer (Lane and Cornell, 2013). Checking these goals on a daily basis helps both the student and the teacher devise learning practice that actually happens in the distracting clinical environment.

Using the Microskill Approach to Help Students Develop Task Mastery

There is increasing evidence that breaking complex tasks into smaller component (micro) skills that can be mastered individually is a more efficient method of teaching than trying to teach an entire task all at once (Neher *et al.*, 1992; Razavi *et al.*, 2010). Cognitive task analysis, a formal method of determining component skills, looks at each decision point in a procedure and determines how experts navigate these points (Wingfield *et al.*, 2015). A less formal method involves having at least three experts write down the steps of a procedure or process, followed by a consensus session in which they discuss why they do what they do. Regardless of how one gets to the component skills, the task for the busy clinician-teacher is to identify which component skills a student needs to practice and to devise a method that enables the student to practice within the clinical environment.

Using the Microskill Approach to Ensure a Focus on Learning

Before focusing on the skills the student needs, the teacher should focus on what skills they need to teach in the hospital. Because the clinic is so distracting for both teachers and students, a number of systems have been developed to help learning occur within the normal flow of a busy practice. These systems break the task of clinical teaching into manageable steps that are easy to remember and master (Baker *et al.*, 2015; Lane and Cornell, 2013; Neher *et al.*, 1992; Pascoe, Nixon, and Lang, 2015; Wolpaw *et al.*, 2012; Wolpaw, Wolpaw, and Papp, 2003). All concentrate on assessing where the student is in their reasoning and helping them to progress. Perhaps best known is the "one-minute manager" or "five microskills" system (see Box 12.2), which can be used at any step of the decision-making process (Neher *et al.*, 1992; Wolpaw *et al.*, 2012).

Getting a commitment starts with asking the right questions ("Which diagnosis do you think is most likely?" "What treatment option are you going to pick?" "What do you think the results of this test are going to be?"). As an example, a student has committed to a tentative diagnosis of neoplasia regarding a young indoor–outdoor male cat presenting with an enlarging painful mass over the right shoulder and a body

Box 12.2: Quick Tip – five microskills for clinical teaching

- Get a commitment
- Probe for supporting evidence
- Teach general rules
- Reinforce what was done right
- Correct mistakes

temperature of 102.9 °F. Once the student has committed to a likely diagnosis, diagnostic plan, treatment plan, or opinion about the case, the teacher then asks for supporting evidence.

The second step should be limited to a few encouraging questions, rather than "grilling" the student to the bottom of her knowledge base. For the teacher, it is a diagnostic step to determine the student's reasoning. The teacher must guard against using this step to get enough data to solve the problem. In our example, the student thinks that neoplasia is most likely because the rapid enlargement of the mass and pain the cat is displaying are most likely to indicate neoplasia. When the clinician asked if the student had any thoughts regarding the body temperature, the student indicated that she thought that it was within normal limits for a painful cat in an exam room.

Once the student has explained her reasoning, the teacher moves to the third step, which is to take the student's specific reasoning and relate it to a more general rule or treatment principle. This is a good place to indicate to the student that we are all learners. In our example, the clinician might say: "The most likely neoplastic cause of a rapidly enlarging mass over the shoulder in a young cat is vaccine-induced fibrosarcoma, but I believe that recommended vaccine sites are more distal. I can't remember the exact recommendations, so you might want to look these up and report back to the group."

The next step is specifically to praise what was done right. In this case the student has conducted a very thorough history, so the clinician might say: "You used your funnel technique very effectively. You went from open-ended questions to close-ended questions. You listened quietly and reflected the client's answers back to him to ensure that you heard correctly."

The final step is to correct mistakes. The best way to correct a mistake is to get the student to correct herself, so the teacher might say: "Can you think of any other conditions that might cause fever, pain, and swelling?" In this case, the teacher has reframed the complaint into a sequence that might help the student remember that infection causes heat, pain, and swelling. If the student says an abscess, then the teacher can say: "Good thought. What can we do to tell these two conditions apart?" If the student remains puzzled, the teacher can say: "What would you like to do to determine if this mass is neoplastic?"

It should be noted that the fifth skill (correct mistakes) was deliberately placed last by the developers of the one-minute manager/five microskills technique. It is common for busy clinicians to use a student as an information conduit to solve clinical problems efficiently (Wolpaw, Wolpaw, and Papp, 2003). Once the information is gathered, the clinician may ask a question or two of the student regarding the case and rapidly correct any misconceptions. This is considered to be teaching on the fly. The good news is that the student does get rapid feedback and, if delivered nonjudgmentally, the feedback is likely to be effective. The problem is that the student has no opportunity to practice framing an idea, supporting that idea, receiving wisdom on how to tie the specific case to general knowledge, receiving feedback on what was done well, correcting herself, and then moving to the next step. Sticking to the five skills reminds the busy clinician to help the student teach herself first and to correct the student second.

Clinical/Critical Thinking Development

In order to be able to teach clinical reasoning, it helps to understand how expert clinicians solve diagnostic and other clinical problems. There is a developing body of research regarding expert diagnosis and how it differs from novice diagnosis (Bordage, Grant, and Marsden, 1990; Custers, 2015; Harasym, Tsai, and Hemmati, 2008; Norman, 2005; Sutkin *et al.*, 2008). The expert uses a highly nuanced "illness script," which is a mental description of the prototypical case with neural connections to memories of exceptions, things to watch out for, and individual case features. This description is temporally sequenced according to the usual information flow and management sequence of the case. The memory of the case is stored in long-term memory and mental processing is very rapid. The diagnosis is often being refined by the expert early in the history-taking process. If the case has no key distinguishing features or there are features that do not fit, the expert goes to a search pattern based on a schema or algorithm, which is still very rapid. If needed, the expert can go to the slower, hypothesis-based reasoning pattern that allows for testing of each case feature against what the expert knows about the pathophysiology of the disease process. The expert primarily uses the illness script to get the diagnosis, but rapidly switches between the other two modes as needed. Experts who use illness script and algorithm-based reasoning to solve diagnostic problems have been shown to be much faster and more accurate than those who use hypothesis-based deductive reasoning for clinical problem-solving.

In contrast, most students come out of their preclinical years reliant on using pathophysiology as the starting point for an undifferentiated list of disease entities and their features (Harasym, Tsai, and Hemmati, 2008; Sutkin *et al.*, 2008). Depending on the curriculum, the "mental storage boxes" for the various disease entities may be based on discipline, system, disease feature, or clinical presentation. The goal of students' teaching hospital experience is to help them build appropriate prototypical illness descriptions and to link them to previous knowledge (Bowen, 2006). This process will allow students to develop rapid, accurate diagnostic abilities and, if needed, "backward" processing to access previously learned basic knowledge. Locating where a student is in their development of diagnostic reasoning requires that the clinician have a system for assessing a student's processing (Baker *et al.*, 2015). Using the five microskills approach in combination with the assessment portion of the **P**roblem-**O**riented **M**edical **R**ecord (POMR; Weed, 1968) will quickly give the clinician an idea of whether the student needs to work on basic knowledge ("I don't know anything about this disease presentation or its pathophysiology"), to develop schemes to manage and use their knowledge ("I do know, here's all of my knowledge, help me prioritize it"), or is at the stage of developing generalized illness descriptions that incorporate pertinent clinical details and relative likelihood of disease.

Once the teacher knows the student's processing level, the challenge is to give the student a learning task that will enable them to move toward the next stage and to bring value to the group processing of the case. The temptation for the expert, who rapidly processes complex case details, is either to bypass the student and teach general knowledge in a rounds session, or to overwhelm the student with rapid details and orders, putting them into a "fetch and do paperwork" role. If the teacher and student have already determined rotational and individual learning goals, these goals can be used to focus learning. The student with a weak knowledge base can be assigned specific "look-up" tasks to report back to the group. The student who needs algorithms or organizational schema can be tasked with finding them and explaining them to the group. All students benefit when the clinician takes a specific case presentation and converts it into a more generalized description. It is much easier for the student to retain the generalized illness description if the teacher uses a contrast-and-compare method when converting a specific case to the general case (Bowen, 2006). As an example, if the case involves a large breed of dog presenting for lethargy and collapse, with a large spleen and a low packed cell volume, whose diagnosis is splenic torsion, the clinician would review the clinical features used to differentiate splenic torsion from hemagiosarcoma or immune-mediated anemia.

Diagnostic reasoning is only one aspect of a clinician's cognitive task. A diagnostic and treatment plan also need to be developed. Again, the temptation when the hospital gets busy is to use rapid mental processing to develop the list of necessary tests or treatments and assign the student to making them happen. Using the five microskills approach regarding diagnostic and treatment plans will help the student own the clinical tasks and will allow the teacher to devise an appropriate learning task. The student with little knowledge is encouraged to review testing details and to report back. The student who already knows the common testing algorithms can be assigned to look at evidence-based treatment options or to consult with other specialists, expanding the knowledge of the entire group. Management decisions can be compared with evidence for efficacy, and the specific choice for the patient can be used as a focal point to discuss how one takes evidence and applies it to a specific case.

The POMR is an essential tool in teaching clinical reasoning (Weed, 1968). By having the student identify each problem and complete **S**ubjective observations, **O**bjective observations, **A**ssessment of, and a **P**lan for each problem (SOAP), the clinician can identify the student's ability to delineate problems, to process each problem, and to propose methods for diagnosis and/or treatment. With the transition to electronic medical records, some teaching hospital services have converted to a medical/legal record, while others maintain the traditional POMR (Friedman, Sainte, and Fallar, 2010; Peled *et al.*, 2009). The most valuable aspect of the SOAP format is the assessment field, which allows the student to discuss their reasoning regarding the specific problem and their rationale for choosing specific diagnostic tests or treatments. If the POMR is to have teaching value, daily, specific, constructive written feedback must be provided to the student regarding their thought processing. Making sure that the electronic record allows student case notes with feedback is critical for students to practice reasoning through cases.

Surgical Teaching

Surgical planning and execution, during which the student is part of a large surgical team, is a common treatment scenario in the teaching hospital. In order to ensure that students' learning needs are addressed in this process, the BID (**B**rief, **I**ntraoperative teaching, **D**ebrief) method was developed (Roberts *et al.*, 2009, 2012). In the Brief session, the surgeon asks the learner about their learning goals for the surgery. Once the goals are established, they guide the teaching within the Intraoperative phase. After the surgery, the Debrief occurs. This has four parts: reflection, rules, reinforcement, and correction (see Box 12.3). Using this system, the surgeon can quickly establish different learning goals for the resident and the

---

 Box 12.3: Focus on the BID system for surgical teaching

Brief

Teacher: "Lisa, I know you have had considerable experience on the mobile unit doing spays and neuters. What are your goals for learning during this intestinal resection/anastomosis?"

Student: "I'd really like to review the anatomy and I would like to place at least one intestinal suture, if possible."

Teacher: "Did you complete the resection/anastomosis exercise in the simulation laboratory?"

Student: "I sure did and I've only had one cup of coffee this morning!"

Teacher: "Sounds like you are ready to help us, provided the tissues aren't too friable."

Intraoperative

Teacher: "Lisa, now that we have the abdomen exposed, how are we going to differentiate the jejunum from the ileum?"

Student: "The ileum is going to have an antimesenteric vessel, while the jejunum does not. Both have arcade vasculature on the mesenteric side."

Teacher: "Since the mass we are removing is in the distal jejunum, how does the arcade vasculature affect the surgery?"

Once the surgeon has completed the mesenteric aspect of the anastomosis, the student places two sutures in an easily accessible portion of the intestine. Her hands are steady and she has good fine motor control.

Debrief

Teacher: "Lisa, what did you find most challenging about placing the intestinal sutures?"

Student: "It was hard to avoid incorporating the mucosa into the suture bite." (Reflection)

Teacher: "It can be difficult to keep the mucosa from rolling out. You can trim it if needed. (Rules) You showed good fine motor control and you placed the suture correctly, exiting the submucosa while avoiding the mucosa. (Reinforcement) You might want to practice torquing your hand a bit more as you place the suture. If the tissues are friable, pushing in a straight line, rather than following a curved motion, can tear the tissues." (Correction)

student, allowing the teaching to be focused on the individual learner's needs.

Other practices (Zundel *et al.*, 2015) that students, residents, and surgeons identify as helpful for learning when the student is not the primary surgeon include the following:

- Familiarize the student with the operating room environment and its rules.
- Talk about team function in the operating room and relate how it contributes to the outcome.
- Make sure that the student has detailed procedural information and time to prepare for a given surgery.
- Assign one person to be in charge of teaching so that the student knows to whom to address questions.
- Talk through the procedure before and while doing it.
- Make sure that the student knows their expected role in the operating room.
- Ask questions of the student.
- Show enthusiasm for student learning in the operating room.

Psychomotor Skills Development

When teaching psychomotor skills in the clinic, there must be a balance between giving the students experience, patient welfare, and the efficiency of the clinic. Clinicians need to establish what skills are to be practiced or demonstrated on the rotation. Rules for patient welfare and efficiency (typically, X tries or X minutes) need to be explained and enforced. As with cognitive skills, the most efficient way to develop expertise is to practice the component skills and then put the entire task together (Razavi *et al.*, 2010; Wingfield *et al.*, 2015). Having a skills video library available allows the clinician/technician to direct the student to the video before performing the task. This step ensures that the student reviews the steps, without taking up the teacher's time. The teacher can then ensure content knowledge and observe the student as the entire task is performed.

After the task is finished, the student is asked to self-critique, the teacher gives praise on the specific things the student did well, and the teacher offers tips for getting to the next level of mastery. If needed, the student is directed to practice of specific component parts of the skill.

Communication Skills Development

There are innumerable opportunities to teach communication in the teaching hospital (Adams and Kurtz, 2012). Developing communication policies and protocols within the hospital ensures that staff and students have a similar understanding of the communication requirements. Creating communication learning outcomes for each rotation ensures that this important skill does not get forgotten. Providing the student with a small laminated patient communication summary sheet, such as the Calgary–Cambridge Communication Process Skills Guide, provides a framework for them to follow (Kurtz *et al.*, 2003).

Teaching of oral communication has traditionally focused on veterinary student–client interactions, such as history taking, phone communication, and giving discharge instructions. If the exam rooms have one-way glass or video cameras, students can practice their communication skills under observation with direct feedback. If the exam rooms are closed to observation, using two students at a time in a room can enable one student to be the communicator and one to be the recorder for peer feedback. A resident or clinician can serve the same role, but that is often more threatening to the student. Another method for getting immediate and direct feedback is to solicit feedback from the client. Experienced clients can often give very helpful suggestions. If the clinician is comfortable with teaching the component skills for client communication, using role play in the rounds setting provides an opportunity for practice and feedback (Nestel and Tierney, 2007). Phone communications are an opportunity to practice more advanced skills, such as talking about money and empathically listening to an anxious client.

As teamwork becomes the norm in veterinary medicine, being overt and mindful about communications within the hospital is a necessary step. It is helpful to students to have clinicians discuss the communication standards and processes within the hospital, rather than simply modeling them. In busy hospitals these communications can involve a plethora of face-to-face, phone, e-mail, text message, and web-based medical record communications. Without agreed upon standards, communications can be less than professional and occur at all hours, regardless of emergent status, under the stress of handling complex cases in a complex environment. Sample rules include that text messages and e-mails are limited to facts; communication between certain hours is limited to a true need-to-know basis; face-to-face communication is on a first-name basis for all team members within a given area; face-to-face communication uses formal names under specified circumstances; no whining about or belittling of other services or their staff members. It helps to have a ready list of examples of professional exchanges for the clinicians to model and the students to practice. Students are very astute at picking up the "hidden curriculum" in the clinic (Birden et al., 2013; Madigosky et al., 2006), and if poor interprofessional communication behaviors are tolerated, they can become very cynical about whether good communication skills really matter.

Veterinary teaching hospitals are getting bigger and the distractions from mobile technology are increasing. As human hospitals increased in size, many adopted formal communication and body-language rules from the hospitality industry (Wu, Robson, and Hollis, 2013), such as "Smile and make eye contact if you are within 20 feet of another person, speak to the person if within 10 feet." Showing students that adopting a few basic communication policies can lead to a better work environment and having students practice colleague interaction skills helps to prepare them for work within both small and large organizations.

Teamwork Skills Development

Medical teams differ by specialty, but those most studied are "action" teams functioning in high-risk settings such as the emergency room, intensive care unit (ICU), surgery, or anesthesia (Fernandez et al., 2008; Manser, 2009; Morey et al., 2002; Morrison, Goldfarb, and Lanken, 2010; Reader et al., 2009; Risser et al., 1999; Salas et al., 2008). Characteristics of highly functional medical teams include dispersed leadership, individual and mutual accountability, defined outcomes that the team needs to accomplish, engaging in open-ended discussion and problem-solving meetings, ability to deliver a collective work product, and ability to discuss, decide, and work together. The role of the senior clinician in the teams with the best performance has been shown to be that of a delegator and flexible process monitor, similar to the Multiplier, who helps every member of the team contribute their best effort to the task at hand (Reader et al., 2009). There are a number of medical staff training protocols that are being adapted for medical student and resident training (Crew Resource Management, MEDTeams, TeamSTEPPS), and the US Accreditation Council for Graduate Medical Education now requires programs to provide this training (Haerkens et al., 2015; Morey et al., 2002; Salas et al., 2008).

Patient safety concerns within human hospitals have resulted in a number of communication protocols designed to prevent errors and improve handoffs between caregiver teams (Haig, Sutton, and Whittington, 2006; Lenert, Sakaguchi, and Weir, 2014; Motley and Dolansky, 2015; Risser et al., 1999; Thompson et al., 2008; Townsend-Gervis, Cornell, and Vardaman, 2014). Teaching these protocols to veterinary students can help develop more precise thinking about the case and can provide opportunities for the practice of basic team communications skills. The most common mnemonic used for case handoffs is SBAR (**S**ituation, **B**ackground, **A**ssessment, **R**ecommendation), though more recently the I-PASS (IIPE-PRIS **A**ccelerating **S**afe **S**ign-outs) has been developed as another aid for standardizing the handoff (Starmer *et al.*, 2012). These remind the communicator to convey the present situation of the patient, background of the patient, assessment of patient problems, and recommendations for problem resolution. While the mnemonic has not solved all deficiencies in the transfer of case information, it has been shown to improve safety and the quality of the transfer information. Other commonly taught team communication skills (Fernandez *et al.*, 2008; Risser *et al.*, 1999) are the following:

- *Closed-loop confirmation*:

  VETERINARIAN CHRIS   "Sally, this 10-year-old FS (female spayed) Labrador Retriever needs a large-bore jugular catheter placed and Lactated Ringer's solution needs to be started at a rate of 10 ml/kg/hr."

  VETERINARY TECHNICIAN SALLY   "Chris, I hear that you want a 10-gauge jugular catheter to be placed in this 10-year-old FS Lab and then you want me to start giving Lactated Ringer's at a rate of 10 ml/kg/hr using that line."

- *Second challenge*:

  VETERINARIAN CHRIS   "Sally, please administer 30 mg/kg of cefoxatin IV to Duffy."

  VETERINARY STUDENT JANET   "Duffy is allergic to amoxicillin. Can he get cefoxitin?"

  VETERINARIAN CHRIS   "Janet, thanks for reminding me. We should give it slowly. The risk of cross-reactivity with second-generation cephalosporins is low, but reactions do happen."

- *Call-out*: This technique is used when team members have assigned roles, as in an acute trauma assessment or cardiac code team. Each team member is assigned to one region or vital sign and calls out the assessment to the recorder. The recorder confirms with closed-loop communication and records the assessment. Assigning a student to the recorder role allows them to practice closed-loop communication and accurate recording.

In each of these examples, all members of the team are on a first-name basis and all have a responsibility to speak up if they think there is a problem, in keeping with safety culture recommendations to develop a flat, nonhierarchical culture.

Professional Identity Development

Students enter veterinary college with an incomplete understanding of the many roles that veterinarians occupy, the skills needed to survive as a veterinarian, and the ethical dilemmas that all veterinarians face at some time in their career. Best evidence suggests that role modeling and mentoring are major methods through which students develop their identities, and that the clinical environment is critical to the student's development of a positive attitude toward the profession and its code of behavior (Birden *et al.*, 2013). The difference between professionalism, which is a prescribed set of successful professional behaviors, and professional identity formation has to be clarified. One definition from medical training is:

> Professional identity formation is the transformative journey through which one integrates the knowledge, skills, behaviors and values of a competent, humanistic physician with one's own unique identity and core values. This continuous process fosters personal and professional growth through mentorship, self-reflection, and experiences that affirm the best practices, traditions and ethics of the medical profession. The education of all medical students is founded on professional identity formation. (Holden *et al.*, 2015, p. 762)

Within both human and veterinary medicine, fairly complete lists of the full task domains and the component skills are available (Burns *et al.*, 2006; Holden *et al.*, 2015; Pelzer, Hodgson, and Werre, 2014). Recently attention has focused on self-care, resilience, and wellness behaviors as being necessary for a fruitful and successful veterinary career (Cake *et al.*, 2015).

Clinicians can foster the development of the student's professional identity by modeling and encouraging self-reflection (Buckley *et al.*, 2009; Driessen, van Tartwijk, and Dornan, 2008; Wald, 2015). This one skill is the means through which a student can integrate the suggested roles, behaviors, skills, and so on into their own sense of themselves. Having this habit has been shown to contribute to personal resilience (Wald, 2015). In its most complete form, teaching of reflection involves developing a mentored portfolio of written reflections on a number of topics. This portfolio gives the student practice in looking a situation, defining the essentials, developing a plan for a similar or alternative plan for the next similar situation, and then trying out a new plan. It allows the clinician-teacher to provide the support and challenge needed to grow the student. Sample topics include ethical dilemmas, management of a case, and behavior toward a co-worker. If time is short, the clinician may only have the opportunity to encourage verbal self-reflection (the five microskills model can be used) or an unmentored personal student blog/journal. Simply discussing the value of the habit and incorporating self-reflection topics into the flow of clinic teaching show the student that the practice is valuable. Perhaps if more students were taught this skill, there would be less despair when veterinarians encountered difficult situations in practice.

Provision of Practice Opportunities

Within the clinic, the development of practice opportunities must be deliberate if the student is reliably to master the skills needed for practice. It is too easy for a student to be a good "worker," performing all designated tasks, yet failing to practice independent decision-making,

identification of learning gaps, or skill mastery. Clinician time should be prioritized for teaching topics that are not taught well by technology, such as debriefing of communications, discussions of ethical dilemmas, or prioritization of complex treatment decisions. As teaching moves more toward a coaching role and away from "professing," time to assess and develop a plan for each student's learning needs must be available. Many resourceful clinicians keep notes on their students similar to those they keep on their cases, allowing them to direct the student to the best use of their clinic experience. Having reliable, readily available web-based learning resources in addition to the more traditional resources (books, articles, preclinical notes) broadens the experience that can be provided in the hospital.

Rounds

Rounds have traditionally been used as the primary mode of teaching in the hospital. Rounds occupy a significant portion of the clinician's time and need to be structured to deliver the most effective learning possible and to include activities that cannot be duplicated by other means (Lane and Cornell, 2013). To maximize benefit, the learning outcome of the rounds session should be stated. Examples are case-based rounds with self-reflection on learning goals; topic-based rounds in which each member of the team will present information at their level; house officer rounds focused on advanced communication skills; role-playing rounds in which communication skills can be practiced; or financial dilemma case-based rounds. Once the learners know what to prepare for, the teacher needs to establish a safe climate for practice and to ensure that all students are heard. Having a system in which the learner presents the case succinctly and then focuses on the uncertainties the case material has generated has been shown to be an effective way to increase the delivery of material that the student actually needs for learning, rather than what the teacher thinks is needed (Wolpaw *et al.*, 2012). If the teacher models prompting ("Keep going, I'd like to hear more"), sharing the spotlight ("I'd like to hear more about what Allen thinks about those laboratory findings"), showing uncertainty ("That's really interesting new information you presented and we will have to consider this in our case management plan"), case extension ("What would you have done if this case had presented to a hospital in which radiographs and non-expert ultrasonagraphy were the only imaging modalities?"), role play ("Let's do some role play to practice how this sensitive information might be conveyed to the owner"), or commitment ("Let's all bet on what the complete blood count is going to look like in this case"), the entire team will often quickly pick up on the active learning style and incorporate it in their presentations (Lane and Cornell, 2013). Incorporating self-reflection into the presentation ("What did you do well in this presentation and what could be improved?") allows the student to become comfortable with feedback. The teacher can coach the other learners as they present feedback to help them learn appropriate, specific language for providing feedback. If needed, the teacher can pull a student aside after rounds to deliver feedback regarding some serious deficiency in a timely, private manner.

Medical Records

The POMR has long been used as a tool to train students in critical reasoning (Weed, 1968). In order to be effective, the written feedback for the student needs to be specific and timely, so that the next problem list, SOAP, or discharge instructions can be used to practice new skills. If the teacher gives the student a few items to practice in the next writing event, the student will have a learning outcome to achieve and the feedback process can proceed with them achieving increasingly difficult goals. Providing the feedback as questions can help students begin to ask themselves the questions, a key element in developing a habit of self-reflection and life-long learning. A common dilemma is whether or not to correct spelling and grammar, which are not the primary focus of the feedback.

Couching these corrections in the context of professionalism and professional respect can help to make these "picky" corrections more palatable. Asking a student to self-correct a sample of their own writing can guide the teacher's coaching. If the student can recognize needed improvements in prioritization, summarization, reasoning, use of appropriate vocabulary, spelling, or grammar, the teacher needs only to get them to focus on practicing the deficient area. If the student cannot recognize deficiencies and self-critique, the teacher must help them understand the standard against which they are being judged and then give them practice in recognizing whether the standard has been met or not. If the POMR reveals a true knowledge deficit, then the teacher can point to resources to help the student acquire the necessary knowledge.

Web-Based Practice

Web-based practice tools are very useful to ensure that each student on a rotation leaves having been exposed to the basic knowledge, skills, and attitudes detailed in the learning outcomes for the rotation. Web practice has been shown to be a successful method for the delivery of image-recognition practice (dermatological photos, ophthalmic photos, neurological videos, orthopedic videos, electrocardiograms, various imaging modalities; Hatala, Brooks, and Norman, 2003; Vandeweerd *et al.*, 2007). Mixing up different types of cases and images has been shown to offer better long-term retention than providing neatly organized images (Cendan and Lok, 2012; Hatala, Brooks, and Norman, 2003). Providing feedback that compares and contrasts the image details for different kinds of cases allows the student to retain the knowledge more easily (Cendan and Lok, 2012).

Web-based case scenarios allow exposure to prototypical cases and can be used to teach clinical reasoning, if appropriate feedback is provided as the student goes through the case. Students prefer cases that take about 15 minutes to complete (Jäger *et al.*, 2014; Kleinsmith *et al.*, 2015) rather than longer cases. Case design can be either linear or branching, but linear cases are much easier to create in most online learning environments. Students who complete virtual cases in pairs, discussing each case decision, perform better in follow-up tests than students who work alone (Jäger *et al.*, 2014). Effect sizes for learning using virtual cases have been shown to be larger for clinical reasoning than for communication or ethics training (Consorti, 2012). By mixing virtual case practice with face-to-face discussion regarding the virtual case, the clinician-teacher can take advantage of the ready pool of material that students have practiced and expand on the areas that need discussion.

Simulations

Simulation training can range from task trainers for isolated skill practice, to stuffed animals with paper case material, to virtual reality cases that respond as a patient and client would (Motola *et al.*, 2013). The most-studied use of simulation training for clinical case material has been in training for emergent scenarios in the emergency department, trauma center, or an anesthesia setting (McGaghie *et al.*, 2010; Steadman *et al.*, 2012). Training using simulation is very effective, because it allows response teams or students to practice repeatedly in a training setting that closely resembles the actual clinical setting. Simulation training in medical schools is now expanding to train students in the management of prototypical cases in various specialties. These high-fidelity virtual reality trainers are very expensive to build, so simulation training of case material in veterinary colleges is likely to be mixed-modality training, in which the simulation provides the case details or dilemma, to which the students then respond, while the teacher directs the mannequin's response. The addition of simulations can turn a routine verbal rounds discussion into an exciting learning setting that involves responding to various clinical presentations, role playing the initial communications, using task trainers to practice the fine motor skills needed for some appropriate intervention,

practicing teamwork using a treatment protocol, and then crafting an appropriate handoff communication.

Actual Clients and Patients

The role of the teaching hospital as the provider of exciting and relevant case material for training students cannot be underestimated. Recently, concern has been expressed that specialty service-based hospitals do not provide adequate case material for training students in entry-level general practice skills (Stone *et al.*, 2012). In response, many colleges have created primary care clinics to provide exposure to general practice cases. Students can readily go back and forth and learn from both complex and primary care cases, as long as teachers are respectful and clear about the difference between being a skilled primary care clinician and being a skilled specialist (May, 2015). In the primary care setting the focus is on wellness, disease prevention, and initial diagnosis and treatment. Chronic patients in this setting have responded to therapy and can be managed by caregivers at home. This setting allows students to get repeated practice in maintaining relationships with long-term clients, in enabling clients to keep animals healthy, and in responding to typical client complaints regarding the health of their animal(s). In the specialty setting, the focus is on diagnosis of cases for whom routine diagnostics and treatment have failed to lead to resolution of disease, and on providing diagnostic and treatment modalities that are beyond the scope of primary care. Learning to process the specialty cases provides the student with repeated practice in diagnostic reasoning, advanced client communication, teamwork, and navigating systems-based medicine. Within the specialty hospital, breaking the case up into components and allowing the student to concentrate on one problem at a time provides practice in problem identification, problem assessment, and prioritization of diagnostic and treatment plans. Limiting the number of cases assigned to a student prevents cognitive overload and exhaustion as the student completes tasks that are very energy intensive (Ericsson, 2008).

Managed well, the teaching hospital provides a rich intellectual environment that allows the student repeatedly to practice cognitive and noncognitive skills in a variety of settings and in the presence of clinician-teachers who care deeply about student learning. The case material provides the stimulus for far-ranging discussions, allowing the student to connect the knowledge and skills being learned to prior learning experiences. The student's attitudes benefit from being modeled on empathic clinicians who gain respect as they practice in a competent and caring fashion.

Assessment on the Clinic Floor

Assessment drives learning because, when time is limited, the student will focus on the specific learning needed to pass a high-stakes test that determines whether or not they will pass the rotation. Unless the assessments are designed to promote learning that achieves the rotation learning outcomes, there will be a "disconnect" between the outcomes and the learning. Writing the outcomes first, then designing the assessments to get the desired outcome, and only then determining the focus of the learning activities on the rotation will ensure alignment. Assessment methods that can be used on the clinic floor are detailed in Part Three, Chapter 13: Learning in Real-World Settings.

An Example: The Multiplier versus the Diminisher

These examples are based on concepts outlined in Wiseman, Bradwejn, and Westbroek (2014) (see Box 12.4 and Box 12.5).

 Box 12.4: Example of the Multiplier

Dr. Multiplier (Dr. M) is responsible for a clinical neurology rotation that involves a dedicated clinical technician, a third-year resident, a first-year resident, two senior students, and a second-year student. On the first day of the block, he meets with the team and goes over the organization of the service and his service philosophy. He tells them that each of them is responsible for the care and safety of the patients, and outlines the procedure if any member of the team has concerns. Dr. M explains how the five microskills system works and states that he expects the students and the residents to use this approach in case presentations.

Dr. M runs receiving by having the senior students see the cases, with the second-year student acting as an observer and peer coach. The senior student presents his case to the resident and the resident uses the five microskills approach to focus the student's learning. The second-year student is consulted regarding her thoughts on the case presentation. Once the resident has seen the case and confirmed or corrected the student's presentation, Dr. M meets the client and models client communication for the resident and the student. The technician and the student admit the case. Dr. M moves on to debrief the next student and resident.

After receiving two seizure cases, an atlanto-axial subluxation case and a progressive chronic paraplegia case, Dr. M send his students to get lunch and confers with the residents and the technician. They determine the necessary orders, which the technician and residents then process. The students return and the residents and technician go to eat. Dr. M eats while he directs case presentation rounds using a positive and nonthreatening questioning technique. He confirms that each student has a learning outcome for their cases. He determines that one of the senior students is overwhelmed by her cases and that the second-year student has a large amount of clinical experience. He suggests that the second-year student might like to work directly with the resident on one of the seizure cases. The second-year student is confident enough to mention that he thought he heard some irregularity in the dog's heart rhythm on the initial physical exam. Dr. M suggests that the student might want to put in a cardiology consult. When the residents return, Dr. M goes over their learning outcomes for the cases they have chosen. The third-year resident wants to be primary surgeon on the atlanto-axial subluxation and needs to visualize the procedure step by step. The first-year resident wants to direct the workup of the chronic paraplegia case because he is unsure of how to approach this case. Dr. M asks him how he would like to pursue the diagnostic workup. Dr. M lets the students know what they can expect for any afternoon diagnostic procedures and tomorrow's surgery day. He suggests that any student not

involved directly in a procedure might want to work on their written records. The focus of the feedback will be on problem identification and prioritization. The general pathophysiology of each problem must be described.

The afternoon workups proceed, the students work on their records, and the team does a quick debrief at 5 p.m. The second-year student excitedly reports that the cardiology consult has determined that the irregular heart rhythm he thought he heard was caused by ventricular premature beats, and the recommendation is to Holter monitor the dog to determine whether the episodes are seizures, syncope, or a combination of the two. The team high-fives him for a great catch. The third-year resident role plays the client communication regarding this fact and, based on the student's performance, decides that the student should make the call, talk to the client, and then hand off the communication to the resident. Despite this excitement, the entire team is out of the hospital by 5.30 p.m.

 Box 12.5: Example of the Diminsher

Dr. Diminisher (Dr. D) is responsible for a clinical neurology rotation that involves a dedicated clinical technician, a third-year resident, a first-year resident, two senior students, and a second-year student. On the first day of the block, he meets with the team and makes it clear that he is the senior clinician and is ultimately responsible for the care and safety of the patients. He outlines the schedule of the service.

Dr. D runs receiving by having the senior students see the cases. He orders the second-year student to follow one of the senior students. The students are told that they will present each case

to him so that he can get the facts, then he and a resident will go into the room and talk to the client.

After receiving two seizure cases, an atlanto-axial subluxation case and a progressive chronic paraplegia case, it is the middle of the afternoon (there has been much waiting for Dr. D). Everyone is really hungry, but is afraid to say so. The technician is missing because she is off taking her required lunch break. Dr. D seems to run on air and sends the students off to see if diagnostic procedures can be arranged for the afternoon. The residents are used to this schedule and have snacks that they grab. They whisper to the students that they had better keep protein bars handy. One of the senior students is overwhelmed, but sees no option but to keep all the cases she has taken in. The second-year student tries to help, but is unsure of his role. The third-year resident wants to be primary surgeon on the atlanto-axial subluxation, but she knows that Dr. D likes to do the surgery himself; she hopes that she will get to assist. The first-year resident is unsure of how to approach the chronic paraplegia case, so he asks Dr. D what to do. Dr. D dictates a plan.

The afternoon workups proceed. At 5.30 p.m., Dr. D sits down with the team for rounds. He begins by directing all the questions regarding each case to the student on the case. He then starts giving a lecture on seizure diagnostics. The second-year student nudges one of the senior students to tell Dr. D that he thought he heard an irregular heart rhythm on physical exam of one of the dogs with seizures. The senior student is brave enough to break into Dr. D's monologue. Dr. D's comment is: "It's probably just a sinus arrhythmia." He proceeds with his lecture. He finishes up at 6.30 p.m. and the students start working on their medical records. They finally head for dinner at about 7.30 p.m.

References

Adams, C.L., and Kurtz, S. (2012) Coaching and feedback: Enhancing communication teaching and learning in veterinary practice settings. *Journal of Veterinary Medical Education*, **39** (**3**), 217–228.

Baker, E.A., Ledford, C.H., Fogg, L., *et al.* (2015) The IDEA assessment tool: Assessing the reporting, diagnostic reasoning, and decision-making skills demonstrated in medical students' hospital admission notes. *Teaching and Learning in Medicine*, **27** (**2**), 163–173.

Birden, H., Glass, N., Wilson, I., *et al.* (2013) Teaching professionalism in medical education: A Best Evidence Medical Education (BEME) systematic review. BEME Guide No. 25. *Medical Teacher*, **35** (**7**), e1252–e1266.

Bolt, D.M., Witte, T.H., and Lygo-Baker, S. (2010) The complex role of veterinary clinical teachers: How is their role perceived and what is expected of them? *Journal of Veterinary Medical Education*, **37** (**4**), 388–394.

Bordage, G., Grant, J., and Marsden, P. (1990) Quantitative assessment of diagnostic ability. *Medical Education*, **24** (**5**), 413–425.

Bowen, J.L. (2006) Educational strategies to promote clinical diagnostic reasoning.

New England Journal of Medicine, **355** (**21**), 2217–2225.

Buckley, S., Coleman, J., Davison, I., *et al.* (2009) The educational effects of portfolios on undergraduate student learning: A Best Evidence Medical Education (BEME) systematic review. BEME Guide No. 11. *Medical Teacher*, **31** (**4**), 282–298.

Burns, G.A., Ruby, K.L., Debowes, R.M., *et al.* (2006) Teaching non-technical (professional) competence in a veterinary school curriculum. *Journal of Veterinary Medical Education*, **33** (**2**), 301–308.

Cake, M.A., Bell, M.A., Bickley, N., and Bartram, D.J. (2015) The life of meaning: A model of the positive contributions to well-being from veterinary work. *Journal of Veterinary Medical Education*, **42** (**3**), 184–193.

Cendan, J., and Lok, B. (2012) The use of virtual patients in medical school curricula. *Advances in Physiology Education*, **36** (**1**), 48–53.

Consorti, F., Mancuso, R., Nocioni, M., and Piccolo, A. (2012) Efficacy of virtual patients in medical education: A meta-analysis of randomized studies. *Computers and Education*, **59**, 1001–1008.

Custers, E.J. (2015) Thirty years of illness scripts: Theoretical origins and practical applications. *Medical Teacher*, **37** (**5**), 457–462.

Driessen, E., van Tartwijk, J., and Dornan, T. (2008) The self critical doctor: Helping students become more reflective. *BMJ*, **336** (**7648**), 827–830.

Ericsson, K.A. (2008) Deliberate practice and acquisition of expert performance: A general overview. *Academic Emergency Medicine*, **15** (**11**), 988–994.

Fernandez, R., Kozlowski, S.W., Shapiro, M.J., and Salas, E. (2008) Toward a definition of teamwork in emergency medicine. *Academic Emergency Medicine*, **15** (**11**), 1104–1112.

Friedman, E., Sainte, M., and Fallar, R. (2010) Taking note of the perceived value and impact of medical student chart documentation on education and patient care. *Academic Medicine*, **85** (**9**), 1440–1444.

Haerkens, M.H., Kox, M., Lemson, J., et al. (2015) Crew resource management in the intensive care unit: A prospective 3-year cohort study. *Acta Anaesthesiologica Scandinavica*, **59** (**10**), 1319–1329.

Haig, K.M., Sutton, S., and Whittington, J. (2006) SBAR: A shared mental model for improving communication between clinicians. *Joint Commission Journal on Quality and Patient Safety*, **32** (**3**), 167–175.

Harasym, P.H., Tsai, T.C., and Hemmati, P. (2008) Current trends in developing medical students' critical thinking abilities. *Kaohsiung Journal of Medical Sciences*, **24** (**7**), 341–355.

Hatala, R.M., Brooks, L.R., and Norman, G.R. (2003) Practice makes perfect: The critical role of mixed practice in the acquisition of ECG interpretation skills. *Advances in Health Sciences Education: Theory and Practice*, **8** (**1**), 17–26.

Holden, M.D., Buck, E., Luk, J., et al. (2015) Professional identity formation: Creating a longitudinal framework through TIME (Transformation in Medical Education). *Academic Medicine*, **90** (**6**), 761–767.

Jäger, F., Riemer, M., Abendroth, M., et al. (2014) Virtual patients: The influence of case design and teamwork on students' perception and knowledge – a pilot study. *BMC Medical Education*, **14**, 137.

Kleinsmith, A., Rivera-Gutierrez, D., Finney, G., et al. (2015) Understanding empathy training with virtual patients. *Computers in Human Behavior*, **52**, 151–158.

Kochevar, D.T., and Peycke, L.E. (2008) Balancing veterinary students' and house officers' learning experiences in veterinary teaching hospitals. *Journal of Veterinary Medical Education*, **35** (**1**), 6–10.

Kurtz, S., Silverman, J., Benson, J., and Draper, J. (2003) Marrying content and process in clinical method teaching: Enhancing the Calgary–Cambridge guides. *Academic Medicine*, **78** (**8**), 802–809.

Lane, I.F., and Cornell, K.K. (2013) Teaching tip: Making the most of hospital rounds. *Journal of Veterinary Medical Education*, **40** (**2**), 145–151.

Lenert, L.A., Sakaguchi, F.H., and Weir, C.R. (2014) Rethinking the discharge summary: A focus on handoff communication. *Academic Medicine*, **89** (**3**), 393–398.

Madigosky, W.S., Headrick, L.A., Nelson, K., et al. (2006) Changing and sustaining medical students' knowledge, skills, and attitudes about patient safety and medical fallibility. *Academic Medicine*, **81** (**1**), 94–101.

Magnier, K.M., Wang, R., Dale, V.H., and Pead, M.J. (2014) Challenges and responsibilities of clinical teachers in the workplace: An ethnographic approach. *Journal of Veterinary Medical Education*, **41** (**2**), 155–161.

Manser, T. (2009) Teamwork and patient safety in dynamic domains of healthcare: A review of the literature. *Acta Anaesthesiologica Scandinavica*, **53** (**2**), 143–151.

May, S. (2015) Towards a scholarship of primary health care. *Veterinary Record*, **176** (**26**), 677–682.

McGaghie, W.C., Issenberg, S.B., Petrusa, E.R., and Scalese, R.J. (2010) A critical review of simulation-based medical education research: 2003–2009. *Medical Education*, **44** (**1**), 50–63.

Morey, J.C., Simon, R., Jay, G.D., et al. (2002) Error reduction and performance improvement in the emergency department through formal teamwork training: Evaluation results of the

MedTeams project. *Health Services Research*, **37** (**6**), 1553–1581.

Morrison, G., Goldfarb, S., and Lanken, P.N. (2010) Team training of medical students in the 21st century: Would Flexner approve? *Academic Medicine*, **85** (**2**), 254–259.

Motley, C.L., and Dolansky, M.A. (2015) Five steps to providing effective feedback in the clinical setting: A new approach to promote teamwork and collaboration. *Journal of Nursing Education*, **54** (**7**), 399–403.

Motola, I., Devine, L.A., Chung, H.S., *et al.* (2013) Simulation in healthcare education: A best evidence practical guide. AMEE guide no. 82. *Medical Teacher*, **35** (**10**), e1511–e1530.

Neher, J.O., Gordon, K.C., Meyer, B., and Stevens, N. (1992) A five-step "microskills" model of clinical teaching. *Journal of the American Board of Family Practitioners*, **5** (**4**), 419–424.

Nestel, D., and Tierney, T. (2007) Role-play for medical students learning about communication: Guidelines for maximising benefits. *BMC Medical Education*, **7**, 3.

Norman, G. (2005) Research in clinical reasoning: Past history and current trends. *Medical Education*, **39** (**4**), 418–427.

Pascoe, J.M., Nixon, J., and Lang, V.J. (2015) Maximizing teaching on the wards: Review and application of the One-Minute Preceptor and SNAPPS models. *Journal of Hospital Medicine*, **10** (**2**), 125–130.

Peled, J.U., Sagher, O., Morrow, J.B., and Dobbie, A.E. (2009) Do electronic health records help or hinder medical education? *PLoS Medicine*, **6** (**5**), e1000069.

Pelzer, J.M., Hodgson, J.L., and Werre, S.R. (2014) Veterinary students' perceptions of their learning environment as measured by the Dundee Ready Education Environment Measure. *BMC Research Notes*, **7**, 170.

Razavi, S.M., Karbakhsh, M., Panah Khahi, M., *et al.* (2010) Station-based deconstructed training model for teaching procedural skills to medical students: A quasi-experimental study. *Advances in Medical Education and Practice*, **1**, 17–23.

Reader, T.W., Flin, R., Mearns, K., and Cuthbertson, B.H. (2009) Developing a team performance framework for the intensive care unit. *Critical Care Medicine*, **37** (**5**), 1787–1793.

Risser, D.T., Rice, M.M., Salisbury, M.L., *et al.* (1999) The potential for improved teamwork to reduce medical errors in the emergency department. The MedTeams Research Consortium. *Annals of Emergency Medicine*, **34** (**3**), 373–383.

Roberts, N.K., Brenner, M.J., Williams, R.G., *et al.* (2012) Capturing the teachable moment: A grounded theory study of verbal teaching interactions in the operating room. *Surgery*, **151** (**5**), 643–650.

Roberts, N.K., Williams, R.G., Kim, M.J., and Dunnington, G.L. (2009) The briefing, intraoperative teaching, debriefing model for teaching in the operating room. *Journal of the American College of Surgery*, **208** (**2**), 299–303.

Salas, E., DiazGranados, D., Weaver, S.J., and King, H. (2008) Does team training work? Principles for health care. *Academic and Emergency Medicine*, **15** (**11**), 1002–1009.

Smith, J.R., and Lane, I.F. (2015) Making the most of five minutes: The clinical teaching moment. *Journal of Veterinary Medical Education*, **42** (**3**), 271–280.

Starmer, A., Spector, N., Srivastava, R., Allen, A., *et al.* (2012) I-PASS, a mnemonic to standardize verbal handoffs. *Pediatrics*, **129** (**2**), 201–204.

Steadman, R.H., Coates, W.C., Huang, Y.M., *et al.* (2006) Simulation-based training is superior to problem-based learning for the acquisition of critical assessment and management skills. *Critical Care Medicine*, **34** (**1**), 151–157.

Stone, E.A., Conlon, P., Cox, S., and Coe, J.B. (2012) A new model for companion-animal primary health care education. *Journal of Veterinary Medical Education*, **39** (**3**), 210–216.

Sutkin, G., Wagner, E., Harris, I., and Schiffer, R. (2008) What makes a good clinical teacher in medicine? A review of the literature. *Academic Medicine*, **83** (**5**), 452–466.

Thompson, D.A., Cowan, J., Holzmueller, C., *et al.* (2008) Planning and implementing a systems-based patient safety curriculum in medical education. *American Journal of Medical Quality*, **23** (**4**), 271–278.

Townsend-Gervis, M., Cornell, P., and Vardaman, J.M. (2014) Interdisciplinary rounds and structured communication reduce re-admissions and improve some patient outcomes. *Western Journal of Nursing Research*, **36** (**7**), 917–928.

Vandeweerd, J.M., Davies, J.C., Pinchbeck, G.L., and Cotton, J.C. (2007) Teaching veterinary radiography by e-learning versus structured tutorial: A randomized, single-blinded controlled trial. *Journal of Veterinary Medical Education*, **34** (**2**), 160–167.

Wald, H.S. (2015) Professional identity (trans)formation in medical education: Reflection, relationship, resilience. *Academic Medicine*, **90** (**6**), 701–706.

Weed, L.L. (1968) Medical records that guide and teach. *New England Journal of Medicine*, **278** (**12**), 652–657.

Wingfield, L.R., Kulendran, M., Chow, A., *et al.* (2015) Cognitive task analysis: Bringing Olympic athlete style training to surgical education. *Surgical Innovation*, **22** (**4**), 406–417.

Wiseman, L., Bradwejn, J., and Westbroek, E.M. (2014) A new leadership curriculum: The multiplication of intelligence. *Academic Medicine*, **89** (**3**), 376–379.

Wolpaw, T., Côté, L., Papp, K.K., and Bordage, G. (2012) Student uncertainties drive teaching during case presentations: More so with SNAPPS. *Academic Medicine*, **87** (**9**), 1210–1217.

Wolpaw, T.M., Wolpaw, D.R., and Papp, K.K. (2003) SNAPPS: A learner-centered model for outpatient education. *Academic Medicine*, **78** (**9**), 893–898.

Wu, Z., Robson, S., and Hollis, B. (2013) The application of hospitality elements in hospitals. *Journal of Healthcare Management*, **58** (**1**), 47–62.

Zundel, S., Wolf, I., Christen, H.J., and Huwendiek, S. (2015) What supports students' education in the operating room? A focus group study including students' and surgeons' views. *American Journal of Surgery*, **210** (**5**), 951–959.

13

Learning in Real-World Settings

Tim J. Parkinson

Institute of Veterinary, Animal & Biomedical Sciences, Massey University, New Zealand

---

 Box 13.1: Key messages

- Real-world settings are an essential part of modern veterinary curricula, which help to prepare students for their work as practicing clinicians.
- Real-world settings can provide programs with access to clinical material that can be difficult to obtain through a traditional veterinary teaching hospital (VTH). Such material particularly includes primary accession/shelter medicine, food animal, and public practice.
- Real-world settings can be provided by the use of nontraditional VTH models, contracted practices, or informal teaching arrangements.

- Real-world settings have to have clear learning and teaching objectives, set clear expectations (assessed) of students' performance, and achieve minimum clinical standards.
- Clinical teachers in real-world settings need to be given training in workplace-based learning and in assessment of students in the workplace.
- Clinical teachers in real-world settings need to be included in the academic community of the parent institution.

Introduction: Real-World Settings as the New Norm of Veterinary Education

Informal schemes for veterinary students to undertake placements in the "real-world" settings of the clinical practice and government service branches of the veterinary profession are long-standing components of veterinary education. However, recent years have seen an unprecedented emphasis on such placements as a formal, critical, and integral part of veterinary curricula. The main themes that have come together to bring real-world placements to the forefront of curricula are the recognition that there are significant areas of veterinary practice that cannot readily be taught within the confines of an academic institution; the need to provide students with a greater scale or scope of clinical opportunities than are available through a university hospital; and constraints on universities' ability to provide a full spectrum of clinical experience to students.

Veterinary Medical Education: A Practical Guide, First Edition. Edited by Jennifer L. Hodgson and Jacquelyn M. Pelzer.
© 2017 John Wiley & Sons, Inc. Published 2017 by John Wiley & Sons, Inc.

There has also been a significant change in the pedagogical environment of medical (and hence veterinary) education over the past two or three decades that has helped to drive clinical teaching toward real-world settings. There has been a substantial shift from didactic instruction and apprenticeship models of clinical instruction toward student-centered, constructivist modes of delivery, and the systematizing of clinical instruction around the competencies required of the newly graduated veterinarian. Furthermore, the competencies that the practicing veterinary profession expects of its new graduates are no longer confined to the areas of declarative knowledge and technical skills, but are also increasingly in the affective domains of communication, professionalism, and interpersonal skills. The profession, in fact, expects that graduates will be able to perform the clinical and technical tasks that will enable them to be effective as revenue earners (e.g., Jaarsma *et al.*, 2008). To meet these new expectations, veterinary schools have had to invest in teaching methods that place greater emphasis on these skills, and, as part of that investment, have had to develop means by which they can be taught in the context of students' real-world aspiration to be clinical practitioners.

Concurrent with these developments has been the opening of a number of new veterinary schools. For the established schools, their veterinary teaching hospitals (VTH) have had a long history of existence and, hence, also have a well-defined place in the veterinary community for their referral services and their needs for case material for clinical teaching. For new schools, setting up clinical teaching facilities has been challenging, as they do not have that history in the veterinary community. Even where there has been a long period of advocacy for a new school, that school, once founded, has to struggle for its "place in the sun" of a share of the local primary or referral caseload. Sometimes the need can be met by the purchase of an existing practice, sometimes there might be a gap in the provision of local/regional veterinary services, and sometimes neither of these options is readily apparent. This is not only the situation for new schools: existing schools may not be able to sustain some components of the teaching practice. Food animals commonly fall into this category: locations that may have provided a broad agricultural hinterland when the school was founded are now covered with urban development, and the rural practice has disappeared (Klee, 2008). Moreover, the effectiveness of clinical learning is also affected by the nature of the clinical practices that universities operate, inasmuch as universities need a cadre of clinical specialists to maintain their impetus in clinical excellence and research. Specialists, who may be operating at the level of secondary or tertiary referral, are not necessarily enthralled by teaching students simple medical or surgical procedures, so tension can ensue between the need for clinical specialisms and the achievement of Day One Competencies.

The net result of all of these trends has been a dramatic evolution of the use of external real-world settings, from the informal arrangements of "seeing practice" into key, core, planned, contractually defined components of the modern veterinary curriculum. Consequently, most veterinary schools have moved some or all of their clinical teaching to some form of distributed teaching model. Development of the distributed model, and the means by which it could be accredited as a means of providing clinical education, was not without controversy (Nelson, 2012), but the outcome of that period of discussion has been a robust model for curriculum delivery beyond the bounds of the veterinary teaching hospital.

Formal Rotations in the Real World

Harden, Sowden, and Dunn (1984), in their seminal review of educational strategies in medical curricula, argued for community-based medicine as a critical curriculum component to supply the needs of practitioners who would subsequently provide primary accession medical services to the community. They noted that the hospital-based approach of medicine "has fostered an 'ivory tower' approach to medicine

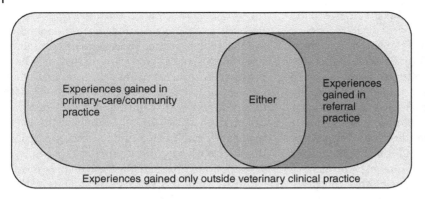

Figure 13.1 Veterinary medicine in primary and referral practices. Source: Harden *et al.*, 1984. Reproduced with permission of Wiley Blackwell.

in which students during their training have little contact, if any, with the community which they are being trained to serve" (p. 291), and that "in hospital-based curricula it is in the process of becoming a doctor that the trend towards specialization has been initiated, intensified and maintained" (pp. 291–292). The large number of veterinary students who take internships as their first postgraduation employment who made that choice during their clinical training (Barbur *et al.*, 2011) and the remarkable growth in veterinary specialty practice (Albers, 2008) may be symptomatic of the same process occurring in veterinary education.

By contrast, community-based training helps students to understand the importance of primary healthcare, provides access to a wide range of clinical material that is seldom seen in a teaching hospital (Figure 13.1), and, if managed well, can provide an intensely active learning environment. Most veterinary schools have recognized the disconnect between the high-level referral practice that typically characterized a VTH and the expectations of Day One Competencies of graduates, and have sought either to diversify back into primary accession care themselves or to obtain real-world placements with private practices. For example, Ohio State University recently re-established an ambulatory large animal clinical facility (Masterson *et al.*, 2004), the University of Florida partnered with a private practice to deliver a small animal emergency medicine rotation (Olson, 2008), and Colorado State University has developed

---

 Box 13.2: Focus on apprenticeship and systematic models of clinical teaching

Apprenticeship

Students are attached to one clinical teacher or unit for a period. What is taught may depend on what patients are available and on the interests of staff concerned. The teaching itself is largely opportunistic and is often based on unpredicted clinical situations as they arise. The hope is that the students will, over a period of time, see a representative sample of medical practice.

Source: Based on Harden, Sowden, and Dunn, 1984.

Systematic

The clinical material that is available for clinical instruction should not be left to chance, but should be planned. The program is designed so that the experiences necessary for the training of all students are covered. The essential components of the course are spelled out clearly to the students, and may include a list of skills to master and conditions that they should have encountered.

a pet hospice program to teach students how to manage the human and animal aspects of terminal care (Bishop *et al.*, 2008).

Harden, Sowden, and Dunn (1984) also compared the modes of instruction during clinical rotations, contrasting the apprenticeship model that characterized traditional clinical curricula with a more systematic approach (see Box 13.2). The use of Day One Competencies to define the graduate outcomes of veterinary curricula has created a concurrent expectation that there will be planned and defined clinical learning experiences; and, since these are the competencies of a general practitioner, many of the competencies need to be learned in the context of primary accession, commercial, clinical practice.

Animal Handling and Husbandry

One of the unique features of veterinary degrees that derive from the British (Royal College of Veterinary Surgeons, RCVS) model of veterinary education is the requirement for students to gain real-world experience of working with animals, particularly livestock, during the vacations of the junior years of their studies (Box 13.3).

The intent of these placements is to "provide the student with all the necessary handling skills and husbandry experience of common domestic species that they need to master before they progress to the clinical components

of the course" and to "develop their animal handling skills across a range of common domestic species … and … their understanding of the practice and economics of animal management systems and animal industries" (RCVS, 2009, pp. 2–3). Using the model presented in Figure 13.1, these placements also engage students with the problems and practicalities of livestock management that they may never encounter in clinical veterinary practice.

The need for students to become familiar with livestock is the key foundational pillar of animal handling and husbandry (AH&H) placements, especially in the face of the decline in familiarity of working with livestock among entrants to veterinary school. The emphasis of AH&H placements has shifted with time: originally conceived as periods of "farm work," these placements are now likely to have specific learning outcomes in terms of both the technical skills of familiarity/confidence with livestock, and gaining understanding of the management and economic factors that underpin livestock enterprises. Students generally have to produce a factual report on the placement, which may also require them to research and discuss in depth some aspect of the farm's activity. Bristol University, for example, sets animal health-related tasks for students to research during their placements, with the expectation that each student will be able to lead a tutorial on that topic when they return to campus.

 Box 13.3: Examples of animal handling and husbandry as an extramural component of veterinary programs

United Kingdom	India
Evidence must be provided that extramural farm animal husbandry practical work is used within the curriculum to complement intramural studies to support students' attainment of comprehensive understanding of livestock and farm systems. (RCVS, 2015, p. 16)	Hands-on training of the students on the overall farm practice of livestock management including cleaning, feeding, watering, grooming, milking, routine healthcare, record keeping, sanitation, housing, fodder production. (Veterinary Council of India, 2008, p. 160)

As with all real-world settings, students need to be adequately underpinned by university courses. Universities commonly provide junior-years courses in animal handling, but these may not be sufficient to meet either the requirements of health and safety authorities, or (perhaps more importantly!) the expectations of farmers. Some universities have therefore added intensive training around livestock/farm safety as a precursor to the AH&H placements. For example, Melbourne University (2015) requires that students undertake "an approved five day residential course in animal handling, environmental safety and management" as a prerequisite for its junior year courses in animal health, while Massey University (New Zealand) requires students to undertake a similar course at an agricultural training organization as the precursor to its AH&H placements.

There is, finally, an increasingly important, but deliberately understated, objective of such placements; namely, the recruitment of students into rural practice. Ensuring positive experiences of students in rural placements is seen as a key step in the development of an interest in a career in rural practice, as it is well documented that students who have had positive rural experiences are more likely to make initial career choices in this direction (Lenarduzzi, Sheppard, and Slater, 2009). In the realm of medical education, it is clear that recruitment into "difficult" areas can be enhanced by exposing students to a program-long, "longitudinal pipeline" of relevant, community-based placements (Quinn et al., 2011), and, in the veterinary context, pre-entry or early-program exposure to the rural sector is critical in orienting students toward future employment in that area (Schmitz *et al.*, 2007). In North American universities, in which AH&H placements are not mandated by accreditation, the importance of high-quality farm exposure is nonetheless well recognized, and such programs have been developed in several universities that serve agricultural hinterlands (e.g., Smith, 2004; Karrier *et al.*, 2008); these programs appear to be effective at recruiting students into food animal tracks.

Real-World Placements as a Key Link from the Preclinical to the Clinical Phases of the Program

In order to "have a realistic and appropriate perspective of the responsibilities of the veterinary profession" (University of California, Davis, 2015), prospective students are usually required to have completed a significant amount of veterinary experience before admission. After admission, regardless of whether a veterinary medical degree program adopts the traditional "preclinical, paraclinical, clinical" model or whether it has a more integrated structure, familiarization and enculturation with clinical practice are a key transition though which students have to progress. Johnson (2015) reviewed the programs of extramural study (EMS) placements in UK veterinary curricula, with the view that early clinical placements were primarily of value in learning the culture of veterinary clinical practice and observing the management of cases.

This process is commonly started at the transition from the junior to the senior years of the program – often at the start of the final year. However, current thinking is that clinical activities need to be incorporated into the program at a very much earlier level, ideally as early as possible. In fact, this is the process that many veterinary schools operate. Early-years clinical experience is important, as it provides context and reality for preclinical studies and, even if brief, such placements are well received. For example, D'Amore *et al.* (2011) describe a one-week placement of first-year medical students in rural Australia as being enjoyable, but also as a vehicle for students to understand the clinical and technical learning that they would need to achieve to be successful in clinical practice. Kaye et al. (2010) had a similar experience of placement of first-year medical students in rural Uganda: "many of the students … were in favor of this being part of their medical training. Some of the reasons given … were that it enables students to understand the medical conditions in rural areas, to see a variety of medical conditions (some of which are not seen in the teaching hospital), and to learn about the management of the health care system." In veterinary education, Stone *et al.* (2012) argued for exposure to companion animal primary care throughout the curriculum as a means of providing interest in primary practice *per se* and of creating context for concurrent studies. Interestingly, they "originally thought that the first-year students could serve as animal handlers, second-year students as receptionists, third-year students as veterinary technicians, and fourth-year students as clinicians. This proved to be fallacious thinking" (p. 212); rather, they found that "junior" students benefitted most when fully incorporated into the "inter-professional team." Likewise, initiatives in the United States and Canada have aimed at stimulating the interest of first- and second-year doctor of veterinary medicine (DVM) students in food animal medicine by getting them involved in real-world problems at the farm, practice, or rural industry level (e.g., Iowa State University: Karrier *et al.*, 2008; Michigan State University: Howard, Lloyd, and Grooms, 2009).

On the other hand, starting clinical practice can be stressful. One way to address this issue is the use of simulators to familiarize students with the clinical material and interpersonal interactions that they will encounter – a process that has been beneficial in nursing and midwifery (McNamara, 2015; Cummins *et al.*, 2015). Likewise, nursing education has emphasized the importance of clear goals and expectations around early-year clinical placements (Andrew *et al.*, 2009). Veterinary curricula similarly need to have clear expectations of students' achievements in early clinical placements (Bell *et al.*, 2010). For example, James Cook University, Queensland, Australia (2015a) has a series of preclinical courses in veterinary professional practice, which structure learning experiences across the early years of the program to create understanding of, and familiarity with, veterinary clinical practice as a precursor to the main block of clinical studies in the final year. Learning outcomes for the early stages

of these placements are largely in the affective domain of communication, workplace ethics, and teamwork, with later placements having a greater emphasis on "clinical" skills such as client communication, history taking, record keeping, and clinical examination.

Real-World Placements in Clinical Practice

In order for veterinary schools to meet the expectations of Day One Competencies in companion animal practice, students need to be exposed to a broad range of primary accession and referral medicine, and (in the terms used in Figure 13.1) to the diseases and problems that are found in the "community," but are not (or not commonly) seen in veterinary practice.

Most aspects of companion animal practice can be taught in external placements, and there are many examples in the literature of such placements. Emergency medicine and terminal care (Bishop *et al.*, 2008) have already been mentioned; and private specialty clinics, wholly or partly owned subsidiaries, and private primary healthcare clinics (Bishop *et al.*, 2008; Lloyd *et al.*, 2008; Olson, 2008; Tyner *et al.*, 2014) have all been used to good effect. There are common threads to the success of these placements, of which the most important appear to be:

- Structured expectations of students' learning.
- The physical and professional resources of the practice.
- A collegial relationship between the university and the practice.

One of the most important aspect of students' learning in the real world is that they are enabled to behave as though they actually are in the real world. In other words, students need to be active participants in the diagnostic workup, clinical procedures, and interactions with clients. However, the problems of prioritizing between the needs of the case (and demands of the animal's owner) and the expectation of the student are well known (e.g., Magnier *et al.*, 2011), and it is equally well known that real-world placements are of marginal value where students are merely observers. Hence, managing the expectations of both the students ("how much I want to do") and the practices ("how much I am prepared to let you do") is an important component in the success of real-world placements. Sometimes students' learning is structured by the university, in terms of, for example, a cadre of technical and/or professional skills that the students are expected to achieve during their placement. Commonly this is managed through a structured logbook (Dale, Pierce, and May, 2013), a list of technical skills, or a series of learning objectives. Alternatively, the objectives for each placement can be negotiated between the student and the university or between the student and the practice. For example, the Royal Veterinary College (RVC, 2014) expects that students arrive with "a reasonable list of objectives for their time spent at that placement. It expects that their students will have a common sense approach to setting out this list of objectives, bearing in mind the stage of the course they have reached and their own level of competence." This process of agreeing outcomes is valuable for all parties, since it allows the "I want to/you can do" discussion to be held at the start of the placement rather than leaving one or other party dissatisfied at its end; and it allows for objective assessment of the student's achievements during the placement.

Development of students' nontechnical skills may, in fact, be one of the most valuable aspects of real-world placements in companion animal practice. Even though there are many useful ways of teaching communication skills in the "safe" setting of the university (e.g., Chun *et al.*, 2009), real communication with clients remains a most demanding skill to learn, and transferring skills learned in the preclinical safe environment into the real-world workplace is critical to the professional development of fledgling clinicians. Consequently, providing opportunity for client interactions, with a focused, sympathetic critique (Adams and Kurtz, 2012), is an area of real-world placements that is undergoing rapid development. The second major nontechnical skill of which students have limited understanding is that of the business of veterinary practice (Bachynsky *et al.*, 2013). Even though students do not necessarily take on board the commercial realities of practice during their clinical year (Rhind et al., 2011), those who are enabled to do so are better equipped for the commercial realities of their postgraduation work. Consequently, greater emphasis is being placed on students' understanding of the business of commercial practice during their placements (particularly during the preclinical/clinical link placements). Interestingly, while early forays into improving students' understanding of veterinary business were largely report based, tracking students' earning potential through actual client charging plans (Roth, Poon, and Hofmeister, 2014) seems to be a way of moving business understanding from theory into students' repertoire of skills.

Shelter Medicine

Shelter medicine can be used to provide access to a wide range of clinical material: large numbers of animals for desexing surgery and other everyday procedures, along with the infectious diseases and "diseases of neglect" that are commonplace in the wider animal-owning community. Stevens and Gruen (2014) summed up the benefits of shelter medicine experience to students as providing "opportunities to practice zoonotic and species-specific infectious disease control, behavioral evaluation and management, primary care, animal welfare, ethics, and public policy issues" (p. 83); for this reason, many veterinary schools have incorporated local animal shelter resources into their clinical teaching. Indeed, for many schools, shelter medicine placements were their first foray into a distributed clinical teaching model. Desexing surgery is, of course, a critical skill for the graduate companion animal veterinarian, and the plentiful supply of animals requiring this surgery in animal shelters makes this a great environment in which students can learn that skill. Moreover, the students themselves can be a resource to the shelter by helping to manage the caseload of desexing surgery, so that there are useful outcomes for the school, the student, and the shelter itself. The mobile desexing service at Purdue University (Freeman *et al.*, 2013), the collaboration between Texas A&M University and the Brazos Animal Shelter (Snowden *et al.*, 2008), and the integration of the People's Dispensary for Sick Animals (PDSA) into the clinical rotations of the RVC (Mahoney and Martin, 2011) are examples of such services. Developed countries may also assist developing countries in a similar way: Massey University sends groups of final-year students annually to the Pacific island nation of Samoa, where the students gain a great deal of experience in desexing surgery, while the country has the benefit of control of its feral dog population. The benefits of shelter medicine go far beyond desexing surgery, since students also have to manage animals with infectious diseases that are unusual in the population of owned, vaccinated animals; in managing these cases, students learn that epidemiological principles can be applied to managing infectious diseases beyond the boundaries of food animal practice.

Food Animal Practice

The use of real-world settings for teaching food animal practice has become an integral part of most universities' food animal programs. Indeed, long before the notions of "distributed model" or "real-world setting" had entered the vocabulary of veterinary education, difficulties of maintaining an adequate caseload through the VTH were forcing schools into developing relationships with private or state-run practices.

The importance of industry exposure as a means of recruiting students' interest in food animal practice is well recognized and so, interestingly, where the model of AH&H EMS is not mandated by accreditation, it may evolve anyway. For example, Michigan State University developed a "summer food systems fellowship program" (Howard, Lloyd, and Grooms, 2009) with the intent of interesting and challenging food animal students in order to "maintain populations of graduates who are willing to seek out job opportunities in the production animal

arena" (p. 280). Immersion experience with the dairy industry is a strong pillar of this initiative. In Cornell University's Summer Dairy Institute (Nydam *et al.*, 2009), there is a strong emphasis on both the farm-level and herd health skills that dairy practitioners will need. Likewise, the University of Minnesota has a partnership with a large-scale dairy farm to provide students with hands-on experience in the management and disorders of cows in the pari-parturient period, as well as in the farm-level and clinician-level decision-making that surrounds such animals (Fetrow *et al.*, 2004). A similar initiative in this arena is the Swine Medicine Education Center, a partnership between Iowa State University and AMVC Veterinary Services, which provides education and experience for veterinary students and graduates in various aspects of the pork industry (Iowa State University, 2015) in the real-world settings of pig farms and clinical practice. The importance of these initiatives is twofold. First, individual universities find it increasingly difficult to maintain faculty recruitment in specialized food animal areas, hence where such centers and immersion activities are managed on a regional or interinstitutional basis, better utilization of scarce faculty resources and stability of programs can be achieved (Moore, 2006). Second, such initiatives are of increasing importance in maintaining an adequate cadre of veterinary graduates entering food animal practice. This is partly due to the benefits of bringing like-minded students together: Nydam *et al.* (2009) recognized that the paucity of students who are interested in food animals in a typical veterinary class can leave those students feeling isolated, so a significant benefit is achieved by bringing students from various veterinary schools together into a situation in which they do not feel like a minority.

More common, however, is the use of private practices to augment (or replace) the cases available through the VTH. The University of Wisconsin, for example, described an integrated program of dairy exposure over its four-year veterinary degree, of which placements with private dairy practice form a prominent component (Cook *et al.*, 2004). During the initial placements, students had experience with the routine cases of individual animal medicine and herd health procedures, but thereafter they could return to undertake further rotations to broaden their experience in more complex aspects of herd health management. Michigan State University, in addition to the farm exposure that has already been mentioned, also described ambulatory food animal/equine rotations based in private practices (Kopcha *et al.*, 2005). Many other examples exist: Nottingham University in the United Kingdom has a fully dispersed clinical teaching model, the RVC contracts practices far away from the suburban sprawl of London to provide food animal clinical training, and most of the schools in Australasia use external practices for a greater or lesser amount of their food animal training (e.g., Windsor, 2009). The objectives of these rotations, which are to "provide students with introductory on-farm experience focusing on examination, diagnosis, treatment, and prevention of common medical and surgical conditions of horses and/or food animals" and "practice management, including management of personnel, inventory, and finances" (Kopcha *et al.*, 2005, p. 355), are typical of the purposes of such real-world placements. In fact, these are probably the main benefits that can be achieved through the use of practices – exposure of

students to large numbers of routine cases and procedures, which give them the technical competence to have confidence to undertake the more complex tasks of herd health management and advice.

The remote location of many rural practices often requires that some form of living accommodation is provided. Melbourne University has partnered with its rural practices to build or rent accommodation at each of its rural practice locations; Ohio State University has provided mobile home accommodation at its rural practices (Masterton *et al.*, 2004); and James Cook University (2015b) has partnered with a private practice to develop a Veterinary Teaching Resource Centre, which provides seminar rooms, computer laboratory, offices, and accommodation facilities.

Veterinary Public Health

Understanding and experience in veterinary public health (VPH), particularly as it relates to meat and livestock products, are key components of the Day One Competencies of veterinary graduates. Some of these expectations, as required by the European Association of Establishments for Veterinary Education (EAEVE), are listed in Box 13.4. Likewise, the more recent Day One Competencies of

---

 Box 13.4: Example of key learning outcomes in veterinary public health

- Know how to carry out ante-mortem inspection on farm or in the abattoir and assess the welfare of the animals concerned.
- Be familiar with veterinary public health and the respective legal regulations.
- Understand post-mortem inspection and possess basic practical skills within the food production business and inspection requirements.
- Understand the importance of risk-based monitoring of the processes (HACCP [hazard analysis and critical control points] concept).

These tasks require a sound knowledge of the pathology, microbiology, parasitology, pharmacology and toxicology of food animals, of epidemiology and of the legal requirements, allowing [graduates] to ensure public health and report back along the food chain to the farmer and to the Competent Authority.

Source: Abridged from European Association of Establishments for Veterinary Education, 2015.

the veterinary graduate developed by the OIE (World Organisation for Animal Health) as minimum standards for veterinary education worldwide define a broad range of competencies in (*inter alia*) food hygiene and the control of zoonoses (OIE, 2012). North American veterinary programs have traditionally placed less emphasis on food hygiene than have European programs, but in consequence, specific "public health" or "food hygiene" pre-entry programs (Hoet *et al.*, 2008), electives (Akers *et al.*, 2008), tracks (see Stoddard and Glynn, 2009), or intercalated degrees (e.g., Olsen and Remington, 2008) have had to be developed to attract students into these areas of the veterinary profession. Which of these approaches yields a graduate with adequate competence in VPH is not clearly established – at least, not according to the criteria of Smulders *et al.* (2012) – but real-world placements in the food-processing industries are an integral part of any VPH educational program.

On the other hand, however desirable real-world placements in VPH may be, they are not always easy to procure. Abattoirs are not necessarily receptive to receiving disinterested students on compulsory placements, nor are there always enough places within the food industry for all students to have adequate placements. Consequently, arrangements have to be made with either the food industry itself or the veterinary/government regulators of that industry for student placements. In Australia and New Zealand, abattoir/food industry placements are organized by the Australian Quarantine and Inspection Service and the Ministry for Primary Industries Verification Service, respectively. These services ensure that students have a level of exposure to food industry processors (ante-mortem examination, red and white meat and dairy processing, quality control) to meet the Day One Competencies, in an educational milieu that promotes students' engagement with the learning outcomes. This approach probably reflects the current role of the veterinary profession in the food industry, although the classic meat inspection placements that form the backbone of some veterinary programs are

well received by students (Lundén, Björkroth, and Korkeala, 2007). As with other real-world experiences, the key to successful VPH placements appears to be well-focused learning outcomes, so that both student and supervisor have a clear understanding of the expectations for the placement.

The EMS Model of Real-World Placements

The 26 weeks of compulsory EMS required by the RCVS for all UK veterinary graduates is a long-established program of real-world placements. The expectations of EMS have developed over the years (Taylor and Barnes, 1998), but since the RCVS review in 2009, clear objectives for students, universities, and provider practices have been laid out, predicated on the principles that students must take responsibility for their own learning during EMS; and that universities and providers must support the students in this process. The aims of EMS (Box 13.5) have much in common with many of the processes and placements that have been developed by individual institutions, but differ in that the core requirements are mandated for all UK veterinary schools. While this may initially seem overly prescriptive, its effect is that issues such as insurance, indemnity, accommodation, and so on are managed in an identical manner by all schools, which simplifies the demands on provider practices. The scheme also differentiates "transition" EMS for students who are moving from the preclinical to clinical phases of the program from the substantive clinical EMS, thus helping to remove misunderstandings about the capabilities of students at different stages of their education. Finally, the scheme indicates the areas in which students should be assessed, which include attitude, professional appearance, communication skills, animal handling skills, knowledge and problem-solving skills, manual skills, contribution to clinical discussion, and understanding of practice management; a list that encompasses most of the objectives of real-world placements.

The main drawback of the EMS scheme is that it requires considerable voluntary effort

Box 13.5: Focus on the aims of clinical EMS

- Work placements should ... allow students to gain an appreciation of ... how veterinary medicine and science operates in "real-life" and commercial environments. Specifically, placements should enable students to:
- Appreciate the importance of herd health and the epidemiological approach to production animal work.
- Develop their understanding of practice economics and practice management.
- Develop their understanding and gain further experience of medical and surgical treatments in a variety of species.
- Develop communication skills for all aspects of veterinary work.

- Expand their experience to those disciplines and species not fully covered within the university.
- Appreciate the importance of animal welfare in animal production and in the practice of veterinary medicine.
- Gain experience to help them appreciate the ethical and legal responsibilities of the veterinary surgeon in relation to individual clients, animals, the community and society.
- Gain experience of a variety of veterinary working environments.

Source: RCVS, 2009.

on the part of the practicing profession: each student has to undertake 26 weeks of EMS in order to complete their degree, with the consequence that demands on practices can be heavy (Morris, 2009). The main advantage of the EMS scheme is that it can very substantially augment the overall clinical exposure of veterinary graduates. The emphasis placed on students taking responsibility for their own learning has led to the development of a range of materials to support their EMS placements. The EMS Driving Licence (Bell, 2011; and see http://www.ems.vet.ed.ac.uk/emsdl/) helps students to understand the expectations of provider practices and to plan their own learning around their clinical placements, and its use improves student outcomes from EMS placements (Bell *et al.*, 2010).

Management of Real-World Placements

Resources

It has been surprisingly difficult to define the requirements around the physical and

professional resources that a practice needs to have to host student placements, particularly in view of the widely varying emphases that different schools place on their real-world components: some universities, for example, have distributed most of their core teaching into private (or quasi-private) practices, others have partitioned compulsory core rotations between the VTH and external providers, and yet others follow the RCVS model of core rotations delivered through a VTH supported by less-structured EMS. Initially, there was an expectation on the part of accrediting bodies that the experience in external practices would replicate that of a VTH, but more recent iterations of accreditation standards have accommodated the breadth of types of placement that are deemed to be acceptable for core clinical rotations (Box 13.6). The guidelines of the American Veterinary Medical Association (AVMA) are helpful in providing an overview of the provisions of core off-campus rotations (AVMA, 2015b). Universities that use off-campus/distributed practices have had to work these accreditation requirements into their own specifications for the practice that

Box 13.6: Example of accreditation standards for off-campus clinical rotations

Clinical educational ... experience can include exposure to clinical education at off-campus sites, provided the college reviews these clinical experiences and educational outcomes. Further, such clinical experiences should occur in a setting that provides access to subject matter experts, reference resources, modern and complete clinical laboratories, advanced diagnostic instrumentation and ready confirmation. (AVMA, 2015a)

Core clinical teaching facilities may be provided on campus or externally. The school must ensure standards of teaching clinics remain comparable with the best available in the private sector, (e.g., for small animal practices, ASAVA hospital standards), through regular review. (AVBC, 2016)

they use. A consensus of these expectations now appears to have emerged, as summarized in Box 13.7 from the guidelines of the Western University of Health Sciences (2013).

One of the key issues that has emerged from the period of developing off-campus instruction as part of the core curriculum is the need for a nominated individual at each practice site who is responsible for both mentoring and assessing each student. For example, Sydney University expects that "One practitioner is nominated as an Extramural Supervisor during the time the student is on placement. The Extramural Supervisor effectively acts as the student's mentor and colleague, even though the student may work with or visit other practitioners during the rotation. At the end of the student's time at a site, the Extramural Supervisor is required to complete a report providing details on the student's educational development and behaviour" (Sydney University, 2015). Interestingly, Baguley (2006) found that the interactions between students and this nominated supervisor, and the feedback received from members of the practice, were regarded as valuable aspects of students' learning during off-campus placements.

Consequently, the relationship between the university and its distributed teaching practices needs to be both contractual and collegial. Accreditation authorities require that there are contractual arrangements in place, at least for core rotations, in order to provide; 1) stability of availability of placement, 2) clear expectations of the placement, particularly around the access of students to case material, and 3) the obligations of both parties with respect to health and safety, indemnity, and student behavior/discipline. However, the collegial relationship between university and practice is at least as important as the contractual relationship. Again, there seems to be some critical aspects to this. Members of the practice need to be acknowledged as part of the university's community – for example, through adjunct appointments, or continuing professional development (CPD) activities to which they have preferential or sole access, or regular visits from faculty members to the practice (and vice versa). The extramural program at Sydney University has required "the teaching staff to develop numerous resources to ensure that students, staff and members of the profession (including extramural supervisors) are able to participate in a 'virtual campus' that supports the needs of each group" (Windsor, 2009, p. 694). This may even extend to joint or shared appointments between the practice and the university. For example, Melbourne University has had a residency program in which university residents are placed in partnering dairy practices; the residents contribute to the clinical activities of the practice, take responsibility for the students during their placements, and act as a conduit between the clinical departments of the university and the practices (Melbourne University, 2016).

Box 13.7: Example of guidelines for off-campus clinical facilities: Western University of Health Sciences

- Off-campus clinical sites must have:
- Sufficient number of veterinarians to provide adequate supervision and direction for the number of students.
- An adequate caseload or number of animals to ensure a rich and varied clinical educational experience for the student.
- Subject matter experts in the area for which the site is approved to host students (such as specialty college diplomates, ABVP [American Board of Veterinary Practitioners] diplomates, general practitioners, researchers).
- Diagnostic and therapeutic service components, including pharmacy, diagnostic imaging, diagnostic support services, dedicated isolation facilities, intensive/critical care, ambulatory/field services vehicles, and necropsy facilities as appropriate for the type of practice/facility.

- On-site reference resources that are available to students.
- Comprehensive and retrievable medical records system.
- Provision for student interaction and discussion in the work-up of patients (including physical examination, diagnosis, diagnostic problem-oriented decision making, and case management decisions through hands-on experiences and discussions with clinicians).
- An environment that allows supervision and monitoring of the student's educational experience; and a designated individual at the site who must provide feedback on student performance to both to the student and the college.

Source: Abridged from Western University of Health Sciences, 2013.

Training in workplace-based teaching and assessment is also an important part of the collegial relationship (Baguley, 2006). Communication skills, which are particularly suitable for teaching in a real-world setting, are also challenging for teacher and assessor: how best to capitalize on the "in the moment" teaching opportunities, the integration of communication with other clinical skills, and the modeling of effective (or ineffective!) communication skills (Adams and Kurtz, 2012). Likewise, learning how to give students valid/helpful feedback on their communication skills (feedback that is more akin to a descriptive problem-solving session than an evaluative lecture) is a key skill that clinical teachers need to learn.

Moreover, as a consequence of better definition of the sociocultural interactions of workplace-based learning in clinical practice, a new understanding of the principles that need to be addressed in assessment is emerging: the relationship between teacher and student is increasingly seen as less a hierarchy and more a professional community (Scholz, Trede, and Raidal, 2013). In fact, the quality of the mentor relationship has been identified as one of the key elements in the success of community placements – not only in terms of the students' outcomes, but also in terms of the maintenance and improvement of the quality of the placement (Thistlethwaite *et al.*, 2013). Importantly in this equation, the clinical teachers need to have a clear idea of what is required of the students, so that they can help the students identify/self-identify the gaps in their knowledge and skills (Magnier *et al.*, 2011).

Assessment

As the use of real-world experiences in teaching veterinary medicine has expanded, there has been a concomitant development of the methods used for assessment. Assessment of

Undertaking these DOPS as stand-alone observations can be time consuming, however, so a most cost-effective way of managing DOPS is to undertake the observations as part of students' routine clinical activities during rotations. Nor do the procedures need to be complex: although some (e.g., desexing surgery of small animals) are both complex and demanding, others (e.g., correctly placing an intravenous catheter) are not. In fact, breaking up the procedural skills into those that need to be assessed holistically (desexing surgery again) and those that do not allows for students to be given an extensive catalog of procedures that they are expected to perform during their final-year rotations. The overhead cost of developing such lists can be relatively low and, provided that care is taken in ensuring that students will have the opportunity to undertake the task and will be assessed at a level commensurate with Day One Competencies, they provide a useful means of ensuring competence across a range of skills. In terms of the "systematic" model of clinical instruction proposed by Harden, Sowden, and Dunn (1984), such lists of skills are particularly useful in ensuring the consistency of students' experience. Thus, for any skill that a student *must* complete, the university *must* ensure that the student has the opportunity to do so, and a systematization of clinical instruction is the consequence. As with the mini-CEX, DOPS can have a formative or summative function and, while the checklist is not the most reliable method of *assessing* DOPS, it is a very good method for providing *feedback* on the procedure. Thus, if a checklist that enumerates the steps required for successful completion underpins the procedure, students can readily be given feedback on the basis that (for example) Steps 1–3 were successfully accomplished, but Step 4 (which could be a "critical failure" step) was not. Moreover, the prescription for the clinical procedure can build in levels of competence, which allows its assessment to be a useful marriage of self-assessment and supervisor assessment. For example, Fuentealba, Mason, and Johnston (2008, p. 36) describe four levels of attainment:

- Level 1: Student has cognitive knowledge of the competency.
- Level 2: Student has observed performance of the competency live or electronically.
- Level 3: Student has performed the competency under supervision.
- Level 4: Student has performed the competency independently.

The current paradigm of clinical instruction is that failure or poor performance is followed by the opportunity for remediation. Whether real-world placements are the ideal environment for remediation is open to question: it may be that the student needs to go back to the VTH to hone their skills before being returned to workplace learning. For example, Michigan University notes that, once a deficiency is recorded, a plan is developed for remediation, and that student needs to spend additional time either at the same practice, at a different practice, or in the university VTH to improve that skill (Kopcha *et al.*, 2005).

Other means of assessing students' learning in practices include reflective journals, portfolios, case logs, and case books. These are all useful for evaluating various aspects of students' learning, as well as giving an indication of the coverage and caseload of individual external practice placements.

Conclusion

Real-world placements have become an integral part of veterinary curricula, in response to increased expectations of the clinical skills of graduates, difficulties in maintaining the full breadth of clinical exposure within a traditional VTH, and universities' need to develop cost-effective methods of clinical instruction. Real-world placements can involve a contractual relationship between the university and provider practices, or can be a contribution of the practicing profession to the education of the next generation of graduates. Regardless, real-world placements require the engagement and cooperation of the practicing profession to provide access to their facilities, expertise, and time for student education. Early models of real-world placements were relatively unstructured, but the learning experience, and the assessment of that learning experience, have become increasingly structured over time – especially in placements that are considered to be part of the core clinical curriculum. In parallel, however, there has also been an increase in the responsibility that students have to take for their learning, so that the outcomes of a placement are as likely to be negotiated between student and supervisor as they are to be dictated by the academic institution. Increasing student numbers and the growing demands of universities for real-world placements are, nevertheless, at risk of placing pressure on the availability of enough placements for all students. Management and support of practices are critical to the success of real-world placements, not only in terms of the logistics of such activities, but also in providing the training that the clinicians require to be effective teachers.

References

Adams, C.L., and Kurtz, S. (2012) Coaching and feedback: Enhancing communication teaching and learning in veterinary practice settings. *Journal of Veterinary Medical Education*, **39**, 217–228.

Akers, J., Payne, P., Holcomb, C.A., *et al.* (2008) Public-health education at Kansas State University. *Journal of Veterinary Medical Education*, **35**, 188–193.

Albers, J.W. (2008) The future of specialty practice. *Journal of Veterinary Medical Education*, **35**, 51–52.

American Veterinary Medical Association (2015a) *Requirements of an Accredited College of Veterinary Medicine*. https://www.avma.org/ProfessionalDevelopment/Education/Accreditation/Colleges/Pages/coe-pp-requirements-of-accredited-college.aspx (accessed November 2015).

American Veterinary Medical Association (2015b) *Off-Campus and Distributive Sites*. https://www.avma.org/ProfessionalDevelopment/Education/Accreditation/Colleges/Pages/coe-pp-off-campus-and-distributive-sites.aspx (accessed November 2015).

Andrew, N., McGuinness, C., Reid. G., and Corcoran, T. (2009) Greater than the sum of its parts: Transition into the first year of undergraduate nursing. *Nurse Education in Practice*, **9**, 13–21.

AVBC (2016) *Accreditation Standards*. Australasian Veterinary Boards Council.

https://avbc.asn.au/wp-content/uploads/documents/public/AVBCStandardsAug2016.pdf (accessed November 30, 2016).

Bachynsky, E.A., Dale, H.M., Kinnison, T., *et al.* (2013) A survey of the opinions of recent veterinary graduates and employers regarding early career business skills. *Veterinary Record*, **172**, 604–609.

Baguley, J. (2006) The role of final year extramural placements in the undergraduate veterinary curriculum. *Australian Veterinary Journal*, **84**,182–186.

Barbur, L., Shuman, C., Sanderson, M.W., and Grauer, G.F. (2011) Factors that influence the decision to pursue an internship: The importance of mentoring. *Journal of Veterinary Medical Education*, **38**, 278–287.

Battistone, M.J., Pendleton, B., Milne, C., *et al.* (2001) Global descriptive evaluations are more responsive than global numeric ratings in detecting students' progress during the inpatient portion of an internal medicine clerkship. *Academic Medicine*, **76** (suppl.), S105–S107.

Bell, C. (2011) Online tool helps students prepare for EMS. *Veterinary Record*, **168**, i. doi:10.1136/vr.g7104

Bell, C., Baillie, S., Kinnison, T., and Cavers, A. (2010) Preparing veterinary students for extramural clinical placement training: Issues identified and a possible solution. *Journal of Veterinary Medical Education*, **37**, 190–197.

Bishop, G.A., Long, C.C., Carlsten, K.S., *et al.* (2008) The Colorado State University Pet Hospice program: End-of-life care for pets and their families. *Journal of Veterinary Medical Education*, **35**, 525–531.

Chun, R., Schaefer, S., Lotta, C.C., *et al.* (2009) Didactic and experiential training to teach communication skills: The University of Wisconsin–Madison School of Veterinary Medicine collaborative experience. *Journal of Veterinary Medical Education*, **36**, 196–201.

Cook, N.B., Eisele, C.O., Klos, R.F., *et al.* (2004) A coordinated teaching program for future dairy practitioners at the University of Wisconsin–Madison, School of Veterinary Medicine. *Journal of Veterinary Medical Education*, **31**, 372–379.

Cummins, A.M., Catling, C., Hogan, R., and Homer, C.S.E. (2015) Addressing culture shock in first year midwifery students: Maximising the initial clinical experience. *Journal of the Australian College of Midwives*, **27**, 271–275.

Dale, V.H.M., Pierce, S.E., and May, S.A. (2013) Benefits and limitations of an employer-led, structured logbook to promote self-directed learning in the clinical workplace. *Journal of Veterinary Medical Education*, **40**, 402–418.

D'Amore, A., Mitchell, E.K.L., Robinson, C.A., and Chesters, J.E. (2011) Compulsory medical rural placements: Senior student opinions of early-year experiential learning. *Australian Journal of Rural Health*, **19**, 259–266.

European Association of Establishments for Veterinary Education (2012) *Guidelines, Requirements and Main Indicators for Stage 1 (Ia) and Stage 2 (Ib)*. http://www.eaeve.org/fileadmin/downloads/sop/SOPs_GA_Budapest_2012_AnnexI-_Revised_in_April_2015.pdf (accessed November 2015).

Fetrow, J., Ames, T., Farnsworth, R., *et al.* (2004) Minnesota's Transition Management Facility: A private–public partnership in dairy veterinary education and applied research. *Journal of Veterinary Medical Education*, **31**, 368–371.

Freeman, L.J., Ferguson, N., Lister. A., and Arighi, M. (2013) Service learning: Priority 4 Paws mobile surgical service for shelter animals.

Journal of Veterinary Medical Education, **40**, 389–396.

Fuentealba, C., and Hecker, K. (2008) Clinical preceptor evaluation of veterinary students in a distributed model of clinical education. *Journal of Veterinary Medical Education*, **35**, 389–396.

Fuentealba, C., Mason, R.V., and Johnston, S.D. (2008) Community-based clinical veterinary education at Western University of Health Sciences. *Journal of Veterinary Medical Education*, **35**, 34–42.

Harden, R.M., Sowden, S., and Dunn, W.R. (1984) Educational strategies in curriculum development: The SPICES model. *Medical Education*, **18**, 284–297.

Hauer, K.E., Holmboe, E.S., and Kogan, J.R. (2011) Twelve tips for implementing tools for direct observation of medical trainees' clinical skills during patient encounters. *Medical Teacher*, **33**, 27–33.

Hecker, K.G., Norris, J., and Coe, J.B. (2012) Workplace-based assessment in a primary-care setting. *Journal of Veterinary Medical Education*, **39**, 229–240.

Hoet, A.E., Caswell, R.J., DeGraves, F.J., *et al.* (2008) A new approach to teaching veterinary public health at the Ohio State University. *Journal of Veterinary Medical Education*, **35**, 160–165.

Howard, E.K., Lloyd, J.W., and Grooms, D.L. (2009) Innovations in food-supply veterinary medicine: The Michigan State University College of Veterinary Medicine Summer Food Systems Fellowship program. *Journal of Veterinary Medical Education*, **36**, 280–283.

Iowa State University (2015) http://vetmed.iastate.edu/news/isu-swine-medicine-center-receives-approval-board-regents (accessed November 2015).

Jaarsma, D.A.D.C., Dolmans, D.H.J.M., Scherpbier, A.J.J.A., and van Beukelen, P. (2008) Preparation for practice by veterinary school: A comparison of the perceptions of alumni from a traditional and an innovative veterinary curriculum. *Journal of Veterinary Medical Education*, **35**, 431–438.

James Cook University (2015a) *Bachelor of Veterinary Science*. https://www.jcu.edu.au/

courses-and-study/courses/bachelor-of-veterinary-science (accessed November 2015).

James Cook University (2015b) *Tableland Veterinary Service*. https://www.jcu.edu.au/college-of-public-health-medical-and-veterinary-sciences/veterinary-sciences/tableland-veterinary-service (accessed November 2015).

Johnson, B. (2015) A fresh look at EMS. *In Practice*, **32**, 207–209.

Karrier, L.A., Ramirez, A., Leuscheng, B., and Harbur, P. (2008) SPIKE and D-PIKE: Innovative experiences that engage students early and position them to succeed in food-supply veterinary medicine. *Journal of Veterinary Medical Education*, **35**, 297–304.

Kaye, D.K., Mwanika, A., Sekimpi, P., *et al.* (2010) Perceptions of newly admitted undergraduate medical students on experiential training on community placements and working in rural areas of Uganda. *BMC Medical Education*, **10**, 47. doi:10.1186/1472-6920-10-47

Klee, W. (2008) Education in buiatrics – now and in the future. *Proceedings of 25th World Buiatrics Congress, Budapest, Hungary; Hungarian Veterinary Journal*, **130**, **Supp. 1**, 62–66.

Kopcha, M., Lloyd, J.W., Peterson, F., and Derksen, F.J. (2005) Practice-based education at Michigan State University. *Journal of Veterinary Medical Education*, **32**, 555–561.

Lenarduzzi, R., Sheppard, G.A., and Slater, M.R. (2009) Factors influencing the choice of a career in food-animal practice among recent graduates and current students of Texas A&M University, College of Veterinary Medicine. *Journal of Veterinary Medical Education*, **36**, 7–16.

Lloyd, J.W., Fingland, R., Arighi, M., *et al.* (2008) Satellite teaching hospitals and public–private collaborations in veterinary medical clinical education. *Journal of Veterinary Medical Education*, **35**, 43–47.

Lundén, J., Björkroth, J., and Korkeala, H. (2007) Meat inspection education in Finnish veterinary curriculum. *Journal of Veterinary Medical Education*, **34**, 205–210.

Magnier, K., Wang, R., Dale, V.H.M., *et al.* (2011) Enhancing clinical learning in the workplace: A qualitative study. *Veterinary Record* **169**, 682–686.

Mahoney, P., and Martin, N. (2011) EMS: Developing a structured approach. *In Practice*, **33**, 38–41.

Masterson, M.A., Welker, B., Midla, L.T., *et al.* (2004) Use of a non-traditional university ambulatory practice to teach large animal medicine. *Journal of Veterinary Medical Education*, **31**, 380–383.

McIlroy, J.H., Hodges, B., McNaughton, N., and Regehr, G. (2002) The effect of candidates' perceptions of the evaluation method on reliability of checklist and global rating scores in an objective structured clinical examination. *Academic Medicine*, **77**, 725–728.

McNamara, N. (2015) Preparing students for clinical placements: The student's perspective. *Nurse Education in Practice*, **15**, 196–202.

Melbourne University (2015) *VETS70006 Applications in Animal Health 1*. https://handbook.unimelb.edu.au/view/2015/VETS70006 (accessed November 2015).

Melbourne University (2016) *Dairy Resident Training Program*. http://www.u-vet.com.au/learning-at-uvet/dairy-resident-training-program (accessed November 2015).

Miller, G.E. (1990) The assessment of clinical skills/competence/performance. *Academic Medicine*, **65**, s63–s67.

Moore, D.A. (2006) Veterinary school consortia as a means of promoting the food-supply veterinary medicine pipeline. *Journal of Veterinary Medical Education*, **33**, 539–542.

Morris, A. (2009) From EMS to the impact of the recession on animal health. *Veterinary Record*, **164**, 673–676.

Nelson, P.D. (2012) Veterinary college accreditation: Setting the record straight. *Journal of the American Veterinary Medical Association*, **240**, 810–814.

Nydam, C.W., Nydam, D.V., Guard, C.L., and Gilbert, R.O. (2009) Teaching dairy production medicine to entry-level veterinarians: The Summer Dairy Institute model. *Journal of Veterinary Medical Education*, **36**, 16–21.

OIE (2012) *OIE Recommendations on the Competencies of Graduating Veterinarians ("Day 1 graduates") to Assure National Veterinary Services of Quality.* http://www.oie.int/fileadmin/Home/eng/Support_to_OIE_Members/Vet_Edu_AHG/DAY_1/DAYONE-B-ang-vC.pdf (accessed November 2015).

Olsen, C.W., and Remington, P.L. (2008) The dual DVM/MPH degree at the University of Wisconsin—Madison: A uniquely interdisciplinary collaboration. *Journal of Veterinary Medical Education*, **35**, 177–181.

Olson, S.A. (2008) Emergency medicine clerkship: A joining of private-practice referral veterinary medicine with an academic institution. *Journal of Veterinary Medical Education*, **35**, 31–33.

Quinn, K.J., Kane, K.Y., Stevermer, J.J., *et al.* (2011) Influencing residency choice and practice location through a longitudinal rural pipeline program. *Academic Medicine*, **86**, 1397–1406.

Rhind, S.M., Baillie, S., Kinnison, T., *et al.* (2011) The transition into veterinary practice: Opinions of recent graduates and final year students. *BMC Medical Education*, **11**, 64.

Roth, I.G., Poon, W.Y.L., and Hofmeister, E. (2014) Examination of factors that influence students' average client transactions in a small-animal primary care clinical environment. *Journal of Veterinary Medical Education*, **41**, 400–405.

Royal College of Veterinary Surgeons (2009) *EMS Recommendations, Policy & Guidance.* http://www.rcvs.org.uk/document-library/ems-recommendations-policy-and-guidance/ (accessed November 2015).

Royal College of Veterinary Surgeons (2015) *Standards and Procedures for the Accreditation of Veterinary Degrees*, RCVS, London.

Royal Veterinary College (2014) *EMS at the RVS.* https://www.rcvs.org.uk/document-library/ems-at-the-rvc/ (accessed November 2015).

Schmitz, J.A., Vogt, R.J., Rupp, G.P., *et al.* (2007) Factors associated with practice decisions of Nebraska veterinarians regarding type of practice and community size. *Journal of Veterinary Medical Education*, **31**, 366–367.

Scholz, E., Trede, F., and Raidal, S.L. (2013) Workplace learning in veterinary education: A sociocultural perspective. *Journal of Veterinary Medical Education*, **40**, 355–362.

Smith, B.P. (2004) The UC Davis early dairy experience program. *Journal of Veterinary Medical Education*, **34**, 340–349.

Smulders, F.J.M., Buncic, S., Fehlhaber, K., *et al.* (2012) Toward harmonization of the European food hygiene/veterinary public health curriculum. *Journal of Veterinary Medical Education*, **39**, 169–179.

Snowden, K., Bice, K., Craig, T., *et al.* (2008) Vertically integrated educational collaboration between a college of veterinary medicine and a non-profit animal shelter. *Journal of Veterinary Medical Education*, **35**, 637–640.

Solarsh, G., Lindley, J., Whyte, G., *et al.* (2012) Governance and assessment in a widely distributed medical education program in Australia. *Academic Medicine*, **87**, 807–814.

Stevens, B.J., and Gruen, M.E. (2014) Training veterinary students in shelter medicine: A service-learning community-classroom technique. *Journal of Veterinary Medical Education*, **41**, 83–89.

Stoddard, R.E., and Glynn, M.K. (2009) Opening the window on public health to veterinary students. *Revue scientifique et technique*, **28**, 671–679.

Stone, E.A., Conlon, P., Cox, S., and Coe, J.B. (2012) A new model for companion-animal primary health care education. *Journal of Veterinary Medical Education*, **39**, 210–216.

Sydney University (2015) *VSIP – Veterinary Student Internship Programme.* http://sydney.edu.au/vetscience/partners/vsip/intro.shtml (accessed November 2015).

Taylor, I., and Barnes, J. (1998) *Supporting Independent Learning in Veterinary Extramural Rotations.* RCVS, London.

Thistlethwaite, J.E., Chong, A.A.L., Dick, M.L., *et al.* (2013) A review of longitudinal community and hospital placements in medical education: BEME guide no. 26. *Medical Teacher*, **35**, e1340–e1364.

Tyner, C.L., Harkness, J., Hoblet, K., *et al.* (2014) University teaching hospital and private clinic collaboration to enhance veterinary educational opportunities at Mississippi State University. *Journal of Veterinary Medical Education*, **41**, 90–95.

University of California, Davis (2015) *Criteria for Admission*. http://www.vetmed.ucdavis.edu/students/admissions/criteria.cfm (accessed November 2015).

Veterinary Council of India (2008) *Minimum Standards of Veterinary Education: Degree Course (B.V.Sc. & A.H.) Regulations, 2008*. www.vci.nic.in/writereaddata/Final%20RegulationsMSVE%20(1).doc (accessed November 2016).

Western University of Health Sciences (2013) *Fourth Year Core Clinical Sites*. http://www.westernu.edu/bin/veterinary/allguidelines/facilitiesguidelines/facilitesguidelines4thyrcore.pdf (accessed November 2015).

Windsor, P. (2009) Can curriculum innovations create incentives for young veterinarians to practise in remote rural areas? *Revue scientifique et technique*, **28**, 689–697.

Part IV

Assessing the Student

14

Concepts in Assessment

Jared Danielson[1] and Kent Hecker[2]

[1] *College of Veterinary Medicine, Iowa State University, USA*
[2] *Faculty of Veterinary Medicine, Cumming School of Medicine, University of Calgary, Canada*

Box 14.1: Key messages

- Expect modest differences in terminology among the many communities that write about education and assessment.
- Assessment can occur at many levels within the educational endeavor, including at the student, classroom, and program levels.
- Assessment can serve both formative and summative purposes.
- Assessment can be norm or criterion referenced. Decisions regarding how or whether or not grades are assigned are independent of the quality of the assessment itself.
- Carefully characterizing what your students need to know or be able to do is fundamental to effective assessment. A taxonomy of learning outcomes and skillfully worded objectives can be helpful.
- High-quality assessment adheres to standards/principles of validity, propriety, utility, and feasibility.

Introduction

The language of education and educational assessment is not uniform, owing in large part to the many backgrounds of those engaged in it. For 2014, the Scimago Journal and Country Rank (Scimago Lab, 2015) listed 914 journals in the category of education. Among the top 50 were general education journals representing a variety of perspectives, including educational psychology, child development, learning sciences, educational technology, and higher education, as well as a variety of discipline-specific journals, including engineering, science, economics, sociology, second-language acquisition, mathematics, and medicine. The remaining 864 indexed education journals were similarly diverse. While critical concepts in assessment are common among these many perspectives, there is inevitable variability in context, emphasis, and language. Where possible, in this chapter we will employ terms that are common across domains, using specific examples from the terms used in health professional education where appropriate. However, do not be surprised if after reading

---

Veterinary Medical Education: A Practical Guide, First Edition. Edited by Jennifer L. Hodgson and Jacquelyn M. Pelzer.
© 2017 John Wiley & Sons, Inc. Published 2017 by John Wiley & Sons, Inc.

this chapter, you encounter new and different language or terminology in subsequent reading.

To assess something is to examine it in order to characterize or quantify attributes of interest, usually for the purpose of making a decision. There are a number of labels that can be applied to assessment of students, such as *testing, evaluation,* or *measurement.* We consider the terms *evaluation* and *assessment* to be synonymous (Scriven, 1991). *Testing* is a specific assessment strategy that involves examinations (as opposed to other assessment strategies such as portfolios). We refer to *measurement* as the specific characteristics of assessment that are most closely tied to the validity of the claims that might be drawn from the assessment, as opposed to other considerations such as utility, feasibility, or propriety.

There are many potential approaches to devising a chapter on assessment. Some assessment texts focus primarily on the role of assessment in the context of an endeavor, such as higher education (Banta *et al.,* 1996; Huba and Freed, 2000). Others focus on the effective use of assessment information (Popham, 2006), or on the process of creating effective assessments (Hopkins, 1998; Secolsky and Denison, 2012). In this chapter we will define and explain key concepts in the context of practical problems that a veterinary educator might face, providing examples where possible. We will frame the chapter in terms of concepts in three general categories: *why* to assess (purposes of assessment), *what* to assess (defining outcomes), and *how* to assess (methodological and practical considerations). We hope that you can use this chapter to guide some specific assessment activities. For instance, we explain the characteristics of effective objectives, in hopes that you will be able to write better objectives after reading that section. However, the primary purpose of the chapter is to provide a conceptual overview for next steps in improving your own assessments, and to provide a foundation for additional reading.

Why: Purposes of Assessment

Levels of Assessment

Assessment can occur at numerous levels of the educational endeavor. At the most fundamental level, we seek to determine what individual students know and/or can do; this constitutes assessment at the *learner* level. Sometimes assessment at the learner level provides insufficient information to answer relevant questions about an educational outcome. Imagine, for instance, that learners in a clinical pharmacology course consistently master what they are taught, but are perennially unprepared to perform common dosage calculations in subsequent courses or clinical experiences. If this were the case, assessment would need to be conducted at the *course level* to determine why students who appeared to be learning the foundational knowledge were subsequently not competent in a key area. Assessment activities at the course level might explore questions such as whether the desired content is being taught at all, whether existing tests are adequately measuring the desired learning outcomes, and/or whether there are adequate opportunities for practice. Some important questions cannot be answered at the student or course level, however. Imagine, for instance, that veterinary students perform well in all of their courses, and that all of their courses prepare them adequately for subsequent courses, but that on graduation they are systematically deficient in a specific area. Such a scenario would reveal the need for assessment at the program level, answering questions such as whether or not knowledge and skills in the deficient area are taught or valued by the institution. One can conceive of important assessment questions at levels other than these three: for instance, it might be appropriate to conduct assessment at the department level, or much more broadly (for example, across a state, province, or country). However, most educational assessments in veterinary medicine can be characterized as being at the level of the learner, course, or program. In this chapter, we will provide concepts that can be applied at any of those levels, although the emphasis will mostly be at the learner level.

Formative versus Summative Assessment

Assessments at any of these levels can be *formative* or *summative* (Bloom, Hasting, and Madaus, 1971). *Formative assessment* is used principally for improvement. At the student level, a scored but ungraded test or other practice activity can provide students with the information they need to make improvements in knowledge or skills, and can help the instructor know what knowledge or skills to emphasize. At the course level, an instructor might ask students to respond to informal or unofficial course or faculty evaluations, or invite a colleague to observe and provide informal input. At the program level, a veterinary school department chair or dean might ask a group of colleagues to conduct a mock accreditation site visit. In all of these instances, the primary purpose of the assessment is to offer the entity being assessed a low- or no-risk opportunity to see how it is doing, and where improvements might be needed. *Summative assessment*, in contrast, is used to inform a decision regarding the future of the entity being assessed, and usually involves important stakes. At the student level, a graded examination is summative, because it results in a score or grade point average that might influence important decisions such as the student's ability to move forward in the curriculum or be placed in a residency program. At the classroom level, faculty and course assessments are summative whenever they are used to make decisions such as whether or not the instructor will continue to be invited to teach, obtain tenure, or receive a raise. Official accreditation site visits and reviews of annual reports to the accrediting body are summative assessments at the program or institution level, because they influence whether or not the institution will enjoy the privileges of accreditation.

Sometimes the terms formative and summative are used as if they were inherent characteristics of assessment instruments or tools. However, the key attribute that distinguishes a formative assessment from a summative one is the purpose for which it is used. The exact same exam is a formative assessment if used as a practice exam, and a summative assessment if used as a final exam. The term *feedback* is occasionally substituted in casual conversation for *formative assessment*, because the primary purpose of feedback is to provide information to the entity being assessed. However, both formative and summative assessments can provide valuable feedback to learners, teachers, and programs.

Grades, Normative versus Criterion-Referenced Assessment, and Rigor

Many faculty assess students, at least in part, so that they can assign a grade. Similarly, some students seem to engage in assessment activities primarily so that they can receive a grade (a good one, they hope). Grades in turn can be reported to external stakeholders, such as directors of residency programs, future graduate programs, or employers, who might use them as one source of evidence regarding what the student has learned or is likely to be able to achieve. Grades and grade point averages can be helpful because they provide a relatively concise mechanism for communicating what a student has learned or can do, relative to others who participated in a similar experience (see Box 14.2). Grades also communicate information about other kinds of issues, such as how good students are at anticipating what professors will ask on tests, how hard they work, how much extra credit work they complete, or whether or not they have unexcused absences. Assessment is not the same as grading. Assessment determines what students know or can do, and grading documents merit or rank in an educational setting. Instructors and institutions can use assessment information for a variety of important purposes, including deciding what to teach next/more/better/less, and when/how/to whom to provide remediation, as well as to assign grades.

Assessments are either *norm referenced* or *criterion referenced*, depending on whether they compare examinees to each other, or to an established standard (Glaser, 1963). Assessments

Box 14.2: Focus on assumptions about grades

Grades are not an inevitable characteristic of assessment, nor do they have to coincide with individual courses. A number of medical education programs use two-interval (pass/fail) grading (Spring *et al.*, 2011) rather than conventional letter grading. Furthermore, some medical programs employ progress testing (Finucane *et al.*, 2010; van der Vleuten, Verwijnen, and Wifnen, 1996), in which assessment occurs at the institution level and not the course level. Available studies suggest that such approaches improve student wellbeing without having an adverse impact on learning (Spring *et al.*, 2011). These strategies focus on ensuring that all students achieve an acceptable level of competence, without excessive concern for sorting or ranking. While students are not assigned a grade, they are, of course, assessed all the same. Determining what students know is essential, whether that knowledge is associated with a letter grade or not.

that are intended to compare examinees to each other are referred to as *norm-referenced* tests, because they reference a group *norm* or average. Some assessment purposes are best served by referencing norms. For example, placement exams like the Graduate Record Examination (GRE) are used by academic programs to select students when filling a limited number of seats. In such cases, programs will admit a full cohort whether those students are remarkably capable academically, or are barely able to meet the minimum standard. Decision-makers seek to admit the most qualified applicants from the available pool.

In other cases, assessment serves to compare examinees to an established standard. Such assessments are *criterion referenced*, because the standard of success references one or more established criteria. Licensing exams are criterion referenced: test designers seek to establish the minimum knowledge and skills required of a competent practitioner in a specific discipline, and to determine whether or not each examinee is minimally competent. Hopefully, all competent examinees will pass the test, and all incompetent examinees will fail it. (For those of you who are suddenly getting flashbacks to your Public Health course, educational assessment is indeed similar to other kinds of assessment, and while educational assessment folks do not use those terms, this use of criterion-referenced

assessments is similar to the use of diagnostic tests in veterinary medicine, and the concepts of sensitivity and specificity certainly apply.)

Bear in mind that it is the inference that is made from the test, and not the test itself, that is either norm or criterion referenced. However, as noted by W. James Popham:

> More often than not, ... if an educational measuring instrument is built to provide norm-referenced inferences, it usually does *not* do a good job in providing criterion referenced interpretations. And, if an educational measuring instrument is originally built to provide criterion-referenced inferences, it usually does *not* do a good job in providing norm-referenced interpretations. (Popham, 2006, p. 35)

We suggest that in most educational settings, it makes more sense to design tests to support criterion-referenced rather than norm-referenced inferences. After all, interested stakeholders, including the students themselves and the public at large, have a greater interest in knowing how well each individual's performance matches a relevant standard than how well it matches the performance of other students.

Rigor is not a precise assessment term such as *validity* or *accuracy*, but is often used in lay language to reference how challenging or difficult an assessment is, with the assumption that a rigorous assessment is able to separate the truly prepared from the more casually prepared. Of course, designing an assessment that does clearly differentiate those who excel from those who do not is helpful. However, instructors are advised not simply to rely on statistical manipulation of test scores to create the appearance of rigor. Some instructors assume that an exam will automatically be rigorous if the grades are normally distributed, with scores being assigned automatically to grades based on where those scores fall in the distribution. Similarly, some instructors assume that the lower the average on a test, the more rigorous the assessment process. However, rigor is not a function of score distribution or grading scale. Rather, a "rigorous" assessment provides valid, useful, sufficiently comprehensive information about what students know, or are able to do with what they have learned. There is nothing inherently wrong with grades being normally distributed, but faculty who are primarily interested in a normal distribution of scores might just as well assess students based on their height, weight, or body temperature. As noted by Bloom, Hastings, and Madaus (1971, p. 45), "There is nothing sacred about the normal curve. It is the distribution most appropriate to chance and random activity. Education is a purposeful activity, and we seek to have the students learn what we have to teach."

Describing What to Measure

If it is important to establish the criteria by which learners will be assessed, it is first necessary to characterize the outcomes of learning accurately and precisely. Taxonomies of learning facilitate this purpose. Just as veterinarians and animal scientists use taxonomies of organisms to learn rules that apply to certain orders, families, or species of animals, and not to others, educational practitioners learn rules that apply to certain types of learning outcomes, and not to others. Most educators are familiar, conceptually, with broad types of learning outcomes; they often hear messages to teach "higher-order" rather than "lower-order" thinking, or to emphasize "critical thinking" rather than "rote memorization." Such ideas can be useful reminders that we would like our students to be able to do things that are important or meaningful, but they are not sufficiently precise to guide specific assessment or teaching decisions. Taxonomies of learning outcomes are intended to help provide more precision. Unfortunately for educators, there is no universally accepted taxonomy of learning outcomes, so it is not uncommon to become familiar with one taxonomy, only to find that colleagues are familiar with another (Alexander, Schallert, and Hare, 1991; de Jong and Ferguson-Hessler, 1996). We will introduce two common taxonomies in hopes that you can apply the principles discussed regardless of the taxonomy you happen to be employing at any particular time.

Bloom's taxonomy, perhaps the best-known classification scheme for learning outcomes, defines three domains of knowledge: *cognitive* (having to do with intellectual or thinking/reasoning skills), *affective* (having to do with attitudes, beliefs, and motivation), and *psychomotor* (having to do with the ability to manipulate tools, objects, or one's own body; Bloom *et al.*, 1956). The cognitive domain, as found in the 2001 revision of Bloom's taxonomy (Anderson *et al.*, 2001), conceptualizes learning outcomes across two dimensions: the cognitive process dimension, which includes *remember, understand, apply, analyze, evaluate*, and *create*; and the knowledge dimension, which includes *factual knowledge, conceptual knowledge, procedural knowledge*, and *metacognitive knowledge*. In this framework, instructional outcomes are classified in terms of both the cognitive process and the knowledge dimension being targeted. This approach is flexible and powerful, but requires more than a casual familiarity with the specific terms and concepts of the taxonomy. Therefore, for veterinary educators with an interest in clearly and effectively classifying educational outcomes, Bloom's taxonomy can provide a valuable approach, but a thorough discussion of it is beyond the scope of this chapter.

Other categorizations of learning outcomes have also been created to facilitate instructional design and evaluation. Among those, Gagné, Briggs, and Wager's (1992) taxonomy has been particularly influential among practitioners who design/evaluate instruction. Smith and Ragan's (2005) adaptation of Gagné's framework is often used to train beginning instructional designers, and is useful because it is relatively concise and involves all three knowledge domains (cognitive, psychomotor, and affective). In Table 14.1, the left-hand columns provide Smith and Ragan's categorization of learned capabilities; the middle column offers a brief definition with examples from a veterinary context; and the right-hand column contains appropriate assessment approaches for the capability. The latter are not meant to be limiting, but to provide the reader with the approaches that most commonly and best match the learned capability. Furthermore, assessment of lower-order knowledge/skills can often be embedded into assessment of higher-order knowledge/skills.

There are at least two important problems that can arise from a fundamental misunderstanding of, or inattention to, kinds of learning outcomes:

- *Outcomes snobbery, and a resulting sloppiness in measurement.* It can be tempting to want to appear to "keep up with the Joneses" when it comes to learning outcomes. Instructors want to be seen as teaching important things like problem-solving or "critical thinking," as opposed to "lesser" outcomes like facts or terms. However, this impulse can be counterproductive. The purpose of using a taxonomy of learning outcomes is not to identify and favor certain learning outcomes while avoiding others, but accurately to characterize what needs to be learned in any given context. "Lower-order" outcomes are often fundamental to more advanced ones. Facts and terms are important building blocks of a discipline; it is not possible to learn advanced

concepts, principles, and so forth without them.
- *Mismatching desired outcomes and assessments.* It is remarkably common for educators to create assessments that seem relatively unrelated to their desired learning outcomes. For instance, an instructor might claim to be testing problem-solving (or "critical thinking") when the test questions themselves primarily measure students' ability to remember definitions of terms. Often such misalignment goes quite unnoticed by the instructor, for lack of having carefully defined the desired learning outcomes in the first place. Considering where the desired learning outcome fits in the context of a taxonomy of learning outcomes can help to prevent this problem.

In addition to general taxonomies of learning outcomes, other frameworks have been suggested for identifying important types of learning outcomes in specific fields. One framework that has gained popularity in medical education is Miller's Framework for Clinical Assessment (Miller, 1990). Miller conceived of this framework in response to the need to document clinical proficiency and the knowledge related to it as it develops during the transformation of novice into independent practitioner. He defined ability at the lowest ("Knows") level of his framework as knowing "what is required in order to carry out … professional functions effectively." The second level ("Knows How") involves "the skill of acquiring information from a variety of human and laboratory sources, to analyze and interpret these data, and finally to translate such findings into a rational diagnostic or management plan." The "Shows How" level involves a student actually demonstrating the ability "when faced with a patient." The "Does" level aims to "predict what a graduate does when functioning independently in a clinical practice" (p. S63). Not intended to be a complete taxonomy of learning outcomes, Miller's framework provides a useful approach for conceptualizing outcomes specific to the task of becoming a medical practitioner. Ultimately,

Table 14.1 Smith and Ragan's adaptation of Gagné's learned capabilities.

Learned capability		Definition with veterinary example	Common assessment approach
Intellectual skills	Problem-solving	Applying known principles or other knowledge/skills to address previously unencountered problems. In veterinary medicine, we often think of diagnostic and clinical decision making as examples of problem-solving.	Examinee solves an authentic problem. Responses can vary from selecting an option in an extended matching or script concordance test, to providing descriptions, differential diagnosis lists, problem lists, treatment protocols, etc. Testing environments can include classroom, clinical, and computer-based settings.
	Procedure	Learning and performing the appropriate ordered steps in a task. Drawing blood, making a blood smear, performing a physical exam, conducting a medical interview, and countless other veterinary tasks all involve procedures.	Examinee performs the procedure while examiner uses an observation protocol to assess the performance.
	Principle	Principles are also called rules, and describe the relationships among concepts or ideas. Understanding mechanisms of disease or health, the action of drugs, and so forth involves principles.	Examinee explains or applies principles in response to open-ended or carefully written multiple-choice items.
	Defined concept	The ability to categorize accurately based on defined or theoretical attributes. Examples of defined concepts are innumerable, and include things such as specific diseases, conditions such as stress or anxiety, and so forth.	Examinees are shown examples and close nonexamples of the target concept(s) and asked to identify the accurate examples, through either multiple-choice or short-answer questions.
	Concrete concept	The ability to categorize accurately based on concrete attributes such as size, shape, and color. Examples are endless, such as surgical instruments, species of animals, and body condition scores (by appearance).	
	Discrimination	Ability to perceive that two things match or do not. For instance, students learning cytology must be able to distinguish subtle differences between the appearance of normal and abnormal cells; students learning abdominal palpation must be able to detect subtle differences in size, firmness, or location of the structures being palpated.	Similar to concepts, examinees choose between examples and nonexamples.

(Continued)

Table 14.1 (Continued)

Learned capability	Definition with veterinary example	Common assessment approach
Declarative knowledge	Knowing "that" something is. Being able to recite information from memory such as facts or labels. There is no assumption of understanding embedded meaning.	Rote production (written or spoken) is necessary to ensure mastery, though multiple-choice-type items are sufficient to ensure recognition.
Cognitive strategies	Strategies that learners/problem solvers employ to manage their own learning/thinking. Rehearsing what one has learned, tying new knowledge to prior knowledge, and so forth.	Not typically assessed in higher education environments; assumed to translate into mastery of other learned outcomes.
Attitudes	Attitudes are affective learning outcomes. An attitude is a mental state that influences what we choose to do. Attitudes have cognitive and behavioral components. When we are tasked with measuring things like "ethical behavior" or "professionalism," we are often trying to measure attitudes.	Attitudinal surveys or observation of behaviors that demonstrate the desired outcome in the absence of a threat for noncompliance.
Psychomotor skills	"Coordinated muscular movements that are typified by smoothness and precise timing" (Smith and Ragan, 2005, p. 82). Many veterinary tasks have psychomotor components, including countless surgical, clinical, or diagnostic techniques such as knot tying, making a blood smear, venipuncture, instrument handling during surgery, and so forth.	Examinee performs the procedure while examiner uses an observation protocol to assess the performance.

that is the purpose of any taxonomy of learning outcomes: to allow the educator to conceptualize specific learning outcomes in ways that facilitate learning and assessment.

Objectives

Critical to defining learning outcomes is creating useful outcomes statements, most commonly and broadly referred to as *objectives* (Anderson *et al.*, 2001). You have likely heard a variety of labels substituted for objectives, some of which include goal, outcome, proficiency, competency, entrustable professional activity, content standard, curricular aim, performance standard, and academic achievement standard (Anderson *et al.*, 2001; Flynn

et al., 2014; Popham, 2006). The term objective itself is sometimes qualified with terms such as *instructional*, *educational*, *global*, or *program* (Anderson *et al.*, 2001). The Council on Education (COE) of the American Veterinary Medical Association (AVMA) refers to its nine clinical proficiency outcomes areas as *competencies* (AVMA COE, 2014); similarly, the Royal College of Veterinary Surgeons (RCVS) refers to its required outcomes of veterinary programs as *Day One Competencies* (RCVS, 2014). The Association of American Medical Colleges (AAMC) recently abandoned the term competency for the required outcomes to enter residencies in favor of *core entrustable professional activity (EPA)*, arguing, among other things, that doing so allowed for framing those outcomes in terms of activities that represent everyday work in clinical settings (Flynn *et al.*, 2014). All of these outcomes labels have as their common ancestor the term *objective*, which is still most commonly associated with carefully worded educational outcomes (Anderson *et al.*, 2001). The characteristics of effective objectives are similar, regardless of the specific emphasis, purpose, or label employed when writing them. In this section we will discuss and illustrate general characteristics of useful outcomes statements, employing the term *objective*, although you may have cause to use other terms and/or to modify your objectives themselves somewhat, depending on the context in which you are writing them.

In general, objectives are helpful for guiding both instruction and assessment only if they are sufficiently detailed for the intended purpose. We will describe a long-used approach to writing detailed objectives using the Instructional Development Institute's acronym ABCD: A = Audience, B = Behavior, C = Condition, and D = Degree (Merrill and Goodman, 1972). Note that objectives fall on a continuum of specificity, from very broad (program or discipline level) to more specific (course, class, or module level). Some educators find excessively detailed objectives to be limiting, causing them to lose sight of the forest for the trees, and leading some to abandon the specification of condition and degree. Furthermore, condition and degree are rarely specified when articulating broad (program- or course-level) outcomes. Nonetheless, if you master this approach, you will be able to provide the right degree of specificity when needed, reducing that specificity by eliminating unnecessary elements as desired.

Audience

Audience refers to the group that will be assessed, and matching the objective to the group being assessed is essential to validity. As educational measurement expert Michael Kane points out, "validity is not a property of the test. Rather, it is a property of the proposed interpretations and uses of test scores" (Kane, 2013, p. 3). Applied to the question of audience, a test might produce valid interpretations and uses when used with one audience or context, and meaningless data when used with another. When writing objectives for tests, it is important to specify the audience in sufficient detail that your questions will not miss their mark. Is the assessment intended for first-year veterinary students, fourth-year veterinary students, first-year residents, fourth-year residents, or graduate students? In our experience, veterinary faculty most commonly miss the mark in terms of audience by writing questions that are too detailed or advanced for the level of their learners.

Behavior

The *behavior* is simply represented by the "verb" in the objective (Anderson *et al.*, 2001). The care and precision with which you describe what your students will do to demonstrate what they have learned will pay great dividends when you design assessments. One common mistake in writing objectives is to choose verbs that are too general to be useful for guiding assessment. Words such as "know," "understand," "appreciate," "recognize that," "see," and "become familiar with" are usually too vague to guide assessment. The Internet abounds with lists of verbs that are helpful for writing objectives, often associated with discussions of Bloom's taxonomy.

Helpful verbs describe what students will do to demonstrate that they have certain knowledge or skills. Helpful objective statements describe tasks that can actually be done in the assessment setting. To illustrate, let us imagine that you want your students to "understand" aseptic technique. To demonstrate their mastery of this technique, students might do any number of things, including the following:

- Given five descriptions of scenarios involving surgery, one of which describes appropriate aseptic technique and four of which describe common critical errors in aseptic technique, select the error-free description.
- Write an accurate definition of aseptic technique.

- Given a description of a situation demanding aseptic technique, describe what steps must be taken to ensure aseptic technique.
- Demonstrate aseptic technique in a simulated surgical setting.
- Demonstrate aseptic technique in an authentic surgical setting.

All of these behaviors are reasonable surrogates for "understand" and all are sufficiently specific to guide assessment. However, they do not all measure the same ability. One of your most important tasks is to determine what your students need to be able to do with the knowledge or skills you are teaching, and then to do your best to make sure that your assessments reflect those needs.

Condition

Helpful objectives adequately describe the *conditions* of assessment. Conditions include the setting and resources that you will need to assess the behavior you have identified. For instance, will the task be done in a classroom setting, lab, or clinical setting? Will it involve a real client/patient or a standardized client/patient? Will students have access to notes/textbooks? It is not uncommon for instructors to write an objective such as "demonstrate aseptic technique" and then measure the objective with a multiple-choice question, because they did not foresee or plan for the resources necessary to observe all of the students performing the task. In such a situation, it would be preferable for the instructor to write a more realistic objective and accurately measure it, than to write an ideal objective and largely ignore it.

Degree

Helpful objectives define important criteria of *degree* such as accuracy, precision, speed, and/or thoroughness. For example, given a specific clinical scenario, must students identify the top five of five likely differential diagnoses, or is it acceptable to identify three of the top five? If performing venipuncture, must the student collect a certain amount of blood with no more than a given number of "sticks"? Can the blood be collected from one of several sites, or must students demonstrate proficiency on multiple sites? Answers to these kinds of questions are often helpful when planning/creating assessments.

Well-written objectives help address the important assessment purpose of ensuring that what the instructor hopes the students know or can do matches what is taught, and in turn matches the assessment. Table 14.2 contains four test questions with an accompanying precise objective for each question. In each objective, the **audience is bolded**, the <u>behavior is underlined</u>, the *condition is in italics*, and the degree is in ALL UPPER CASE. Each of the four test questions could accompany the excessively broad objective: "Understand hemostasis." Each question tests a quite different intellectual skill from the others. The instructor's task is to decide what skill is most important to measure, and to write an assessment that does so.

Sometimes it can be difficult and time consuming to articulate objectives that adequately express the desired behavior, condition, and/or degree. However, once you develop the habit, you will find that it is almost as easy – and considerably more worthwhile – to write helpful objectives than unhelpful ones.

How to Measure (Principles)

As explained in the previous section, accurately determining where your desired learning outcomes fit in a taxonomy of learning outcomes and writing clear objectives both provide important clues to how you might want to conduct an assessment. In other words, carefully characterizing *what* you intend to measure has implications for *how* you intend to measure it. There are other important considerations as well. Texts written with educational measurement professionals in mind detail a variety of considerations when creating educational measures, and we recommend those for readers who wish to make a serious study of educational measurement. The following "big ideas" are

Table 14.2 Potential assessment items with corresponding objective statements for the excessively general objective "understand hemostasis".

Assessment item	Related objective/explanation
Question 1. In the process of primary hemostatic plug formation, exposed subendothelium, vWF, GPlb, receptor, and collagen resulting from vessel injury lead <u>most immediately</u> to which of the following processes? a. Vessel spasm b. Platelet adhesion and shape change* c. Thrombus consolidation d. Fibrin meshwork	**Objective:** *Given 4 potential sequences of hemostatic blood formation processes,* **first-year veterinary students** will <u>recognize the correct sequence,</u> FOR ANY TWO NONCONTIGUOUS PROCESSES, WITHOUT REFERENCE MATERIALS. **Discussion:** Note that because this is a multiple-choice item, the students cannot actually construct a response. All multiple-choice questions, at the end of the day, require recognition and selection, and not construction of an answer. It would be tempting, but inaccurate, to use the verb "list" or "order" in an objective for this particular assessment. We have chosen "recognize the correct sequence," since respondents do not actually produce a list or form a sequence, they simply remember a sequence. The essential condition is that the student will be shown potential sequences of hemostatic blood formation processes. The objective does not dictate a format other than that, although in this case the question has been written in a standard multiple-choice format. The instructor has specified that this task should be done from memory, and, recognizing that it might be a little too tricky/picky to have students distinguish between two contiguous processes that might overlap, instead chooses processes that are at least two steps apart from each other, hence the reminder of "noncontiguous." This item measures either recognition of verbal information and sequence, or mastery of concepts and principles, depending on whether the student has learned the information in a rote way or a principle-based way.
Question 2. Describe the process of hemostatic plug formation, including all fundamental processes in accurate order.	**Objective:** *Given a paper and pencil,* **first-year veterinary students** will <u>describe the process of hemostatic plug formation,</u> INCLUDING AT LEAST 10 OF THE 13 FUNDAMENTAL PROCESSES, IN ACCURATE ORDER. **Discussion:** The behavior for this objective is pretty straightforward. It does not matter whether students use pencil and paper, a computer, or something else to answer, but the condition should be clear enough to ensure that it matches the test environment and is a good fit to what the students will be asked to do. A good degree statement is particularly important with a question in which students will need to produce a constructed response (such as a description of a process, in this case), because this will be very helpful to whomever is tasked with grading the responses. Good degree statements make it much easier to write *response characteristics*, which are detailed criteria used to evaluate responses. This item measures either recall of verbal information, or mastery of concepts and principles, depending on whether the student has learned the information in a rote way or a principle-based way.

(Continued)

Table 14.2 (Continued)

Assessment item	Related objective/explanation
Question 3. The arrest of bleeding by the physiological properties of vasoconstriction and coagulation or by surgical means is known as a. Hemostasis* b. Anemia c. Polycythemia d. Coagulation	**Objective:** *Given the definition of hemostasis and four terms related to hematology, including hemostasis,* **first-year veterinary students** will <u>select the term that matches the definition,</u> WITHOUT USING REFERENCE MATERIALS. **Discussion:** This particular item only measures recognition of verbal information (a definition), and so would probably not be appropriate for veterinary students.
Question 4. You are presented with Buddy, a 5-year-old male neutered Doberman pinscher. Buddy's owner reports that he has been increasingly listless over the past month, and seems to get occasional nosebleeds. The owner is unaware of Buddy eating anything unusual, and reports that Buddy has not experienced any trauma. On examination you notice that Buddy has pale mucus membranes. List your top three differentials, and the most appropriate diagnostic approach for ruling each of them in or out.	**Objective:** *Given a written scenario describing a patient suffering from an abnormality that causes bleeding,* **first-year veterinary students** <u>will list</u> three of the five most likely differentials, and the most appropriate diagnostic approach for addressing each differential. **Discussion:** This item almost certainly requires students to remember and apply concepts and principles that were learned earlier, and hence seems to involve problem-solving.

Note: In each objective, the **audience is bolded**, the <u>behavior is underlined</u>, the *condition is in italics*, and the degree is in ALL UPPER CASE.

derived from published standards (Gullickson, 2003; AERA, APA, and NCME, 2014) for those professionals, and are useful for anyone seeking to engage in educational assessment.

Validity

"Validity refers to the degree to which evidence and theory support the interpretations of test scores for proposed uses of tests" (AERA, APA, and NCME, 2014, p. 11). Most veterinary educators are very familiar with the concept of validity. For example, valid scores from diagnostic tests identify diseases or conditions when they are present, and fail to identify them when they are absent. Similarly, a score from a valid educational test will identify expertise, or ability, when it is present, and will fail to identify it when it is absent, and scores are often expected to distinguish accurately between levels of expertise or ability. The validity of uses of test scores or other educational assessment scores is particularly important when the stakes are high. Board examinations, entrance examinations,

and professional aptitude tests are assembled with great care, and considerable attention is given to the validity of test interpretations, because very high-stakes decisions (such as whether or not someone will be licensed or accepted into a program of study) are made based on those test scores.

The 2014 Standards for Educational and Psychological Testing (AERA, APA, and NCME, 2014, p. 23) direct test developers that "clear articulation of each intended test score interpretation for a specified use should be set forth, and appropriate validity evidence in support of each intended interpretation should be provided." Associated with that overarching standard are 25 supporting standards, including factors such as the existence or absence of support for various interpretations of the test, constructs measured by the test, likely interpretations or uses of a test that have not been validated, the intended population for the test, the composition of test takers from which validity evidence was obtained, internal structure of the test, relationships between test scores and other related constructs, and more. The design and interpretation of professional tests involve teams of content experts and psychometricians, as well as expertise that is often not available to veterinary educators engaged in everyday assessment activities such as writing questions for midterm or final exams, or designing an objective structured clinical examination (OSCE) station. However, there are several simple questions that anyone can ask to help safeguard the validity of the interpretation of their assessments.

Are my Measures Aligned with my Objectives?

If you have written the objectives carefully, and constructed your test items with your objectives in mind, then you have made the first and most essential step in ensuring that they are aligned. It is easy to misalign measures inadvertently, as the following two examples illustrate.

When I (JD) was a Master's student, I taught English as a Second Language (ESL) to middle-school students. My students' other teachers and I would occasionally meet to coordinate our efforts. During one such meeting, the math teacher produced a sample of one of my student's math assignments and criticized it at length, suggesting that the student should receive a poor grade because of the large size and sloppiness of the writing. I asked if the answers were correct. My colleagues charitably attributed my question to my innocent and well-intentioned ignorance of the importance of neatness, and the conversation moved on with the implied understanding that this assignment (and all such assignments) deserved a low grade, regardless of the accuracy of the answers. On another occasion, I was teaching a workshop to graduate students regarding how to write effective multiple-choice questions. I explained that test-wise students use strategies such as "convergence" to guess the correct answer without understanding the content. A bright student raised his hand and asked whether it was a good idea to write a test that purposefully leads test-wise students toward wrong answers.

Both of these examples illustrate how everyday teaching and assessment situations provide instructors with attractive opportunities unwittingly to compromise validity. In the first case, while it is not wrong to hold students responsible for producing neat work, our student (and his parents) needed to understand that the score he received on that assignment supported a (hopefully) valid interpretation of his neatness, but it did not support a valid interpretation of his math ability. Similarly, in the second example, if instructors choose to use test-taking strategies to purposefully ensnare test-wise students, they are choosing to measure students' test-wiseness, in addition to (or rather than) their knowledge of the content. Clearly, if the goal of the assessment is to measure ability in the content area being taught, such strategies undermine that goal, introducing systematic variation in scores that is unrelated to the ability of interest. These two examples illustrate the importance of aligning measures with objectives as a simple matter of meeting minimum validity standards. As we will see in a subsequent section, such testing approaches also compromise the propriety of the assessment.

What is the Relationship between Scores on my Assessment and Performance on Other Related Assessments?

Often, you are not the only individual testing students' ability in the disciplinary area in which you teach; usually, their ability is measured again in subsequent courses, or even on standardized examinations. For instance, the Veterinary Education Assessment (VEA; NBVME, 2015) produced by the International Council for Veterinary Assessment" (ICVA) in the United States provides scores in anatomy, physiology, pharmacology, pathology, and microbiology. Comparing the scores that students receive in similar content areas across exams can provide an estimate of the extent to which what is being measured is consistent. Theoretically, significant correlations between scores on various exams in the same disciplinary area can provide evidence that the knowledge/skills being tested by one test draw on the same ability/knowledge base, or indicate preparation for, another test.

What Do Other Experts Think about my Assessments?

Frequently other experts can see problems or ambiguities in our questions that we do not. They can also help us ensure that our tests are accurate and consistent with what is being taught elsewhere, providing a source of evidence regarding validity. A variety of expert opinions are helpful, including opinions from those with expertise in our own content area, teachers of courses for which ours are prerequisite, and experts in education and assessment.

What are the Psychometric Properties of my Assessment?

Most automatic multiple-choice scoring systems produce estimates of the overall *internal* *consistency* (one estimate of reliability) of the exam, and also estimate the discrimination of each item. Such reports also typically show how many students chose each option of each question, and the extent to which higher- or lower-scoring students selected each option. Instructors can quickly and easily use these kinds of item analyses to identify questions that pose measurement problems. There are important measurement questions involved in scored performance-based examinations (such as essays, short-answer questions, or clinical skills) as well. For instance, are scoring rubrics carefully designed and employed to ensure that multiple raters score similarly to each other, or that a single rater is consistent over time? If multiple raters are used, are efforts taken to train raters, and to estimate and improve (as needed) interrater reliability?

Box 14.3: Focus on common questions about validity and what contributes to grading

Faculty often ask whether it is okay to consider factors other than relevant knowledge or skills when assigning grades. For instance, should grades be influenced by attendance, effort, participation in discussions, attitude, peer scores, completion of homework, and so forth? Such strategies employ grades to incentivize behavior that improves learning and/or classroom climate. This can be an appropriate use of grading, and is quite commonly employed. However, this issue illustrates one of the reasons that grades, in and of themselves, are not adequate indicators of knowledge and/or skills, and why both students and the institution (college/university/accrediting body) need more precise estimates of competence than just grades. For students, we call this information "feedback," and it can come in many forms. Ideally, every time a veterinary student is observed or assessed, they will receive useful and timely feedback about their performance.

Box 14.4: How to obtain student's test scores

Note that policy or other ethical considerations might make it difficult to obtain your students' scores on examinations outside of your class. However, any institution should have faculty or staff who are authorized to access scores across courses. Those staff could obtain the scores for you, combine them with your data, and give them back to you in a de-identified form. They might even do the analysis for you.

some of the most common assessment pitfalls. We hope that you are able to use these ideas as a foundation for creating and improving educational assessments in your veterinary education classroom, and as a basis for future learning about educational assessment.

References

AERA, APA, and NCME (2014) *Standards for Educational and Psychological Testing*, American Educational Research Association, Washington, DC.

Alexander, P.A., Schallert, D.L., and Hare, V.C. (1991) Coming to terms: How researchers in learning and literacy talk about knowledge. *Review of Educational Research*, **61** (**3**), 315–343. doi:10.3102/00346543061003315

Anderson, L.W., Krathwohl, D.R., Airasian, P.W., *et al.* (2001) *A Taxonomy for Learning, Teaching, and Assessing: A Revision of Bloom's Taxonomy of Educational Objectives*, Addison Wesley Longman, New York.

AVMA COE (2014) *Accreditation Policies and Procedures of the AVMA Council on Education: March 2014.* American Veterinary Medical Association Council on Education. https://www.avma.org/ProfessionalDevelopment/Education/Accreditation/Colleges/Documents/coe_pp.pdf (accessed November 8, 2016).

Banta, T.W., Lund, J.P., Black, K.E., and Oblander, F.W. (1996) *Assessment in Practice: Putting Principles to Work on College Campuses*, Jossey-Bass, San Francisco, CA.

Bloom, B.S., Engelhart, M.D., Furst, E.J., *et al.* (1956) *Taxonomy of Educational Objectives: The Classification of Educational Goals: Handbook 1 Cognitive Domain*. Longmans, Green, New York.

Bloom, B.S., Hasting, T., and Madaus, G. (1971) *Handbook of Formative and Summative Evaluation of Student Learning*, McGraw-Hill, New York.

de Jong, T., and Ferguson-Hessler, M.G.M. (1996) Types and qualities of knowledge. *Educational Psychologist*, **31** (**2**), 105–113. doi:10.1207/s15326985ep3102_2

Finucane, P., Flannery, D., Keane, D., and Norman, G. (2010) Cross-institutional progress testing: Feasibility and value to a new medical school. *Medical Education*, **44** (**2**), 184–186. doi:10.1111/j.1365-2923.2009.03567.x

Flynn, T., Call, S., Carraccio, C., *et al.* (2014) *Core Entrustable Professional Activities for Entering Residency: Curriculum Developers' Guide.* Association of American Medical Colleges, Washington, DC.

Gagné, R.M., Briggs, L.J., and Wager, W.W. (1992) *Principles of Instructional Design*, 4th edn, Harcourt Brace Jovanovich, Fort Worth, TX.

Glaser, R. (1963) Instructional technology and the measurement of learning outcomes: Some questions. *American Psychologist*, **18**, 519–521.

Gullickson, A.R. (2003) *The Student Evaluation Standards: How to Improve Evaluations of Students*, Corwin Press, Newbury Park, CA.

Hopkins, K.D. (1998) *Educational and Psychological Measurement and Evaluation*, 8th edn, Allyn and Bacon, Needham Heights, MA.

Huba, M.E., and Freed, J.E. (2000) *Learner-Centered Assessment on College Campuses: Shifting the Focus from Teaching to Learning*, Allyn and Bacon, Boston, MA.

Kane, M.T. (2013) Validating the interpretations and uses of test scores. *Journal of Educational Measurement*, **50** (**1**), 1–73.

Merrill, M.D., and Goodman, R.I. (1972) *Selecting Instructional Strategies and Media: A Place to Begin*, National Special Media Institutes, Washington, DC.

Miller, G.E. (1990) The assessment of clinical skills/competence/performance. *Academic Medicine*, **9** (Sept. suppl.), S63–S67.

NBVME (2015) *Veterinary Educational Assessment (VEA)*. National Board of Veterinary Medical Examiners. https://www.nbvme.org/other-nbvme-exams/qualifying-examination-vea/ (accessed August 27, 2015).

Popham, J.W. (2006) *Assessment for Educational Leaders*, Pearson Education, Boston, MA.

RCVS (2014) *Day One Competences*. Royal College of Veterinary Surgeons. https://www.rcvs.org.uk/document-library/day-one-competences/ (accessed November 8, 2016).

Scimago Lab (2015) *Scimago Journal and Country Rank*. www.scimagojr.com (accessed August 27, 2015).

Scriven, M. (1991) *Evaluation Thesaurus*, 4th edn, Sage, Newbury Park, CA.

Secolsky, C., and Denison, D.B. (eds) (2012) *Handbook on Measurement, Assessment, and Evaluation in Higher Education*, Routledge, Taylor and Francis, New York.

Smith, P.L., and Ragan, T.J. (2005) *Instructional Design*, 3rd edn, John Wiley & Sons, Inc., Hoboken, NJ.

Spring, L., Robillard, D., Gehlbach, L., and Simas, T.A. (2011) Impact of pass/fail grading on medical students' well-being and academic outcomes. *Medical Education*, **45** (**9**), 867–877. doi:10.1111/j.1365-2923.2011.03989.x

van der Vleuten, C.P., Verwijnen, G.M., and Wifnen, W.H.F.W. (1996) Fifteen years of experience with progress testing in a problem-based learning curriculum. *Medical Teacher*, **18** (**2**), 103–109.

15

Written Assessment

Jared Danielson[1] and Kent Hecker[2]

[1] *College of Veterinary Medicine, Iowa State University, USA*
[2] *Faculty of Veterinary Medicine, Cumming School of Medicine, University of Calgary, Canada*

Box 15.1: Key messages

- Written assessments can be completed without access to anything other than the assessment itself, including the medium (e.g., paper or computer) used to administer it.
- Written assessments can require either selected or constructed responses. Selected-response items offer advantages in testing feasibility, efficiency, and reliability. Constructed-response items offer greater authenticity.

- There are a number of simple rules that, if followed, will greatly improve the validity of written test items.
- Effective written tests are carefully planned to consider factors such as content, format, length, and scoring.
- Item analysis provides a helpful tool for evaluating the effectiveness of your written assessments.

Introduction

Traditionally, written assessments are thought of as pencil-and-paper tests. However, many such tests today are completed using a computer, with little or no "writing" (and lots of "clicking"). Therefore, it is helpful to think of written assessments as those that can be completed without access to anything other than the assessment itself, including the medium used to administer it (paper, computer, etc.). Written assessments are generally used to measure knowledge/skills in the cognitive domain. The purposes of this chapter are to help you write effective assessment items in several common

formats; design effective written tests; and evaluate the quality of your tests and items.

Creating Written Assessment Items

Individual test questions are referred to as *items*, which come in two varieties: *selected response* and *constructed response*. As implied by the names, selected-response items require examinees to select among two or more potential answers, and constructed-response items require them to construct an answer. Common selected-response formats include

---

Veterinary Medical Education: A Practical Guide, First Edition. Edited by Jennifer L. Hodgson and Jacquelyn M. Pelzer.
© 2017 John Wiley & Sons, Inc. Published 2017 by John Wiley & Sons, Inc.

true–false, multiple choice, and matching, with more than one variety of each. Common constructed-response formats include short answer and essay.

Selected-Response versus Constructed-Response Formats

When planning any written item, whether it requires a selected or a constructed response, the test designer must consider what stimulus (item stem) the students will respond to and how they should respond (the correct answer). With selected-response items, the stimulus is the item stem, and the response is the choice of an option. With constructed-response formats, the stimulus is an item stem (question) and the response is something else, like an essay or short answer (see Box 15.2).

The advantage to selected-response formats is that they are easy to grade, because the judgment regarding what constitutes a correct answer is made prior to the students taking the test. Selected-response items also tend to have good psychometric properties, because there

is no variation in answer format, and thus no variability in judging answers across respondents. The advantage to constructed-response formats is that they can provide students with more realistic tasks than just a selection of options. For instance, in the "real world" a veterinarian is more likely to produce a list of differential diagnoses than to choose from a list that someone else has created. All things considered, the advantages of selected-response items in terms of practicality and statistical validity make it worth the effort of carefully designing high-quality selected-response items that provide the most authentic task possible. Constructed-response items are best reserved for testing that cannot be done with selected-response items.

Selected-Response Items

There are many varieties of selected-response items. The following discussion provides basic rules of selected-response item design, and shows how to create two common types of items: one-correct-answer multiple choice and extended matching.

 Box 15.2: Where's the evidence?

What do the experts say regarding when to use selected-response versus constructed-response items? Consider these two quotes:

> "Selected-response items are the most appropriate item format for measuring cognitive achievement or ability, especially higher order cognitive achievement or cognitive abilities, such as problem solving, synthesis, and evaluation." (Downing, 2006, p. 288)

> "Selected-response items are not appropriate for measuring students' abilities to synthesize ideas, to write effectively, or to perform certain types of problem-solving operations." (Popham, 2006, p. 215)

Hopefully, Popham (Emeritus Professor in the Graduate School of Education at University of California, Los Angeles) and Downing (Associate Professor of Medical Education at the University of Illinois at Chicago) would not object to our juxtaposing these two quotes. We do so simply to illustrate that it is not easy to find an incontrovertible rule associating certain learning outcomes with particular testing formats. Our recommendation is that you consider the specific knowledge or ability you wish to measure, and choose the format that seems to you to provide the most authentic measure of that task, taking into account factors such as validity, reliability, and practicality, as described in Part Four, Chapter 14: Concepts in Assessment.

Multiple-Choice (One-Correct-Answer) Questions

Figure 15.1 illustrates what a basic multiple-choice item looks like, and provides labels for basic question components: stem, options, answer, and distractors. Because many veterinary educators have taken many multiple-choice tests in their academic careers, and because on the surface multiple-choice questions all basically look the same, it is easy to assume that multiple-choice items are easy to write. However, multiple-choice questions, especially those that measure outcomes like principles or problem-solving, are actually quite difficult to write well. This section explains basic rules of writing effective multiple-choice items, and highlights some of the most common item flaws.

Good Multiple-Choice Questions Measure Stated Learning Objectives from the Course

It is easy inadvertently to measure superfluous skills, such as knowledge of test-taking strategies, that do not address your learning objectives. The following strategies will help you reduce this threat to the validity of your questions:

- Avoid using obviously wrong "freebee" distractors, just for fun or because you ran out of plausible options. (If you want to use a "fun" distractor, make it an additional option, ensuring that you still have two to four distractors in which you have some confidence.)
- Avoid writing items that purposefully disadvantage students who know a lot about multiple-choice tests and thus are "test-wise." Strategies used by test-wise students will be discussed more in the next section.
- Avoid including questions regarding material that is trivial or obscure, which is sometimes done to produce the illusion of difficulty and/or a normal distribution of scores. Your goal is to provide a valid measure of student ability, not to produce a particular distribution of scores (see Part Four, Chapter 14: Concepts in Assessment).
- Think carefully about the appropriate difficulty of your distractors. Most of the time distractors are not "completely" wrong, and frequently the answer is not correct to the exclusion of all other potentially correct answers; rather, answers fall on a continuum from very wrong to very right. As seen in Figure 15.2, your task is to come up with an answer that is clearly correct to prepared students, and distractors that are clearly wrong to prepared students, but attractively plausible to the unprepared. Figure 15.3 illustrates this rule with a practical example. The correct answer is the technique that most commonly produces the error, but the "kind

---

Your friend complains that every time s/he tries to make a diagnostic blood smear, the resulting smear is too thick (lacking a monolayer of cells with a feathered edge), and only covers a small portion of the slide. What is most likely causing the problem?

← Stem

a. the spreader slide is cracked or dirty
b. the angle of the spreader slide is too steep
c. the angle of the spreader slide is not steep enough
d. the blood is not allowed to spread along the entire edge of the spreader slide before the spreader slide was advanced
e. too much downward pressure or jerky, uneven motions are used on the spreader slide

← Options

– The correct option is called the answer (in bold).

– The incorrect options are called distractors.

Figure 15.1 The anatomy of a multiple-choice item.

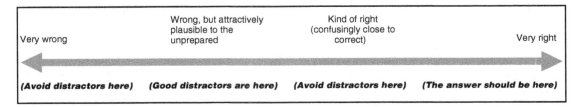

Figure 15.2 Continuum of "rightness" to "wrongness" of multiple-choice options.

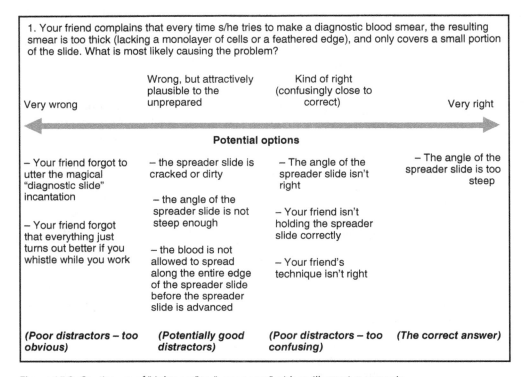

Figure 15.3 Continuum of "rightness" to "wrongness" with an illustrative example.

of right" distractors are unnecessarily tricky because they are also right, but less specific than the right answer. The "wrong, but attractively plausible to the unprepared" distractors are clearly wrong, but are common errors that create problems when making blood smears, and therefore are plausible to those who did not prepare. The "very wrong" options are obviously "throw-away" distractors. Students may find them entertaining, but even the least-prepared student would not choose them. It can be very difficult to come up with three or four compelling distractors for any given item. If this occurs, take comfort in the knowledge that three options (the answer and two good distractors) are typically sufficient for appropriate statistical properties, and that few items, even professionally written and edited ones, have more than two "functional" distractors (meaning that they are chosen by more than a handful, maybe 5%, of respondents; Downing, 2006).

not only are the questions in a confusing order, but one is given in the form of a range, and they vary in terms of how they employ decimals. Keep in mind that if using electronic testing with this sort of question, you will want to disable features that automatically scramble option order.

Examples:

6) How many mg of Enrofloxacin are needed for a 20 kg dog if the dose is 2.5 mg/kg?
   a) 60 mg
   b) 30 mg
   c) 40 mg
   d) **50 mg.**
7) How much does a 58 lb dog weigh in kg?
   a) **26.3**
   b) 27
   c) 20–30
   d) 0.26
   e) 2.63.

6   Avoid Using None of the Above

Questions that employ *none of the above* as an option are problematic, because students can usually imagine some better correct answer than the best one on the list, and are left to decide whether you wish them to choose the best one on the list, or the better option you might be thinking of. If you use *none of the above*, be sure that all the alternatives are clearly, unambiguously, and completely incorrect. In the case of Question 8, option a is a recommended approach, but there are several other options that many would consider as good or preferable, so it is not clear whether a or e is the best answer.

8) You are conducting a study to determine which of two approaches to teaching surgery produces superior learning gains. As part of the study, two blinded raters score each student's performance. Which statistical test would you use to compare the raters' scores in order to estimate reliability?
   a) intraclass correlation
   b) linear regression
   c) analysis of variance

   d) t-test
   e) none of the above.*

7   Avoid Using All of the Above

Using *all of the above* is problematic for two reasons. First, students only have to rule out one of the other distractors to know that *all of the above* is incorrect. Second, if *all of the above* is the intended correct answer, all of the other options should be clearly right, and equally right. If some of the other options are more right than others, students are forced to determine whether you intend them to choose the one best answer, or all plausible answers. In Example 9, all three strategies could address the problem, although options a or c seem most promising. Prepared students will spend an inordinate amount of time trying to guess what the item writer was thinking.

9) You are practicing creating blood smears that will make the faculty and staff in the pathology lab happy, but you keep producing smears that cover the entire slide and do not show a feathered edge. What would be the best strategy for solving this problem?
   a) Use a smaller drop of blood for making your smear.
   b) Make sure you are not moving your spreader slide too slowly.
   c) Make sure you are not holding your slide lower than a 30° angle.
   d) All of the above.*

8   Avoid Absolute or Vague Terms

There are plenty of problems with Example 10, including the fact that both a and c are plausible options. However, test-wise students will be fairly confident that options b and d are wrong, simply because they employ the term *always*, and in any case involving judgment the terms *always* and *never* are (almost) always wrong. The terms *generally* and *in most cases* (along with other vague terms) are problematic because they will be interpreted differently by different people, including different experts. This item would be much improved by simply specifying the blade itself in each option, removing the additional verbiage, and substituting a different (and less appropriate) blade choice in place of No. 10 or No. 22.

10) You need to make a large incision in the skin of a medium-sized dog. Which scalpel blade will you choose?
    a) Generally choose a No. 10 blade.*
    b) Always choose a No. 11 blade.*
    c) In most cases, a No. 22 blade would be appropriate.*
    d) Always choose a number 12 blade.*

Extended-Matching Questions

Conceptually, extended-matching questions simply expand the multiple-choice format by providing more options from which the student can choose, and by providing an option list that can be used for multiple stems (see also Boxes 15.3 and 15.4). This format was shown in a large-scale study involving a board exam to demonstrate superior psychometric properties to conventional multiple-choice (one-best-answer) items, presumably because students must engage in the more difficult task of comparing the merits of many options,

and test writers do not always accurately predict which answers will function as effective distractors (Case and Swanson, 1993). This section will provide a brief introduction to extended-matching items. Those wanting to employ these items in their testing are encouraged to read Case and Swanson's *Constructing Written Test Questions for the Basic and Clinical Sciences* (2002), which is freely available on the Internet and contains many examples of effective questions, themes, and option lists.

Extended-matching items comprise:

- a theme
- an option list
- a lead-in statement
- two or more item stems.

Extended-matching items have the advantage of requiring examinees to select one best answer, while weighing multiple plausible options. As is the case with regular multiple-choice items, one option should be clearly preferable to the others. Alternatively, credit can be given for more than one option, as long as the number of correct options is specified (the Pick N Items format; Case and Swanson. 2002).

 Box 15.3: Example of an extended matching question

Theme: Statistical Tests

Options:
A. ANCOVA	F. Multiple Regression
B. ANOVA	G. Paired Samples t-test
C. Cronbach's Alpha	H. Path Analysis
D. Independent Samples t-test	I. Rasch Analysis
E. Linear Regression	J. Repeated Measures ANOVA

Lead-In: *For each research scenario described below, select the most appropriate statistical test.*

Stems:
1. An instructor is interested in determining whether students perform better on his final exam when they chew bubble gum or when they do not. He wants to have one section of his course chew bubble gum during the final, while the other section does not, and compare the average final exam scores between sections.
ANS: D

2. The same instructor mentioned in Question 1 would like to find out whether students score better under either of two different lighting conditions. He proposes to have all of his students answer some questions in dim lighting and answer other questions in bright lighting, and then compare students' average scores achieved under dim lighting conditions with their average scores achieved under bright lighting conditions.
ANS: G

Box 15.4: Example of an extended-matching question

1. Major causes of regenerative anemia.

Options: Condition A: Blood-loss anemia   Condition D: Portosystemic shunt
Condition B: Extravascular hemolytic anemia   Condition E: Urinary tract obstruction
Condition C: Intravascular hemolytic anemia

For each of the following patients, select the single most likely condition.

1. You are presented with a 5-year-old female neutered Labrador. When the owner left for work yesterday evening the dog was normal. On return from a night shift, he found the dog collapsed. The dog is up to date on vaccines, and the only drug therapy is routine parasite control. On physical exam, mucus membranes are pale with capillary refill (CPR)>2 seconds. Heart rate is 150 bpm; a soft systolic murmur is heard. Respiratory rate is 50 bpm. Abdominal palpation is unremarkable. During the examination a small volume of red urine is passed.

2. You are presented with a 7-year-old female entire mixed-breed dog. The owner reports the dog has been "off color" for about 2 weeks. She has slowed down on walks. She is slightly picky about food and has started drinking more. He considers she is urinating and defecating normally. She is fully vaccinated, receives routine flea and tick control, and phenylpropanolamine for urinary incontinence at a dose adjusted by the owner according to clinical signs. On physical exam, she is quiet, alert, and responsive. Mucus membranes are pale with a slightly yellow tinge. CPR>2 seconds. Heart rate is 120 bpm. Respiratory character is panting. Hepatosplenomegaly is palpable.

Source: Example courtesy of Unity Locke.

Extended-matching items generally follow the same rules as regular multiple-choice items. However, the following specific rules will make extended-matching items effective:

- All four components (theme, options, lead-in, and stems) are essential.
- Options should be homogenous (all from the same theme).
- The stem should be long; options short.
- Options should include single words or short phrases; they can also include labeled areas in visual material.
- Options should contain no verbs.
- Effective stems are scenario based, not simple triggers for verbal recall.

Option lists can include anything about which you wish to test. Some ideas include cell types, structures, diagnoses, enzymes, toxins, pathological processes, diagnostic tests, elements of a feed lot, causes of clinical signs, and so forth. For instance, the options in Box 15.4 are causes of regenerative anemia.

Constructed-Response Formats

Despite our best efforts to create valid recognition items, in some cases they just will not measure what needs to be measured. When the necessary artifact of learning is a written explanation, the constructed written answer provides a good solution. It is tempting to assume that constructed-response formats produce inherently valid testing results because they require students to engage in authentic activities. On the contrary, however, constructed-response items introduce an additional source of potential error: the judgment employed in scoring. Therefore, considerable care must be taken to assure the validity of constructed-response scores.

Response Characteristics

Response characteristics describe the ideal response to a question, as well as likely incorrect or partially correct responses and/or other important considerations unique to the specific question (Smith and Ragan, 2005b). They include information such as desired content to be included in the answer (facts, concepts, principles, and so forth) and important criteria for correctness, such as importance (or not) of correct spelling, percentage of required information that is acceptable, and so on. Often response characteristics are codified in the form of rubrics or checklists. For example, Table 15.1 is a fragment of a rubric designed by Amanda Fales-Williams and Jared Danielson to assess lengthy and involved case reports, more complicated but similar to what might be produced in an essay response to a test question

Table 15.1 Rubric fragment: Assessing the case correlation assignment (report).

	Item	Good	Adequate	Marginal	Unacceptable
Thoroughness of correlation	1. Did the case author connect the ante-mortem abnormalities to findings at necropsy, and/or isolate inconsistent findings?	Each abnormality has a logical and readable explanation that is clearly tied to the necropsy findings. Or, the case author identifies all inconsistencies between ante-mortem and post-mortem data, or states (accurately) that no inconsistencies were present. (10)	The primary abnormalities are explained correctly, but secondary changes are ignored or are incorrectly explained. Or, all abnormalities are explained, but the explanations are somewhat vague or incomplete. The case author identifies most discrepancies between ante-mortem and post-mortem data. (7)	Some attempt is made to explain the abnormalities, but explanations are incomplete, illogical, or unclear. The case author identifies less than half (but at least one) of the existing inconsistencies between ante-mortem and post-mortem data. (5)	The case author fails to show how the abnormalities are related to the necropsy findings, or explanations are incorrect or difficult to understand. The case author does not identify any existing inconsistencies between ante-mortem and post-mortem data. (0)
	2. Rationality of theories for connections or unanswered questions	The case author constructs a logical, clearly stated explanation for the connections/discrepancies; this theory is reasonable given the data. (5)	The explanations for connections/inconsistencies between ante-mortem and post-mortem data are either partially inaccurate or incomplete. (4)	The explanations for connections/inconsistencies between ante-mortem and post-mortem data contain major inaccuracies or conceptual omissions. (2.5)	No explanation is given for inconsistencies between ante-mortem and post-mortem data. (0)
	3. Support for theories on connections and discrepancies	The case author thoroughly supports the explanations by citing specific examples from the case record and from recent literature. (10)	The case author refers to the case record, but support might be vague or imprecise. Citations from the literature leave unanswered questions. (7.5)	The case record data are underutilized or are used incorrectly in support of the explanation. There is minimal or inappropriate citation of literature. (5)	Theories are unsupported by either case record data or literature. (0)

addressing the following objective: "Given a description of a hospital case involving a common disease in a common domestic animal, and including ante- and post-mortem data, explain the findings, correlating ante- and post-mortem data and explaining any inconsistencies or discrepancies."

When deciding how to assess the task, the lead instructor (Dr. Fales-Williams) identified 5 overall categories of performance that were important, with a total of 21 subcategories. Table 15.1 shows three subitems associated with one of the main categories. The first row of that table illustrates that for a response to be considered "good," it must clearly tie all ante-mortem data abnormalities to the necropsy findings, or identify and explain any inconsistencies between ante-mortem and post-mortem data. Criteria are also established for adequate, marginal, and unacceptable performance, and points (in parentheses) are associated with each level of performance. This rubric provides insight into what the instructor deemed essential for understanding the material. For the response characteristics, the "good column" represents the right answer; the adequate, marginal, and unacceptable columns represent the common errors or omissions that the instructor foresaw the students making; and there are suggested points assigned to each level of performance. Such an involved rubric might be unnecessarily complicated for many constructed-response items. Response characteristics might be as simple as a list of desired and unacceptable characteristics, as seen in Table 15.2.

Designing accurate and helpful response characteristics can be time consuming. However, rewards are reaped in time saved and increased consistency while grading.

Item Stem (the Question)

Item stems should provide the prepared student with all the information needed to give a correct and complete answer. Problematic stems are often too vague. The following examples show effective and less-effective stems for two different objectives.

Objective 1

"Given a description of a hospital case involving a common disease in a common domestic animal, and including ante- and post-mortem data, explain the findings, correlating ante- and post-mortem data for all available information, and explaining any inconsistencies or discrepancies in the data." (Note that a stem for this objective would have to be accompanied by a sufficient amount of material describing a hospital case. That material is not provided as part of this example.)

- *Example 1* (less effective): For the case information provided, give your best analysis of the data.

- *Example 2* (more effective): For the case information provided, carefully analyze the data. List any inconsistencies or discrepancies between what was identified pre and post mortem. Describe those inconsistencies,

Table 15.2 A simple "response characteristics" table.

Objective: *Describe key characteristics and uses of common scalpel blades*
Format: *Constructed response*

Necessary elements	1. At least three of the following blades must be included: No. 10, 11, 12, 15, 22.
	2. Descriptions must include general shape and at least one common use for each blade.
	3. Purpose must match description; partial credit awarded if purpose matches description, but blade number remembered inaccurately.
Penalized errors	1. Providing an inaccurate description.
	2. Omitting the most common use.
	3. Including an inappropriate use.
Nonpenalized errors	1. Spelling/grammatical errors.

and report what you would have expected to see. Describe any additional information you would need to gather in order to resolve the inconsistencies that you found.

Objective 2

"Describe key characteristics and uses of common scalpel blades."

- *Example 1* (less effective): List and describe several common scalpel blades.
- *Example 2* (more effective): List three of the five most common scalpel blades used in veterinary surgery. For each blade, describe and/or sketch its shape, and briefly describe at least one common use.

Both of the less effective examples are too general to provide students with the information they need to write a complete and correct answer. In other words, prepared students could answer the questions as asked and still do poorly. In both of the effective examples, sufficient detail is provided that a prepared student who answers the question completely, as asked, should receive full credit for their response. These examples illustrate why it is helpful to write response characteristics prior to creating the item stem itself.

Test Specifications

Prior to this point in the chapter we have focused our attention on creating effective written assessment items. Effective items are essential, but not sufficient to ensure that the test will be effective. Items must be part of a carefully designed set of questions, commonly referred to as a test. Creating test specifications helps you design a test that adequately addresses your course's most important objectives within the available timeframe.

The nature of test specifications and the amount of detail they include can vary considerably depending on the context. For those who design examinations for a living, test specifications include "purpose and intended uses of test, as well as detailed decisions about content, format, test length, psychometric characteristics of the items and test, delivery mode, administration, scoring, and score reporting" (AERA, APA, and NCME, 2014, p. 76). A thorough discussion of the factors influencing each of these decisions is beyond the scope of a single chapter. We will discuss four of the most common specifications: content, format, length, and scoring.

Content

The test's content should align with its purpose; in the classroom, that means aligning content with course objectives. High-stakes examinations are built on complex, rigorous, and technical content-definition processes. For example, the content of the North American Veterinary Licensing Examination (NAVLE) is based on a thorough job analysis of practicing veterinarians. Individual course instructors lack the resources to do such a comprehensive content analysis, but any classroom assessment should be based on the instructor's best efforts to determine which specific knowledge and skills are most important to teach and test, and how much attention each deserves. Webb (2006) described four alignment criteria for planning the content of an examination: categorical concurrence, depth-of-knowledge consistency, range-of-knowledge correspondence, and balance of representation.

Categorical concurrence refers to the extent to which standards and tests "address the same content categories or topics" (Webb, 2006, p. 163). This is another way of saying that your test should address the same content categories as your instructional objectives. If you have designed your course independent of others, then you likely established those objectives yourself. In other cases, your course may be responsible for meeting some external standard(s) (such as curricular program objectives or the standards set by a professional society).

Depth-of-knowledge consistency refers to the extent to which the level(s) of desired learning outcome is/are reflected on the test. For instance, if the desired learning outcomes for a unit primarily involve clinical problem-solving, the test for that unit should primarily be designed to measure problem-solving, and not

the content being tested, while those who fail have not. Similarly, you may be interested in ensuring that cutoffs between grades seem purposeful and defensible rather than arbitrary or capricious. The process of assigning a certain evaluative judgment to a given test score is referred to as *standard setting*. Standards may be norm or criterion referenced (see Part Four, Chapter 14: Concepts in Assessment). Criterion-referenced standards are considered appropriate and norm-referenced standards inappropriate for decisions such as licensure, graduation, or passing/failing a course, because the practical importance of such decisions reflects standards of competence rather than comparison with other examinees (Hambleton and Pitoniak, 2006). The Standards for Educational and Psychological Testing (AERA, APA, and NCME, 2014) include a variety of standards that are relevant to standard setting. Among those, the following important considerations seem particularly relevant to veterinary medical education:

- Well-qualified individuals should use defensible and well-described processes for setting standards.
- Conditional standard errors of measurement should be reported at each performance standard (cutoff).
- The rationale for establishing cut scores, and empirical evidence justifying specific cut scores, should be presented.
- The level of performance for passing a credentialing test should reflect the knowledge or skills required for competence, and not be used to regulate the number of individuals passing the test.

There are many standard-setting methods (Hambleton and Pitoniak, 2006; Cizek, 2012) and they generally involve several days of work by panels of content experts. Common standard-setting procedures include the Nedelsky, Anghoff, and Ebel methods for selected-response items and the Modified Anghoff, Modified Ebel, and Bookmark methods for constructed-response items. Despite the fact that rigorous standard-setting processes are usually not feasible for the typical classroom test, some standard-setting concepts may be helpful to you in your everyday creation of written tests:

- Panelists are used to make judgments concerning individual test items. They are asked to perform tasks such as estimating the likelihood that a borderline examinee would answer each item correctly or not. Great care is taken to ensure that panels represent relevant perspectives. You may not have access to an external panel, but you certainly have access to colleagues who would review your questions and let you know whether they seem appropriate for your audience.
- You will have more confidence in your cutoff scores if you base them on an analysis of items rather than an arbitrary grading scale. We recommend that you associate the probability of success on each item with a level of mastery. You can then use those estimations to help you in setting your grading scale (or at least your pass/fail scale). Your scale may not be perfect, but you will have greater confidence in the grading decisions that you make.

Evaluating the Test

In this section we will briefly describe how to interpret the analyses that typically accompany automated scoring of selected-response exams. The approach we describe here is commonly available from item-scoring services provided by universities using classical test theory methods. Another common approach to item analysis is item response theory (IRT; see for example Yen and Fitzpatrick, 2006). However, because IRT analysis is seldom available to the university instructor, we do not discuss it in this chapter. Note that while item analysis results can be helpful to you in estimating the reliability of your test overall and the performance of each selected-response item, they are insufficient for making validity claims regarding the use of your test. Other considerations, such as the reliability of scoring of constructed-response items, and the extent to which your students' test scores predict or are in some other way associated with their subsequent success, are also important for evaluating the appropriateness of your test for its intended purpose.

Overall Reliability

Test analysis reports typically include an overall estimate of reliability, often the Kuder-Richardson -20 (KR-20) or Cronbach's alpha, which estimate internal consistency. Cronbach indicated that alpha "estimates the proportion of the test variance due to all common factors among the items. That is, it reports how much the test score depends upon general and group rather than item specific factors" (Cronbach, 1951, p. 320). If a test has high internal consistency, students who score better on most items also score better on the test overall, and vice versa. Reliability scores can range from 0 to 1, a value of 1 indicating that there are no random errors of measurement and a value of 0 indicating that all variance in scores is random. There are no universally accepted standards for reliability, but generally a score of at least 0.70 is considered necessary to support valid measurement (Pedhazur and Schmelkin, 1991). Test developers often seek higher reliability, especially for high-stakes examinations. For instance, the mean reliability for the 2013–2014 administration of the NAVLE was 0.91 (NBVME, 2014).

Item Discrimination

The discriminating power of an item refers to the extent to which it distinguishes between examinees who scored well and those who scored poorly on the test overall. If an item has good discrimination, examinees who answer the item correctly tend to do well on the test overall, and vice versa. There are several approaches to estimating item discrimination. One common approach is the point-biserial correlation, which is the correlation between test takers' scores on the test overall, and their scores on a specific item (Livingston, 2006). Another approach is to calculate the difference between the proportion of the top test performers who

answered the item correctly and the proportion of the bottom test performers who answered the item correctly (Hopkins, 1998). Discrimination can range from -1 to 1. Items with negative discrimination are answered correctly more frequently by lower-performing students than by higher-performing students. Hopkins (1998, p. 261) identifies discrimination values of .40 and up as excellent, .30 to .39 as good, and .10 to .29 as fair. Note that sometimes you may choose to include test items even if they have poor discrimination. For example, some very easy items might have low discrimination, but accurately measure knowledge or skills that are essential for all students to master.

Difficulty

An item's difficulty (referred to as its p-value) is the percentage of respondents answering that item correctly (Livingston, 2006). To provide some context, the average difficulty of all NAVLE items (2013–2014 administration) was 0.71 (NBVME, 2014). Typically, classroom exams would be less difficult than high-stakes certification exams.

Using Item Analysis to Improve your Items

Many item analysis reports for multiple-choice items include the percentage of respondents who selected each option (the correct answer and any distractors), as well as the point-biserial correlation for each option. Analysis at this level can be helpful for determining specific problems with individual items. The following common patterns might be useful to you in interpreting results regarding specific items:

- *High discrimination, high difficulty* (e.g., missed by 50%+ of respondents). The content was likely not taught as effectively as it could have been, or the content was too advanced for the class.
- *Low discrimination, high difficulty*. The item might be tricky or was coded incorrectly. If a distractor shows better discrimination than the correct answer, make sure that the distractor is not actually the right answer miscoded, or that the question is not confusing or poorly worded. If the question looks okay,

Box 15.5: Examples of additional resources

There are many excellent and detailed resources for developing written assessments. The following are some of our favorites.

Item writing

Case, S., and Swanson, D. (2002) *Constructing Written Test Questions for the Basic and Clinical Sciences*, 3rd edn, National Board of Medical Examiners, Philadelphia, PA. This excellent and highly readable guide to writing test questions in the medical sciences is full of excellent examples and nonexamples of multiple-choice, extended-matching, and similar item formats.

Haladyna, T.M. (2004) *Developing and Validating Multiple-Choice Test Items*, 3rd edn, Lawrence Erlbaum Associates, Mahwah, NJ. An in-depth treatment of multiple-choice test items, how to write them, and potential pitfalls.

Raymond, M., and Roeder, C. (2012) *Writing Multiple Choice Questions: An Introductory Tutorial*. National Board of Medical Examiners. http://download.usmle.org/IWTutorial/intro.htm (accessed November 9, 2016). This excellent item-writing tutorial from the National Board of Medical Examiners is freely available online and is actually fun (really!) to take.

Test development

Baillie, S., Warman, S., and Rhind, S. (2014) *A Guide to Assessment in Veterinary Medical Education*. University of Bristol. http://dbms.ilrt.bris.ac.uk/media/user/260731/A_Guide_to_Assessment_in_Veterinary_Medicine.pdf (accessed November 9, 2016). This concise guide provides a handy introduction to methods of assessment in veterinary medical education, with many relevant references for additional reading.

Cizek, G.J. (2012) *Setting Performance Standards: Foundations, Methods, and Innovations*, 2nd edn, Routledge, New York. An excellent resource for those who would like to know more about standard setting.

Hopkins, K.D. (1998) *Educational and Psychological Measurement and Evaluation*, 8th edn, Allyn & Bacon, Needham Heights, MA. Hopkins's classic introduction to measurement and evaluation in education has been a standard textbook in educational measurement for decades – and with good reason. It is a robust and accessible introduction to educational measurement.

Lane, S., Raymond, M.R., and Haladyna, T.M. (2016) *Handbook of Test Development*, 2nd edn, Taylor & Francis, New York. A comprehensive treatment of test development from A–Z.

---

then try to figure out how and where in the curriculum so many good students developed the same misconception.

- *Low discrimination, low difficulty.* Very easy questions do not discriminate well, but if an easy item measures something essential, there is no reason to change it based solely on the item analysis.
- *Distractors.* It is not uncommon for well-performing items to have only two functional distractors. If your item is otherwise performing well, there is no need to worry excessively about one or two unused distractors.

These basic concepts should be helpful to you in evaluating your tests. Of course, there is much more that can be done to evaluate tests than we have described here, and the interested reader is encouraged to explore the additional resources described in Box 15.5.

Conclusion

Because written assessment is so common in educational settings, especially in the preclinical years of veterinary school, and because most instructors have seen (and taken) so many tests, it is easy to assume that anyone with content knowledge can easily develop an effective test. We hope we have convinced you that time spent acquainting yourself with and following the

principles of effective test development is time well spent. Your best efforts to design effective tests will positively influence your students and many others within the present and future scope of their influence.

References

AERA, APA, and NCME (2014) *Standards for Educational and Psychological Testing*, American Educational Research Association, Washington, DC.

Anderson, L.W., Krathwohl, D.R., Airasian, P.W., et al. (2001) *A Taxonomy for Learning, Teaching, and Assessing: A Revision of Bloom's Taxonomy of Educational Objectives*, Addison Wesley Longman, New York.

Case, S.M., and Swanson, D.B. (1993) Extended-matching items: A practical alternative to free-response questions. *Teaching and Learning in Medicine*, **5** (**2**), 107–115.

Case, S.M., and Swanson, D.B. (2002) *Constructing Written Test Questions for the Basic and Clinical Sciences*, 3rd edn, National Board of Medical Examiners, Philadelphia, PA.

Cizek, G.J. (2012) *Setting Performance Standards: Foundations, Methods, and Innovations*, 2nd edn, Routledge, New York.

Cronbach, L.J. (1951) Coefficient alpha and the internal structure of tests. *Psychometrika*, **16**, 297–334.

Downing, S.M. (2006) Selected-response item formats in test development, in *Handbood of Test Development* (eds S.M. Downing and T.M. Haladyna), Lawrence Erlbaum Associates, Mahwah, NJ, pp. 287–302.

Gagné, R.M., Briggs, L.J., and Wager, W.W. (1992) *Principles of Instructional Design*, 4th edn, Harcourt Brace Jovanovich, Fort Worth, TX.

Hambleton, R.K., and Pitoniak, M.J. (2006) Setting Performance Standards, in *Educational Measurement* (ed. R.L. Brennan), Praeger, Westport, CT, pp. 433–470.

Hopkins, K.D. (1998) *Educational and Psychological Measurement and Evaluation*, Allyn and Bacon, Boston, MA.

Kolen, M.J. (2006) Scaling and norming, in *Educational Measurement* (ed. R.L. Brennan), Praeger, Westport, CT, pp. 155–186.

Livingston, S.A. (2006) Item analysis, in *Handbook of Test Development* (ed. S.M. Downing and T.M. Haladyna), Lawrence Erlbaum Associates, Mahwah, NJ, pp. 421–441.

NBVME (2014) *2013–2014 Technical Report: North American Veterinary Licensing Examination*, National Board of Veterinary Medical Examiners, Bismarck, ND.

Pedhazur, E.J., and Schmelkin, L.P. (1991) Reliability, in *Measurement, Design and Analysis: An Integrated Approach* (eds E.J. Pedhazur and L.P. Schmelkin), Lawrence Erlbaum Associates, Hillsdale, NJ, pp. 81–117.

Popham, W.J. (2006) *Assessment for Educational Leaders*, Pearson Education, Boston, MA.

Smith, P.L., and Ragan, T.J. (2005a) Instructional analysis: Analyzing the learning task, in *Instructional Design* (eds P.L. Smith and T.J. Ragan), John Wiley & Sons, Inc., Hoboken, NJ, pp. 75–102.

Smith, P.L., and Ragan, T.J. (2005b) *Instructional Design*, 3rd edn, John Wiley & Sons, Inc., Hoboken, NJ

Webb, N.L. (2006) Identifying content for student achievement tests, in *Handbook of Test Development* (eds S.M. Downing and T.M. Haladyna), Lawrence Erlbaum Associates, Mahwah, NJ, pp. 155–180.

Yen, W.M., and Fitzpatrick, A.R. (2006) Item response theory, in *Educational Measurement* (ed. R.L. Brennan), Praeger, Westport, CT, pp. 111–154.

16

Performance and Workplace-Based Assessment

Kirsty Magnier and Matthew Pead

Royal Veterinary College, UK

 Box 16.1: Key messages

- The authentic contextualized environment of the workplace appears to be the best environment in which to assess the complex blend of skills required in graduates from professional veterinary courses.
- Performance-based methods such as the objective structured clinical examination (OSCE) offer a fair and reliable method of assessing clinical skills.
- Assessment methods such as the mini clinical evaluation exercise (mini-CEX), direct observation of procedural skills (DOPS), multisource feedback (MSF), and the portfolio are valid for assessing and stimulating student learning in the workplace.

- A main benefit of workplace-based assessment methods is the provision of immediate feedback to contribute to students' development and progress, and they offer the opportunity for more complex aspects of competence such as professionalism to be captured.
- A number of challenges in implementing workplace-based assessment methods are recognized, which include questions over reliability, feasibility, and faculty/staff training.
- The way forward for those designing veterinary courses appears to be to employ a suite of assessments, preferably ones that have a basis in the peer-reviewed educational literature.

Introduction

Those on courses related to working in the veterinary professions require a wider variety of assessments than most students. They have a considerable span of learning outcomes to fulfill in the cognitive domain, but in addition must achieve a variety of psychomotor and affective outcomes that can be seen as measures of performance or competence in skills related

to their professional life. Such skills and competencies are often learned in the workplace, and may be assessed there too. Thus, assessment on veterinary courses must provide feedback, motivation, and an understanding of achievement against outcome across a great variety of learning outcomes. In addition, assessment of the future veterinary professional must also satisfy the demands of public accountability, government, and regulatory bodies, and ulti-

---

mately must safeguard veterinary medicine as a profession with an assurance that graduates are "safe to practice."

Traditional assessment methods focus on what a student knows and can recall about a concept or topic, but do not always address more complex professional constructs. Over the last 20 years there has been a recognition that formats like long- and short-answer questions and multiple-choice tests have many issues with reliability and validity in assessing the more complex issues of competence and performance in a professional framework, and thus are not fit for this purpose. This has generated new assessment methods aimed at addressing these issues, which in turn has increased the range of assessment formats used in veterinary courses.

Miller (1990) developed a pyramidal framework for describing levels of competence within a hierarchy of knowledge, application, and performance, with associated methods of assessment (Holsgrove, 2003). The bottom level of the pyramid, entitled "Knows," refers to the recall of factual knowledge. The second level, "Knows how," refers to the ability to apply the factual knowledge in a particular context. It implies that there is more to competence than knowledge alone. The third level, "Shows," relates to the ability to demonstrate competence in a practical, "simulated" environment; what a professional actually does in the workplace is at the top and fourth level of the pyramid, "Does." This model sets a framework for a succession of levels of competence that can guide the implementation of assessment on veterinary courses. However, there are some important additional considerations that the model does not fully describe. The workplace is rightly at the peak of the pyramid, representing the ultimate goal of a course or perhaps a capstone assessment. However, there is an implication that as assessment comes closer to the workplace, its volume may reduce. In reality, workplace-based assessment represents the skills most relevant to professional life, and the point at which numerous component skills learned on a course are combined into clinical reasoning and professional competence. As these are the ultimate goals of most clinical courses, course design should take into account that workplace-based assessment may need to be a larger or even dominant volume of the assessment that students experience. Perhaps Miller's pyramid needs to be drawn like a spinning top (Figure 16.1) – an appropriate metaphor for the careful balance of skills that the modern caring professional requires. In addition, as it has been demonstrated that students' abilities assessed in a simulated environment do not always predict their performance in the workplace (Rethans *et al.*, 1991), assessment of performance at one level of the pyramid needs to be carefully harnessed to the next stage.

The workplace has benefits in terms of learning and feedback over a more conventional didactic environment. Assessment in an authentic clinical setting is a strong motivator for learning (Spencer, 2003). Learners are better at reproducing and applying knowledge

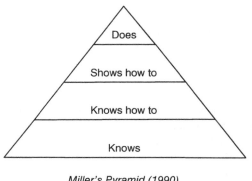

Miller's Pyramid (1990)

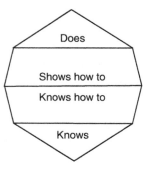

The Magnier-Pead Top

Figure 16.1 Miller's pyramid establishes a hierarchy of skills capped by a student demonstrating competence in the workplace. When considering the design of learning and assessment, it may be useful to think of this hierarchy encompassed in the shape of a top, with the emphasis more on workplace-based assessments than on simple knowledge recall.

and skills if the context in which they have to perform resembles the context in which the knowledge and skills were first learned (Regehr and Norman, 1996). This relates to the "encoding and context specificity principle," which states that information is learned within a context and that the context within which the memory has been developed is stored as well as the memory (Schuwirth and van der Vleuten, 2004). It is also relevant to the concept of "situated learning," which plays a critical role in the development of health professionals (Lave and Wenger, 1991). The workplace is an excellent opportunity for an almost continuous stream of feedback, since junior professionals are often teamed with a range of experienced practitioners whom they can use as role models and sources of information. However, the most problematic facet of the workplace in assessment is the variable experience of each individual. This means that it is often difficult to ensure that each student has a chance to learn and demonstrate a very specific skill, although there are generic skills, particularly those in the affective domain, that everyone in the workplace experiences, and so these are the ones that can be most reliably assessed.

In the purest sense, the most valid place to assess how a student will perform in practice is in the workplace, and the logical extension of this would be to assess all the competency outcomes required at the end of a professional course in this fashion. However, there are issues of practicality and reliability that make this difficult to achieve, and in many cases such an assessment would not completely satisfy the regulatory burden with which many courses work. Most veterinary courses that have performance-based outcomes need to pick assessments appropriate both to those outcomes and to the resources of the institution from a palette of peer-reviewed assessment vehicles. This chapter provides an overview of performance and workplace-based assessment methods as currently used in veterinary and medical education, and establishes some of the challenges that are associated with their use, particularly for undergraduate students.

Performance-Based and Workplace-Based Assessment Methods

This section presents a chronological overview of the progress of assessment from traditional classroom environments (a "contextual vacuum") to authentic settings such as the workplace, and why this was needed. The focus in this part of the chapter will be on the methods and their impact, including long-case and clinical evaluation exercise (CEX) assessment, objective structured clinical examination (OSCEs), mini clinical evaluation exercises (mini-CEX), direct observation of procedural skills (DOPS), multi-source feedback (MSF), and portfolios.

Earlier written assessment methods such as essays, multiple-choice questions, and short-answer questions were designed to assess recall of knowledge, but are not suitable for assessing the application of knowledge in a practical/clinical environment. Written or single-answer questions have been extended by the use of vehicles such as open-book exams, extended-matching questions, and script concordance tests to move the outcome measured by an assessment toward clinical reasoning. Clinical reasoning is a higher cognitive skill requiring the collation of objective and subjective information relating to a patient, and the subsequent synthesis of an appropriate plan for further diagnosis or treatment. It is an essential method for clinical professionals, especially those working at a junior level, where their lack of experience means that they have little recourse to pattern recognition to solve clinical problems. However, these formats are still devoid of all the practical considerations of the workplace, leaving a gap for assessment methods to address. The long case and the CEX were among the first vehicles developed to evaluate undergraduate and graduate students' clinical skills in a workplace setting.

Long Case and Clinical Evaluation Exercise

The long case has been used to evaluate undergraduate students' clinical skills for the last

30 years. The student is given "observed" time with a real patient in a clinical setting, gathers information about their problem, and performs a physical examination. The student then relays information to the examiners, who ask about the patient and related topics, enabling them to judge the quality of the student's performance (Norcini, 2001).

Strengths of the long case include its authenticity: the student is able to perform an examination on a real patient in the workplace. However, it is an assessment that is fraught with concern over reliability. Wilson *et al.* (1969) discussed how a candidate being assessed via the long case was scored differently by different examiners, thus reaffirming the issues with interrater reliability (Davis *et al.*, 2001). As well as examiner effects, case specificity (intercase reliability) can be a problem, and therefore this method should not be used solely to summatively assess a student's clinical skills (Norcini, 2001). Modifications to the assessment may increase the reliability, such as increasing the number of encounters the students have to face, examiner training, and increasing the number of examiners present (Ponnamperuma *et al.*, 2009). Although this may improve the reliability of the assessment method, it will not raise it to a level that supports its use in a high-stakes examination (Wass, Jones, and van Vleuten, 2001).

In 1962, the traditional clinical examination exercise was developed with a purpose to assess clinical skills in doctors in postgraduate training, and it eventually replaced the oral examination for certification in the United States (Searle, 2008). The assessment is of two hours' duration, and involves a senior staff member observing a medical graduate (candidate) taking a history and performing a physical examination on a patient, then assessing their performance on it directly afterward (Durning *et al.*, 2002). The CEX uses direct observation of candidates, thus giving them the opportunity for immediate feedback. The use of a real patient instead of a standardized patient means that the exercise is feasible and not costly (Norcini *et al.*, 1995).

However, the CEX was criticized for the length of time it took to complete each assessment, limited reliability due to the few assessments happening with the candidate (one CEX per year), and only being observed by one examiner. This eventually led to its replacement in the curriculum by the mini-CEX (Durning *et al.*, 2002), which is reviewed later in the chapter.

There was recognition that the long case and the CEX had reliability issues, which brought a new and innovative phase in the history of assessment. This saw a progression from subjective assessments (long case, CEX) in the 1960s toward a more objective, structured format (OSCE) in the 1970s, with a greater emphasis on achieving a minimum acceptable level of reliability and validity (Rhind, 2006).

Objective Structured Clinical Examination

Over 30 years ago the OSCE was introduced into medical education by Harden *et al.* (1975) as a format that evaluates the performance of undergraduate and graduate clinical skills in an objective, structured, and simulated learning environment. This method examined a number of clinical competencies across a range of problems and comprised a circuit of individual stations, each of which is 5–10 minutes in duration, around which the candidates rotate. In each station a student is examined on a single competency on a one-to-one basis by an examiner. Students are assessed on their clinical, history-taking, problem-solving, and communication skills in an objective and structured format, and may be required to interact with a patient (simulated or real). This method assesses at the third level, "Shows," of Miller's pyramid (Miller, 1990).

The strengths of this format lie in the standardization that occurs: it allows a fair comparison between candidates. Each station has a different examiner recording the candidate's progression through a checklist of steps, ensuring the objectivity of the examination. On entering a station, each candidate is given the same amount of information about the task, keeping to a structured format. A weakness of the OSCE is that it is set in an artificial, "simulated" environment, which may not mirror the constraints or freedoms of a real workplace. The simulated environment limits the type of scenario that the student will be able to encounter (Smee, 2003). The feasibility of the method also needs to be considered, since OSCEs are resource intensive in terms of the extensive preparation and costs involved, principally staff being fully trained to be observers and then taking time out of their other duties.

Scoring of an OSCE is either "analytical," through a tick box, checklist-rating format (yes/no), or "holistic," with a global ratings scale (GRS) that reviews performance using a Likert-scale approach (Read *et al.*, 2015). The checklist approach is more commonplace within veterinary education, but a number of systems also incorporate a global assessment/judgment at the end, which is used for the purposes of standard setting and not to influence the mark of an individual candidate. The checklist approach is considered reductionist and may not consider the sum of all the different parts of the performance during the session, whereas the global rating scales appear to allow the assessor to accommodate the more qualitative elements of the performance, since the examiner is required to make a judgment along a scale that is continuous (Regehr and Norman, 1996). Regehr and Norman's (1996) was one of the first studies to compare the different approaches for scoring a candidate's performance; their results revealed that global rating scales scored by experts showed higher interstation reliability, better construct validity, and better concurrent validity than checklists. They used experts as their examiners, which brings up the issue of training for this approach in order to avoid subjectivity and low reliability in the judgments. More recent research from Read *et al.* (2015) found that there was no significant difference in observer scores of student performance between institutions using checklists and global rating scales.

The OSCE was perceived to be groundbreaking and innovative in the 1970s to 1980s

and remains a respected and commonly used method in medicine, as it has enabled the assessment of individual competencies in a controlled and simulated environment (Hodges, 2006). Its development and acceptance in veterinary education occurred around the beginning of 2003 and a new term has been used to describe the format that is more specific to certain aspects and areas of the veterinary profession: OSPVE (objective structured practical veterinary examination). This was coined by a project at the Royal Veterinary College in 2002 that was exploring new methods of assessment, a major part of which was the development of the OSPVE. The two terms are used interchangeably.

Figure 16.2 shows a typical OSCE assessment form.

Mini Clinical Examination Exercise

In the 1990s the authenticity of the learning environment began to be recognized as important, with assessment methods shifting from educational classroom environments to real-life settings in the workplace, ensuring a balance between reliability and validity. Authentic assessment methods were designed on the principle that people are better at reproducing and applying knowledge and skills if the context in which they have to do so resembles the context in which the knowledge and skills were first learned (Regehr and Norman, 1996). Interest in assessment of graduates in the workplace was renewed with the evolution of the mini-CEX and DOPS. The majority of these workplace-based assessment methods originated and are primarily used within the graduate curriculum in medicine, but are being adapted by some medical and veterinary medical schools in Europe and the United States for their undergraduate programs.

The CEX was mentioned as an earlier method of assessment of clinical skills, but has been replaced by the mini-CEX due to its questionable reliability. The latter method was developed to capture performance in the workplace at the "Does" (highest) level of Miller's

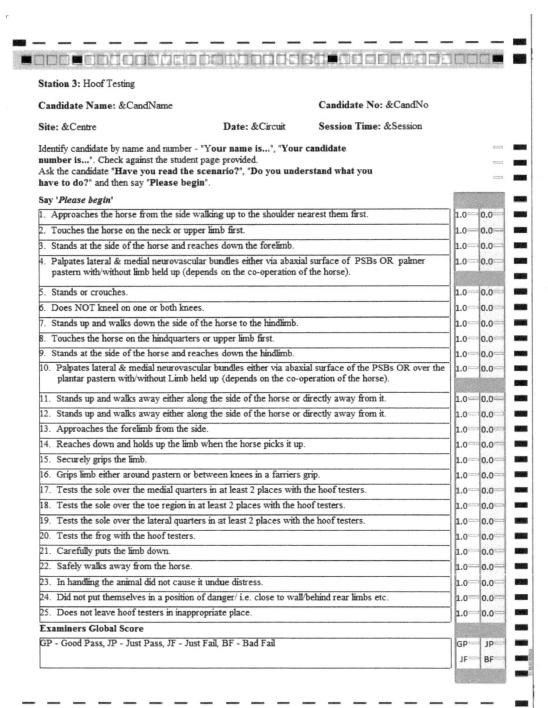

Station 3: Hoof Testing

Candidate Name: &CandName   **Candidate No:** &CandNo

Site: &Centre   **Date:** &Circuit   **Session Time:** &Session

Identify candidate by name and number - "**Your name is...**", "**Your candidate number is...**". Check against the student page provided.
Ask the candidate "**Have you read the scenario?**", "**Do you understand what you have to do?**" and then say "**Please begin**".

Say '*Please begin*'

1. Approaches the horse from the side walking up to the shoulder nearest them first.	1.0	0.0
2. Touches the horse on the neck or upper limb first.	1.0	0.0
3. Stands at the side of the horse and reaches down the forelimb.	1.0	0.0
4. Palpates lateral & medial neurovascular bundles either via abaxial surface of PSBs OR palmer pastern with/without limb held up (depends on the co-operation of the horse).	1.0	0.0
5. Stands or crouches.	1.0	0.0
6. Does NOT kneel on one or both knees.	1.0	0.0
7. Stands up and walks down the side of the horse to the hindlimb.	1.0	0.0
8. Touches the horse on the hindquarters or upper limb first.	1.0	0.0
9. Stands at the side of the horse and reaches down the hindlimb.	1.0	0.0
10. Palpates lateral & medial neurovascular bundles either via abaxial surface of the PSBs OR over the plantar pastern with/without Limb held up (depends on the co-operation of the horse).	1.0	0.0
11. Stands up and walks away either along the side of the horse or directly away from it.	1.0	0.0
12. Stands up and walks away either along the side of the horse or directly away from it.	1.0	0.0
13. Approaches the forelimb from the side.	1.0	0.0
14. Reaches down and holds up the limb when the horse picks it up.	1.0	0.0
15. Securely grips the limb.	1.0	0.0
16. Grips limb either around pastern or between knees in a farriers grip.	1.0	0.0
17. Tests the sole over the medial quarters in at least 2 places with the hoof testers.	1.0	0.0
18. Tests the sole over the toe region in at least 2 places with the hoof testers.	1.0	0.0
19. Tests the sole over the lateral quarters in at least 2 places with the hoof testers.	1.0	0.0
20. Tests the frog with the hoof testers.	1.0	0.0
21. Carefully puts the limb down.	1.0	0.0
22. Safely walks away from the horse.	1.0	0.0
23. In handling the animal did not cause it undue distress.	1.0	0.0
24. Did not put themselves in a position of danger/ i.e. close to wall/behind rear limbs etc.	1.0	0.0
25. Does not leave hoof testers in inappropriate place.	1.0	0.0

Examiners Global Score

GP - Good Pass, JP - Just Pass, JF - Just Fail, BF - Bad Fail	GP JP JF BF

Figure 16.2 A typical OSCE assessment form.

pyramid, although its utility is still in its infancy (Miller, 1990).

The purpose of the mini-CEX is to formatively assess the clinical skills of graduates in the workplace. The examiner observes an encounter of 15–20 minutes with a patient that may be conducted in a variety of settings (inpatient, emergency room, and outpatient), then gives immediate feedback to the candidate. This format entails an assessment sheet that the examiner uses to assess the candidate's competency in history taking, physical examination tools, clinical decision-making, professionalism, counseling, organization, and overall clinical competence (Malhotra, Hatala, and Courneya, 2008). Traditionally, examiners in this method included faculty staff and clinical specialists, but nurses and those in appropriate allied health professions can also act as examiners in certain situations. Teachers perceived it to be a useful and feasible method for promoting "direct observation" and "constructive feedback" (Alves de Lima *et al.*, 2010). The study by Alves de Lima *et al.* (2010) found that residents in medical education perceived the mini-CEX to be a useful method that promoted reflection and a constructive approach to learning. The perceived acceptability and validity of the method were also reported by Hill *et al.* (2009) from the experience of staff and students using it.

In order to achieve significant interrater reliability, the assessment is undertaken over a period, several times a year, and with a number of different examiners, resulting in a reliable measure of an individual's performance. There is variability about how many times a student needs to be observed, ranging from 7 to 14 encounters per year and by multiple raters, which can create organizational and feasibility issues (Norcini, 2005; Sidhu, McIlroy, and Regehr, 2005; Alves de Lima *et al.*, 2010; Williams, 2003). These weaknesses raise the issue about the method's use as a formative or summative piece of assessment, and whether it can be employed in isolation. It is not recommended for summative high-stakes assessment.

The mini-CEX is primarily used in medicine, but variations of the method are being piloted and used formatively in veterinary education. The Faculty of Veterinary Medicine at Utrecht University (Netherlands) instigated a new assessment program in 2010 that includes a modified mini-CEX with its undergraduate veterinary students (Jaarsma *et al.*, 2010; Bok *et al.*, 2013). The University of Glasgow (Scotland) has piloted the Veterinary Clinical Assessment Tool (VCAT), which is based on the mini-CEX (Hammond, 2010). This formative assessment method involves a candidate being observed by an examiner in an encounter with a patient (consultation) around a skill such as history taking. The candidate receives immediate feedback about the encounter based on their performance, in nine specific areas of clinical and professional competence (history taking, animal handling, physical examination, communication, practical skills, clinical judgment, professionalism, organization/efficiency, overall clinical care). Ontario Veterinary College at the University of Guelph (Canada) uses a modified mini-CEX with its students in a small animal clinical rotation (Hecker, Norris, and Coe, 2012).

Directly Observed Procedural Skills

The DOPS assessment method was developed in the United Kingdom in 2002 by the Royal College of Physicians, as there was no suitable assessment method for observing and examining a procedure carried out by graduates (Wilkinson, Campbell, and Judd, 2008). Its premise is similar to the mini-CEX in that graduates are observed with real patients, but instead the focus is on evaluating their procedural skills in the workplace (Prescott *et al.*, 2002). Candidates have opportunities to learn and practice their skills in the workplace and elect to take their DOPS when they feel they are proficient in the task specified. They are given 15 minutes to perform a common procedure under observation, and then spend 5 minutes receiving specific feedback from the observer on their procedural skills. It is expected that students will be observed several times a year by a number of different examiners to ensure reliability. The examiners normally use a checklist or rating scale to record their observations during the encounter (Figure 16.3).

Similar to the mini-CEX, faculty, clinical specialists, and senior nursing staff in the appropriate area observe the procedure. The immediate feedback that they give to the candidate is perceived as a strength of the format. This enables candidates to identify their areas of weakness and improve on them for future practice (Cohen, Farrant, and Taibjee, 2009). Adequate time and resources are required for the successful implementation of this method (Wilkinson *et al.*, 2008). From an examiner's perspective, the difficulty around organization of this format was noted as a weakness. Candidates also commented on the perceived stress of being observed (Cohen, Farrant, and Taibjee, 2009). Research from Bindal, Wall, and Goodyear (2011, p. 925) suggests that both graduates and examiners perceive the method "as a tick box exercise that has limited educational impact." This negativity toward workplace-based assessments was reiterated by Massie and Ali (2015), who reviewed the literature and identified studies examining graduate and examiner perceptions of workplace-based assessments, where criticisms related to insufficient time available to undertake them and inadequate training of trainers.

DOPS are primarily used in the postgraduate medical education curriculum, although a number of institutions are currently trialing or implementing this method at the undergraduate level in medical and veterinary education (Wilkinson *et al.*, 2008). The University of Nottingham (United Kingdom) uses DOPS with its final-year students on clinical rotations. Students initially sign themselves off independently as being competent in a certain area before being assessed by an examiner (Cobb *et al.*, 2013). The Royal Veterinary College approved the method in 2011 and it is being used as a checkpoint to assess the animal-handling capabilities of third-year veterinary students. Students have to pass DOPS to continue their

undergraduate course. The method is also used to assess undergraduates in the Faculty of Veterinary Medicine at Utrecht University (Bok *et al.*, 2013). One of the principal benefits of the system is the way in which it values the subjective views of the skilled examiner in feedback.

Multisource Feedback

Although the previous methods have included humanistic aspects such as professionalism and communication in their assessment format, their purpose focused more on the clinical and technical aspects of learning in the workplace. The use of multisource feedback (MSF) is a recognized method for assessing clinical and nonclinical parameters by utilizing a number of judgments from different members of staff about a student's behavior (professionalism, communication, teamwork). Assessment by members of a clinical team with whom the student works can provide useful data in assessing their capacity for teamwork and their interprofessional behavior with patients and clients (Violato and Lockyer, 2003; Dannefer *et al.*, 2005). This format is collated via a number of structured questionnaires completed by staff members (faculty, nurses, clinical specialists) about a trainee and reflects routine performance rather than a single encounter (Norcini and Burch, 2007; Wilkinson *et al.*, 2008). The examiner or the student's supervisor will interpret the responses and provide individual feedback. As with the mini-CEX and DOPS, MSF is regarded as an effective method for providing feedback to students about their clinical and nonclinical performance in the workplace (Donnon *et al.*, 2014). Feedback needs to be delivered in a productive and timely manner for the process to progress and to be constructive for students (Norcini, 2003). This is considered to be one of the better methods, focusing on the "humanistic aspects" of the clinical encounter such as communication and professionalism, which are particularly hard to measure (Violato and Lockyer, 2003). In order to achieve significant reliability, the performance of the student is judged over a number of encounters.

Station 2: DOPs Assessment Sheet

Candidate Name: **Candidate No:**

Site: **Date:**   **Session Time:**

Assessor to confirm:
- Candidate Name & Number
- Candidate understands what they have to do

(EE=Exceeds Expectations, M=Meets Expectations, BF=Borderline Fail, BE=Below Expectations)

Health and Safety of Self and Other Participants (NOT ANIMALS)	EE	M
- Biosecurity measures heeded	BF	BE
- Is appropriately dressed (no jewellery, hair not obstructive, nails short & undecorated, no strong scents used)		
- Does not put self or others at risk		

Animal Welfare	EE	M
- Animal is not unduly stressed	BF	BE
- Animal is not handled roughly		
- Animal is handled in a calm, confident manner		

Technical Ability	EE	M
- Carries out physical skills effectively	BF	BE
- Does not lose control of the animal at any point		
- Animal is handled in a calm, confident manner		

Communication	EE	M
- Communicates effectively with assessor	BF	BE
- Communicates with animal in approriate manner dependant on species		
- Body language towards animal to be taken into account (student not nervous/overly cautious)		

Assessor Comments on areas of weakness and strengths

Overall Result

C = Competent (only 1 BF or better) N = Not Yet Competent (2 or more BFs **OR** any BEs)	C	N
Please ensure you actively seek further opportunities to practice ☐ (Tick if applicable)		

Figure 16.3 A typical DOPS assessment form.

MSF can be further classified into specific versions that institutions are using with their students. Graduates in medical education in hospitals in Sheffield in the United Kingdom have used the Sheffield Peer Review Assessment Tool (SHEFFPAT; Archer, Norcini, and Davies, 2005). Results from the study showed the method to be reliable, valid, and feasible. Newer peer-rating methods have since been introduced, including Team Assessment of Behaviour (TAB), which is now used in foundation program training with the Mini Peer Assessment Tool (mini PAT) in the UK medical education system (Whitehouse *et al.*, 2007).

Although MSF is valued, there are a number of problems associated with the method from the perspective of staff using it. The dissemination and collection of all the feedback from all staff is perceived as time consuming and an administrative burden (Cohen, Farrant, and Taibjee, 2009). It is a method that has been used in the graduate medical curriculum in medicine on the Modernising Medical Careers (MMC) foundation program to assess doctors' performance in the workplace in the United Kingdom. The Faculty of Veterinary Medicine at Utrecht University also uses MSF within an e-portfolio in its undergraduate assessment program (Jaarsma *et al.*, 2010; Bok *et al.*, 2013).

Portfolios

Portfolios are a tool used to support and assess competence development in the workplace (Driessen, 2009). They are not viewed as an assessment method, but as a "vessel" that contains evidence of a student's performance and progression in attaining competencies (Baillie and Rhind, 2008). They provide an assessment of a student's performance that stimulates learning from experience (Driessen, 2009), and are associated with the belief that adults are capable of engaging in self-directed learning (Timmins and Dunne, 2009). When portfolios were first introduced into medicine in 1991, their format was similar to an artist's portfolio, an accumulation of documents relating to a work placement (Driessen, 2009). With further development,

portfolios were organized to allow students to provide a record or piece of evidence for individual competencies (Bird, 1990).

A secondary purpose is portfolios' use as a reflective tool: when students periodically look back on their cases, they consider their knowledge, planning, and diagnosis of a case and reflect on alternative courses of actions. Student reflections are underpinned by the material enclosed in the portfolios, essays, short-answer questions, clinical encounters, or procedural encounters (Driessen *et al.*, 2003). To ensure a portfolio's effective use for reflective practice, a mentor is required to aid discussion and provide support (Goldberg *et al.*, 1996).

The use of portfolios in medical and veterinary education has met with mixed reports of success (Driessen *et al.*, 2007). By 2000–2003, portfolios were being implemented in medical schools in undergraduate universities across the United States, United Kingdom, and Europe (Driessen *et al.*, 2003; Snadden and Thomas, 1998). The Universities of Liverpool and Nottingham recently implemented portfolios with their veterinary undergraduate students from Year 1, providing the students with a record of evidence that displays their knowledge, skills, and professional attitudes in a competency framework. The validity of a portfolio is high if the records include accurate real-life activities that provide evidence of a competency being achieved (Baillie and Rhind, 2008).

Issues arising with portfolios relate to the perceptions held by both staff (mentors) and students. The relevance of the portfolio needs to be addressed thoroughly; furthermore, members of staff who are mentors need to be fully committed to this method of assessment if it is to be implemented. Students need to see how the portfolio will eventually benefit them, by developing their reflective skills for lifelong learning. If the purpose of the portfolio is unclear, then its value will be superficial (Driessen *et al.*, 2003). The mentor will assist the student in helping to recognize their learning needs, validate the material, and ensure that the professional aspects of working on a case will become part of the learning process (Driessen *et al.*, 2003). Mossop and Senior (2008) state that peer support sessions need to be formally scheduled, allowing students to reflect on their placements in light of what their peers have experienced. Training of the mentor is crucial and can take many different forms; for example, training before and during a program of study, and the inclusion of discussion groups with other mentors to learn from each other, have proved beneficial (Dekker *et al.*, 2009).

Provision of Feedback

There are a number of elements in workplace-based assessment methods that make them valid for assessing and stimulating students' learning related to their place in an authentic learning environment. This allows for more complex aspects of competency such as professionalism to be captured, and it provides a number of opportunities for feedback. One of the main purposes and values of workplace-based assessment methods is the provision of immediate feedback. All of the methods mentioned in the previous section afford immediate feedback, a necessity in driving learning and reflection (Cohen, Farrant, and Taibjee, 2009; van der Vleuten, 1996). The workplace is an environment where providing feedback can be difficult, since most clinical staff will be trying to balance their clinical and teaching responsibilities, which may have an indirect impact on the amount and quality of the feedback (Wilkinson *et al.*, 2008). Although it depends on the method, feedback should be provided directly after assessment whenever possible; it should be specific and focused on the needs of the student and their performance to have maximum effect (Cantillon and Sargeant, 2008). It should identify areas in which the student has shown excellence as well as areas that require improvement, in order for students to understand their weaknesses as well as their strengths. If feedback is vague or too critical this may demotivate students, making them less likely to change or improve on their practice (Sargeant, Mann, and Ferrier, 2005). There is also a case for a more

reflective type of feedback. Assessment in the workplace has a valuable function in providing a collection of snapshots of a student's performance in an authentic environment. If these are collected in a learning diary, students can reflect on them on their own, or with a tutor, to provide them with a more holistic perspective on their progress and their preparation for the tasks they will be undertaking every day in practice.

Practicalities of an Authentic, Complex Learning Environment

The veterinary clinical workplace is a complex and unpredictable learning environment where students can actively put into practice their clinical and professional knowledge and skills (Magnier *et al.*, 2011). In most countries the regulations under which veterinary professionals work afford the student great opportunities to work in an authentic environment with the "safety net" of supervision by a qualified practitioner, who is ultimately responsible for the care and welfare of the patients. The authenticity of the clinical setting and active participation in professional practice have been identified as critical motivators for students' learning (Spencer, 2003). Assessment is an important part of this, and the closer an assessment is placed to the environment in which the skill being assessed really takes place, the more valid the assessment becomes.

The capacity of the clinical workplace to provide learning and assessment opportunities for students to develop their technical and nontechnical competencies is sometimes compromised by its variability (Magnier *et al.*, 2011). The number and type of cases presented in clinics cannot be controlled by clinical staff, yet teaching, learning, and assessment opportunities in a clinical setting are dependent on the cases that come through the door (Lane and Strand, 2008). A busy or overstretched clinical service may be compromised in terms of the time staff have available to spend with students, whereas having too few clinical cases equates to a loss of learning opportunities. Clinical staff have to balance the student's desire to practice and be assessed on clinical skills on the cases presented against the wishes of the client and the welfare of the patient. In a course that comprises a number of visits to different clinical units, it will normally be possible for students to experience an appropriate number of learning opportunities in skills that can be generalized, such as communication and professionalism, but requirements for experience in specific skills or situations may not always be possible to meet with a variable caseload. In these cases, the course design needs to include other opportunities to learn and assess such skills so that students can meet all their outcome requirements.

Assessment of Professional Skills

When learning and assessment are situated in practice, clinical skills cannot be divorced from professional skills. One of the great strengths of workplace-based assessment methods is their ability to document the humanistic aspects of a clinical encounter. According to Ginsburg *et al.* (2002), this aspect can only be fully developed in such clinical settings. For instance, through witnessing professional decision-making and encountering their own challenges, medical students can come to develop their own "professional judgment." Ginsburg *et al.* (2002) argue that professional judgment cannot be adequately learned from lectures or by rote, nor can it be assessed by written examinations alone. Students, as novices, acquire and apply professionalism through specific instances, and their professionalism must be taught and assessed in a clinical setting.

Challenges of Workplace-Based Veterinary Assessment

There are a number of challenges associated with the implementation of the methods that have already been mentioned, including reliability, requirement for competency, faculty training, and preparation for the workplace, and these should be reflected on in the process of assessment.

Reliability and Case Specificity

Van der Vleuten (1996) developed the "utility index," which includes five criteria against which assessment methods are reviewed: reliability, validity, acceptability, feasibility, and educational impact. Each criterion is important, and optimization of any assessment method is about balancing the different elements of the utility index. Although all of these criteria are important, it is recognized that no assessment method can score uniformly high on all five criteria. A tradeoff occurs and is necessary to ensure that the purpose of assessment is achieved when selecting an assessment method (Wass, Jones, and van der Vleuten, 2001; Wass, Bowden, and Jackson, 2007).

All the workplace-based assessment methods mentioned have high validity and educational impact due to the authenticity of their setting, their capacity to provide significant feedback, and students' belief in the importance of that setting in relation to their future career (face validity). Most of these methods have significant questions over their reliability and feasibility, however. Problems relating specifically to reliability include the number of encounters, number of examiners, and conflict in the role of a supervisor who is facilitating the learner, but who is also involved in the examination process. Reliability can be improved with an emphasis on the assessment of learners in a greater variety of settings, including an increased number of encounters and examiners (Schuwirth and van Der Vleuten, 2003). The importance of assessing learners in different settings relates to the property of competence being specific to certain clinical contexts and not a generic ability, but it does require more assessment and so raises problems of feasibility in many courses (McKimm and Swanwick, 2009).

Requirements for Veterinary Day One Competencies

Graduates from veterinary programs require a much larger range of Day One skills than those from medical programs. This places a much larger burden of assessment, particularly in specific skills, on veterinary courses; and this burden is exacerbated by the requirement to demonstrate to professional and regulatory bodies that each student is competent in a full range of the required skills. In addition, most of the modern structures for workplace-based assessment have been developed for medical postgraduate trainees. These learners are normally working in clinical teams, where more senior colleagues who can share the burden of acting as observer/assessors outnumber the trainees. This relationship of observers to students rarely exists in veterinary undergraduate assessment. The result of this is that in general veterinary courses have more competencies to assess and fewer people to do it, and frequently the only feasible strategy is to select the attributes that are best assessed in the workplace, and find a compromise that samples the remainder of the required skills. Thus, the traditional theme in professional course assessment of coverage and sampling widely across the content of the curriculum remains important, and the challenge is to keep this assessment as close to the workplace as is feasible.

Training of Staff as Assessors

Workplace-based assessment methods rely on judgments by qualified professionals. There is a widely held assumption that qualified professionals will be able to assess students in their area of expertise, but this is not necessarily true (Murphy, 1999). There is often excessive variability within the ratings by qualified professionals: there is the potential that assessors mark consistently lower or higher than others, known as "hawks and doves," respectively; that candidates benefit from the "halo effect," where existing information about a candidate may bias the assessor's judgment; or the phenomenon of the assessor having a good/bad day – all of which may affect the reliability of the assessment (Hays, 2006; Cohen, Manion, and Morrison, 2000; Swanwick and Chana, 2007). Performance ratings will also be influenced by the assessor's

expertise, which may have an impact on the feedback given to trainees and on the accuracy of performance ratings (Lievens, 2001; Kerrins and Cushing, 2000). Newer research has focused on the cognitive processes that are used to make these social judgments, suggesting that assessors make inferences during a clinical assessment (Gingerich *et al.*, 2014).

Implementing training to counter these possibilities requires extensive time, resources, and acceptability to staff. Implementation of one-off training sessions may not be appropriate for the development of professional judgment and decision-making; this requires long-term support, coaching, and feedback, as well as reflection on the strategies used in judging performance (Anders Ericsson, 2008). There is a limit to what formal training sessions can do, as an assessor's expertise seems to develop through real-world experience (Govaerts, 2011; Govaerts *et al.*, 2011).

Preparing Students Before They Even Reach the Workplace

The transition to the clinical workplace is widely viewed as stressful and anxiety inducing (Radcliffe and Lester, 2003; Alexander and Haldane, 1979; Teunissen and Westerman, 2011). Magnier *et al.* (2011) reported students' perceived inadequacies in terms of interacting with colleagues and a lack of "working knowledge" of what their role should be, as well as a lack of confidence relating to prior knowledge and the ability to perform relevant skills competently; this is consistent with findings in other studies (O'Brien, Cooke, and Irby, 2007; Godefrooij, Diemers, and Scherpbier, 2010). Students have to adjust to being part of a team and are required to display values and attitudes associated with being a professional in an everyday capacity (Prince *et al.*, 2005). While a moderate level of stress is considered beneficial for students to perform well, a high stress level can be counterproductive and inhibitive to learning and assessing in the workplace (van Hell *et al.*, 2008). Should we be thinking about preparing our students for the workplace in regard to their learning and being assessed?

Future of Veterinary Workplace-Based Assessment

The authentic contextualized environment of the workplace appears to be the best environment in which to assess the complex blend of skills required in graduates from professional veterinary courses. Difficulties with reliability, sampling, and feasibility restrict the use of this area in many courses to those skills that are most suited to the environment or most difficult to properly assess elsewhere. Inevitably, assessment programs use a number of methods, and some of these suffer in terms of validity because of their distance from the workplace. One way to overcome this difficulty is to coordinate assessments over the life of a course in a system of program assessment. This holistic approach to assessment is advocated by van der Vleuten and Schuwirth (2005; Schuwirth and van der Vleuten, 2011). The approach proposes that methods have stronger potential if they are used as part of an overall assessment program, and allows for compensation for the weaknesses of some methods reconciled by the strengths of other methods, which may result in a "diverse spectrum of complementary measurement instruments that can capture competence as whole" (Dijkstra, van der Vleuten, and Schuwirth, 2010). It uses the assessment of students in their actual workplace as an opportunity to gather just as much information as is required to certify their ability and to build up a final picture of them in an authentic learning environment.

The way forward for those designing veterinary courses appears to be to employ a suite of assessments, preferably ones that have a basis in the peer-reviewed educational literature. Contextualizing assessment in relation to the workplace, and interlinking individual methods in a program-based approach, help support the validity of the assessments and compensate for some of the difficulties with their feasibility.

References

Alexander, D.A., and Haldane, J.D. (1979) Medical education: A student perspective. *Medical Education*, **13**, 336–341.

Alves de Lima, A.E., Conde, D., Aldunate, L., and van der Vleuten, C.P. (2010) Teachers' experiences of the role and function of the mini clinical evaluation exercise in post-graduate training. *International Journal of Medical Education*, **1**, 68–73.

Anders Ericsson, K. (2008) Deliberate practice and acquisition of expert performance: A general overview. *Academic Emergency Medicine*, **15**, 988–994.

Archer, J.C., Norcini, J., and Davies, H.A. (2005) Use of SPRAT for peer review of paediatricians in training. *British Medical Journal*, **330**, 1251–1253.

Baillie, S., and Rhind, S. (2008) A Guide to Assessment Methods in Veterinary Medicine. Royal College of Veterinary Surgeons. http://www.live.ac.uk/Media/LIVE/PDFs/ assessment_guide.pdf (accessed November 9, 2016).

Bindal, T., Wall, D., and Goodyear, H.M. (2011) Trainee doctors' views on workplace-based assessments: Are they just a tick box exercise? *Medical Teacher*, **33**, 919–927.

Bird, T. (1990) The schoolteacher's portfolio: An essay on possibilities, in *The New Handbook of Teacher Evaluation: Assessing Elementary and Secondary School Teachers* (eds J. Millman and L. Darling-Hammond), Corwin Press, Newbury Park, CA.

Bok, H.G.J., Teunissen, P.W., Favier, R.P., et al. (2013) Programmatic assessment of competency-based workplace learning: When theory meets practice. *BMC Medical Education*, **13**, 123.

Cantillon, P., and Sargeant, J. (2008) Giving feedback in clinical settings. *BMJ*, **337**, 1292–1294.

Cobb, K.A., Brown, G., Jaarsma, D.A.D.C., and Hammond, R.A. (2013) The educational impact of assessment: A comparison of DOPS and MCQs. *Medical Teacher*, **35**, e1598–e1607.

Cohen, L., Manion, L., and Morrison, K. (2000) *Research Methods in Education*, Routledge Falmer, London.

Cohen, S.N., Farrant, P.B.J., and Taibjee, S.M. (2009) Assessing the assessments: U.K. dermatology trainees' views of the workplace assessment tools. *British Journal of Dermatology*, **161**, 34–39.

Dannefer, E.F., Henson, L.C., Bierer, S.B., et al. (2005) Peer assessment of professional competence. *Medical Education*, **39**, 713–722.

Davis, M.H., Ben-David, M.F., Harden, R.M., et al. (2001) Portfolio assessment in medical students' final examinations. *Medical Teacher*, **23**, 357–366.

Dekker, H., Driessen, E., Braak, E.T., et al. (2009) Mentoring portfolio use in undergraduate and postgraduate medical education. *Medical Teacher*, **31**, 903–909.

Dijkstra, J., van der Vleuten, C., and Schuwirth, L. (2010) A new framework for designing programmes of assessment. *Advances in Health Sciences Education*, **15**, 379–393.

Donnon, T., Al Ansari, A., Al Alawi, S., and Violato, C. (2014) The reliability, validity, and feasibility of multisource feedback physician assessment: A systematic review. *Academic Medicine*, **89**, 511–516.

Driessen, E. (2009) Portfolio critics: Do they have a point? *Medical Teacher*, **31**, 279–281.

Driessen, E., van Tartwijk, J., van der Vleuten, C., and Wass, V. (2007) Portfolios in medical education: Why do they meet with mixed success? A systematic review. *Medical Education*, **41**, 1224–1233.

Driessen, E., van Tartwijk, J., Vermunt, J., and van der Vleuten, C. (2003) Use of portfolios in early undergraduate medical training. *Medical Teacher*, **25**, 18–23.

Durning, S.J., Cation, L.J., Markert, R.J., and Pangaro, L.N. (2002) Assessing the reliability and validity of the mini-clinical evaluation exercise for internal medicine residency training. *Academic Medicine*, **77**, 900–904.

Gingerich, A., Kogan, J., Yeates, P., et al. (2014) Seeing the "black box" differently: Assessor cognition from three research perspectives. *Medical Education*, **48**, 1055–1068.

Ginsburg, S., Regehr, G., Stern, D., and Lingard, L. (2002) The anatomy of the professional lapse: Bridging the gap between traditional frameworks and students' perceptions. *Academic Medicine*, **77**, 516–522.

Godefrooij, M., Diemers, A., and Scherpbier, A. (2010) Students' perceptions about the transition to the clinical phase of a medical curriculum with preclinical patient contacts; a focus group study. *BMC Medical Education*, **10**, 10–28.

Goldberg, L.R., McCormick Richburg, C., and Wood, L.A. (2006) Active learning through service – learning. *Communication Disorders Quarterly*, **27**, 131–145.

Govaerts, M.J. (2011) Climbing the pyramid: Towards understanding performance assessment. PhD thesis, University of Maastricht.

Govaerts, M.J., Schuwirth, L., van der Vleuten, C., and Muijtjens, A.M. (2011) Workplace-based assessment methods: Effects of rater expertise. *Advances in Health Sciences Education: Theory and Practice*, **16**, 151–165.

Hammond, J. (2010) In clinic assessment in veterinary education: Adapting the Mini CEX to create a veterinary clinical assessment tool. Poster presented at Association for Medical Education in Europe (AMEE), Glasgow.

Harden, R.M., Stevenson, M., Downie, W.W., and Wilson, G.M. (1975) Assessment of clinical competence using objective structured examination. *BMJ*, **1**, 447–451.

Hays, R. (2006) Teaching and learning in clinical settings, in *Teaching and Learning in Clinical Settings* (ed. R. Hays), Radcliffe Publishing, Oxford, pp. 125–146.

Hecker, K.G., Norris, J., and Coe, J.B. (2012) Workplace-based assessment in a primary-care setting. *Journal of Veterinary Medical Education*, **39**, 229–240.

Hill, F., Kendall, K., Galbraith, K., and Crossley, J. (2009) Implementing the undergraduate mini-CEX: A tailored approach at

Southampton University. *Medical Education*, **43**, 326–334.

Hodges, B.D. (2006) The objective structured clinical examination: Three decades of development. *Journal of Veterinary Medical Education*, **33**, 571–577.

Holsgrove, G.D. (2003) Assessment in the foundation programme, in *Assessment in Medical Education and Training: A Practical Guide* (eds N. Jackson, A. Jamieson, and A. Khan), Radcliffe Publishing, Oxford, pp. 41–51.

Jaarsma, A.D.C., Bok, G.J., Theyse, L.F.H., et al. (2010) One assessment program for an undergraduate veterinary master curriculum. Poster presented at Association of Medical Education in Europe (AMEE), Glasgow.

Kerrins, J.A., and Cushing, K.S. (2000) Taking a second look: Expert and novice differences when observing the same classroom teaching segment a second time. *Journal of Personnel Evaluation in Education*, **14**, 5–24.

Lane, I.F., and Strand, E. (2008) Clinicial veterinary education: Insights from faculty and strategies for professional development in clinical teaching. *Journal of Veterinary Medical Education*, **35**, 397–407.

Lave, J., and Wenger, E. (1991) *Situated Learning: Legitimate Peripheral Participation*, Cambridge University Press, Cambridge.

Lievens, F. (2001) Assessor training strategies and their effects on accuracy, interrater reliability, and discriminant validity. *Journal of Applied Psychology*, **86**, 255–264.

Magnier, K., Wang, R., Dale, V.H.M., et al. (2011) Enhancing clinical learning in the workplace: A qualitative study. *Veterinary Record*, **169**, 682.

Malhotra, S., Hatala, R., and Courneya, C. (2008) Internal medicine residents' perceptions of the mini-clinical evaluation exercise. *Medical Teacher*, **30**, 414–419.

Massie, J., and Ali, J. (2015) Workplace-based assessment: A review of user perceptions and strategies to address the identified shortcomings. *Advances in Health Sciences Education*, **21**, 455–473.

McKimm, J., and Swanwick, T. (2009) Assessing learning needs. *British Journal of Hospital Medicine*, **70**, 348–351.

Miller, G.E. (1990) The assessment of clinical skills/competence/performance. *Academic Medicine*, **65**, S63–S67.

Mossop, L.H., and Senior, A. (2008) I'll show you mine if you show me yours! Portfolio design in two UK veterinary schools. *Journal of Veterinary Medical Education*, **35**, 599–606.

Murphy, R. (1999) Principles of assessment: A reminder, in *Success and Failure in Professional Education* (ed I.M. Ilott), Whurr Publishers, London.

Norcini, J.J. (2001) The validity of long cases. *Medical Education*, **35**, 720–721.

Norcini, J.J. (2003) Peer assessment of competence. *Medical Education*, **37**, 539–543.

Norcini, J.J. (2005) Current perspectives in assessment: The assessment of performance at work. *Medical Education*, **39**, 880–889.

Norcini, J.J., Blank, L.L., Arnold, G.K., and Kimball, H.R. (1995) The mini-CEX (clinical evaluation exercise): A preliminary investigation. *Annals of Internal Medicine*, **123**, 795–799.

Norcini, J., and Burch, V. (2007) Workplace-based assessment as an educational tool: AMEE guide no. 31. *Medical Teacher*, **29**, 855–871.

O'Brien, B., Cooke, M., and Irby, D.M. (2007) Perceptions and attributions of third-year student struggles in clerkships: Do students and clerkship directors agree? *Academic Medicine*, **82**, 970–978.

Ponnamperuma, G.G., Karunathilake, I.M., McAleer, S., and Davis, M.H. (2009) The long case and its modifications: A literature review. *Medical Education*, **43**, 936–941.

Prescott, L.E., Norcini, J.J., Mckinlay, P., and Rennie, J.S. (2002) Facing the challenges of competency-based assessment of postgraduate dental training: Longitudinal evaluation of performance. *Medical Education*, **36**, 92–97.

Prince, K.J.A.H., Boshuizen, H.P.A., van der Vleuten, C.P.M., and Scherpbier, A.J.J.A. (2005) Students' opinions about their preparation for clinical practice. *Medical Education*, **39**, 704–712.

Radcliffe, C., and Lester, H. 2003. Perceived stress during undergraduate medical training: A qualitative study. *Medical Education*, **37**, 32–38.

Read, E.K., Bell, C., Rhind, S., and Hecker, K.G. (2015) The use of global rating scales for OSCEs in veterinary medicine. *PLoS One*, **10**, e0121000.

Regehr, G., and Norman, G.R. (1996) Issues in cognitive psychology: Implications for professional education. *Academic Medicine*, **71**, 988–1001.

Rethans, J.J., Sturmans, F., Drop, R., and van der Vleuten, C. (1991) Assessment of the performance of general practitioners by the use of standardized (simulated) patients. *British Journal of General Practice*, **41**, 97–99.

Rhind, S.M. (2006) Competence at graduation: Implications for assessment. *Journal of Veterinary Medical Education*, **33**, 172–175.

Sargeant, J., Mann, K., and Ferrier, S. (2005) Exploring family physicians' reactions to multisource feedback: Perceptions of credibility and usefulness. *Medical Education*, **39**, 497–504.

Schuwirth, L.W.T., and van der Vleuten, C.P.M. (2003) The use of clinical simulations in assessment. *Medical Education*, **37**, 65–71.

Schuwirth, L.W., and van der Vleuten, C.P. (2004) Changing education, changing assessment, changing research? *Medical Education*, **38**, 805–812.

Schuwirth, L.W.T., and van der Vleuten, C.P.M. (2011) Programmatic assessment: From assessment of learning to assessment for learning. *Medical Teacher*, **33**, 478–485.

Searle, G.F. (2008) Is CEX good for psychiatry? An evaluation of workplace-based assessment. *Psychiatric Bulletin*, **32**, 271–273.

Sidhu, R.S., Mcilroy, J.H., and Regehr, G. (2005) Using a comprehensive examination to assess multiple competencies in surgical residents: Does the oral examination still have a role? *Journal of American College of Surgeons*, **201**, 754–758.

Smee, S. (2003) ABC of learning and teaching in medicine. Skill based assessment. *BMJ*, **326**, 703–706.

Snadden, D., and Thomas, M.L. (1998) Portfolio learning in general practice vocational training – does it work? *Medical Education*, **32**, 401–406.

Spencer, J. (2003) ABC of learning and teaching in medicine: Learning and teaching in the clinical environment. *BMJ*, **326**, 591.

Swanwick, T., and Chana, N. (2007) Workplace-based assessment for general practice training, in *Assessment in Medical Education and Training* (eds N. Jackson, A. Jamieson, and A. Khan), Radcliffe Publishing, Oxford, pp. 74–85.

Teunissen, P.W., and Westerman, M. (2011) Opportunity or threat: The ambiguity of the consequences of transitions in medical education. *Medical Education*, **45**, 51–59.

Timmins, F., and Dunne, P.J. (2009) An exploration of the current use and benefit of nursing student portfolios. *Nurse Education Today*, **29**, 330–341.

van der Vleuten, C.P.M. (1996) The assessment of professional competence: Developments, research and practical implications. *Advances in Health Science Education*, **1**, 41–67.

van der Vleuten, C.P., and Schuwirth, L.W. (2005) Assessing professional competence: From methods to programmes. *Medical Education*, **39**, 309–317.

van Hell, E.A., Kuks, J.B.M., Schönrock-Adema, J., et al. (2008) Transition to clinical training: Influence of pre-clinical knowledge and skills, and consequences for clinical performance. *Medical Education*, **42**, 830–837.

Violato, C., and Lockyer, J. (2003) Multisource feedback: A method of assessing surgical practice. *BMJ*, **326**, 546–548.

Wass, V., Bowden, R., and Jackson, N. (2007) The principles of assessment design, in *Assessment in Medical Education and Training* (eds N. Jackson, A. Jamieson, and A. Khan), Radcliffe Publishing, Oxford, pp. 11–26.

Wass, V., Jones, R., and van der Vleuten, C. (2001) Standardized or real patients to test clinical competence? The long case revisited. *Medical Education*, **35**, 321–325.

Whitehouse, A., Hassell, A., Bullock, A., et al. (2007) 360 degree assessment (multi source feedback) of UK trainee doctors: Field testing of team assessment of behaviours (TAB). *Medical Teacher*, **29** (**2-3**), 171–176.

Wilkinson, T.J., Campbell, P.J., and Judd, S.J. (2008) Reliability of the long case. *Medical Education*, **42**, 887–893.

Wilkinson, J., Crossley, J.G.M., Wragg, A., et al. (2008) Implementing workplace-based assessment across the medical specialties in the United Kingdom. *Medical Education*, **42**, 364–373.

Williams, A. (2003) Informal learning in the workplace: A case study of new teachers. *Educational Studies*, **29**, 207–219.

Wilson, G.M., Lever, R., Harden, R.M., et al. (1969) Examination of clinical examiners. *The Lancet*, **293** (**7584**), 37–40.

17

Feedback

Karen K. Cornell

College of Veterinary Medicine & Biomedical Sciences, Texas A&M University, USA

 Box 17.1: Key messages

- Feedback is the process by which information is provided to a learner with the goal of influencing future performance.
- Individual characteristics and preferences of the learner affect the action taken after receiving feedback.
- Culture, as it relates to feedback, influences the learner's seeking and reception of feedback.
- Educators' responsibilities in providing feedback include creating and communicating clear goals and objectives, providing feedback at different levels conforming to the learner's needs, and conveying specific suggestions for how to improve future performance.
- Use of a framework for the delivery of the feedback message aids in reducing instructors' anxiety related to feedback.
- Feedback is critical for the development of reflective knowledge-building for the learner.

Introduction

The term feedback was utilized first in the 1860s industrial revolution to describe the process by which output signals of energy, or momentum, are returned to the point of origin within a system to modulate future performance of that system. In these systems, the returning signal immediately influenced future output. Review of this original use of the term is valuable to remind one of the ultimate goal of feedback, which is to influence future performance. A critical difference between feedback in medical education from that within a mechanical system is the human influence on the process. The characteristics of the provider of feedback, the individual receiving the feedback, and the culture or environment within which the feedback is given greatly affect the ability of feedback to influence future performance. An additional objective of feedback in medical education is again related to the human portion of the feedback process, and is the reinforcement of feedback-seeking behavior. Feedback-seeking, defined as the conscious devotion of effort toward determining the correctness and adequacy of one's behaviors for attaining valued goals, facilitates the lifelong learning required of veterinarians (Ashford, 1986).

Defining Feedback

There are many important dimensions within the definition of feedback. The components of effective feedback in medical education include provision of information regarding prior performance, promotion of positive and desirable learner development, resultant action taken by the learner, facilitation of refinement of the learner's self-assessment skills, and promotion of future feedback-seeking. It is important to differentiate between feedback and evaluation. Feedback is intended to be instructional, providing information for the learner regarding the gap between current performance and desired performance, and is forward looking, specific, and descriptive. Feedback is not always corrective, and may be employed to reaffirm performance that requires no modification, using specific examples for clear illustration. In contrast, evaluation is focused on the past and is a judgment of past performance. While some evaluations include feedback, the simple attainment of a "B+" gives a learner little information regarding how to improve their knowledge or application of knowledge. Winne and Butler (1994, p. 5740) defined feedback as "information with which a learner can confirm, add to, overwrite, tune, or restructure information in memory, whether that information is domain knowledge, meta-cognitive knowledge, beliefs about self and tasks, or cognitive tactics and strategies." A key point is that this definition includes the need for learner self-assessment, and it requires the learner to confirm the accuracy of feedback received, or tune it to their own beliefs. In addition to addressing a specific task or act, this process aids in the development of the learner's self-assessment skills (see Box 17.2).

There are many common assumptions regarding feedback. These include that all feedback is good feedback, more feedback is better,

feedback is a one-way flow of information, feedback is complete when the message is delivered, and one model of feedback is effective for all learners and all situations. It is important for veterinary medical educators to move beyond these assumptions. The goal of this chapter is to provide the background information and scaffolding to assist in making that move.

Impact of Feedback

Hattie, Biggs, and Purdie (1996) report that the influence of feedback on student achievement is highest in situations in which the student has demonstrated prior cognitive ability; direct instruction was provided; there was reciprocal teaching; or direct feedback was offered. While the impact of feedback varies, the greatest demonstrated effect was reported when feedback was provided regarding a specific task and how to perform that task more effectively. Multiple studies in medical education have demonstrated that individuals in an environment with feedback have greater confidence and motivation, interpersonal skills, learner satisfaction, clinical performance, accuracy of self-assessment, and patient satisfaction (see Box 17.3; Crommelinck and Anseel, 2013; Boud and Molloy, 2013; Thomas and Arnold, 2011; Clynes and Raftery, 2008; Davis *et al.*, 2006). Conversely, individuals who do not receive feedback are more likely to overestimate their abilities, lack reinforcement of effective performance, fail to correct poor performance, and receive a false positive impression (Davis *et al.*,

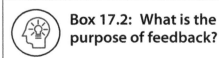

Box 17.2: What is the purpose of feedback?

Information provided to a learner with which they can confirm, add to, overwrite, or restructure memory to improve future performance and further refine self-assessment skills.

Box 17.3: Where's the Evidence? Impact of effective feedback in medical education

- Increased confidence and motivation
- Increased interpersonal skills
- Increased learner satisfaction
- Increased clinical performance
- Increased accuracy of self-assessment

2006; Ende, Pomerantz, and Erickson, 1995; Laidlaw *et al.*, 2006; Waitzkin, 1985; Spickard *et al.*, 2008; Cantillon and Sargeant, 2008).

Timing of Feedback

Numerous studies have been done to assess the effect of the timing of feedback as it relates to academic achievement. Results vary and are challenging to quantify. There are many factors related to timing that influence the effectiveness of feedback, including the difficulty or complexity of the task and the amount of processing required to complete it (Schroth, 1992). Delayed feedback may be better for supporting the transfer of knowledge, whereas immediate feedback may be more effective in the short term for supporting the development of procedural skills (Schroth, 1992).

The Role of the Feedback Recipient

Positive or Negative Feedback

Whether feedback is reinforcing or corrective in nature may influence its impact on the learner's ability to enact change. In some instances overly critical feedback can have a negative impact on learning (Kluger and DeNisi, 1996; Hattie and Timperley, 2007).

On average, positive and negative feedback are similar in their effects on performance, but it is well documented that feedback that threatens

the self is likely to debilitate recipients (Kluger and van Dijk, 2010; Sargeant *et al.*, 2008). For this reason, feedback is best received and acted on if the learner's preferences regarding feedback are considered. Because the individual receiving the feedback must be able to decode and utilize the information provided, it must be considered that each learner brings to the interaction their own thoughts, experiences, and self-assessments. In situations in which the learner seeks feedback, it is important to consider the types or features of the feedback that they are seeking. Some learners seek appreciation in order to gain motivation and encouragement, some seek coaching so that they may move their own performance closer to the desired performance, and others truly seek evaluation so that they know their location relative to the standards or performance of others. This desire for evaluation also facilitates the alignment of their expectations and informs their decision-making (see Box 17.4; Stone and Heen, 2014).

Archer (2010, p. 101) states that "educators must acknowledge the psychosocial needs of the recipients while ensuring that feedback is both honest and accurate."

Promotion or Prevention Focus

Kluger and van Dijk's 2010 study suggests that the benefit of positive or negative feedback is dependent on the regulatory focus of the learner: promotion or prevention (see Box 17.5).

Box 17.4: Focus on the types of learner-sought feedback

- *Appreciation* – to gain motivation or encouragement
- *Coaching* – instruction to move current performance to desired performance
- *Evaluation* – knowledge of current location as it relates to standards or performance of others

Box 17.5: Outcomes of prevention or promotion focus feedback

Prevention focus	Promotion focus
• Avoidance of pain or punishment	• Regulated by the achievement of pleasure or reward
• Things done because "we have to"	• Things done because "we want to"
• – feedback results in ↑ performance	• – feedback results in ↓ performance
• + feedback results in ↓ performance	• + feedback results in ↑ performance

Learners, and the tasks with which they are confronted, may be prevention or promotion focused (Watling *et al.*, 2012). A prevention focus indicates that all actions are directed toward avoiding poor outcomes or punishment, and as a result learners do things because they perceive they must do them. For instance, completing a calculation for a constant-rate infusion might be considered a prevention-focused task, since the penalty for failure or error is very high. In this example, achieving the correct answer is met with relief and is not likely to change performance in the future, while a negative outcome is likely to change future performance drastically. A promotion focus indicates that actions are directed toward the achievement of reward or pleasure, thus it involves goals that are desires and things the learner wants to do. An example of a promotion-focused task might be the assignment to develop innovative ways to distribute personnel in order to cover work shifts. If the feedback regarding the innovative plans includes the comment that they are appropriate, effective, and helpful, the learner is likely to be motivated to contribute more. If, however, the ideas are received negatively, the learner may be inclined to abandon attempts to improve. In healthcare, promotion and prevention foci become complicated to differentiate. As veterinary healthcare professionals we are required to be aware of potential mistakes and their impact, for instance the failure of a ligature resulting in hemorrhage, while also thinking "outside of the box" in diagnosis and treatment, for example performing a muscle biopsy for an unusual weakness presentation (Kluger and van Dijk, 2010).

Learners' Perception of Feedback

Learners' perception of feedback is also important to understand. In a study of medical students, 96% considered it important to receive feedback, yet only 59% felt that they received enough feedback (Murdoch-Eaton and Sargeant, 2012). Perhaps the most disturbing finding of this study was that only 36% of students reported that they knew where to seek additional feedback. This lack of knowledge of where to seek feedback is counterintuitive, since these were students in training programs; it seems they should have known to ask their teachers. Perhaps this has more to do with the features of the possible providers of feedback than a true lack of knowledge of where to seek it.

Another key feature of the learner is an understanding of where they are in the learning process for the task in question. Eva *et al.* (2012) report a paradox in student response to feedback, with the finding that individuals need to achieve a level of comfort, experience, and confidence prior to being prepared to ask for or receive corrective feedback. In practice, this means that we must give the student time and space to make attempts at a task or behavior before providing immediate feedback. For example, immediately correcting the student's grip of needleholders before they begin suturing for the first time is likely to frustrate them more and result in less long-term impact than allowing them to recognize the difficulties of utilizing the incorrect grip and then providing suggestions for improvement.

The Role of the Feedback Provider

As mentioned earlier, medical students desire feedback and do not believe that they receive enough feedback (Murdoch-Eaton, 2012). Why do they not ask? Studies in human and veterinary medical education indicate that students, and residents for that matter, are reluctant to seek feedback (Eva *et al.*, 2012; Bok *et al.*, 2013; Delva *et al.*, 2013; Reddy *et al.*, 2015). Encouragement of feedback-seeking, or "the conscious devotion of effort towards determining the correctness and adequacy of one's behaviors for attaining valued goals" as defined by Ashford (1986, p. 466), requires that several characteristics of a feedback provider are met.

Based on a study by Crommelinck and Anseel (2013), characteristics of the feedback provider that influence feedback-seeking behavior are the history of a provider already giving feedback to the learner, the accessibility of the feedback provider to the learner, and the perceived level of expertise associated with the provider as it relates to the task at hand. In a separate study of faculty and residents in human medicine, Delva *et al.* (2013) reported that the lack of quality of the feedback provided, the lack of direct observation, and the provision of infrequent feedback were factors that discouraged feedback-seeking by residents in training. Bok *et al.* (2013) reported that veterinary students sought feedback more when they perceived that the feedback provider had good communication skills, the provider could give feedback on directly observed learner performance, and there was a longer history of working together. The duration of time working together was also reported as an important factor in feedback behaviors by both faculty and residents in Delva *et al.*'s (2013) study. Feedback is best received, and therefore acted on, when it is perceived as being provided from a position of beneficence

Box 17.6: Focus on characteristics of feedback providers that promote feedback-seeking behavior

- Direct observation of the learner
- Quality feedback regularly provided from a perceived position of beneficence
- Accessible to the learner
- Expertise in the task at hand
- Time working with the learner

by an individual with whom the learner has developed a relationship of respect during the experience (Watling *et al.*, 2012; Boud and Molloy, 2013). The characteristics of feedback providers that promote feedback-seeking behaviors are included in Box 17.6.

Targeting Feedback at a Specific Level

As someone delivering feedback, it is important to understand that feedback may be provided to the learner at different levels, and that the level at which feedback is provided affects the ability of the learner to receive that feedback (Hattie and Timperley, 2007). Feedback may be focused at one of four levels – task level, process level, self-regulation level, and personal level – each of which may have a different impact on the learner (Figure 17.1).

Task-Level Feedback

Task-level feedback focuses on how a specific task is accomplished or performed. For instance, feedback regarding the tying of a square knot or choosing the correct answer from incorrect answers is task-level feedback. This is the most common form of feedback provided by teachers in classrooms (Airasian, 1997). When providing feedback at the level of a task, it has most impact when it corrects faulty interpretation of data

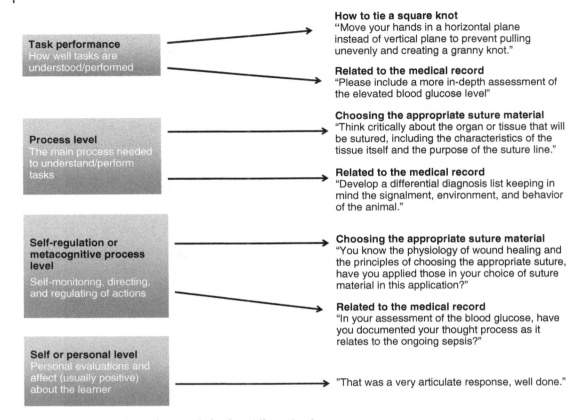

How to tie a square knot
"Move your hands in a horizontal plane instead of vertical plane to prevent pulling unevenly and creating a granny knot."

Related to the medical record
"Please include a more in-depth assessment of the elevated blood glucose level"

Task performance
How well tasks are understood/performed

Choosing the appropriate suture material
"Think critically about the organ or tissue that will be sutured, including the characteristics of the tissue itself and the purpose of the suture line."

Related to the medical record
"Develop a differential diagnosis list keeping in mind the signalment, environment, and behavior of the animal."

Process level
The main process needed to understand/perform tasks

Choosing the appropriate suture material
"You know the physiology of wound healing and the principles of choosing the appropriate suture, have you applied those in your choice of suture material in this application?"

Related to the medical record
"In your assessment of the blood glucose, have you documented your thought process as it relates to the ongoing sepsis?"

Self-regulation or metacognitive process level
Self-monitoring, directing, and regulating of actions

Self or personal level
Personal evaluations and affect (usually positive) about the learner

"That was a very articulate response, well done."

Figure 17.1 Feedback may be provided at four different levels.

rather than a lack of data. The student who does not have knowledge of more than one type of diabetes receives less benefit from a discussion of why a patient has Type I diabetes rather than Type II diabetes than a student who knows of the two types, but has misinterpreted the data or incorrectly applied it to the clinical case. Lack of information is best addressed by additional instruction rather than feedback alone.

A meta-analysis of 74 studies of feedback reported the effect or impact of different forms of feedback on educational achievement (Hattie, Biggs, and Purdie, 1996). The study found that feedback regarding a task and how to complete it more effectively had the highest effect sizes. The effect of task-related feedback (0.95) was greater than the effect of punishment (0.20), praise (0.14), or reward (0.31). It was

hypothesized that praise has a lesser effect because it provides little specific information regarding successful or unsuccessful performance of the task. Feedback at the task level is most effective for goal-related, challenging tasks that are not complex. Feedback provided at the task level is both more easily given and received, as the ability to do either is not closely related to the receiver's value of self. It is, however, possible to provide too much feedback if it is focused only at the task level (Kluger and DeNisi, 1996). Task-directed feedback alone has the potential to direct attention at an immediate goal, detracting from focus on a broader, high-performance goal. Task-related feedback in its simplest form does not promote broad application of the acquired knowledge or proficiency. A student who receives feedback regarding technical aspects of knot-tying without understanding why the type of knot they are mastering is important does not transfer information to other applications or similar problems. Therefore, an overarching goal of task-related feedback is to move students beyond the task level to the processing level, and ultimately to the self-regulation level.

Processing-Level Feedback

Feedback at the processing level is related to learners' understanding of the underlying "how" or "why" associated with tasks or processes. At this level, feedback is related to students' understanding of meaning, and the relationships between tasks, cognitive processes, and transference of knowledge to more difficult or untried tasks. Feedback at this level is also aimed at increasing students' abilities to detect their own errors. Feedback at the process level enhances deeper learning than feedback at the task level (Balzer, Doherty, and O'Connor, 1989). Building on the previous example of diabetes, applying the physiology of insulin resistance to acromegaly in cats would be taking this knowledge to the processing level, and therefore feedback at this level would address how to better understand the underlying process. For instance, rather than simply learning to give more insulin to an acromegalic cat, a student provided with processing-level feedback might better understand why patients other than this particular cat do not respond to insulin. Feedback at the process level, which includes a student's ability to understand a task or concept, is increasingly close to self-identity, and is therefore more challenging for the learner to receive than task-related feedback.

Self-Regulation Level Feedback

Self-regulation includes the ability of the student to self-assess and create internal feedback, their willingness for and proficiency in seeking and responding to feedback, and their attributions regarding success or failure. In short, it

is the way in which learners monitor, direct, and regulate actions toward the learning goal. Learners who are less effective in these skills are more dependent on external inputs for feedback and rarely seek feedback in ways that effectively enhance future learning. Hattie and Timperley (2007, p. 94) report that "students' willingness to invest effort in seeking and dealing with feedback information relates to the transaction costs invoked at the self-regulatory level." Transaction costs include the effort necessary for the search for feedback, the effect of having others evaluate them, and the impact of having evaluated their own performance wrongly. Delva *et al.* (2013) reported that medical residents' willingness to seek feedback was related to the perceived cost and the perceived value of the possible feedback. Factors influencing the perceived cost included the time spent interacting with faculty, the quality of the feedback provided by faculty, and the emotional risk of receiving negative feedback (Delva *et al.*, 2013). Feedback that aids in self-regulation helps to clarify what good performance is, facilitates the development of self-assessment/reflection in learning, delivers high-quality information to students about their learning, encourages teacher and peer dialogue around learning, fosters positive motivational beliefs and self-esteem, and provides opportunities to close the gap between current and desired performance. Feedback at the self-regulation level might include: "I followed your thought process in your medical record and noted that you applied your knowledge of the physiology of diabetes to reassess your initial diagnosis of Type I diabetes in your patient. It seems as if the writing of your thoughts in the medical record led to a deeper understanding of the disease and a reassessment of your own application of knowledge. Is that correct?" Feedback targeted at the self-regulation level is yet another step closer to self than task- or process-related feedback, and therefore can be the most challenging form of feedback to deliver and receive. At the self-regulation level, commitment to goals is a major mediator of effectiveness of feedback (van Dijk and Kluger, 2004, 2011).

Self- or Personal-Level Feedback

Feedback on this level is a personal evaluation of the learner and their affect. This type of feedback generally contains little task-related information and rarely increases learner self-regulation or process-level performance. Multiple studies have demonstrated low effects of praise on student achievement (Kluger and DeNisi, 1998; Wilkinson, 1981). The exception to these findings is when praise is directed at the effort, self-regulation, engagement, or processes related to the task and its performance. For instance, "You displayed very good effort in researching diabetes, applying the information you gathered to this case, and documenting it in your medical record." This type of praise can improve self-efficacy and therefore have an impact on task performance in the future.

The Process of Feedback

Hattie and Timperley (2007) propose a process for feedback that requires three distinct phases. The Feed-Up phase occurs prior to student performance and includes the process of establishing and refining learning goals. The Feedback phase includes the actual delivery of the feedback regarding student performance. The Feed-Forward phase provides information for the student regarding ways to alter the performance in order to approach the goal, as well as plans for next steps in feedback.

Feed-Up: Defining the Goal or Target

In the Feed-Up process, students and instructors establish learning goals. When done well, the instructor-established goals are provided through written materials such as the syllabus, in combination with additional dialogue depending on the setting. Proactive students establish their own goals based on the information provided by the instructor, in conjunction with their own learning foci. Instructor-defined objectives that are clear and specific with obvious importance relative to future student aspirations facilitate students' incorporation of these objectives into self-defined, personally meaningful goals. When the intended goal is clear and there is a high degree of belief that eventual success is achievable, students demonstrate increased effort and a high level of commitment to achieving the goal. Lack of clarity around the intended goal or unclear expectation has been reported to increase student anxiety (Siqueira Drake *et al.*, 2012) and may result in reduced or less effective effort. In some cases this goal-setting may require a facilitated discussion with the instructor, so that the student may understand why learning specific information is meaningful to their future. Goals may be performance or learning oriented. Performance-oriented goals are related to the learners' desire to demonstrate competence to others and to be positively evaluated. Learning-oriented goals demonstrate the desire to develop new skills and master new situations. Performance-oriented individuals believe that intelligence is innate, and therefore are characterized by a tendency to give up more easily and have less interest in difficult, challenging tasks in which success is less likely. Learning-oriented individuals reflect the belief that intelligence is malleable, and therefore tend to continue despite failure and to pursue challenges. To aid the student in achieving long-term success, it is beneficial for instructors to offer assistance in gaining an understanding of the need for learning-oriented goals.

Additionally, clear goals allow more directed feedback and focus students' attention. Therefore they are more effective than general or nonspecific goals (Locke and Latham, 2002). Students committed to specific goals are more likely to seek and receive feedback (Locke and Latham, 2002). When feedback is provided, it should be given in context related to a specific goal.

Feedback: Delivering the Message

As we as educators strive to help our learners become better in their chosen pursuits, it is important to recognize the need for the learner to self-assess, process additional feedback that is received, compare the two inputs, and make adjustments to future performance. In order to encourage this self-assessment or reflection, the delivery of feedback is best initiated by requesting the student's own self-assessment. In addition to providing insight into the student's perspective on their performance, it helps to establish the feedback session as a conversation rather than a one-sided delivery of information. Self-assessment enables instructor understanding of the student's perception of performance and identifies a starting point for the instructor. Students who are accurate with their self-assessments may only require confirmation of those assessments, with additional related examples or observations. Students who are overly harsh with their self-assessments may require examples of things done well in order to encourage further learning. The self-assessment may also identify gaps between instructor-desired goals and student-set goals. All of this information provides the educator with a more informed view as to the most appropriate focus of the feedback message. The self–assessment may also be helpful to the provider of feedback as they determine whether directive or facilitative feedback would be most beneficial for the learner (see Box 17.7). Directive feedback provides information on what requires correction. Facilitative feedback provides comments and suggestions to facilitate self-revision. This encourages subsequent reflective knowledge-building.

Reflective knowledge-building is a process in which students are given the opportunity to reflect on and evaluate their own work in relation to feedback input from others. Students then use the results of this evaluative process to build a better understanding as they progress (Boud and Molloy, 2013; Roscoe and Chi, 2008).

Many providers of feedback view the creation and delivery of the message as the most challenging phase of the feedback process. Much of this difficulty is related to concerns regarding the reaction of the learner to the message, as well as a feeling of lack of training in how to deliver the message (Delva *et al.*, 2013). A simple scaffolding of the process may help instructors to become more comfortable with it. The model proposed here – Context–Behavior–Impact–Next steps (CBIN), adapted by the Institute for Healthcare Communication from the Situation Behavior Impact model from the Center for Creative Leadership – allows the instructor to think through the portions of the message in a logical progression, and to present the information in a manner in which the learner can accurately receive it (see Figure 17.2). The first step is a description of the *context* in which the information was gathered. Here the provider of feedback must be as specific as possible. Evoking a defensive response from the learner does not promote self-refection or effective processing of the information. For example, a description of context might include "this morning when I observed you in the exam room with Mrs. Smith" or "last Monday when we were performing joint taps in the treatment room." The next step is to describe the *behavior*. Specific and nonjudgmental description is essential. In this portion of the feedback process it is critical for the instructor to have an understanding of the level of feedback being provided. The effectiveness of feedback increases as its focus moves further from self and more toward a specific task (Kluger and DeNisi, 1996). The impact of the student's action may be as simple as "when the suture ends were pulled unevenly as the square knot was tightened it became a half-hitch or granny knot," or as complex as "when it was pointed out to Mrs. Jones that she was late for her appointment, I saw her drop her eyes and noted that she

Box 17.7: What's the meaning of directive and facilitative feedback

- *Directive feedback* provides information on what requires correction.
- *Facilitative feedback* provides comments and suggestions to facilitate self-revision.

did not speak again until we asked questions of her in the exam room." As this feedback message unfolds, it is important to engage the learner in discussion around the observations and again seek their thoughts regarding the information.

The final step of the CBIN scaffold is to provide the learner with *next* steps. This might include specific strategies for improving the performance, for example "apply tension evenly on both ends of the suture as the knot is tied so it tightens down as a square knot." While this need for the provision of strategies to improve performance seems the obvious thing to do, only 50% of feedback encounters in one study of medical education included strategies for how the learner could improve (Fernando *et al.*, 2008).

Feed-Forward: Where to Go from Here

The final phase of the feedback process involves providing students with information that expands their learning opportunities. More than simply further refinement of a single task or area of knowledge, quality feedback challenges students to expand their self-assessment skills, strive for deeper understanding or broader

application of knowledge, and improve their self-regulation abilities.

Feedback-Seeking and Reflective Knowledge-Building

Boud and Molloy (2013, p. 148) state that "the process of feedback might be prompted by what teachers say or write, but the process is not concluded until action by the student occurs." Establishing a culture in which students have an active role in the feedback process instead of assuming the role of passive recipients of information is essential, as the learner is the only one who can ultimately act to change performance. Once established, a feedback-encouraging culture will support students' development of the skills necessary to seek feedback, self-evaluate, and then interpret the internal and external judgments in order to change future actions. While it is clear from the literature that feedback is expected and valued by learners and instructors, barriers still exist to establishing a culture of feedback. Most reported barriers are related to the time required to provide feedback, the concern about an emotional response from the learner, and the lack of confidence on the part of the instructor in the skill set necessary to deliver feedback.

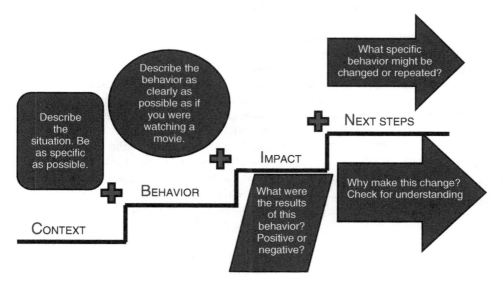

Figure 17.2 The CBIN model for providing feedback. Source: Institute for Healthcare Communication. Reproduced with permission.

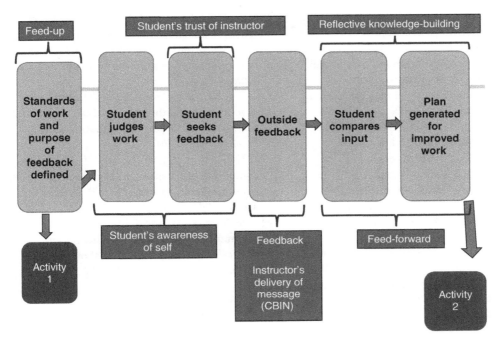

Figure 17.3 The complex process of feedback that when done well results in improved performance and increased reflective knowledge building. Source: Adapted from Boud and Malloy, 2013.

Conclusion

Figure 17.3 provides an overview of the many components of the complex feedback process outlined here. We as educators must gain a deeper understanding of feedback and the skills necessary to provide it in order to aid our students in developing a process that facilitates their becoming skilled, self-aware learners capable of lifelong learning.

References

Airasian, P.W. (1997) *Classroom Assessment*, 3rd edn, McGraw-Hill, New York.

Archer, J.C. (2010) State of the science in health professional education: Effective feedback. *Medical Education*, **44**, 101–108.

Ashford, S.J. (1986) Feedback-seeking in individual adaptation: A resources perspective. *Academy of Management Journal*, **29**, 465–487.

Balzer, W.K., Doherty, M.E., and O'Connor, R. (1989) Effects of cognitive feedback on performance. *Psychological Bulletin*, **106**, 410–433.

Bok, H.G., Teunissen, P.W., Spruijt. A., *et al.* (2013) Clarifying students' feedback-seeking behaviour in clinical clerkships. *Medical Education*, **47**, 282–291.

Boud, D., and Molloy, E. (2013) *Feedback in Higher and Professional Education: Understanding It and Doing It Well*, Routledge, New York.

Cantillon, P., and Sargeant, J. (2008) *Teaching Rounds: Giving Feedback in Clinical Settings*. British Medical Association, London.

Clynes, M.P., and Raftery, S.E.C. (2008) Feedback: An essential element of student learning in clinical practice. *Nurse Education in Practice*, **8**, 405–411.

Crommelinck, M., and Anseel. F. (2013) Understanding and encouraging feedback-seeking behaviour: A literature review. *Medical Education*, **47**, 232–241.

Davis, D.A., Mazmanian, P.E., Fordis, M., *et al.* (2006) Accuracy of physician self-assessment compared with observed measures of competence. *Journal of the American Medical Association*, **296**, 1094–1102.

Delva, D., Sargeant, J., Miller, S., *et al.* (2013) Encouraging residents to seek feedback. *Medical Teacher*, **35**, e1625–e1631.

Ende, J., Pomerantz, A., and Erickson, F. (1995) Preceptors' strategies for correcting residents in an ambulatory care medicine setting: A qualitative analysis. *Academic Medicine*, **70**, 224–229.

Eva, K.W., Armson, H., Holmboe, E., *et al.* (2012) Factors influencing responsiveness to feedback: On the interplay between fear, confidence, and reasoning processes. *Advances in Health Sciences Education: Theory and Practice*, **17**, 15–26.

Fernando, N., Cleland, J., McKenzie, H., and Cassar, K. (2008) Identifying the factors that determine feedback given to undergraduate medical students following formative mini-CEX assessments. *Medical Education*, **42**, 89–95.

Hattie, J., Biggs, J., and Purdie, N. (1996) Effects of learning skills interventions on student learning: A meta-analysis. *Review of Educational Research*, **66**, 99–136.

Hattie, J., and Timperley, H. (2007) The power of feedback. *Review of Educational Research*, **77**, 81–112.

Kluger, A.N., and DeNisi, A. (1996) The effects of feedback interventions on performance: A historical review, a meta-analysis, and a preliminary feedback intervention theory. *Psychological Bulletin*, **119**, 254–284.

Kluger, A.N., and DeNisi, A. (1998) *Feedback Interventions: Toward the Understanding of a Double-Edged Sword*, Cambridge University Press, Cambridge.

Kluger, A.N., and van Dijk, D. (2010) Feedback, the various tasks of the doctor, and the feedforward alternative. *Medical Education*, **44**, 1166–1174.

Laidlaw, T.S., Kaufman, D.M., MacLeod, H., *et al.* (2006) Relationship of resident characteristics, attitudes, prior training and clinical knowledge to communication skills performance. *Medical Education*, **40**, 18–25.

Locke, E.A., and Latham, G.P. (2002) Building a practically useful theory of goal setting and task motivation: A 35-year odyssey. *American Psychologist*, **57**, 705–717.

Murdoch-Eaton, D. (2012) Feedback: The complexity of self-perception and the transition from "transmit" to "received and understood." *Medical Education*, **46**, 538–540.

Murdoch-Eaton, D., and Sargeant, J. (2012) Maturational differences in undergraduate medical students' perceptions about feedback. *Medical Education*, **46**, 711–721.

Reddy, S.T., Zegarek, M.H., Fromme, H.B., *et al.* (2015) Barriers and facilitators to effective feedback: A qualitative analysis of data from multispecialty resident focus groups. *Journal of Graduate Medical Education*, **7**, 214–219.

Roscoe, R., and Chi, M. (2008) Tutor learning: The role of explaining and responding to questions. *Instructional Science*, **36**, 321–350.

Sargeant, J., Mann, K., Sinclair, D., *et al.* (2008) Understanding the influence of emotions and reflection upon multi-source feedback acceptance and use. *Advances in Health Sciences Education*, **13**, 275–288.

Schroth, M.L. (1992) The effects of delay of feedback on a delayed concept-formation transfer task. *Contemporary Educational Psychology*, **17**, 78–82.

Siqueira Drake, A.A., Hafen, M., Rush, B.R., and Reisbig, A.M. (2012) Predictors of anxiety and depression in veterinary medicine students: A four-year cohort examination. *Journal of Veterinary Medical Education*, **39**, 322–330.

Spickard, A., Gigante, J., Stein, G., and Denny, J.C. (2008) Automatic capture of student notes to augment mentor feedback and student performance on patient write-ups. *Journal of General Internal Medicine*, **23**, 979–984.

Stone, D., and Heen, S. (2014) *Thanks for the Feedback: The Science and Art of Receiving Feedback Well*. Viking Penguin, New York.

Thomas, J.D., and Arnold, R.M. (2011) Giving feedback. *Journal of Palliative Medicine*, **14**, 233–239.

van Dijk, D, and Kluger, A.N. (2004) Feedback sign effect on motivation: Is it moderated by regulatory focus? *Applied Psychology*, **53**, 113–135.

van Dijk, D, and Kluger, A.N. (2011) Task type as a moderator of positive/negative feedback effects on motivation and performance: A regulatory focus perspective. *Journal of Organizational Behavior*, **32**, 1084–1105.

Waitzkin, H. (1985) *Information Giving in Medical Care*, American Sociological Association, Washington, DC.

Watling, C., Driessen, E., van der Vleuten, C.P.M., *et al.* (2012) Understanding responses to feedback: The potential and limitations of regulatory focus theory. *Medical Education*, **46**, 593–603.

Wilkinson, S.S. (1981) The relationship of teacher praise and student achievement: A meta-analysis of selected research. *Dissertation Abstracts International*, **41**, 3998.

Winne, P., and Butler, D. (1994) Student cognition in learning from teaching, in *International Encyclopaedia of Education*, 2nd edn (eds P. Peterson, E. Baker, and B. McGaw), Pergamon, Oxford, pp. 5738–5745.

18

Academic Standards and Progression

Kristin P. Chaney, Kenita S. Rogers and Virginia Fajt

College of Veterinary Medicine & Biomedical Sciences, Texas A&M University, USA

 Box 18.1: Key messages

- Academic standards are often a collection of expectations that attempt to address the needs of accrediting bodies, stakeholders within the profession, and faculty curriculum committees.
- In the modern professional education setting, standards must address not only academic coursework requirements, but also competence in technical skills, nontechnical skills, and professional behaviors.
- Academic standards need to be consistent, fair, well communicated, and above legal reproach.

- Measures to identify at-risk students early in the program allow additional opportunities for intervention and remediation.
- The rigor and purpose of remediation procedures should be carefully developed both to ensure appropriate standards and to allow individual progression as standards are met.
- Academic standards are a pivotal benchmark for program quality, and each institution should carefully engage on a regular basis with faculty and administration regarding the development of best practices.

Introduction

Developing and adhering to academic standards for progression is a critical component of highly successful veterinary programs. Academic standards often represent a collection of expectations that attempt to address the needs of accrediting bodies, stakeholders within the profession, faculty, members of curriculum committees, and students. In the modern professional education setting, standards must address academic coursework requirements, as well as competence in technical skills, nontechnical skills, and professional behaviors.

Academic standards need to be consistent, fair, well communicated, and above legal reproach. In the veterinary profession, standards for progression are determined at the program level, and therefore often reflect institutions' individuality.

Defining Academic Standards and Progression

Since the establishment of the first veterinary college in Lyon, France in 1761, professional

---

Veterinary Medical Education: A Practical Guide, First Edition. Edited by Jennifer L. Hodgson and Jacquelyn M. Pelzer.
© 2017 John Wiley & Sons, Inc. Published 2017 by John Wiley & Sons, Inc.

veterinary medical education has continually evolved. There are several publications detailing the historical establishment of veterinary schools, evolution of curricula, and increasing diversity in student bodies (Smith, 2010, 2011a, b, 2013; Smith and Fenn, 2011; Fletcher, Hooper, and Schoenfeld-Tacher, 2015; Kochevar, 2015; Greenhill *et al.*, 2015). However, despite their importance to ensuring quality within the profession, academic standards are infrequently mentioned in the literature. Both human and veterinary medical education programs have a clear obligation to society to deliver competent healthcare professionals, and defining standards for academic progression is where most programs begin. All programs have at-risk students who are more likely than others to fail to graduate, either through dropout or dismissal. Their academic performance lies at the threshold or below the standards of acceptable competence as determined by relevant institutions (Winston, van der Vleuten, and Scherpbier, 2010). This subset of students remains the primary focus of discussion related to setting standards, assessing competence, and providing remediation opportunities.

In many allied health science fields, including medicine, pharmacy, and nursing, governing bodies play an integral role in the establishment of standards and guidelines to ensure the quality of individual graduates (Poirier, Kerr, and Phelps, 2013; Giddens, Keller, and Liesveld, 2015). The American Veterinary Medical Association Council on Education (AVMA-COE) holds veterinary programs to high standards for accreditation, requiring evidence that students are observed and assessed for attaining competence in nine specific areas. It recently updated the standards to require that processes be in place to remediate students who do not demonstrate competence in these prescribed areas. Regardless, the creation of academic standards for individual student progression is left to the independent discretion of veterinary education programs. With the wide variety of educational models, this customized independence allows each program to define its own academic standards for progression, recognizing that without sufficiently rigorous standards it would be possible to graduate students who were not uniformly qualified, and making a discussion of veterinary academic standards relevant and necessary.

Who Determines the Standards for Each Program?

In veterinary medical education, standards for academic progression are determined by a wide variety of stakeholders. Each veterinary college must uphold programmatic standards as established by the AVMA-COE to maintain accreditation. For example, programs are required to maintain specific passing rates for the national licensing examination (NAVLE), although direct individual student standards for progression are left to the discretion of each program. In allied health fields, governing bodies often presume a more intensive role in the academic progression of students. The current Accreditation Council for Pharmacy Education (ACPE) requires schools to provide individualized assistance to students with academic difficulty. As of 2016, this governance by the ACPE extends to include language for "identifying and intervening when students have academic difficulty" (Moser *et al.*, 2015). Many veterinary programs meet additional standards for accreditation defined at the university level by higher education commissions. Contributions to standards are also created by faculty, curriculum committees, administration, and legal counsel at each institution. To ensure that the integrity of the standards is maintained, faculty members must receive administrative support. Administrative personnel should understand the academic standards for their institution, be willing to adhere to those standards, and support faculty to ensure that standards are consistently applied and upheld. Without intentional demonstration of administrative support, faculty may find it difficult to maintain the standards for individual students (Poirier, Kerr, and Phelps, 2013). Upholding academic standards requires diligence and consistency across the entire educational program (Irby and Milam, 1989). In summary, academic standards need to be consistent, fair, well communicated, and above legal reproach.

What Areas Should Have Standards Assessed?

As a discipline, veterinary educators should consider the following areas on which to base standards for academic progression: foundation knowledge, technical skills, nontechnical skills (communication, leadership, and teamwork), professional behaviors (ethical/moral reasoning, personal decision-making), and clinical rotation assessments.

Foundation Knowledge

Foundation knowledge is the critical educational component that allows students to grow academically and clinically, and supports their ability to problem-solve and think critically. Important tactics for the promotion of student progression in this setting include employing instructional techniques that focus on the student-learner and assessment strategies that highlight critical thought and reasoning skills. Students' grade point average (GPA) is the most frequently used means of assessing their mastery of foundation knowledge and, as such, is commonly employed as an academic standard. An interesting study from Kansas State University explored grade inflation in veterinary medicine. It suggested that "a change in academic standards and student evaluation of teaching may have contributed to relaxed grading standards and technology in the classroom may have led to higher (earned) grades as a result of improved student learning" (Rush, Elmore, and Sanderson, 2009, p. 107). This concept is not unique to veterinary education and has been identified as a concern in other health professions (Shoemaker and DeVos, 1999; Speer, Solomon, and Fincher, 2000).

Technical Skills

Technical skills are an inherent component of veterinary competence, so many programs are engaging in skills assessments that can be considered an academic standard or barrier to progression. Numerous programs have employed directed examinations, including objective structured clinical examinations (OSCEs), as a required assessment for progression.

Nontechnical Skills

The NAVMEC report (NAVMEC Board of Directors, 2011) confirmed the importance of business acumen, leadership, multicultural awareness, and interpersonal skills to successful veterinary careers. Historically, nontechnical skills have been neglected in favor of instruction in foundation knowledge and technical skills, but many programs now recognize the need to intentionally instruct students in these skills and have them woven into veterinary curricula. Indeed, these skills must be repeatedly practiced throughout the program to ensure that students achieve confidence and understanding (Burns et al., 2006). Practicing nontechnical skills from the earliest point within a curriculum promotes stronger veterinary graduates, making it important to consider the relevance of such skills as an academic standard for progression.

Professional Behaviors

Some students admitted to professional programs are fully capable of negotiating the academic challenges associated with veterinary education, but may still struggle in the consistent demonstration of appropriate professional behaviors. Behaviors such as time management, suitable dress, personal hygiene, and moral/ethical reasoning may be innate characteristics of the ideal student, but for some these behaviors must be learned and practiced. This is also recognized in human medical education, and published work has shown an association between lack of professional behaviors in the educational program and disciplinary actions against physicians following graduation (Papadakis *et al.*, 2005). A study of human medical students demonstrated that those with difficulty on clerkships in the third and fourth years of the program often manifested problematic behaviors earlier in medical school, where remediation may have been successful at improving their professional behaviors (Papadakis, Loeser, and Healy, 2001). This remains an important consideration for veterinary education programs, since regardless of career choice, professional behaviors are central to success. There are many doctor of veterinary medicine (DVM) programs that combine professional behaviors with nontechnical skills as a measure of academic performance and progression for students on clinical rotations during their final years. However, these behaviors should be assessed from the earliest possible time point in the curriculum to encourage early remediation if necessary.

Clinical Rotation Assessments

There are many different models of education under the AVMA umbrella, all of which include clinical rotations in the final year(s) of the program. Assessment of performance on clinical rotations serves as an important academic standard for progression and graduation. Clinical rotations act as the final opportunity for students to apply their foundation and clinical knowledge in real-life situations. Students' performance on clinical rotations, termed "workplace-based assessments" in many programs, should include assessments of nontechnical skills including leadership and communication, as well as professional behaviors (Hecker, Norris, and Coe, 2012; Weijs, Coe, and Hecker, 2015).

Options for Assessing Academic Standards

Numerous assessment options are available, with no single method being appropriate or useful for all standards (Vandeweerd *et al.*, 2014),

although some are better suited to specific types of activities. Options for assessment include letter grading, pass/fail grading, OSCEs, Day One Competencies/skills lists, capstone experiences, barrier exams, proficiency scales/rubrics, professional behavior evaluations, and standardized examinations.

Letter and Pass/Fail Grading

Most letter grading schemes are based on a 10-point scale with designations of A through F. In some cases a plus/minus system is also used in an attempt to discriminate further between student performance levels. Of interest is a recent publication in the veterinary literature that describes various methods of reporting calculated grades, and questions whether grades truly represent what a student knows or can do (Royal and Guskey, 2015). This issue is pivotal to defining and maintaining academic standards, and demonstrates the challenges associated with making judgments regarding student progression. If a program utilizes individual course grades as an assessment for meeting standards, each program must identify the accumulated number of unsatisfactory grades, typically Ds or Fs, that triggers remediation or results in dismissal. In a recent survey of pharmacy schools with published guidelines for academic standards, a wide range of criteria for progression (or dismissal) were reported: "cumulative GPA or specific GPA post-probation or suspension; number of times on probation; certain number of F, D, or combination of F and D grades; failing a course more than once; failing two advanced pharmacy practice experiences; or exceeding the matriculation time limit" (Poirier, Kerr, and Phelps, 2013, p. 3).

Changing from letter to pass/fail (P/F) grading has been shown to increase medical students' wellbeing without having an impact on performance in licensing examinations (Bloodgood *et al.*, 2009; Reed *et al.*, 2011; Spring *et al.*, 2011). In dental education, research has shown no difference in the results of dental board examination pass rates when switching to P/F systems, and even demonstrated support for the use of such systems to increase self-regulated and lifelong learning. This study also suggested that specific (letter) grades are not important for maintaining standards (Leske and Ripa, 1985). White and Fantone (2010, p. 469) found that "Pass-fail grading can meet several important intended outcomes, including 'leveling the playing field' for incoming students with different academic backgrounds, reducing competition, fostering collaboration among class members, and more time for extracurricular interests and personal activities." In other reports, moving to P/F grading in medical education has not been beneficial (Gonnella, Erdmann, and Hojat, 2004) or has shown mixed results (McDuff *et al.*, 2014). An online discussion held among Association of American Veterinary Medical Colleges (AAVMC) associate deans related to schemes of P/F versus letter grading for clinical-year rotations revealed 17 out of 20 responding schools reporting letter grading, and 3 schools reporting use of a P/F or satisfactory/marginal/fail scheme.

Objective Structured Clinical Examinations

OSCEs and mini clinical examinations (mini-CEX) are used in professional programs in both North America and elsewhere. Many veterinary schools have adapted this type of structured clinical examination for use in both preclinical and clinical programs. The most valuable aspects of OSCEs and mini-CEX are the ability to standardize the assessment, provide students with a timed clinical experience, and incorporate additional nontechnical skills into the assessment. There is scientific support for both the validity and the reliability of OSCEs, and some programs include this type of examination as a barrier to progression. If OSCEs are introduced into a curriculum, additional components that must be incorporated to ensure academic progression include opportunities for student practice in preparation for examinations, and appropriate remediation measures for students who are unsuccessful. There is evidence in the medical literature to suggest that the most effective remediation measures include not

only review of the material (i.e., practice), but also self-reflection and self-assessment. When these measures are combined, students have demonstrated improved performance on subsequent clinical examinations (White, Ross, and Gruppen, 2009).

Day One Competencies/Skills Lists

Many veterinary education programs use Day One Competencies/skills lists as an academic standard for progression. Typically, these are lists of the technical skills and experiences that students are expected to encounter during the training program. Early in the DVM program, students receive a booklet or online resource for maintaining skills records. At Texas A&M University (TAMU), students must complete a rigorous number of skills during the three-year preclinical program. Performance of individual skills is validated by faculty and/or support staff through an e-mail database. This system requires a student to log in and select the skill(s) performed and the instructor(s) who guided the experience. An automatic e-mail is generated and sent to the instructor, requesting that the skill be either accepted or denied. These skills were previously used as a barrier to graduation, but completion of the skills list is now a requirement for entry into fourth-year clinical rotations. Moving this requirement was in concert with the introduction of a new system of scoring technical skills on clinical rotations in order to focus more intentionally on individual student competence in commonly performed procedures.

Proficiency Scales/Rubrics

While many programs use skills lists as a requirement for student progression, it is important to distinguish "exposure" to a clinical skill from "proficiency" in skill performance. To better ensure TAMU students' competence, clinical skills performed by all fourth-year students are individually assessed in real time using a proficiency scoring rubric (see Table 18.1). Each time a student performs one of the five required skills for each clinical rotation, a score

Table 18.1 Proficiency scoring rubric for clinical skills.

Much below minimum expectations	Below minimum expectations	Expected performance	Exceeds expectations	Excellent	Score
1	2	3	4	5	
Even with intense supervision, student is unable to successfully perform the procedure.	Requires supervision for success in performing the technical skill. Student is unable to perform independently.	Able to perform procedure without supervision, but requires additional experience to build confidence. May take more than one attempt, but student is successful.	Readily performs skill independently. Student needs no instruction or support. Typically achieves success on first attempt.	Complete mastery of skill. Student needs no additional training or experience to become competent or confident. Capable of performing and teaching the procedure.	

is assigned and feedback awarded. Students appreciate the immediate feedback from the score and tips on improving their technical performance. Faculty appreciate the more intentional mechanism for scoring students on routinely performed tasks. The proficiency scoring rubric is used as a barrier assessment, since students must score 3 out of 5 or better for each of five clinical skills per rotation. Students failing to meet this requirement undergo remediation with the individual clinical service to improve technical proficiency.

Capstone Experiences and Barrier Examinations

There are examples of programs in allied health fields that use individual courses as "capstone" experiences for progression. In nursing education, one study described a capstone experience where students were required to achieve a certain grade in a particular course to ensure academic progression. An association between grades in the capstone course and student retention in nursing education was demonstrated (Jeffreys, 2007). A few veterinary programs use capstone courses and barrier examinations as a student standard for progression. The development of entrustable professional activities (EPAs) is a concept originally introduced in 2005 and "can be defined

as a unit of professional practice that can be fully entrusted to a trainee, as soon as he or she has demonstrated the necessary competence to execute this activity unsupervised" (ten Cate *et al.*, 2015, p. 983). Successful execution of EPAs requires multiple competencies, including foundation knowledge, technical abilities, and professional skills. "To give a simple example: if an EPA is 'taking a history', clearly both medical knowledge and communication skill are competencies that, in an inseparable combination, must be present. Both should be assessed before a trainee is trusted to enact the EPA without supervision or confirmation of collected history information" (ten Cate et al., 2015, p. 985). While many allied health professions and some veterinary programs have fully defined EPAs for students to achieve as a benchmark or barrier for progression, in truth clinical rotations are a system of EPAs inherently nested within every veterinary educational program.

Professional Behaviors

Medical students' professional behaviors have been identified as a barrier to progression (Papadakis, Loeser, and Healy, 2001). A system of evaluation was described in this study whereby any student in the first two years of the program would receive a physicianship evaluation form if they received less than a satisfactory rating on any clerkship. These forms were submitted to the academic affairs dean, and if two or more forms were received for an individual student, the dean would include this information in the residency application for that student. In addition, "the student may be eligible for academic dismissal from school even if he or she has passing grades in all courses" (p. 1100). This research group identified that students who demonstrated poor professional behaviors, such as "unnecessary interruptions in class, inappropriate behaviors in small groups both with peers and faculty, unacceptable timing of requests for special needs for taking examinations" (p. 1101), were in need of remediation early in the program. A specific course was identified in the first years of the curriculum for which student evaluations were often linked to deficiencies in physicianship skills later in the program. Based on evaluations from this course, faculty began to recognize opportunities for students to receive early remediation for improving behaviors (Papadakis, Loeser, and Healy, 2001). In a follow-up study, these researchers further described increased risk of disciplinary action by medical boards for physicians demonstrating previously documented unprofessional behavior in medical school (Papadakis *et al.*, 2005). This lends support for the inclusion of nonprofessional behaviors as a barrier or standard for academic progression in veterinary education programs.

Standardized Examinations: Veterinary Educational Assessment, State Boards, and National Licensing Examination

A passing score on the NAVLE is a requirement to practice clinical medicine. According to the AVMA-COE (AVMA, 2016), 80% of students sitting for the NAVLE are expected to have a passing score by the time of graduation. Programs that fail to uphold this standard may be placed on limited accreditation, or terminal accreditation if pass rates are not improved and maintained, so there is a substantial incentive to maintain NAVLE pass rate

standards. In the veterinary literature several publications demonstrate the association of student variables and NAVLE pass rate, including Veterinary Educational Assessment (VEA) scores, undergraduate and veterinary school GPAs (Danielson *et al.*, 2011), Graduate Record Examination (GRE) scores, DVM class rank, and annual DVM GPAs (Roush *et al.*, 2014). The VEA is a 200-item, web-based examination used as a standardized assessment of basic science knowledge for students in veterinary school (NBVME, 2015). This examination is created by experts in specialty fields and administered by the National Board of Veterinary Medical Examiners (NBVME), which is also responsible for administration of the NAVLE. The VEA has been described as similar to the US Medical Licensing Exam (USMLE) Step 1 for medical students, since both examinations focus on foundation science subjects: anatomy, physiology, pharmacology, microbiology, and pathology. As the USMLE Step 1 examination has been proven to be a predictor of success in clinical clerkships and licensing exams, there is similar data to support use of the VEA for student success on the NAVLE (Danielson *et al.*, 2011).

How Are Academic Standards Used?

After development of a consistent set of academic standards that assess the student's abilities, they may be used in a variety of ways. Standards are developed with the primary focus of determining whether the student should progress through each step of the curriculum, but in reality they are also employed to evaluate the strength of a program, by both accrediting bodies and other stakeholders. Standards are the academic institution's obligation to society, ensuring the quality of graduates at least to the level of Day One competence. They also represent an obligation to the student, ensuring that they will have the opportunity to be successful.

The relative success with which a student masters academic standards is also frequently used in a variety of high-stakes decisions, including competitive scholarships and postgraduation education programs such as internships, residencies, and graduate degrees. With recognition that graduation with a DVM or equivalent degree is the ultimate goal, many training programs are also using academic standards to guide students in prioritizing their extracurricular activities. For example, some programs have a minimum overall GPA that students must attain to become elected class officers, corporate representatives, or eligible for certain extracurricular activities.

Informing Students about Academic Standards

For standards to be useful and fair, they must be communicated in a clear, unambiguous manner. Anyone who has been responsible for developing and implementing standards will appreciate how difficult this can be. In truth, standards change over time as new circumstances arise and as they are reviewed and updated by faculty, administration, and legal counsel.

In most programs, a student handbook has been developed to share important information with students and faculty regarding expectations, including academic standards. This information is often shared in print and/or with a web-site link. An early part of the curriculum is typically dedicated to discussing this information with students so that expectations are deliberately communicated for understanding. Changes in academic standards are typically published on a yearly basis. The process for changing standards varies, but often involves faculty and administrative input, as well as the advice of legal counsel. It is important that each change, as well the entire document on a periodic basis, be reviewed by legal counsel so that any consequences of an inability to meet standards will withstand challenge. It is extremely important that published standards be consistently applied and deemed to be fair and necessary for a professional student.

Consequences of Failing to Meet Standards

The most obvious consequence of failure to meet standards is that the student is not allowed to progress through the curriculum. In most circumstances, particularly when the failure to meet standards is academic or related to technical and nontechnical skills, students are allowed an opportunity to remediate the deficiency. How this is accomplished is dependent on the timing of the course, type of remediation required, extenuating circumstances associated with failure, previous failures, available resources, and whether the reason for failure is correctable. Appropriate remediation can require substantial resources, specifically faculty time and support materials. From the student's standpoint, the issues will include time required for remediation, impact on timely progression through the program, financial implications, and resulting personal/emotional difficulties. Mental health issues and learning disabilities may play a role in placing students at risk, and must be effectively addressed for the long-term success of remediation efforts.

Remediation of a didactic course may occur during the summer between academic years or with the next matriculating class. If difficulties are identified early, appropriate support measures such as tutoring or counseling are indicated. Clinical rotation remediation can often be accomplished in a timely manner, since most rotations are repeated throughout the year. If only clinical skills require remediation, the program may utilize OSCEs or other similar means to demonstrate competence.

Effective remediation of professional attributes can be even more complex, as this may involve addressing issues as disparate as poor personal choices or academic dishonesty or illegal activities. The failure to demonstrate appropriate professional behaviors may be unrelated to academic standards, so the process for addressing professionalism may be quite different and include Honor Code Council hearings or even immediate dismissal. Probation requirements may also be different depending on whether the issues are academic or professional. Finally, if the program has policies allowing appeal for readmission after academic dismissal, the student may be required to remediate each area that is viewed as a weakness in order to optimize their chances for ultimate success.

Thoughts on Remediation

The most important role for examinations that determine progress is to ensure that students proceed to the next level only after achieving the intended learning outcomes of the current level. Educators have a duty to help students understand their strengths and weaknesses and to guide improvement (Hays, 2012), so having a clear understanding of the goals of remediation is critical.

Programs deciding to take a proactive approach to helping students develop the necessary skills to prevent academic difficulties should be prepared for a range of potential issues. Problems can be related to testing (test taking, test anxiety), materials (time management, organization/integrating information, formulating learning issues, tutoring requirements, course remediation), noncognitive areas (anxiety, stress, lack of concentration or motivation), cognitive issues (critical thinking, problem-solving, reading comprehension), and/or disabilities (screening, accommodations; Paul *et al.*, 2009). Effective remediation policies should include early detection of problems in academic performance, strategies to help students develop better approaches for academic success, and facilitation of self-directed learning (Maize *et al.*, 2010). Remediation approaches can include exam remediation, course repetition, individualized remediation plans, summer restudy programs, reduced course-load programs, competency lists, and clinical practice remediation.

It should also be recognized that most learners have more than one deficit, and that deficits may vary by academic level of the learner, with

medical knowledge, clinical reasoning, and professionalism being most common (Guerrasio *et al.*, 2014). In one study, remediation of clinical reasoning and communication deficits took the most faculty time, but increased faculty time significantly reduced the odds of a negative student outcome. Learners who struggled with mental wellbeing required significantly more faculty time than other learners, as these issues often slowed the pace at which they could acquire new information because of a more limited ability to remain on task while studying and learning.

Failing an early examination two weeks into medical school was strongly predictive of later student difficulty (Winston, van der Vleuten, and Scherpbier, 2014). These authors found that an examination in the first two weeks of medical school was an early predictor for the target population of students likely to struggle, confirming the notion that close similarity between the predictor task and target task provides sufficient accuracy for targeted early interventions. Further, in the prevention of failure, as with remediation, the type and details of intervention are likely to matter. Importantly, it is essential that systemic issues, such as workload and curricular flexibility, are addressed if there is to be maximal support of increasingly diverse student populations. Under the usual system of remediation (assessment-focused revision program and then reassessment), the majority of poorly performing students fail to improve in clinical assessments. In other words, the poorly performing subgroup achieves only short-term success with traditional remediation and retest models, and, critically, shows an absence of longitudinal improvement. Therefore, following poor performance, remediation should be embedded in the subsequent program (Pell *et al.*, 2012).

Most remediation interventions in medical education focus on improving performance to the standard required to pass resit or retake, rather than to support the development of effective lifelong learning skills (Cleland *et al.*, 2013). Generally, interventions represent "more of the same," such as additional or intensive knowledge or skills teaching. The likely critical factor in short-term improved performance is individual analysis of performance and feedback. Early remediation interventions have the potential to stop the cycle of underperformance that is characteristic of many struggling students. Typically, these students have low self-efficacy beliefs and negative feelings about learning that directly influence their motivation to persist with difficult learning tasks. They need to experience success as soon as they are identified as having difficulties so that they can feel a sense of control over their learning and performance. Intervention may require a substantial time commitment from faculty, including multiple meetings, a flexible curriculum that allows a decelerated track to at-risk students, experienced and mindful faculty facilitators, emotionally supportive relationships, sufficient academic rigor, and timely, constructive feedback in order for students to develop and apply their skills over time (Cleland *et al.*, 2013).

A Few Best Practices for Maintaining Academic Standards

- Students should be well informed about their deficiencies. At TAMU, Progress Committee meetings are held twice per semester in addition to individual meetings with students by instructors, assigned mentors, and members of the academic dean's office. Counseling appointments are available with an onsite counselor as well as on campus. Letters detailing deficiencies are shared with students as well as placed in their academic file.
- There should be easy access to student handbooks that are updated on a regular (yearly) basis, with input from students, faculty, administration, and legal counsel. The academic dean's office should keep good records of issues that arise throughout the year that are not expressly addressed in the handbook,

so that language can be developed to "close loopholes" in the future.
- The faculty should be engaged in continual reassessment of the curriculum and standard-setting to ensure that educational objectives are being met. TAMU faculty meet for a yearly curriculum retreat to discuss important academic issues that affect the program.
- Remediation procedures and content should be faculty driven but administratively supported.
- One aspect of maintaining standards is to afford the student an opportunity to appeal a grade that they feel was assigned unfairly. The process is typically managed administratively, with the protocol for overturning a grade being a determination that the grade was assigned in a capricious or discriminatory manner. For traditional didactic classes, the accrued evidence may be different than in clinical rotations, where the grading is often more subjective. Using scoring rubrics and careful event documentation can help to provide support for a low score. The process usually has two or three levels of appeal, which may include the faculty member, department head, associate dean, and dean or college committee.
- Readmission appeals are utilized after a student has been dismissed from the program, typically for academic reasons. In this case, the appropriate faculty committee hears evidence and decides whether the student should be readmitted to the training program, and, if so, where and under what conditions.
- Students can have a role in the development and dissemination of information regarding standards. At TAMU, students are voting members of the Curriculum Committee and comprise the membership of the Honor Code Council.
- Ideally, individuals with a substantive role in disciplinary action or the appeal process should be separate from student engagement activities such as active mentor groups, in order to avoid the appearance of bias or a conflict of interest.

References

AVMA (2016) Accreditation Policies and Procedures of the AVMA Council on Education (COE). *American Veterinary Medical Association*. https://www.avma.org/ProfessionalDevelopment/Education/Accreditation/Colleges/Pages/coe-pp-requirements-of-accredited-college.aspx (accessed Jan 25, 2017).

Bloodgood, R.A., Short, J.G., Jackson, J.M., and Martindale, J.R. (2009) A change to pass/fail grading in the first two years at one medical school results in improved psychological well-being. *Academic Medicine*, **84** (**5**), 655–682.

Burns, G.A., Ruby, K.L., Debowes, R.M., et al. (2006) Teaching non-technical (professional) competence in a veterinary school curriculum. *Journal of Veterinary Medical Education*, **33** (**2**), 301–308.

Cleland, J., Leggett, H., Sandars, J., et al. (2013) The remediation challenge: Theoretical and methodological insights from a systematic review. *Medical Education*, **47**, 242–251.

Danielson, J.A., Wu, T.F., Molgaard L.K., and Preast, V.A. (2011) Relationships among common measures of student performance and scores on the North American Veterinary Licensing Examination. *Journal of the Veterinary Medical Association*, **238** (**4**), 454–461.

Fletcher, O.J., Hooper, B.E., and Schoenfeld-Tacher, R. (2015) Instruction and curriculum in veterinary medical education: A 50-year perspective. *Journal of Veterinary Medical Education*, **42** (**5**), 489–500.

Giddens, J., Keller, T., and Liesveld, J. (2015) Answering the call for a Bachelors-prepared nursing workforce: An innovative model for academic progression. *Journal of Professional Nursing*, **31** (**6**), 445–451.

Gonnella, J.S., Erdmann, J.B., and Hojat, M. (2004) An empirical study of the predictive validity of number grades in medical school using 3 decades of longitudinal data: Implications for a grading system. *Medical Education*, **38**, 425–434.

Greenhill, L., Elmore, R., Stewart, S., et al. (2015) Fifty years in the life of veterinary students. *Journal of Veterinary Medical Education*, **42** (**5**), 480–488.

Guerrasio, J., Garrity, M.J., and Aagaard E.M. (2014) Learner deficits and academic outcomes of medical students, residents, fellows, and attending physicians referred to a remediation program, 2006–2012. *Academic Medicine*, **89** (**2**), 352–358.

Hays, R.B. (2012) Remediation and re-assessment in undergraduate medical school examinations. *Medical Teacher*, **34**, 91–92.

Hecker, K.G., Norris, J., and Coe, J.B. (2012) Workplace-based assessment in a primary-care setting. *Journal of Veterinary Medical Education*, **39** (**3**), 229–240.

Irby, D.M., and Milam, J.D. (1989) The legal context for evaluating and dismissing medical students and residents. *Academic Medicine*, **64**, 639–643.

Jeffreys, M.R. (2007) Tracking students through program entry, profession, graduation, and licensure: Assessing undergraduate nursing student retention and success. *Nurse Education Today*, **27**, 406–419.

Kochevar, D.T. (2015) Fifty years of evolving partnerships in veterinary medical education. *Journal of Veterinary Medical Education*, **42** (**5**), 403–413.

Leske, G.S., and Ripa, L. (1985) Comparison of dental students' academic performance using honors/pass/fail and letter grades. *Journal of Dental Education*, **49** (**3**), 176–178.

Maize, D.F., Fuller, S.H., Hritcko, P.M., et al. (2010) A review of remediation programs in pharmacy and other health professions. *American Journal of Pharmaceutical Education*, **74** (**2**), 25.

McDuff, S.G.R., McDuff, D., Farace, J.A., et al. (2014) Evaluating a grading change at UCSD school of medicine: Pass/fail grading is associated with decreased performance on preclinical exams but unchanged performance on USMLE step 1 scores. *BMC Medical Education*, **14** (**127**), 1–9.

Moser, L., Berlie, H., Salinitri, F., et al. (2015) Enhancing academic success by creating a community of learners. *American Journal of Pharmaceutical Education*, **79** (**5**), 70.

NAVMEC Board of Directors (2011) The North American Veterinary Medical Education Consortium (NAVMEC) looks to veterinary education for the future: Roadmap for veterinary medical education in the 21st century: Responsive, collaborative, flexible. *Journal of Veterinary Medical Education*, **38** (**4**), 320–327.

NBVME (2015) Veterinary Educational Assessment. *National Board Report*, November, 4. https://www.nbvme.org/image/cache/NBVME_November_2015_National_Board_Report.pdf (accessed November 10, 2016).

Papadakis, M.A., Loeser, H., and Healy, K. (2001) Early detection and evaluation of professionalism deficiencies in medical students: One school's approach. *Academic Medicine*, **76** (**11**), 1100–1106.

Papadakis, M.A., Teherani, A., Banach, M.A., et al. (2005) Disciplinary action by medical boards and prior behavior in medical school. *New England Journal of Medicine*, **353**, 2673–2682.

Paul, G., Hinman, G., Dottl, S., and Passon, J. (2009) Academic development: A survey of academic difficulties experienced by medical students and support services provided. *Teaching and Learning in Medicine*, **21** (**3**), 254–260.

Pell, G., Fuller, R., Homer, M., and Roberts, T. (2012) Is short-term remediation after OSCE failure sustained? A retrospective analysis of the longitudinal attainment of underperforming student in OSCE assessments. *Medical Teacher*, **34**, 146–150.

Poirier, T.I., Kerr, T.M., and Phelps, S.J. (2013) Academic progression and retention policies of colleges and schools of pharmacy. *American Journal of Pharmaceutical Education*, **77** (**2**), 25.

Reed, D.A., Shanafelt, T.D., Satele, D.W., et al. (2011) Relationship of pass/fail grading and curriculum structure with well-being among preclinical medical students: A multi-institutional study. *Academic Medicine*, **86** (**11**), 1367–1373.

Roush, J.K., Rush, B.R., White, B.J., and Wilkerson, M.J. (2014) Correlation of pre-veterinary admissions criteria, intra-professional curriculum measures, AVMA-COE professional competency scores, and the NAVLE. *Journal of Veterinary Medical Education*, **41** (**1**), 19–26.

Royal, K.D., and Guskey, T.R. (2015) Does mathematical precision ensure valid grades? What every veterinary medical educator should know. *Journal of Veterinary Medical Education*, **42** (**3**), 242–244.

Rush, B.R., Elmore, R.G., and Sanderson, M.W. (2009) Grade inflation at a North American college of veterinary medicine: 1985–2006. *Journal of Veterinary Medical Education*, **36** (**1**), 107–113.

Shoemaker, J.K., and DeVos, M. (1999) Are we a gift shop? A perspective on grade inflation. *Journal of Nursing Education*, **38** (**9**), 394–398.

Smith, D.F. (2010) 150th anniversary of veterinary education and the veterinary profession in North America. *Journal of Veterinary Medical Education*, **37** (**4**), 317–327.

Smith, D.F. (2011a) 150th anniversary of veterinary education and the veterinary profession in North America: Part 2, 1940–1970. *Journal of Veterinary Medical Education*, **38** (**1**), 84–99.

Smith, D.F. (2011b) 150th anniversary of veterinary education and the veterinary profession in North America: Part 3, 1970–2000. *Journal of Veterinary Medical Education*, **38** (**3**), 211–227.

Smith, D.F. (2013) Lessons of history in veterinary medicine. *Journal of Veterinary Medical Education*, **40** (**1**), 2–11.

Smith, D.F., and Fenn, M.S. (2011) 150th anniversary of veterinary education and the veterinary profession in North America: Part 4, US veterinary colleges in 2011 and the distribution of their graduates. *Journal of Veterinary Medical Education*, **38** (**4**), 338–348.

Speer, A.J., Solomon, D.J., and Fincher, R.M.E. (2000) Grade inflation in internal medicine clerkships: Results of a national survey.

Teaching and Learning in Medicine, **12** (3), 112–116.

Spring, L., Robillard, D., Gehlbach, L., and Simas, T.A. (2011) Impact of pass/fail grading on medical students' well-being and academic outcomes. *Medical Education*, **45**, 867–877.

ten Cate, O., Chen, H.C., Hoff, R.G., et al. (2015) Curriculum development for the workplace using Entrustable Professional Activities (EPAs): AMEE guide no. 99. *Medical Teacher*, **37**, 983–1002.

Vandeweerd, J.M., Cambier, C., Desbrosse, F., et al. (2014) Competency frameworks: Which format for which target? *Journal of Veterinary Medical Education*, **41** (1), 27–36.

Weijs, C.A., Coe, J.B., and Hecker, K.G. (2015) Final-year students' and clinical instructors' experience of workplace-based assessments used in a small-animal primary-veterinary-care clinical rotation. *Journal of Veterinary Medical Education*, **42** (4), 382–392.

White, C.B., and Fantone, J.C. (2010) Pass-fail grading: Laying the foundation for self-regulated learning. *Advances in Health Sciences Education*, **14**, 469–477.

White, C.B., Ross, P.T., and Gruppen, L.D. (2009) Remediating students' failed OSCE performances at one school: The effects of self-assessment, reflection, and feedback. *Academic Medicine*, **84** (5), 651–654.

Winston, K., van der Vleuten, C.P.M., and Scherpbier, A.J.J.A. (2010) At-risk medical students: Implications of students' voice for the theory and practice of remediation. *Medical Education*, **44**, 1038–1047.

Winston, K., van der Vleuten, C.P.M., and Scherpbier, A.J.J.A. (2014) Prediction and prevention of failure: An early intervention to assist at-risk medical students. *Medical Teacher*, **36**, 25–31.

Part V

Assessing the Program

19

Assessing Teaching Effectiveness

Susan M. Rhind and Catriona E. Bell

Royal (Dick) School of Veterinary Studies, University of Edinburgh, UK

Box 19.1: Key messages

- Decide on the purpose of the evaluation before planning which data or evidence to collect.
- A portfolio approach incorporating multiple sources of data should be used to develop an optimum method to assess teaching effectiveness.
- Student evaluations of teaching effectiveness are an important element of the assessment and should ideally have psychometrician input into their design.

- Peer or other faculty observation should also always form part of the evaluation, supported by appropriate training and mentorship.
- Assessments of outcomes can be difficult to relate directly to individuals, but can be incorporated if practical and possible.
- Teaching scholarship can contribute to an overall portfolio of evidence, but does not necessarily directly relate to teaching effectiveness.

The accuracy of faculty evaluation decisions hinges on the integrity of the process and the reliability and validity of the evidence that is collected. (Berk, 2005)

Defining Teaching Effectiveness

Teaching effectiveness is a term that abounds in the literature, yet it is remarkably difficult to find a concise definition of it. Many articles launch into descriptions of the pros and cons of different strategies to measure teaching effectiveness, yet fail to define the construct that is being measured. The *Oxford English Dictionary* definition of effectiveness is "The degree to which something is successful in producing a desired result"; the question in the context of teaching is: what is the "desired result"?

For the purposes of this chapter, we define teaching effectiveness in veterinary education as "teaching that succeeds in enhancing student learning."

Furthermore, we restrict this definition to that of the *individual teacher*, rather than assessment at overall course or curriculum level, by which point it becomes very difficult to disentangle the myriad of factors that contribute to overall achievement and the student experience. Such curriculum-level assessment of overall teaching effectiveness would tend to be covered in the context of overall outcomes

Veterinary Medical Education: A Practical Guide, First Edition. Edited by Jennifer L. Hodgson and Jacquelyn M. Pelzer.
© 2017 John Wiley & Sons, Inc. Published 2017 by John Wiley & Sons, Inc.

assessment, for instance for the purposes of accreditation.

The terms "assessment" and "evaluation" of teaching effectiveness are often used interchangeably. In the context of students, Cook (2010) proposes the distinction that assessment focuses on the learner, whereas evaluation focuses on programs. Although not directly parallel, for the purposes of this chapter we adopt the term assessment as it applies to specific methods to gather data about the teaching, whereas evaluation is the more global process whereby this assessment information is used to make an overall judgment.

Why Assess Teaching Effectiveness?

As with student assessment, assessing teaching effectiveness at the individual level can be considered as either formative or summative (Brown and Ward-Griffin, 1994; Berk, 2013). Formative assessment contributes to the ongoing improvement and development of an individual's teaching over time. Summative assessment may be for the purposes of annual review, or may be used to inform promotion and tenure decisions (Berk, 2013). In addition to this "teacher-centered" rationale, a robust system of assessment of teaching effectiveness is a prerequisite to ongoing institutional enhancement of student learning and the student experience.

What to Assess?

Ramsden (2003) describes six principles of "effective teaching" in higher education. In Figure 19.1 we align these to the three stages of "preactive," "interactive," and "postactive" described by O'Neill (1988), who, through a systematic review process, identified a "top 20" of factors influencing teaching effectiveness that could be grouped into one of the three categories. O'Neill reviews the evidence for various factors falling into each of his three categories, with examples such as the following:

- *Preactive stage*: planning, preparation, and clear learning objectives.

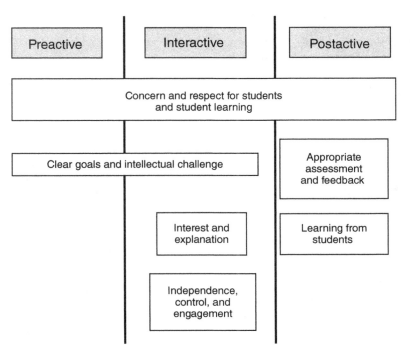

Figure 19.1 Principles of effective teaching mapped to O'Neill's three categories. Source: Based on O'Neill, 1988.

- *Interactive stage*: teacher enthusiasm and creation of a supportive learning environment, management of classroom dynamics.
- *Postactive stage*: feedback to students. In addition, although not included in O'Neill's review, we would also include reflection on feedback *from* students, which in turn can inform the preactive and interactive stages in the future.

An additional framework specific to the context of clinical teaching is that used in the Stanford Faculty Development Program (SFDP; Litzelman *et al*., 1998, 1999). The SFDP "has sought to study and define the components of effective clinical teaching" (Litzelman *et al*., 1998, p. 688) and has been widely used, validated, and accepted within healthcare professions education. The framework is based around seven categories relating to observable teaching behaviors, and these can be used to help define clear objectives for an evaluation of teaching effectiveness within an individual school. Each of these elements also maps to the model illustrated in Figure 19.1. The seven categories are:

- Establishing a positive learning climate (interactive).
- Control of the teaching session (interactive).
- Communicating goals (preactive and interactive).
- Promoting understanding and retention (interactive and postactive).
- Evaluation of learner's achievement of desired goals (postactive).
- Providing feedback to learners (interactive and postactive).
- Promoting self-directed learning (preactive, interactive, and postactive).

All three models discussed emphasize that the effective teacher is much more than an individual who can "perform" well in the classroom or other teaching setting. Hence, any process to assess teaching effectiveness should aim to capture evidence mapped to each of these broad domains in order to gain a holistic overview of teaching effectiveness.

How to Assess Teaching Effectiveness

As with all forms of assessment, it is important to use reliable, valid, and feasible methods (Snell *et al*., 2000). This becomes even more important where the assessment contributes to career decisions for faculty (Beckman *et al*., 2004; Berk, 2013). A poor assessment tool will at best lead to unhelpful, and at worst inaccurate, results. Berk (2013, p. 19) comments that most home-grown rating scales for assessing teaching effectiveness in higher education "do not meet even the most basic criteria for psychometric quality required by professional and legal standards… the serious concern is that decisions about the careers of faculty are being made with these instruments."

Similarly, if we adopt general principles of outcomes-based education and assessment, the purpose of the teaching effectiveness assessment exercise or the decision that will result from it should be defined from the outset, and should then inform the types of evidence that are gathered rather than this working in the opposite direction, as shown in Figure 19.2.

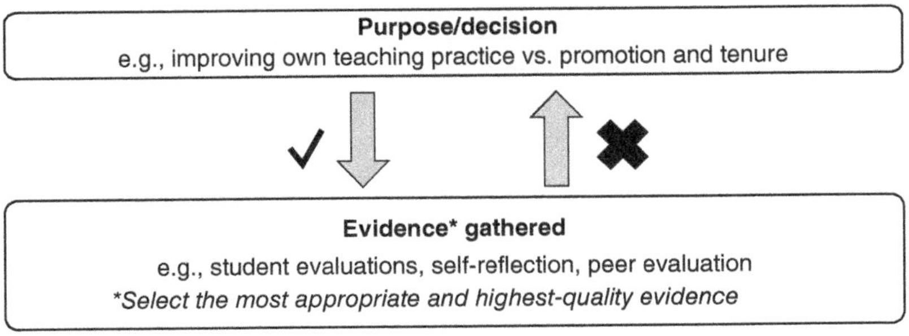

Figure 19.2 Recommended direction of planning a teaching effectiveness assessment exercise using "outcomes-based" principles.

Purpose/decision
e.g., improving own teaching practice vs. promotion and tenure

Evidence* gathered
e.g., student evaluations, self-reflection, peer evaluation
*Select the most appropriate and highest-quality evidence

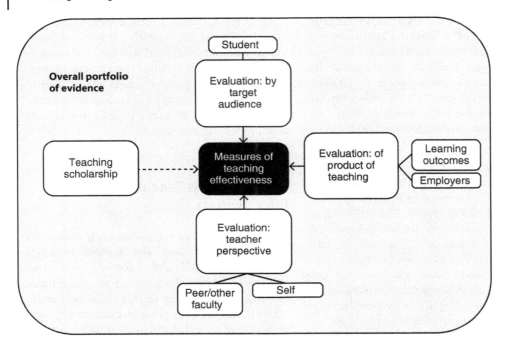

Figure 19.3 The categories of evidence that may be gathered to contribute to an overall portfolio of evidence. Solid lines represent measures that can directly relate to teaching effectiveness, a dotted line indicates no proven direct relationship.

Who Does the Evaluation?

Up to 15 potential sources of evidence relating to teaching effectiveness have been described (Berk, 2005, 2013). These can essentially be grouped into three categories, as illustrated in Figure 19.3:

- Evaluation by the target audience, i.e., the students (or residents).
- Evaluation from the teacher perspective, e.g., self-evaluation, evaluation by peers or other colleagues.
- Evaluation of the product of the teaching, e.g., evaluation of students' abilities at certain stages of the curriculum by faculty, evaluation of graduates by employers.

It is recommended that multiple sources of evidence, and a minimum of three (Berk, 2013), are used to inform a comprehensive evaluation, with information being triangulated

from multiple summative and formative sources (Brown and Ward-Griffin, 1994; Blackmore, 2005; Siddiqui, Jones-Dwyer, and Carr, 2007; Berk, 2013), and that principles of 360° multi-source feedback (in which feedback is elicited from a variety of perspectives) be adopted (Boerboom *et al.*, 2011b; Berk, 2013). The model illustrated in Figure 19.3 provides a global overview of the broad categories of evidence from four different domains; ideally, an overall teaching portfolio would address items from each of the four domains.

These domains can be considered in the context of the well-known model for evaluating educational outcomes by Kirkpatrick (1994). This model has been adapted for use by researchers conducting systematic reviews in order to classify various levels of evidence. We present a simple version of the model in Table 19.1 adapted to the context of assessing teaching effectiveness.

Table 19.1 An adaptation of Kirkpatrick's hierarchy to the context of assessing teaching effectiveness.

	Description	Examples
Level 1	Reaction	Student evaluations of teaching effectiveness, e.g., surveys. Peer evaluation
Level 2	Learning	Learning outcome measures, e.g., summative assessments, North American Veterinary Licensing Examination (NAVLE)
Level 3	Behavior	Transfer of learning to workplace, e.g., employer evaluation
Level 4	Results/impact	Impact on society (e.g., clients) and the profession

Source: Based on Kirkpatrick, 1994.

As noted by Steinert *et al.* (2006), the usefulness of this model is to consider it not necessarily as a hierarchy, but to look for different kinds of evidence that provide a more comprehensive overview of the area in question. Similarly, Yardley and Dornan (2012, p. 105) emphasize that "the purpose to which evidence is put influences its trustworthiness and the best way of synthesising it" – although their context is the appraisal of interventions in medical education, the conclusions are equally appropriate for our consideration of evidence as it relates to teaching effectiveness.

When considering measures of teaching effectiveness, in moving from Level 1 to Level 4 in Table 19.1, the less objective the measures tend to become, then the less definitive one can be that any observed change (for example in behavior) can be clearly linked to one factor, which, for the purposes of this chapter, is the teacher.

Evaluation: Target Audience Perspective

Student Evaluations of Teaching Effectiveness

Student evaluations of teaching effectiveness (SETE) are the most obvious source of data to inform an assessment of teaching effectiveness. Despite receiving a "mixed press" in the literature, they are undoubtedly a cornerstone of the evaluation armory (Surgenor, 2011) and are the first item that should be addressed in any assessment of teaching effectiveness.

The major argument against putting too much weight on SETE relates to the potential for them to be viewed as a "popularity or personality contest," which may have no direct link to student achievement. Various studies have demonstrated the potential impact of factors such as providing chocolate to students before filling in evaluations or faculty personality (Felton, Mitchell, and Stinson, 2004; Youmans and Jee, 2007; Surgenor, 2011), as well as links with examination satisfaction, difficulty, and results (Schiekirka and Raupach, 2015). Many publications emphasize that SETE should not be used as the sole measure for the evaluation. For instance, Sproule (2002, p. 287) notes that "the exclusive use of the student evaluation of teaching data in the determination of instructor performance is tantamount to the promotion and practice of pseudoscience."

Despite these reservations, there is no doubt that SETE are an essential component of any evaluation of teaching effectiveness (Berk, 2005; Marsh, 2007; Surgenor, 2011). Berk (2005, p. 50) comments: "Student ratings are a necessary source of evidence of teaching effectiveness for both formative and summative decisions, but not a sufficient source for the latter. Considering all of the polemics over its value, it is still an essential component of any faculty evaluation system."

Berk (2013) emphasizes the fact that many "home-grown" rating scales are flawed and lack both reliability and validity. In a review of the situation relating to these rating scales, he describes the situation as "ugly," and recommends psychometrician input into both the design and the analysis of the data generated by these evaluations. In reality, for many veterinary schools this may provide a challenge due to size and resources, but nevertheless as a minimum faculty must be aware of the limitations of in-house evaluations that have had no such

Table 19.2 Checklist for student evaluations.

Suggested criteria	Y/N
If items are developed in house, have they been reviewed by a psychometrician?	
If "no" to above, have you considered using validated items from other surveys?	
Are the evaluations released/administered at the same time in the course (e.g., relative to assessments)?	
Are identical instructions given to students for each evaluation?	
Are students given the same (short) window to complete the evaluations?	
Have faculty had input into these decisions?	
Is it possible to have one administrator coordinating the whole process for consistency?	

Source: Adapted from Berk, 2013.

input from relevant experts. A checklist for SETE is presented in Table 19.2.

An additional important point relates to response rates to the evaluations, which it is recommended should be at least 60% (Richardson, 2005). This point should be facilitated by robust and consistent administrative support, as detailed in Table 19.2.

The Place for SETE

What is clear is that while the use of SETE as the *exclusive* measure of assessment of teaching effectiveness is not advisable, it would be a rare institution indeed that did not have a robust system of student evaluations forming a significant component of overall quality assurance processes. Indeed, accreditation and overall quality assurance mechanisms would be impossible without a significant component of student evaluation being built in. A linked point relates to what happens to the data once gathered. It has been shown, for example, that student evaluations in combination with individual consultations with faculty members are more powerful in terms of changing teaching behaviors than faculty merely receiving student evaluations alone (Wilkerson and Irby, 1998).

In addition to standard post-course surveys as a method for SETE, face-to-face student meetings and focus groups can also be valuable in gathering more qualitative data to explore themes that may emerge from survey data analysis.

Teaching Awards

It is generally considered that teaching awards provide relatively low-level evidence of effective teaching (Berk, 2005), and can be seen as a popularity contest rather than recognition of effective teaching *per se*. A review by Huggett *et al.* (2012) encompassing not only health professions education, but also professional and higher education, concluded that limited evidence exists on the design and utility of teaching awards. The review also highlighted potential negative (e.g., reactions from peers) as well as positive (e.g., personal satisfaction and prestige) consequences for recipients. The consequences are very dependent on institutional culture, and while it would be inappropriate to weight it too heavily, this type of evidence can certainly be built into an overall portfolio of evidence and, if supported by other evidence, can be an indicator of committed and excellent teaching.

Evaluation: Teacher Perspective

Peer Evaluation Methods

Peer evaluation can be used to assess and improve teaching, and has been incorporated into faculty development programs since the 1980s (Irby, 1983). The literature shows that a number of related terms exist, including peer observation of teaching, peer review of teaching, reflective partnerships, and peer coaching for teaching improvement. All of these describe activities in which colleagues evaluate and give feedback on areas for improvement and identification of the existing strengths of another individual's teaching based on their observations and judgments, usually in a reciprocal fashion. However, within these models there can be considerable variation in terms of the status, background, and number of observers and what it is that they observe or judge. For example, some models involve one or more observers at a time, from a range of potential backgrounds, such as department colleague, subject expert, or educationalist (Siddiqui, Jones-Dwyer, and Carr, 2007), undertaking a range of activities that may include reviewing course documentation and materials, direct or video-based observation of teaching in the classroom or clinic, and peer discussion and reflection on sources of evidence such as student evaluations or video recordings of teaching sessions (Irby, 1983; Brown and Ward-Griffin, 1994; Wilkerson and Irby, 1998; Yon, Burnap, and Kohut, 2002; Siddiqui, Jones-Dwyer, and Carr, 2007; Boerboom *et al.*, 2011b; Ruesseler *et al.*, 2014).

Utility of Peer Evaluation Methods

The appropriateness of adopting peer evaluation methods to augment student evaluations and other measures of teaching effectiveness has been controversial at times, but can be argued by the fact that colleagues are better placed than students to comment on the curriculum content, instructional methods, and appropriateness of standards for excellence in that subject (Irby, 1983; Brown and Ward-Griffin, 1994). The utility of peer evaluation for summative and formative decisions has been debated, although a review of nursing literature strongly advocated that peer evaluation should be used only for formative purposes (Brown and Ward-Griffin, 1994). The overall consensus in the literature appears largely to concur that peer evaluation is particularly valuable for providing an opportunity to reflect on and improve teaching practice, rather than for informing summative decisions such as promotion and tenure.

Benefits of and Barriers to Implementing Peer Evaluation Methods

Peer evaluation methods can benefit all faculty members involved in the activity, with reviewees potentially showing enhanced reflective skills, improvements in teaching practices, and even positive impacts on promotion outcomes, for instance for medical faculty who

emphasized teaching as a main activity (Irby, 1983), while peer reviewers themselves may be reenthused and motivated to reinvigorate their own teaching practices (Siddiqui, Jones-Dwyer, and Carr, 2007).

There are a number of potential barriers to implementing peer evaluation of teaching, which include a perceived lack of objectivity or reliability; lack of consensus on appropriate criteria for evaluating teaching; lack of time, money, or energy; scheduling conflicts; and the need for a trusting but nonfriendship-based relationship between colleagues (Irby, 1983; Brown and Ward-Griffin, 1994; Blackmore, 2005; Siddiqui, Jones-Dwyer, and Carr, 2007). It is important to select the observer carefully, and mutual expectations should be discussed and agreed in advance (Siddiqui, Jones-Dwyer, and Carr, 2007). Peer evaluations should be based around clearly defined criteria (Irby, 1983) and categorized behavioral objectives (Brown and Ward-Griffin, 1994), and undertaken by trained peer evaluators where possible (Yon, Burnap, and Kohut, 2002; Blackmore, 2005; Warman, 2015). Their reliability can be improved if evaluations are based on direct classroom observations of teaching rather than simply reviewing curriculum documentation and course materials (Irby, 1983). In addition, observers should never intervene during a teaching observation, and confidentiality should be maintained at all times by those involved (Siddiqui, Jones-Dwyer, and Carr, 2007).

Planning a Peer Evaluation

Brown and Ward-Griffin (1994, p. 304) summarize five key criteria that contribute to a successful peer evaluation process:

- Overall approach and criteria developed by local faculty with administrative support – must be relevant to local context.
- Peer evaluation only one component of overall faculty evaluation process, with main purpose to be formative – improvement of teaching and learning.
- Ensure system is equitable and fair – need to be cognizant of importance of mutual trust and support.

- Need trained observers undertaking multiple observations and including constructive feedback in their evaluations.
- Should only use summatively (e.g., promotion and tenure) if information is "carefully gathered, promptly reported and judiciously interpreted."

Referring back to O'Neill's (1988) levels in Figure 19.1, it would also seem sensible that any peer evaluation of teaching effectiveness adopts similar principles and comprises three key domains in terms of preactive, interactive, and postactive dimensions:

- An initial meeting to clarify the purpose and scope.
- An in-class observation.
- A feedback/debriefing session.

This approach is also endorsed in models such as the Integrated Assessment of Teaching (IAT) described by Osborne (1998).

Several studies of peer evaluation methods and tools in the medical/healthcare literature have been published, and these are summarized succinctly by Berk (2013). In contrast, limited evidence exists in the veterinary medical education literature, although one study did describe and evaluate the use of peer reflection meetings in combination with a validated evaluation instrument, the Maastricht Clinical Teaching Questionnaire (MCTQ), which combines self-reflection and student ratings, and addresses the domains of climate, modeling, coaching, articulation, and exploration (Boerboom *et al.*, 2011b, 2012). This study demonstrated that student ratings of the domains in the MCTQ were valid indicators of teaching performance for veterinary clinical faculty (Boerboom *et al.*, 2012), and that the addition of peer reflection meetings led to deeper reflection among faculty and aided in the translation of student feedback into "concrete alternatives for teaching" (Boerboom *et al.*, 2011b, p. e620). This concurs with other healthcare studies showing that peer evaluation can promote changes in reflective practice and the development of teaching methods (Siddiqui, Jones-Dwyer, and Carr, 2007).

The Place for Peer Evaluation

We consider that peer evaluation is an essential component of any program to assess teaching effectiveness. An additional benefit of peer evaluation is that it can also result in positive role modeling by faculty for students in terms of seeking, receiving, and acting on feedback (Brown and Ward-Griffin, 1994). However, ultimately in order to be successful a peer evaluation program needs strong support from the dean and heads of department (Irby, 1983), in addition to "faculty involvement, short but objective methods, trained observers, constructive feedback for faculty development, as well as open communication and trust" (Brown and Ward-Griffin, 1994, p. 299).

Self-Evaluation Methods

Self-evaluation is a less commonly used measure of teaching effectiveness, and while concerns have been expressed that such methods may not be completely reliable (Hartman and Nelson, 1992; Boerboom *et al.*, 2009), some have been shown to be effective and valid methodologies using relatively robust study designs (Skeff, Stratos, and Bergen, 1992; Hewson, Copeland, and Fishleder, 2001; Cole *et al.*, 2004).

Traditional post self-evaluation (Srinivasan *et al.*, 2007) and pre/post self-evaluation (Steinert, Naismith, and Mann, 2012) of teaching competencies before and after completion of a faculty development program may be used. However, retrospective pre/post self-evaluation methods have actually been shown to be more valid measures of self-reported changes in teaching competencies (Skeff, Stratos, and Bergen, 1992; Hewson, Copeland, and Fishleder, 2001). Useful descriptors from a validated rating tool for self-assessment of competencies may range from "1 (I do not do this) to 5 (I'm highly competent at doing this)," while the corresponding tool for retrospective assessment of improvements in teaching may include descriptors such as "1 (no change [includes I would not want to do this or I was already highly effective at doing this]) to 5 (great deal of change or now I regularly do this)" (Hewson, Copeland, and Fishleder, 2001, p. 155).

Review of video-based and audio-based recordings of teaching sessions can also be incorporated into self-evaluation methodologies, with faculty initially reviewing recordings of their own teaching, before moving on to incorporate peer evaluation and discussion of the same materials with their colleagues (Elliot, Skeff, and Stratos, 1999). These and other self-assessment methodologies that include reflective elements can be a useful component of an assessment of teaching effectiveness, and can particularly be used for formative purposes, such as promoting the enhancement of teaching competencies (Cole *et al.*, 2004; Boerboom *et al.*, 2011b).

Objective Structured Teaching Exercises

A tool that has been described for use by either peers or (more commonly) faculty development staff, based on the well-known objective structured clinical examination (OSCE) for objective assessment of clinical skills, is the objective structured teaching exercises or OSTE (Morrison *et al.*, 2003; Stone *et al.*, 2003; Julian *et al.*, 2012).

OSTE checklists typically look for evidence aligned to the phases of preactive, interactive, and postactive illustrated in Figure 19.1. Boillat *et al.* (2012) have published 12 tips on using the OSTE, which include clarifying the goal and target audience, identifying what teaching skills to focus on, and training "standardized learners" who will be taught during the OSTE. Integrating the OSTE into the local context is also emphasized, and almost all of the tips would be appropriate for any evaluation method.

However, while the OSTE may be worth considering, given the many opportunities that exist for fully contextualized, "real-life" observations of teaching to take place in veterinary schools, it is arguable whether it really adds significantly to the armory for assessing teaching effectiveness.

Evaluation: The Product of Teaching Perspective

Learning Outcome Measures

While in an ideal world a tool to link teacher effectiveness with the highest-level changes in Kirkpatrick's (1994) model would be desirable, clearly this is fraught with difficulty. Perhaps Level 2 is the highest at which we can expect to be able to gather evidence that links to individual teacher effectiveness. Even at this level, as Jones (1989, p. 552) reflects, "it is doubtful whether any tertiary institution would have the resources and expertise – or the will – to produce a fair system of summative teacher evaluation based upon student learning outcomes." There are very polarized views on this aspect; for example, Emery, Kramer, and Tian (2003, p. 45) state: "An evaluation of teaching effectiveness must be based on outcomes. Anything else is rubbish." We would argue that a middle ground of utilizing such measures where appropriate (and feasible) to contribute to an overall portfolio of evidence is sensible if practical. Berk (2005) urges caution in their use and we would concur with this view, since cause and effect can become increasingly difficult to prove the further away from the teaching encounter the evaluation occurs.

Graduate and Employer Surveys

We touch on graduate and employer surveys as an important overall outcome measure, but from the point of view of assessing individual teaching effectiveness, often they are not sufficiently granular to be helpful in terms of feedback at the level of the individual teacher. Anecdotally, however, it is not uncommon for graduates of particular schools to have a reputation as being strong in particular areas, because of the recognized profile and expertise of inspirational teachers in given disciplines.

Teaching Scholarship

Completing the categories of evidence illustrated in Figure 19.3 is teaching scholarship. This includes evidence of engagement with pedagogy – either engaging with and/or producing peer-reviewed educational publications or resources (such as those in MedEdPORTAL; Crites *et al.*, 2014). Crites *et al.* (2014, p. 657) advocate that "all scholarship should be guided and judged by Glassick's six core principles of excellence for scholarship," namely, clear goals, adequate preparation, appropriate methods, significant results, effective presentation, and reflective critique (Glassick, 2000). This framework can be helpful when evaluating evidence relating to an individual's teaching scholarship, either in terms of peer-reviewed publications or at the level of adopting a scholarly approach to teaching, as illustrated in Box 19.2. While scholarship underpins many committed teachers' work, and is included by Berk (2013) as evidence of a "teacher scholar," it may of course bear no relation to an individual's actual performance as a teacher. Nevertheless, with this caveat we include it in our overall schema as evidence that should contribute to an overall portfolio of evidence when evaluating teaching effectiveness. After all, we would not consider an effective clinician to be one who was not engaged with current best practice in their discipline. and it should be no different for our educators.

Existing Tools or Instruments

Various tools have been published that may be useful to consult when planning an assessment of teaching effectiveness within a veterinary school. A selection of relevant examples are summarized in Table 19.3. These tools are supported by published factor analysis and reliability data.

Most of these tools have been used in healthcare professions education, with many focusing on the assessment of clinical teaching effectiveness; only one tool has been validated within veterinary medical education (Boerboom *et al.*, 2011a). Further useful information can be found in Beckman *et al.*'s (2004) detailed summary of the key features, domains, validation methods used, and psychometric properties of 21 validated instruments for the assessment of clinical teaching by learners in the healthcare professions. It should be noted, however, that these authors conclude that even when the reliability and validity of clinical assessment instruments have been demonstrated, limitations may still exist in terms of their generalizability to other settings, since assessments of teaching effectiveness should align with the teaching philosophy of the individual institution. This concurs with issues previously discussed in this chapter.

 Box 19.2: Focus on a scholarly approach to teaching

Requirements of a scholarly approach to teaching (Crites *et al.*, 2014):

- Define clear goals for teaching interactions
- Prepare using best practices from the literature

- Select suitable instructional methods and materials
- Use sound educational theories
- Measure the outcomes and impact of teaching
- Demonstrate continual improvement of one's work as a teacher

Table 19.3 Examples of published tools/instruments for assessing teaching effectiveness, plus their key features in terms of discipline and evaluator perspective.

Name of tool	Discipline	Evaluator perspective	Reference(s)
EFFECT instrument (Evaluation and feedback for effective clinical teaching)	Clinical teaching (medicine)	Target audience: resident	Fluit *et al.* (2012)
MCTQ (Maastricht Clinical Teaching Questionnaire)	Clinical teaching (medicine)	Target audience: student Teacher: peer, educationalist	Stalmeijer *et al.* (2008)
	Veterinary education	Target audience: student	Boerboom *et al.* (2011a)
MTEF (Mayo Teaching Evaluation Form)	Various	Teacher: peer	Beckman *et al.* (2003)
SFDP scale (Stanford Faculty Development Program)	Medicine	Target audience: resident and student	Litzelman *et al.* (1998)
Evaluation of Teaching Performance Questionnaire (CEID)	Psychology	Target audience: student	Moreno-Murcia, Silveira Torregrosa, and Belando Pedreño (2015)
Unnamed Teaching Effectiveness Instrument (from Cleveland Clinic Foundation)	Medicine	Teacher: self Target audience: residents and students	Hewson, Copeland, and Fishleder (2001)
SEEQ (Students' Evaluation of Educational Quality)	Various	Teacher: self Target audience: student	Marsh (2007)

Toward an Overall Portfolio of Evidence

As in the context of student assessment, the term "portfolio" can mean many and varied things. However, regardless of individual variation in institutional approach, teaching portfolios typically contain information on work done and any associated feedback, reflection on progress made, and plans for future development. The aims and content areas required in a portfolio must be clear, and mentoring support should also be part of the process (van Tartwijk and Driessen, 2009; van Schaik, Plant, and O'Sullivan, 2013; Crites *et al.*, 2014).

Returning to Figure 19.3, the minimum elements to include in a portfolio addressing teaching effectiveness are student evaluations and evidence from peer or other staff evaluation processes. If possible, other outcome measures of the "product" of the teaching can be included, although the strength of this evidence may be more difficult to relate directly to the individual teacher, as discussed earlier in this chapter. Increasingly, evidence of teaching scholarship by engagement with the educational literature should also be included – in particular emphasizing a reflective approach to teaching practice by linking the evidence to the individual's own teaching practice. Gusic *et al.* (2013) have published an online peer-reviewed Toolbox for Evaluating Educators, which provides extremely detailed criteria and templates for evaluating a teaching portfolio, and is available through the MedEdPORTAL online repository (Gusic *et al.*, 2013).

A final point relating to the overall teaching portfolio again resonates with its use in the context of student assessment; that is, being very clear about what elements are essentially private, what may be discussed with a mentor, and what may be viewed ultimately by a manager or others for promotion and tenure decisions. This multifaceted use is entirely appropriate for a portfolio as long as it is completely clear from the outset where the boundaries lie (van Tartwijk *et al.*, 2007; van Tartwijk and Driessen, 2009; van Schaik, Plant, and O'Sullivan, 2013).

Conclusion

Clearly, there is no one perfect system for the holistic assessment of teaching effectiveness. The overall importance of the necessity of aligning any system with the philosophy of the school or institution has been emphasized (Snell *et al.*, 2000; Beckman *et al.*, 2004). The purpose of the assessment (or the decision that will result from it) must be clearly defined at the outset, and then used to inform which types of evidence are gathered. In addition, multiple sources of evidence should be collated, and methods should be reviewed with faculty "at the table" to decide the next steps and agree which combination of sources is most appropriate for the context of an individual faculty. Such a process is likely to increase ownership, acceptance, and buy-in by faculty, and reduce suspicion and any insecurity or fears.

References

Beckman, T., Lee, M., Rohren, C., and Pankratz, V. (2003) Evaluating an instrument for the peer review of inpatient teaching. *Medical Teacher*, **25**, 131–135. doi:10.1080/0142159031000092508

Beckman, T.J., Ghosh, A.K., Cook, D.A., *et al.* (2004) How reliable are assessments of clinical teaching? *Journal of General Internal Medicine*, **19**, 971–977. doi:10.1111/j.1525-1497.2004.40066.x

Berk, R.A. (2005) Survey of 12 strategies to measure teaching effectiveness. *International Journal of Teaching and Learning in Higher Education*, **17**, 48–62.

Berk, R.A. (2013) Top five flashpoints in the assessment of teaching effectiveness. *Medical Teacher*, **35**, 15–26. doi:10.3109/0142159X.2012.732247

Blackmore, J.A. (2005) A critical evaluation of peer review via teaching observation within higher education. *International Journal of Educational Management*, **19**, 218–232. doi:10.1108/09513540510591002

Boerboom, T.B.B., Dolmans, D.H.J.M., Muijtjens, A.M.M., *et al.* (2009) Does a faculty development programme improve teachers' perceived competence in different teacher roles? *Medical Teacher*, **31**, 1030–1031. doi:10.3109/01421590903183779

Boerboom, T.B.B., Dolmans, D.H.J.M., Jaarsma, A.D.C., *et al.* (2011a) Exploring the validity and reliability of a questionnaire for evaluating veterinary clinical teachers' supervisory skills during clinical rotations. *Medical Teacher*, **33**, E84–E91. doi:10.3109/0142159X.2011 .536277

Boerboom, T.B.B., Jaarsma, D., Dolmans, D.H.J.M., *et al.* (2011b) Peer group reflection helps clinical teachers to critically reflect on their teaching. *Medical Teacher*, **33**, E615–E623. doi:10.3109/0142159X.2011 .610840

Boerboom, T.B.B., Mainhard, T., Dolmans, D.H.J.M., *et al.* (2012) Evaluating clinical teachers with the Maastricht clinical teaching questionnaire: How much "teacher" is in student ratings? *Medical Teacher*, **34**, 320–326. doi:10.3109/0142159X.2012.660220

Boillat, M., Bethune, C., Ohle, E., *et al.* (2012) Twelve tips for using the objective structured teaching exercise for faculty development. *Medical Teacher*, **34**, 269–273. doi:10.3109/0142159x.2011.599891

Brown, B., and Ward-Griffin, C. (1994) The use of peer evaluation in promoting nursing faculty teaching effectiveness: A review of the literature. *Nurse Education Today*, **14**, 299–305. doi:10.1016/0260-6917(94)90141-4

Cole, K.A., Barker, L.R., Kolodner, K., *et al.* (2004) Faculty development in teaching skills: An intensive longitudinal model. *Academic Medicine*, **79**, 469–480.

Cook, D.A. (2010) Twelve tips for evaluating educational programs. *Medical Teacher*, **32**, 296–301. doi:10.3109/01421590903480121

Crites, G.E., Gaines, J.K., Cottrell, S., *et al.* (2014) Medical education scholarship: An introductory guide: AMEE guide no. 89. *Medical Teacher*, **36**, 657–674. doi:10.3109/0142159X.2014.916791

Elliot, D.L., Skeff, K.M., and Stratos, G.A. (1999) How do you get to the improvement of teaching? A longitudinal faculty development program for medical educators. *Teaching and Learning in Medicine*, **11**, 52–57. doi:10.1207/S15328015TLM1101_12

Emery, C.R., Kramer, T.R., and Tian, R.G. (2003) Return to academic standards: A critique of student evaluations of teaching effectiveness. *Quality Assurance in Education*, **11**, 37–46. doi:10.1108/09684880310462074

Felton, J., Mitchell, J., and Stinson, M. (2004) Web-based student evaluations of professors: The relations between perceived quality, easiness and sexiness. *Assessment and Evaluation in Higher Education*, **29**, 91–108. doi:10.1080/0260293032000158180

Fluit, C., Bolhuis, S., Grol, R., *et al.* (2012) Evaluation and feedback for effective clinical teaching in postgraduate medical education: Validation of an assessment instrument incorporating the CanMEDS roles. *Medical Teacher*, **34**, 893–901. doi:10.3109/0142159X.2012.699114

Glassick, C.E. (2000) Boyer's expanded definitions of scholarship, the standards for assessing scholarship, and the elusiveness of the scholarship of teaching. *Academic Medicine*, **75**, 877–880. doi:10.1097/00001888-200009000-00007

Gusic, M.A.J., Baldwin, C., Chandran, L., *et al.* (2013) *Using the AAMC Toolbox for Evaluating Educators: You Be the Judge!* MedEdPORTAL Publications. doi:10.15766/mep_2374-8265.9313

Hartman, S.L., and Nelson, M.S. (1992) What we say and what we do: Self-reported teaching behavior versus performances in written simulations among medical school faculty. *Academic Medicine*, **67**, 522–527.

Hewson, M.G., Copeland, H.L., and Fishleder, A.J. (2001) What's the use of faculty development? Program evaluation using retrospective self-assessments and independent performance ratings. *Teaching and Learning in Medicine*, **13**, 153–160. doi:10.1207/S15328015TLM1303_4

Huggett, K.N., Greenberg, R.B., Rao, D., *et al.* (2012) The design and utility of institutional teaching awards: A literature review. *Medical Teacher*, **34**, 907–919. doi:10.3109/0142159X.2012.731102

Irby, D. (1983) Peer review of teaching in medicine. *Journal of Medical Education*, **58**, 457–461.

Jones, J. (1989) Students' ratings of teacher personality and teaching competence. *Higher Education*, **18**, 551–558. doi:10.1007/BF00138747

Julian, K., Appelle, N., O'Sullivan, P., *et al.* (2012) The impact of an objective structured teaching evaluation on faculty teaching skills. *Teaching and Learning in Medicine*, **24**, 3–7. doi:10.1080/10401334.2012.641476

Kirkpatrick, D.L. (1994) *Evaluating Training Programs: The Four Levels*, Berrett-Koehler, San Francisco, CA.

Litzelman, D.K., Stratos, G.A., Marriott, D.J., and Skeff, K.M. (1998) Factorial validation of a widely disseminated educational framework for evaluating clinical teachers. *Academic Medicine*, **73**, 688–695.

Litzelman, D.K., Westmoreland, G.R., Skeff, K.M., and Stratos, G.A. (1999) Student and resident evaluations of faculty – how reliable are they? *Academic Medicine*, **74**, S25–S27.

Marsh, H. (2007) Students' evaluations of university teaching: Dimensionality, reliability, validity, potential biases and usefulness, in *The Scholarship of Teaching and Learning in Higher Education: An Evidence-Based Perspective* (eds R. Perry and J. Smart), Springer, Dordrecht. doi:10.1007/1-4020-5742-3_9

Moreno-Murcia, J.A., Silveira Torregrosa, Y., and Belando Pedreño, N. (2015) Questionnaire evaluating teaching competencies in the university environment. Evaluation of teaching competencies in the university. *New Approaches in Educational Research*, **4**, 54–61. doi:10.7821/naer.2015.1.106

Morrison, E.H., Rucker, L., Boker, J.R., *et al.* (2003) A pilot randomized, controlled trial of a longitudinal residents-as-teachers curriculum. *Academic Medicine*, **78**, 722–729.

O'Neill, G.P. (1988) Teaching effectiveness: A review of the research. *Canadian Journal of Education / Revue canadienne de l'éducation*, **13**, 162–185. doi:10.2307/1495174

Osborne, J.L. (1998) Integrating student and peer evaluation of teaching. *College Teaching*, **46**, 36–38. doi:10.1080/87567559809596231

Ramsden, P. (2003) *Learning to Teach in Higher Education*, Routledge, London.

Richardson, J.T.E. (2005) Instruments for obtaining student feedback: A review of the literature. *Assessment and Evaluation in Higher Education*, **30**, 387–415. doi:10.1080/02602930500099193

Ruesseler, M., Kalozoumi-Paizi, F., Schill, A., *et al.* (2014) Impact of peer feedback on the performance of lecturers in emergency medicine: A prospective observational study. *Scandinavian Journal of Trauma, Resuscitation and Emergency Medicine*, **22**, 71. doi:10.1186/s13049-014-0071-1

Schiekirka, S., and Raupach, T. (2015) A systematic review of factors influencing student ratings in undergraduate medical education course evaluations. *BMC Medical Education*, **15**, 30. doi:10.1186/s12909-015-0311-8

Siddiqui, Z.S., Jonas-Dwyer, D., and Carr, S.E. (2007) Twelve tips for peer observation of

teaching. *Medical Teacher*, **29**, 297–300. doi:10.1080/01421590701291451

Skeff, K.M., Stratos, G.A., and Bergen, M.R. (1992) Evaluation of a medical faculty development program: A comparison of traditional pre/post and retrospective pre/post self-assessment ratings. *Evaluation and the Health Professions*, **15**, 350–366. doi:10.1177/016327879201500307

Snell, L., Tallett, S., Haist, S., *et al.* (2000) A review of the evaluation of clinical teaching: New perspectives and challenges. *Medical Education*, **34**, 862–870. doi:10.1046/j.1365-2923.2000.00754.x

Sproule, R. (2002) The underdetermination of instructor performance by data from the student evaluation of teaching. *Economics of Education Review*, **21**, 287–294. doi:10.1016/S0272-7757(01)00025-5

Srinivasan, M., Pratt, D.D., Collins, J., *et al.* (2007) Developing the master educator: Cross disciplinary teaching scholars program for human and veterinary medical faculty. *Academic Psychiatry*, **31**, 452–464. doi:10.1176/appi.ap.31.6.452

Stalmeijer, R.E., Dolmans, D.H.J.M., Wolfhagen, I.H.A.P., *et al.* (2008) The development of an instrument for evaluating clinical teachers: Involving stakeholders to determine content validity. *Medical Teacher*, **30**, E272–E277. doi:10.1080/01421590802258904

Steinert, Y., Mann, K., Centeno, A., *et al.* (2006) A systematic review of faculty development initiatives designed to improve teaching effectiveness in medical education: Beme guide no. 8. *Medical Teacher*, **28**, 497–526. doi:10.1080/01421590600902976

Steinert, Y., Naismith, L., and Mann, K. (2012) Faculty development initiatives designed to promote leadership in medical education. A Beme systematic review: Beme guide no. 19. *Medical Teacher*, **34**, 483–503. doi:10.3109/0142159x.2012.680937

Stone, S., Mazor, K., Devaney-O'Neil, S., *et al.* (2003) Development and implementation of an objective structured teaching exercise (OSTE) to evaluate improvement in feedback skills following a faculty development workshop.

Teaching and Learning in Medicine, **15**, 7–13. doi:10.1207/S15328015TLM1501_03

Surgenor, P.W.G. (2011) Obstacles and opportunities: Addressing the growing pains of summative student evaluation of teaching. *Assessment and Evaluation in Higher Education*, **38**, 363–376. doi:10.1080/02602938.2011.635247

van Schaik, S., Plant, J., and O'Sullivan, P. (2013) Promoting self-directed learning through portfolios in undergraduate medical education: The mentors' perspective. *Medical Teacher*, **35**, 139–144. doi:10.3109/0142159X.2012.733832

van Tartwijk, J., Driessen, E., van der Vleuten, C., and Stokking, K. (2007) Factors influencing the successful introduction of portfolios. *Quality in Higher Education*, **13**, 69–79. doi:10.1080/13538320701272813

van Tartwijk, J., and Driessen, E.W. (2009) Portfolios for assessment and learning: AMEE guide no. 45. *Medical Teacher*, **31**, 790–801. doi:10.1080/01421590903139201

Warman, S.M. (2015) Challenges and issues in the evaluation of teaching quality: How does it affect teachers' professional practice? A UK perspective. *Journal of Veterinary Medical Education*, **42**, 245–251. doi:10.3138/jvme.0914-096R1

Wilkerson, L., and Irby, D. (1998) Strategies for improving teaching practices: A comprehensive approach to faculty development. *Academic Medicine*, **73**, 387–396. doi:10.1097/00001888-199804000-00011

Yardley, S., and Dornan, T. (2012) Kirkpatrick's levels and education "evidence." *Medical Education*, **46**, 97–106. doi:10.1111/j.1365-2923.2011.04076.x

Yon, M., Burnap, C., and Kohut, G. (2002) Evidence of effective teaching: Perceptions of peer reviewers. *College Teaching*, **50**, 104–110. doi:10.1080/87567550209595887

Youmans, R.J., and Jee, B.D. (2007) Fudging the numbers: Distributing chocolate influences student evaluations of an undergraduate course. *Teaching of Psychology*, **34**, 245–247. doi:10.1080/00986280701700318

316

20

Assessing the Assessment Process

Kent Hecker[1] and Jared Danielson[2]

[1] Faculty of Veterinary Medicine, Cumming School of Medicine, University of Calgary, Canada
[2] College of Veterinary Medicine, Iowa State University, USA

 Box 20.1: Key messages

- Evaluating your assessment processes provides evidence to improve the assessment *of* and *for* student learning and ultimately your educational program.
- Assessment of student performance should not be considered as a discrete event. As such, assessing your assessment methods should take into consideration the domains of interest being evaluated not only within each assessment method, but across assessment methods.
- Evaluating your assessment process requires evidence. Sources of validity evidence include content evidence, response process evidence, internal structure evidence, relations with other variables evidence, and consequences evidence.
- Various evaluation frameworks can be utilized to assist with collecting and disseminating assessment information. Two of the more familiar frameworks in health professional education are Kirkpatrick's four-level evaluation model and the Context/Input/Process/Product (CIPP) model.

Introduction

Whether at work or in school, we are assessed continuously regarding our performance. In a school environment, assessment is primarily thought of in the context of student performance and learning, typically referred to as "assessment of student learning" and "assessment for student learning." However, "assessment" can also be thought of in terms of course-, curriculum-, program-, or institutional-level evaluation. This chapter builds on the concept of student assessment and casts a reflective lens on evaluating the assessment process that has been put in place, whether within a course, across the clinical year(s), or across the curriculum. We also provide information about why and how a formal and explicit assessment structure should be created and ultimately evaluated. Note that while efforts are occasionally made to differentiate between "evaluation" and "assessment," we follow the convention of treating these as equivalent and will use them interchangeably throughout the chapter (Scriven, 2003).

Veterinary Medical Education: A Practical Guide, First Edition. Edited by Jennifer L. Hodgson and Jacquelyn M. Pelzer.
© 2017 John Wiley & Sons, Inc. Published 2017 by John Wiley & Sons, Inc.

Definitions of Assessment

To provide context for the chapter, we begin by providing two definitions of assessment. Assessment of student learning has been defined as follows:

> Assessment is the process of gathering and discussing information from multiple and diverse sources in order to develop a deep understanding of what students know, understand, and can do with their knowledge as a result of their educational experiences; the process culminates when assessment results are used to improve subsequent learning. (Huba and Freed, 2000, p. 8)

Assessment of a course, curriculum, program, or institution in higher education has been defined as follows:

> Assessment is the process of providing credible evidence of:
>
> - Resources
> - Implementation actions, and
> - Outcomes
>
>   Undertaken for the purpose of improving the effectiveness of
>
> - Instruction
> - Programs, and
> - Services
>
>   in higher education. (Banta and Palomba, 2015, p. 2)

Accountability in Assessment Practices

This chapter is also meant to provide ideas about how best to capture information and evidence to answer questions regarding your assessment practices. Accountability in relation to how and why we assess our students is not a bad thing; by documenting our processes we provide transparency regarding our decisions, and the ability to reflect and improve on our assessment practices for the betterment of our students and schools. Questions that can be asked when evaluating assessment methods/programs include:

- Do the assessment methods capture data relevant to the course/program objectives/competencies of interest?
- Are the assessment methods organized/utilized in an effective manner to capture student performance?
- Are summative and formative assessments utilized?
- Do the assessment methods allow for the provision of feedback to the learner? In other words, in the assessment cycle, can performance information be provided to students to foster learning?
- Are assessment questions linked to specific course/program outcomes?
- Are the assessment methods feasible? Can all stakeholders understand and use the methods as they were intended given their respective constraints?
- Are scores from the assessment methods reliable and valid? Stated differently, is there evidence to support decisions (e.g., pass/fail, promotion, remediation, removal) made from the assessment scores?
- What are the perceptions of the participants involved in the assessment process? How do students, raters, and instructors perceive what is assessed, how assessment occurs, and how feedback is provided?

Evaluation of Assessment Practices

In order to begin the evaluation/assessment process, one of the authors (KH) starts by creating a document like the one provided in Table 20.1. This captures the evaluation questions of interest (which later can be ranked or revised), identifies the information required, where the information comes from, what method will capture the data, how sampling will occur (if required), the schedule, and the

Table 20.1 Template for evaluation questions, sources of data, and proposed analyses.

	EVALUATION QUESTION	INFORMATION REQUIRED	SOURCE OF INFORMATION	METHOD	SAMPLING	SCHEDULE	ANALYSIS
				Assessment questions			
1	Are OSCE scores predictive of clinical rotation performance?	OSCE performance in Years 1, 2, and 3 and clinical rotation performance scores	Raters, students, and clinical preceptors	Exam data from the respective years, clinical rotation information	All students in the DVM program	Exam data for each year and clinical rotation data from the final year	Descriptive, inferential, and multivariate
2	What clinical rotation-based assessments will be acceptable by faculty, students, and clinical partners?	Scores from the mini clinical examination (mCEX), direct observation of procedural skills (DOPS), and the in-training evaluation reports (ITERS)	Clinical rotation instructors, students, raters	Data from the clinical rotation assessment tools, surveys, and interviews	Clinical rotation instructors	Preliminary survey work	Descriptive, inferential, and qualitative
				Impact of assessment on student learning			
3	What is the impact of simulation and virtual training on learning clinical and professional skills?	Performance on simulations and final performance data across courses and clinical rotations	Student performance data	Comparison study of performance using different high-fidelity and low-fidelity simulations	All DVM students	To be determined	Descriptive and inferential; multivariate once there is a number of cohorts to analyze
4	How satisfied are the UCVM students with the assessment program and what are the strengths and weaknesses?	Student perceptions of their undergraduate experience	Students	Interview	Focus groups	As required by the Office of the Associate Dean Curriculum	Qualitative analyses to determine common themes
5	How satisfied are the UCVM faculty with the assessment program and what are the strengths and weaknesses?	Faculty perceptions of the assessment of student performance	Faculty	Survey or interview	Focus groups	As required by the Office of the Associate Dean Curriculum	Qualitative analyses to determine common themes

proposed analyses. Further columns can be included that reflect the validity evidence that we think is being collected, or the evaluation framework categories that are being targeted. These topics will be covered in this chapter.

How to Use Assessment Data

Data from the assessment of student performance is used differently given the interests of each group (for instance, students, instructors, or administrators). For students, assessment is about how they performed, whether against their peers and/or against a set program standard. Ultimately, the output of student assessments (marks) is meant to demonstrate students' achievement and learning; this leads to a recognition that the necessary knowledge, skills, and attitudes have been attained so that they can practice independently, or, more specifically, are licensed to practice in veterinary medicine.

For instructors, assessment data provides information on how students are performing within and across courses. Course coordinators and primary lecturers use performance measures from various assessment methods to gauge students' knowledge, skills, and attitudes for both formative and summative decisions, influenced by students' abilities and course performance. As indicated in Part Four, Chapter 14: Concepts in Assessment, formative assessment is meant to provide performance indicators to both instructor and student in order to assist with future student learning. Summative assessment measures provide data to make decisions about student progression, whether in a course or a program. Formative and summative data can also be used by course coordinators and instructors to assess how well material is being taught and learned in the course. If best practices are used in test development (as shown in Part Four, Chapter 15: Written Assessment) where test specifications and blueprints are created, instructors can also use student performance to determine which topics are best understood and at which level of learning based on which learning taxonomy was used. For

instance, in an anatomy course, if there was a written test on the musculoskeletal system where instructors identified that 10 of the 50 questions were meant to assess the application of knowledge, and a large cohort of students got that subset of questions wrong, instructors can begin to drill down deeper as to why. Were the questions incorrectly worded, miskeyed, or misleading? Was the topic covered to the depth that was expected? If this was a section of the course that multiple instructors covered, was there miscommunication regarding the expectations of the unit?

For administrators (associate dean academic/curriculum and deans), assessment data provides information regarding individual students' performance and curricular performance, which can be used to assess strengths and gaps within and across years.

The components required to evaluate the accuracy of your assessment methods are relatively straightforward, yet the process, infrastructure, and workforce necessary to complete the task can be daunting. The following builds on suggested practices of analysis in order to determine how best to put in the infrastructure needed to assess the assessment process.

Programs of Assessment

Before discussing how to evaluate your assessment process, there needs to be a framework regarding what is being assessed and when. In health professional education, mostly medicine, there has been a recent push to create "programs of assessment" (van der Vleuten and Schuwirth, 2005). It has long been acknowledged that there is no one best assessment method for knowledge, skills, and attitudes. In other words, each assessment method is fallible, with its own inherent strengths and weaknesses. As a result, assessment methods should be purposefully selected and judiciously used so that the combination of scores can be employed to better justify performance-related feedback to students, and rationalize decisions made regarding progression through veterinary school (van der Vleuten *et al.*, 2015). For further reading on developing a program of assessment, refer to Part Four, Chapter 14: Concepts in Assessment and van der Vleuten *et al.* (2015).

To justify decisions regarding assessment practices, two components are typically required: *evidence* to support the decisions and actions that are taken (passing a student, continuation of an assessment method, etc.); and an *evaluation framework* in which the collected evidence can be collated and disseminated in order to justify decisions. In the remainder of this chapter, we will discuss, first, the kinds of evidence that might be required to justify assessment practices; and, second, several helpful frameworks for collating and disseminating assessment information.

Sources of Evidence to Support Decisions and Actions

Ultimately, what is required is validity evidence (as implied by the first part of Banta and Palomba's 2015 definition provided earlier) to support the decisions for the use of each assessment method; the use of the combination of assessment methods; and the use of the data from the assessment methods to determine student performance and competence for progression, remediation, or removal. "Validity refers to the degree to which evidence and theory support the interpretations of test scores for proposed uses of tests" (AERA *et al.*, 2014, p. 11). In this chapter, we will use this definition to mean both the proposed uses of individual tests and the use of proposed uses of multiple assessments in order to justify the intended consequences of an assessment program. So, what is required to create an argument for the validity of the decisions being made from assessment scores? There are five sources of validity evidence that provide data for the use and interpretation of scores. These sources are content evidence, response process evidence, internal structure evidence, relations to other variables evidence, and consequences evidence (Table 20.2; AERA *et al.*, 2014).

Content Evidence

Content evidence refers to the collection of evidence regarding how assessments were developed and reviewed. If multiple domains are assessed, whether knowledge, skills or attitudes, competencies, or professional activities, justification is required as to why they are being assessed and how items/assessment methods were selected. Content evidence for a single test could include information regarding item generation, test blueprinting, exam committee review, and rater training (if required). Content evidence for an assessment program would be documentation regarding how assessment methods were chosen for each course, set of competencies, or professional activities. This would be considered the development of a "master plan" (van der Vleuten *et al.*, 2015), which provides documentation for the reasons why assessment methods were chosen, the weighting of each assessment method for student performance decisions, whether it was for formative or summative decisions, whether the assessment methods were aligned with specific competencies, whether standard-setting methods were used to set performance cut scores for each assessment method, and so on.

Response Process Evidence

Response process evidence refers to how well participants' responses align with the domains being assessed, and whether participants (students and/or raters) understand which domains items are trying to assess. It then follows that evidence required for the assessment process would include data regarding participants' understanding of what the assessment methods are trying to evaluate. For instance, response process evidence could include student, instructor, and/or rater comments regarding the utility of workplace-based assessment – such as a mini clinical evaluation examination (mini-CEX) and/or multiple-choice questions (MCQs) – to assess students' performance on taking a history with a difficult client/patient during their small animal rotation. Documentation would be required regarding why you would use an MCQ

Table 20.2 Types of validity evidence.

Type of validity evidence	Definition	Sources of data
Content	Evidence regarding how items/assessments were developed and reviewed to measure constructs of interest	*Course or class level* Test blueprint, item-writing process, and experience of raters *Program level* Evaluation matrix outlining how various assessment methods align
Response process	How well participants' responses align with the domains being assessed	*Course or class level* Quality control of testing situations, rater training protocols, data from pilot testing of items *Program level* Program documents outlining what domain is being assessed and when, think-aloud protocols with participants to assess understanding
Internal structure	Degree to which individual test items or items from various assessment methods measure the underlying domain of interest	*Course or class level* Item analyses, reliability analyses *Program level* Correlation analyses between scores from different assessment methods Factor analysis
Relations to other variables	Analyses between scores and other measures, including measures that are conceptually the same or different to support the use of the items/scores	*Course, class, and program levels* Assessing relationships with measures theoretically similar and different
Consequences	Information that outlines the impact (anticipated or unintended) of the assessment methods on stakeholders	*Course, class, and program levels* Evidence of the impact of the assessment program on participants, which could include self-reported consequences or observed changes in participants' behaviors

in this situation, since it can test for, at best, the application of knowledge.

Internal Structure Evidence

Data gathered to provide evidence for internal structure includes documentation/analyses regarding the relationship of assessment items within the method (are there items meant to assess similar/different knowledge domains or taxonomies with a respective test?), those relationships across methods, and how the relationships support the objective/competency/construct being measured. Internal structure evidence within method typically takes the form of a reliability analysis,

whether across items (i.e., in an MCQ test), or raters (i.e., in a multisource feedback assessment), or stations (i.e., within an objective structured clinical examination, OSCE). To provide internal structure analyses across methods, the empirical evidence that could be gathered is correlational, showing convergent and/or discriminant relationships between scores from assessment methods or scores for specific attributes across assessment methods. For instance, end of clinical rotation assessments, such as an in-training evaluation report (ITER), are typically broken down into competency domains, such as clinical skill ability, clinical reasoning, and communication skills.

Strong correlations between communication skills scores across a small animal and large animal rotation would be evidence of convergent validity (measuring the same construct), whereas weaker correlations between communication skills scores and clinical reasoning scores would provide evidence of discriminant validity, meaning that we are measuring two different (although potentially overlapping) competencies. Other empirical evidence could also be provided through factor analysis or multitrait, multimethod matrices.

Relations with Other Variables Evidence

Evidence for this category comes primarily from statistical analyses between scores from a variety of measures. Because performance on clinical tasks is generally considered to be the most important indicator of clinical competence, scores on assessments in other settings would primarily be compared with variables captured within the clinical years, licensure exams, and/or alumni data. This could include but not are not limited to NAVLE results, choice of practice, performance within practice (i.e., owner's assessment of graduate's performance), and so on.

Consequences Evidence

The least well-reported and understood source of evidence, the category of consequences evidence probably has the greatest impact on the decisions that are made based on performance scores (Cook and Lineberry, 2016). This category details how scores are used in determining student progression through a curriculum. In other words, consequences evidence outlines the impact (anticipated or unintended) of the assessment methods on stakeholders. For example, it documents decisions such as pass/fail points for examinations, remediation plans for students, and so forth.

Evaluation Frameworks

Assessment (or evaluation) of the assessment process needs a framework within which to

collect, collate, and report the necessary information. There are numerous evaluation frameworks that can be used, the choice of which is dependent on contextual factors within schools, not to mention resource and expertise requirements. When a framework is adapted/adopted, it is best to justify the decision, articulating the framework's strengths and limitations. Common frameworks (models) used within health professional education are Kirkpatrick's four-level evaluation model (Kirkpatrick and Kirkpatrick, 2006) and the Context/Input/Process/Product (CIPP) model (Stufflebeam and Shinkfield, 2007). For broader discussions regarding program evaluation and evaluation models within healthcare professions and their theoretical underpinnings, refer to Cook (2010) and Frye and Hemmer (2012).

Kirkpatrick's Four-Level Evaluation Model

Use of Kirkpatrick's model for evaluation emanates from its logical focus on evaluating program outcomes and gathering/categorizing data into four hierarchical levels. These four categories are (Kirkpatrick and Kirkpatrick, 2006):

- *Participant satisfaction or reaction*: how stakeholders (learners, raters, instructors, etc.) react to the assessment program (requires content evidence).
- *Measures of learning*: for students this consists of assessing knowledge gained, skills improved, and attitudes changed as a result of an assessment program; for instructors it could consist of attitudes changed or knowledge obtained regarding assessment best practices (requires content, internal structure, and possibly response process evidence).
- *Changes in learner/instructor/rater behavior*: whether stakeholders are accepting of the assessment program, complying with the requirements, and changing their performance (requires internal structure, response process, and relationship to other variables evidence).
- *Program's final results*: the outcomes of the assessment process (requires response to

other variables and consequences validity evidence).

To collect information regarding the respective levels, evaluators would categorize evaluation questions into the respective categories and then determine where and from whom to gather the necessary information. This information would then be consolidated and categorized based on the hierarchy and the program outcomes that were being addressed.

Context/Input/Process/Product (CIPP) Model

The CIPP model is built from four complementary evaluation methodologies, and is meant to collect and provide information regarding program/course/curricula improvement, not just reporting information regarding defined outcomes. These four studies (methodologies) include a context evaluation study, an input evaluation study, a process evaluation study, and a product evaluation study. These four components can be implemented independently or synchronously and to varying degrees, dependent on the evaluation questions being asked and the stage of the program.

For instance, a *context* evaluation study (defined as a process to assess needs, opportunities, and effects to determine goals, objectives, and potentially outcomes) could be performed when a program/course/curricula is being planned, or modified. Data collected here would correspond to content evidence as outlined in the evidence of validity section earlier.

An *input* evaluation study (defined as a process to study and evaluate various "inputs" to a program to assess effectiveness) may be appropriate when ascertaining whether or not the suite of assessment methods is required to determine the competence of students, whether within courses or within programs. This allows developers/evaluators, given the context, to justify the use of assessment methods, the timing of assessment methods, and the desired consequences of the scores or student advancement. This again would provide content evidence validity for the proposed uses of the assessment methods.

A *process* evaluation study (a study to determine how a program was delivered/implemented) would provide response process validity evidence, where participants are engaged to determine the extent to which they understand/agree with what is being measured and by whom. Further, information is gathered regarding program implementation, both in relation to how the program was intended to be implemented and how it was actually implemented. When evaluating an assessment program or group of assessment methods, data would be gathered from student performance as well as qualitative components, where participants are asked questions such as "Are the assessment methods/program running efficiently?" or "Do the assessment methods/programs collect the necessary information given the stated goals of the program?" The final study, a *product* evaluation study, focuses on the assessment of outcomes. In the case of evaluating an assessment program, this could entail identifying whether or not the stated competencies are being assessed properly, whether students are being evaluated fairly/objectively, whether or not a program is identifying those students in need of remediation, and so on. This type of study is considered summative in nature, where data are used for decisions regarding sustainability and use of assessment methods. Therefore, these studies require validity evidence from multiple sources, including internal structure, relationships with other variables, and consequences.

Conclusions

Building an explicit program of assessment provides a framework of what to assess and where to assess it. The content of this chapter attempts to close the loop by assessing the assessment process to provide the "how well are we assessing" component. If done properly, the information collected and compiled can be used to make evidence-informed decisions to improve the assessment both of and for student learning, and ultimately improve educational programs.

References

AERA, APA, NCME, and Joint Committee on Standards for Educational and Psychological Testing (2014) *Standards for Educational and Psychological Testing*, American Educational Research Association, Washington, DC.

Banta, T.W., and Palomba, C.A. (2015) *Assessment Essentials: Planning, Implementing, and Improving Assessment in Higher Education*, Jossey-Bass, San Francisco, CA.

Cook, D.A. (2010) Twelve tips for evaluating educational programs. *Medical Teacher*, **32**, 296–301.

Cook, D.A., and Lineberry, M. (2016) Consequences validity evidence: Evaluating the impact of educational assessments. *Academic Medicine*, **91**, 785–795.

Frye, A.W., and Hemmer, P.A. (2012) Program evaluation models and related theories: AMEE guide no. 67. *Medical Teacher*, **34**, E288–E299.

Huba, M.E., and Freed, J.E. (2000) *Learner-Centered Assessment on College Campuses: Shifting the Focus from Teaching to Learning*, Allyn and Bacon, Boston, MA.

Kirkpatrick, D.L., and Kirkpatrick, J.D. (2006) *Evaluating Training Programs: The Four Levels*, Berrett-Koehler, San Francisco, CA.

Scriven, M. (2003) *Evaluation Thesaurus*, Sage, Newbury Park, CA.

Stufflebeam, D.L., and Shinkfield, A.J. (2007) *Evaluation Theory, Models, and Applications*, Jossey-Bass, San Francisco, CA.

van der Vleuten, C.P.M., and Schuwirth, L.W.T. (2005) Assessing professional competence: From methods to programmes. *Medical Education*, **39**, 309–317.

van der Vleuten, C.P.M., Schuwirth, L.W.T., Driessen, E.W., *et al.* (2015) Twelve tips for programmatic assessment. *Medical Teacher*, **37**, 641–646.

21

Institutional Benchmarking

Paul C. Mills[1] and Rosanne M. Taylor[2]

[1] *School of Veterinary Science, University of Queensland, Australia*
[2] *Sydney School of Veterinary Science, University of Sydney, Australia*

 Box 21.1: Key messages

- Benchmarking is a collaborative, structured process of comparing performance and processes, through an agreement to conduct peer review.
- It informs self-evaluation and can be an effective approach to driving change and a focus on quality.

- Delineation of the scope, process, benchmarks, and reporting on outcomes and confidentiality is essential before commencing.
- Benchmarking can contribute to effective outcomes assessment for accreditation.
- While benchmarking is widespread in veterinary education, it has received only limited scientific review.

Introduction and Definitions

Benchmarking is a process by which many aspects of an educational program can be compared between similar institutions. Although this term arises from the practice of cobblers (see Box 21.2), the definition of benchmarking that is more familiar today was developed in the early 1980s at the Xerox Corporation in response to increased competition and a rapidly declining market (Camp, 1989). Universities adopted benchmarking to improve administrative processes and instructional models through comparison with peer institutions (Chaffee and Sherr, 1992; Clark, 1993) as part of an ongoing and systematic process of improvement (Kempner, 1993). Benchmarking has become an

important driver of continuous improvement in universities across the western world, and is now firmly on the agenda for veterinary education (AAVMC, 2011, recommendation 6.2).

A review of the benchmarking literature shows that there are four kinds of benchmarking: internal, competitive, industry, and best

---

 Box 21.2: What is a benchmark?

The term benchmark arises from the practice of cobblers of measuring feet by placing the foot on a bench and creating a template for the shoes.

Veterinary Medical Education: A Practical Guide, First Edition. Edited by Jennifer L. Hodgson and Jacquelyn M. Pelzer.
© 2017 John Wiley & Sons, Inc. Published 2017 by John Wiley & Sons, Inc.

in class. Internal benchmarking can occur at large, decentralized institutions where there are several organizational units that conduct similar processes. Competitive benchmarking analyzes processes against peer institutions that are competing in similar markets. Industry benchmarking extends competitive benchmarking to a larger, broadly defined group of competitors (Rush, 1994). Best-in-class benchmarking uses the broadest application of data collection from different industries to find the best practices available (e.g., for delivery of information technology support). The selection of benchmarking type depends on the desired outcomes, the process(es) being analyzed, and the availability of data and expertise at the institution. (It should be noted throughout this chapter that we consider institutions, higher education institutions, universities, and organizations as interchangeable terms in describing the parent entity and as reflecting the wide scope and applicability of benchmarking.) The increase in all types of university benchmarking in the past two decades has been made possible by the exponential increase in data collection and management within universities.

Benchmarks and standards are commonly understood terms with a particular meaning in higher education (Judd and Keith, 2012; Judd, Pondish, and Secolsky, 2013). A benchmark is used to measure performance against a specific indicator of outcomes (e.g., staff–student ratios, minority student attrition, graduate employment rates), providing a metric of institutional achievement of its mission. A broad definition (Wikipedia, 2016) suggests that businesses benchmark by comparing their processes and performance measures with similar companies, with an objective to improve specific productivity metrics, such as quality, time, and profit margin. Strategic management initiatives can then be instituted to improve performance and productivity against benchmarks.

In contrast, a standard is a predetermined minimum level of acceptable performance (Judd, Pondish, and Secolsky, 2013). A standard is based on judgment and experience, yet can be validated by external experts, including accreditation agencies (Judd and Keith, 2012). In universities, student success is determined once individual standards are met or exceeded (e.g., "Day One" veterinary surgical competencies), while the percentage of successful students in each cohort could be a criterion by which institutions benchmark performance. Veterinary accreditation bodies, such as the American Veterinary Medical Association (AVMA, 2016) and the Royal College of Veterinary Surgeons (RCVS, 2016), seek evidence that the curriculum equips students with entry-level professional competence, and that all graduates achieve the required standard (Yorke, 1999). The standards-based comparisons used in accreditation have attracted criticism for stifling innovation in veterinary education (Eyre, 2011). In contrast, lenient interpretations of the AVMA Council on Education (COE) standards for veterinary clinical education and research, and the lack of a learning environment focused on high-quality contemporary science in teaching and research, are key criticisms leveled at new distributed models, which some commentators believe to threaten veterinary educational outcomes (Marshak, 2011). The peak international veterinary education accreditation bodies have increased their role in defining standards over the past two decades, and commenced a voluntary process of international harmonization of standards and processes, with a high level of agreement in the Day One skills joint accreditation site visits from 2010, and an international standards rubric adopted in 2014 (Massey University, n.d.). However, accreditation does not compare institutional performance, therefore there is a place for systematic competitor benchmarking to drive continuous improvement in veterinary education.

University rankings are now influential proxy measures of quality, driving the choices of potential students and employers, and influencing government and university priorities. The first subject-specific global ranking for veterinary schools, the QS World University Ranking (QS, 2015a), was released in 2015. University rankings emphasize research metrics (i.e., citation impact of publications, grant income) and prestige (e.g., number of Nobel laureates), with little bearing on education quality. The most respected include Shanghai Jiao Tong University Academic Ranking of World Universities (ARWU, 2016), The *Times Higher Education* (2016) World University Rankings, and the National Taiwan University Ranking (NTU Ranking, 2016). The QS World University Ranking balances citation impact and productivity with a broader emphasis on graduate outcomes and reputation with employers and peers. The first QS veterinary school ranking reported a spread of top 50 performance across the United Kingdom, United States, Canada, Australia, New Zealand, and Europe, with all top 20 schools accredited by RCVS, AVMA, Australasian Veterinary Boards Council (AVBC, 2016), European Association of Establishments for Veterinary Education (EAEVE, 2016), or multiple bodies (QS, 2015b). Benchmarking is a more powerful tool than the pursuit of rankings for improving veterinary education, because it drives a proactive, constructive focus on achieving the best performance appropriate to the mission of the university (Marmolejo, 2016).

Improved research performance has been fostered in the United Kingdom (the Research Assessment Exercise, now the Research Excellence Framework) and Australia (Excellence in Research Australia, ERA; Australian Research Council, 2016) through government benchmarking, with rewards for top-performing disciplinary groups. Benchmarking activities across all areas of university operations are undertaken by members of elite research universities, such the Group of Eight in Australia, the American Public Land-Grant Universities, and the Russell International Excellence Group in the United Kingdom (Russell Group, 2016). Leading institutions foster a culture of "research-led" teaching, seeking to ensure that students realize benefits from engagement with research and leading researcher groups. However, the relationship between quality teaching and research, while often promoted, is not direct and requires institutional strategies to be effective (Schapper and Mayson, 2010). Student and employer

stakeholders in veterinary education place the greatest emphasis on professional competence and perceive less relevance in research. Top veterinary schools have responded to the rewards for research productivity and quality in the United Kingdom (HEFCE, 1997) and Australia, and to international rankings, with capacity-building investments in facilities, staff, and programs. This shift in focus and resources could threaten high-cost disciplines such as veterinary science, and limit the capacity of veterinary educators to improve continuously on educational outcomes (Camp, 1989).

This chapter will describe the process of benchmarking and what factors should be considered prior to undertaking a benchmarking exercise in veterinary education, with a focus on curriculum, learning, and student outcomes. Models of benchmarking for quality learning and student outcomes are used to illustrate the processes and procedures required, the tools and support available, examples of their use, and the ways in which benchmarking findings can best drive reflection and improvement.

How Has Benchmarking Been Used in Higher Education?

Benchmarking, as a collaborative, structured process of comparing performance and processes as a means of self-evaluation and self-improvement, was first used in industry as a mechanism to enhance productivity (Camp, 1989) and is now widely applied in higher education. Experiences in the United Kingdom suggest that academics assume a process of regulatory benchmarking, whereby academic standards are referenced to a subject benchmark toward self-assessment and, hence, self-improvement (Jackson, 2001). However, while UK academics are required to internalize and maintain the national subject standards for their discipline, benchmarking can also be an open and collaborative process aimed at identifying and sharing best practice. Known as collaborative benchmarking (see the section on "Developing a benchmark"), this strategy

Table 21.1 Comparison of quality assurance and quality enhancement.

	Standards	Review process	Benchmarks
Quality assurance (QA)	Minimally acceptable, unchanging	Mandatory review by external agencies	Independently verifiable markers set
Quality enhancement (QE)	Agreed, aspirational, progressive	Voluntary self-evaluation	Leading, learning, lagging indicators agreed

can be applied between higher education institutions to improve curricula and enhance student learning through a focus on key processes, as well as outcomes. This (collaborative) focus on parity of standards was adopted by UK government bodies for quality assurance (QA, defined later) based on an outcomes process model (Henderson-Smart *et al.*, 2006). However, quality enhancement (QE), with its focus on continuous improvement of outcomes, particularly student outcomes, is now replacing QA (Biggs and Tang, 2011; see Table 21.1).

Early benchmarking in US education resembled the model used in industry, with higher education providers using benchmarking outcomes to position themselves on a competitive basis. This was less concerned with learning and more about preparation for higher education as a growth "industry," but it did emphasize the need to have collaborative partners outside education (Epper, 1999). In the late 1990s, an international benchmarking consortium was established, the National Association of College and University Business Officers (NACUBO; Kempner, 1993). Again, this focused primarily on the administrative, statistical, and financial aspects of institutions, but did permit some comparisons globally (Garlick and Pryor, 2004). In response to the Spellings Commission's (Spellings, 2006) focus on access, affordability, quality, innovation, and stakeholder accountability, organizations of public universities in the United States (the Association of Public and Land-Grant Universities and the American Association of State Colleges and Universities) developed a Voluntary System of Accountability (VSA), and tested new broad measures of student achievement and graduate outcomes. However, the tests adopted are considered unable to recognize the diversity, breadth, and depth of discipline-specific knowledge and learning (Lederman, 2013), so have experienced limited uptake (Lederman, Loayza, and Soares, 2001). In contrast, the veterinary accrediting agencies, such as AVMA COE, responded with increased focus on these priorities, but have also come under intense scrutiny, requiring changes to their processes, structure, and decision-making.

Why Not Benchmark?

Despite the majority of positive recommendations for using benchmarking and successful examples of its current use, there are critics of its applicability to higher education. There is an opportunity cost in time and resources. Critics argue that it marginally improves existing processes, is applicable only to administrative processes, is a euphemism for copying and stifles innovation, and can expose institutional weaknesses (Brigham, 1995; Dale, 1995). These concerns are largely unfounded, because benchmarking can radically change processes (if warranted), apply to both administration and teaching, and adapt not "adopt" best practices; furthermore, if a benchmarking code of conduct is followed, confidentiality concerns can be reduced. The American Productivity and Quality Center Code of Conduct (APQC, 2016a) calls for benchmarking practitioners to abide by stated principles of legality, exchange, and confidentiality.

What About Veterinary Education Benchmarking?

Collaborative benchmarking commences with agreement on what to benchmark and which processes to adopt. It starts with the end in mind: the common goals of university education for the veterinary profession. These are defined in each school's statements of the intended knowledge, skills, and attitudes of graduating veterinarians, known as program learning outcomes (Biggs and Tang, 2011). They are designed to address the accreditation curriculum standards, and the national and international competencies – for example, NAVMEC (2011) and the OIE (2012) Core Curriculum and "'Day One Graduates" Competencies – situated within the context and mission of the individual institution. Review of curriculum maps reveals the underpinning design and instruction methods used to achieve the intended learning outcomes. Curriculum structure is central to education quality, because comprehensive, effective development of program learning outcomes is essential in professional disciplines like veterinary science. Employers expect that all graduates will be competent in solving veterinary problems through the application of scientific knowledge, technical skills, and professional behaviors (McNally, 1999; Heath and Mills, 2000).

Benchmarking of achievement in the complex, scientifically dense veterinary curriculum is a challenge, particularly in professional, ethical, humanistic domains. The danger is to concentrate on aspects amenable to measurement, neglecting those that are hard to evaluate reliably, despite their importance for professional success. Examples of successful curriculum benchmarking and development projects in Australia and New Zealand have engaged all disciplinary leaders in animal welfare, pharmacology (Office for Learning and Teaching, 2013a), and communication (Office for Learning and Teaching, 2013b), as a group, to review and develop best practice curriculum resources (e.g., veterinary pharmacology, "one welfare") collaboratively. Veterinary accreditation has increased the requirements for comprehensive assessment of students' application and integration of knowledge, skill, and behavior through direct observation measures, particularly in clinical disciplines, for instance objective structured clinical examinations (OSCE; Wikipedia, 2016b), direct observation of procedural skills (DOPS; RCPCH, 2016) or mini clinical examples (mCEX; Baillie and Rhind, 2008).

How Is the Curriculum Benchmarked?

When looking specifically at the curriculum, there are several approaches that may be used to benchmark. Specifically, standards-based benchmarking seeks to determine how good student performance needs to be to meet the learning outcomes (see Stake, 2004). To answer how much is good enough requires that a point on the skill or ability continuum is determined that represents proficient attainment for students or graduates for QA (e.g., the COMPASS tool, which benchmarks speech pathology skills, reported by McAllister *et al.*, 2011). For intra-institutional benchmarking of student learning outcomes, defining such a benchmark requires some form of standard-setting. The field of standard-setting in educational measurement is based on judgment and in some rare instances can be empirical, employing different methodologies to accomplish this purpose (see Pitoniak and Morgan, 2012). It should also be noted that accreditation bodies are increasingly setting the skills that students must attain before graduation (Day- One Competencies) and defining the level of competence required for graduation (UGC, n.d.).

A second type of curriculum benchmarking establishes a criterion of performance growth or progress over time using baselines (ASQ, 2011). A third type of curriculum benchmarking can assess indirect measures of student learning, such as the National Survey of Student Engagement (NSSE, 2016). The relationships identified between students' experience of learning and the quality of their learning are important to recognize, because engagement is vital if students are to transform their knowledge and understanding during their studies. As a consequence, student engagement is an important leading measure in predicting the future impact of curricula and teaching on student achievement.

How Do Accreditation and Benchmarking Differ?

Standards of veterinary training are monitored in Australia and New Zealand by the veterinary registration bodies that oversee accreditation (AVBC, 2016). There is a national standard, the Australasian veterinary graduate attributes (GA), on which each institution bases its program learning outcomes, and these reference RCVS and OIE Day One skills. Prior to the AVMA's introduction of outcomes assessment (Simmons, 2004), accreditation visits had a focus on inputs, including teaching hours, curriculum structure, facilities, access to animals, and caseload for practical experience. Accreditation has shifted to the evaluation of program, student, and institutional outcomes, although the requirement to report on inputs continues for AVBC/RCVS. Effective outcomes assessment requires evidence of review, which can take the form of benchmarking and then effective action to address identified deficits, with ongoing monitoring. Accreditors now seek evidence of graduate "fitness for purpose," including indicators of employment, career impact, and professional retention. An International Accreditation Working Group was formed to harmonize standards and support the demand for "global" accreditation visits of RCVS, AVBC, AVMA, and EAVE, and it developed a rubric for site visit assessments.

Support and Tools Available for Benchmarking

There are a number of resources available to support and/or undertake benchmarking, many of which are online. The American Productivity and Quality Center benchmarking user's guides are available via an online portal (APQC, 2016b), although this is more targeted at business than educational institutions. Benchmarking tools were designed by the US National Association

of College and University Business Office (NACUBO, 2016) for educational institutions (Kempner, 1993). Benchmarking can also be performed independently by an external service provider, such as the European Association for International Education (EAIE, 2014). Subject external examiners with internationally recognized expertise review courses and moderate assessment within their field, following a set of guidelines at University College Dublin (UCD, n.d.). This is a form of direct outcomes assessment, sought by professional accreditation bodies, which will also identify areas requiring improvement compared to external benchmarks.

A comprehensive benchmarking manual developed for the Australian Commonwealth Department of Education, Training and Youth Affairs (McKinnon, Walker, and Davis, 2000) provides a robust set of tools to ascertain university performance trends and to initiate continuous self-improvement activities. The benchmarking metrics use a "lagging, leading, and learning" framework and permit universities to ascertain their competitive position relative to others. McKinnon, Walker, and Davis (2000) proposed 67 benchmarks for higher education institutes, but admitted that these may be unwieldy to monitor on a regular basis and suggested a list of 25 core benchmarks. In practice, many institutions routinely report on 15 or fewer key performance indicators, and fewer than 5 of these relate to students' learning. The Tertiary Education Quality and Standards Agency Guidance Note on Benchmarking (TEQSA, n.d.) has been adapted by most Australian universities.

Developing a Benchmark

Classifications of Benchmarking

Classifications are useful to define the scope and outcomes anticipated from benchmarking (Jackson and Lund, 2000). The processes that characterize benchmarking for best practice in education are described in what follows (Jackson, 2001; Schofield, 1998, 2000) (see also Box 21.3).

Box 21.3: Quick tips on benchmarking: Before you benchmark

Before you benchmark you should have clear definitions of the scope and outcomes you anticipate. A well-defined model or guidelines facilitates the process, simplifies future benchmarking, and defines the approach used and information required.

Implicit or Explicit

Benchmarking can be implicit, a by-product of information gathering by an external agency (e.g., the Australian Graduate Destination Survey of veterinary graduate employment rates), or explicit, using a structured process to gather data not currently available, but important to the institution's goals (e.g., reporting on the success of initiatives to foster resilience in graduating veterinarians).

Independent or Collaborative

Independent benchmarking compares performance against information within a customized database or the public domain (e.g., the performance of veterinary graduates in the US National Veterinary Board examinations or student attrition rates) to determine whether they meet external standards. A more usual process involves collaborative benchmarking between institutions that agree to compare performance in a formal and structured manner (e.g., students' competence level in core manipulative skills in bovine pregnancy diagnosis) against an agreed standard.

Internally or Externally Focused

Internal benchmarking uses comparisons between units, courses, schools, or centers within a university without an external standard (e.g., academic board reviews of colleges). External benchmarking may be competitive, where performance is compared against competitors – for example the Asia Pacific University ranking – or collaborative, involving comparison between universities with a focus on quality assurance – for example reviews by TEQSA (2016), formerly the Australian Universities Quality Agency (AUQA, 2006), or VSA in the United States.

Vertical and Horizontal Processes

Vertical benchmarking compares the performance of a defined functional area (e.g., College of Veterinary Medicine), focusing on the entire process, whereas horizontal benchmarking compares across several functional areas (e.g., student academic misconduct). A further example of process-focused benchmarking may involve selecting activities representative of the higher education institution that are compared with similar activities in other institutions (e.g., admissions processes).

Quantitative and Qualitative Approaches

The qualitative approach involves an informed discussion process, which may be facilitated by an independent consultant and is usually collegiate and developmental (e.g., comparison of veterinary public health curricula when commencing an OIE twinning program). The quantitative approach involves a more defined, systemic approach using agreed measures of performance to compare processes and achievements (Akhlagi, 1997). Quantitation relies on measurement of performance against agreed indicators, which may be lagging (e.g., student progress rates or graduate employment rates, which indicate past performance), learning (e.g., student perceptions of learning, which reflect current performance), or leading (e.g., learning and teaching plans, which anticipate future performance; McKinnon, Walker, and Davis, 2000). The selection of prospective quality enhancement measures for monitoring and driving change is essential.

How to Undertake a Benchmarking Review

Benchmarking can be conducted in a way that is problem based or process based (Stewart, 1996). Problem-based benchmarking investigates problems as they occur, for instance arising from feedback or cost–benefit analysis, and can be largely *ad hoc.* In contrast, process-based benchmarking is a management strategy to incorporate regular review and improvement practices. Stewart (1996) defined steps for continuous improvement in higher education, building on the initial process model described by Spendolini (1992) and Henderson-Smart *et al.* (2006). We have adapted these steps for veterinary education using the Australian TEQSA model.

Step 1: Scope or Goals

Specify what is to be benchmarked. Focus on key processes that are central to the success of the institution's mission. Some examples include preclinical student performance in medical schools (O'Mara *et al.*, 2015), the COM-PASS speech pathology competency-based assessment tool (McAllister *et al.*, 2011), and outcomes from university teacher training (Weeks, 2000).

Step 2: Establish Benchmarking Partnerships

Select a range of benchmarking partners, including some that are perceived to be "better" and some "not as good" in order better to identify aspects of process that actually enhance standards (see Box 21.4). Good partnerships start with an agreement on purpose, a commitment to shared learning, and collaboration rather than competition. Partners define terms and agree on confidentiality, distribution of findings, and possible authorship, if publication is anticipated.

Step 3: Design, Plan, and Secure Resources

Form a benchmarking team in each university, incorporating process owners into the team. Where the activity is embedded in the routine processes and data collection of the institutional administration team, it is more easily managed and more likely to be incorporated in business as usual. The team establishes a schedule, allocates tasks, identifies data sources, and agrees on a systematic, unbiased collection methodology and communications plan.

Step 4: Self-Review

Identify stakeholders to answer particular sections, then collect the data, triangulate it where possible, and analyze it, with the benchmarking team documenting its own internal processes for collection and analysis.

Step 5: Peer Review

The benchmarking partner universities meet to review data and analysis, compare and validate processes, and together identify best practices and focus areas for improvement. A workshop format assists participants in interpretation, learning, and skills development from the exercise.

 Box 21.4: Quick tips on benchmarking: Getting started

A simple approach to benchmarking is to establish contact with colleagues teaching a similar discipline at different institutions. Share and discuss learning objectives, teaching activities, assessment tasks, and outcomes (grades, student satisfaction, staff workloads) to determine which aspects are enhancing student learning. Sharing resources and collaborating on resource development are excellent approaches to improving student outcomes and staff satisfaction, while limiting the impact of curriculum renewal on workloads.

Step 6: Communicate and Implement Change

Prepare a report identifying improvement opportunities and proposing an action plan, and submit it to academic leaders. This will include future iterations of the benchmarking exercise and a series of milestones for when any changes should be introduced.

Step 7: Reflect, Evaluate, and Review

The benchmarking partners reflect on the impact and outcomes of the benchmarking exercise and may share their learning.

Using Benchmarks

Once benchmarks have been identified, the focus can turn to what legitimate uses can be made of benchmarking data on student learning outcomes. Before this question can be answered adequately, there are a number of obstacles that need to be overcome, especially if decisions made based on benchmarking data can be used to effect change. Foremost is that faculty development initiatives may be needed to overcome resistance to the process or outcomes of benchmarking, particularly where curriculum change is proposed after a long period of stasis. Resistance can also result from politically charged comparisons with peer institutions that operate within different contexts. Outcomes assessment has traditionally meant closing the loop after an

intervention has taken place. This can take up to a decade, for instance for curriculum or admissions changes to have an impact on graduate employment. However, benchmarking can close this loop earlier by monitoring leading as well as lagging performance indicators, accelerating progress in improving student outcomes.

Conclusion

Benchmarking is a powerful mechanism to inform curriculum renewal and future development. It provides a potent stimulus for change and, importantly, can identify proven strategies for improvement. It can be used in a focused manner, such as a specific discipline within a curriculum, or to provide an overview of the quality of the entire curriculum, encompassing student learning and outcomes. Benchmarking should be seen as a pathway to improve rather than merely a comparison between cognate institutions, and, as such, should be part of institutional management to ensure best practice. Veterinary educators are benchmarking more frequently at a global level than ever before, in defining the expectations for veterinary graduate capability. The rise in veterinary education as a discipline and in benchmarking projects to improve veterinary education has been remarkable in the past decade, but there remains a dearth of literature describing the processes and outcomes of benchmarking.

References

AAVMC (2011) *Roadmap for Veterinary Medical Education in the 21st Century – Responsive, Collaborative, Flexible*. http://www.aavmc.org/NAVMEC/NAVMEC-Final-Report-Roadmap-for-the-Future-of-Veterinary-Medical-Education.aspx (accessed November 11, 2016).

Akhlaghi, F. (1997) How to approach process benchmarking in facilities management: Catering services in the UK National Health Service. *Facilities*, **15** (**3/4**), 57–61.

APQC (2016a) *Benchmarking Code of Conduct*. https://www.apqc.org/knowledge-base/documents/benchmarking-code-conduct-0 (accessed November 11, 2016).

APQC (2016b) Open Standards Benchmarking. https://www.apqc.org/benchmarking-portal/users-guide (accessed November 11, 2016).

ARWU (2016) *World Top 500 Universities*. http://www.shanghairanking.com/ (accessed November 11, 2016).

ASQ (2011) *Criteria for performance excellence 2011–2012*. American Society for Quality. National Institute of Standards and Technology, Gaithersberg, MD.

AUQA (2006) *Australian Universities Quality Agency: Quality Audit*. Australian Universities Quality Agency, Perth.

Australian Research Council (2016) *Excellence in Research for Australia*. http://www.arc.gov.au/excellence-research-australia (accessed November 11, 2016).

AVBC (2016) *Australasian Veterinary Boards Council Inc*. https://www.avbc.asn.au/ (accessed November 11, 2016).

AVMA (2016) *Veterinary Education*. https://www.avma.org/ProfessionalDevelopment/Education/Pages/default.aspx (accessed November 11, 2016).

Baillie, S., and Rhind, S. (2008) *A Guide to Assessment Methods in Veterinary Medicine*. http://www.live.ac.uk/Media/LIVE/PDFs/assessment_guide.pdf (accessed November 11, 2016).

Biggs, J.B., and Tang, C. (2011) *Teaching for Quality Learning at University*, Open University Press/McGraw-Hill, Buckingham.

Brigham, S. (1995) *Benchmarking*. HEPROC CQI-L Archive. American Association for Higher Education, Washington, DC.

Camp, R.C. (1989) *Benchmarking: The Search for Industry Best Practices That Lead to Superior Performance*, ASQC Quality Press, Milwaukee, WI.

Chaffee, E.L., and Sherr, L.A. (1992) Quality transforming postsecondary education. *ASHE-ERIC Higher Education Report*, **21** (3), 59–78.

Clark, K.L. (1993) Benchmarking as a global strategy for improving instruction in higher education, XI International Conference on New Concepts in Higher Education, December 5–9, Phoenix, AZ.

Dale, B. (1995) Practical benchmarking for colleges and universities. *ASHE-ERIC Higher Education Report*, **24** (5), 19–38.

EAEVE (2016) *The Association: Foundation, Mission and Objectives*. http://www.eaeve.org/about-eaeve/mission-and-objectives.html (accessed November 11, 2016).

EAIE (2014) *Benchmarking Your University*. European Association for International Education, Amsterdam. http://www.eaie.org/blog/benchmarking-your-university/ (accessed November 11, 2016).

Epper, R. (1999) Applying benchmarking to higher education. *Change*, November, 24–31.

Eyre, P. (2011) All-purpose veterinary education: A personal perspective. *Journal of Veterinary Medical Education*, **38**, 328–337.

Garlick, S., and Pryor, G. (2004) *Benchmarking the University: Learning about Improvement. A Report for the Department of Education, Science and Training*. Commonwealth of Australia, Canberra.

Heath, T.J., and Mills, J.N. (2000) Criteria used by employers to select new graduate employees. *Australian Veterinary Journal*, **78**, 312–316.

HEFCE (1997) *Response by the Higher Education Funding Council for England to the Report of the National Committee of Inquiry into Higher Education*. http://webarchive.nationalarchives.gov.uk/20120118171947/http:/www.hefce.ac.uk/pubs/hefce/1997/m18_97.htm (accessed November 11, 2016).

Henderson-Smart, C., Winning, T., Gerzina, T., *et al.* (2006) Benchmarking learning and teaching: Developing a method. *Quality Assurance in Education*, **14** (2), 143–155.

Jackson, N. (2001) Benchmarking in UK HE: An overview. *Quality Assurance in Education*, **9**, 218–235.

Jackson, N., and Lund, H. (2000) Introduction to benchmarking, in *Benchmarking for Higher Education* (eds N. Jackson and H. Lund), Open University Press, Buckingham, pp. 3–12.

Judd, T., and Keith, B. (2012) Student learning outcomes at the program and institutional levels, in *Handbook on Measurement, Assessment, and Evaluation in Higher Education* (eds C. Secolsky and D.B. Denison), Routledge, New York, pp. 31–46.

Judd, T.P., Pondish, C., and Secolsky, C. (2013) Issues in institutional benchmarking of student learning outcomes using case examples. *Research in Higher Education Journal*, **20**, 1–15. http://www.aabri.com/manuscripts/121397.pdf (accessed November 11, 2016).

Kempner, D.E. (1993) The pilot years: The growth of the NACUBO Benchmarking Project. *NACUBO Business Officer*, **27** (**6**), 21–31.

Lederman, D. (2013) Public university accountability 2.0. *Inside Higher Ed*, May 6. https://www.insidehighered.com/news/2013/05/06/public-university-accountability-system-expands-ways-report-student-learning (accessed November 11, 2016).

Lederman, D., Loayza, N., and Soares, R.R. (2001) *Accountability and Corruption: Political Institutions Matter*. World Bank, Washington, DC. doi:10.1596/1813-9450-2708

Marmolejo, F. (2016) Is benchmarking more useful than ranking? *University World News*, January 15. http://www.universityworldnews.com/article.php?story=20160113012615813 (accessed November 11, 2016).

Marshak, R.R. (2011) Veterinary school accreditation: On a slippery slope? *Journal of the American Veterinary Medical Association*, **239**, 1183–1187.

Massey University (n.d.) AVMA Clinical Competencies/RCVS Day One Skills. http://www.massey.ac.nz/massey/fms/Colleges/College%20of%20Sciences/IVABS/vetschool/IVMA%20/AVMA-RCVS%20LO.pdf (accessed November 11, 2016).

McAllister, S., Lincoln, M.I., Ferguson, A., *et al.* (2011) *The Benchmarking COMPASS Database: A Confidential Interactive Web Based Strategy to Benchmark Learning Outcomes*. Australian Universities Quality Forum: Demonstrating Quality, Melbourne. http://www.olt.gov.au/resource-establishing-infrastructure-and-collaborative-processes-cross-institutional-benchmarking-st (accessed November 11, 2016).

McKinnon, K.R., Walker, S.H., and Davis, D. (2000) *Benchmarking: A Manual for Australian Universities*. Department of Education, Service and Training, Commonwealth of Australia, Canberra.

McNally, J.M.K. (1999) Working in groups and teams. In *Using Group-Based Learning in Higher Education* (eds L. Thorley and R. Gregory), Kogan Page, London. pp. 113–122.

NACUBO (2016) *Getting Started on Benchmaking*. National Association of College and University Business Officers, Washington, DC. http://www.nacubo.org/Research/Benchmarking_Resources.html (accessed November 11, 2016).

NAVMEC (2011) *Roadmap for Veterinary Medical Education in the 21st Century: Responsive, Collaborative, Flexible*. North American Veterinary Medical Education Consortium, Washington, DC. http://www.aavmc.org/data/files/navmec/navmec_roadmapreport_web_booklet.pdf (accessed November 11, 2016).

NSSE (2016) *National Survey of Student Engagement*. http://nsse.indiana.edu/ (accessed November 11, 2016).

NTU Ranking (2016) *Performance Ranking of Scientific Papers for World Universities*. http://nturanking.lis.ntu.edu.tw/ (accessed November 11, 2016).

Office for Learning and Teaching (2013a) *Resource Library: Pharmacology*. http://www.olt.gov.au/resource-library?text=pharmacology (accessed November 11, 2016).

Office for Learning and Teaching (2013b) *Resource Library: Veterinary Communication*. http://www.olt.gov.au/resource-library?text=veterinary+communication (accessed November 11, 2016).

OIE (2012) *OIE Recommendations on the Competencies of Graduating Veterinarians ("Day 1" Graduates) to Assure National Veterinary Services of Quality*. World Organisation for Animal Health, Paris. http://www.oie.int/fileadmin/Home/eng/Support_to_OIE_Members/Vet_Edu_AHG/DAY_1/DAYONE-B-ang-vC.pdf (accessed November 11, 2016).

O'Mara, D.A., Canny, B.J., Rothnie, I.P., *et al.* (2015) The Australian Medical Schools Assessment Collaboration: Benchmarking the preclinical performance of medical students. *Medical Journal of Australia*, **202**, 95–99.

Pitoniak, M., and Morgan, D. (2012) Setting and validating cutscores for tests, in *Handbook on*

Measurement, Assessment, and Evaluation in Higher Education (eds C. Secolsky and D.B. Denison), Routledge, New York, pp. 343–366.

QS (2015a) *Top Universities.* http://www.topuniversities.com/ (accessed November 11, 2016).

QS (2015b) *New Ranking of the World's Top Veterinary Schools.* http://www.topuniversities.com/university-rankings-articles/university-subject-rankings/new-ranking-worlds-top-veterinary-schools (accessed November 11, 2016).

RCPCH (2016) *Directly Observed Procedural Skills (DOPS).* Royal College of Paediatrics and Child Health, London. http://www.rcpch.ac.uk/training-examinations-professional-development/assessment-and-examinations/assessment-tools/directly (accessed November 11, 2016).

RCVS (2016) *Education.* http://www.rcvs.org.uk/education/ (accessed November 11, 2016).

Rush, S.C. (1994) Benchmarking – How good is good? in *Measuring Institutional Performance in Higher Education* (eds J.W. Meyerson and W.F. Massey), Petersons, Princeton, NJ, pp. 83–97.

Russell Group (2016) *About.* http://www.russellgroup.ac.uk/about (accessed November 11, 2016).

Schapper, J., and Mayson, S.E. (2010) Research-led teaching: Moving from a fractured engagement to a marriage of convenience. *Higher Education Research and Development*, **29**, 641–651.

Schofield, A. (ed.) (1998) *Benchmarking in Higher Education: An International Review*, Commonwealth Higher Education Management Service, London. http://www.temarium.com/wordpress/wp-content/documentos/Schofield.-Benchmarking-in-HE-an-International-Review.pdf (accessed November 11, 2016).

Schofield, A. (2000) The growth of benchmarking in higher education. *Lifelong Learning in Europe*, **5**, 100–105.

Simmons, D. (2004) The American Veterinary Medical Association Council on Education (COE) Accreditation. *Journal of Veterinary Medical Education*, **31**, 92–95.

Spellings, M. (2006) *A Test of Leadership: Charting the Future of U.S. Higher Education.* U.S. Department of Education, Jessup, MD. http://www2.ed.gov/about/bdscomm/list/hiedfuture/index.html (accessed November 20, 2016).

Spendolini, M.J. (1992) *The Benchmarking Book*, American Management Association, New York.

Stake, R.E (2004) *Standards-Based and Responsive Evaluation*, Sage, Thousand Oaks, CA.

Stewart, R.G. (1996) Key process benchmarking for continuous improvement in higher Education. Master's thesis, Faculty of the Department of Technology, East Tennessee State University.

TEQSA (n.d.) *TEQSA Guidance Note on Benchmarking.* Tertiary Education Quality and Standards Agency, Melbourne. http://www.teqsa.gov.au/sites/default/files/BenchmarkingGNFinal_0.pdf (accessed November 11, 2016).

TEQSA (2016) *Welcome to TEQSA.* http://www.teqsa.gov.au/ (accessed November 11, 2016).

Times Higher Education (2016) *World University Rankings.* http://www.timeshighereducation.co.uk/world-university-rankings (accessed November 11, 2016).

UCD (n.d.) *Guidelines for UCD Staff on the Subject Extern Examiner Process.* University College Dublin. http://www.ucd.ie/registry/assessment/staff_info/subjectexternguidelinesstaff.pdf (accessed November 11, 2016).

UGC (n.d.) *Accreditation System for Veterinary Schools by Australasian Veterinary Boards Council (AVBC), American Veterinary Medical Association (AVMA) and Royal College of Veterinary Surgeons (RCVS).* University Grants Committee of the Hong Kong Special Administrative Region, Hong Kong. http://www.ugc.edu.hk/eng/doc/ugc/publication/report/vstfreport/accreditation.pdf (accessed November 11, 2016).

Weeks, P. (2000) Benchmarking in higher education: An Australian case study. *Innovations in Education and Training International*, **37**, 59–67.

Background

Accreditation may be defined as a recognition status granted to an educational institution (institutional accreditation) or college or school within an institution or an educational program (specialized accreditation) that maintains suitable standards of education. One goal of accreditation is "educational improvement through enforcement of quality educational practices" (Simmons, 2004, p. 89).

Accreditation of higher education institutions or educational programs assures the quality of institutions and programs. An accreditation system differs from an internal review system, as the accreditor protects the interests of the public, universities who accept course work in transfer from other institutions, licensing authorities, employers, and students, by assuring that educational programs meet acceptable levels of quality delivery of curriculum, learning, and student outcomes. In the United States, federal and state governments rely on the accreditation status of institutions to determine whether they are eligible to receive grants and loans. For example, in order for institutions to be eligible to receive Title IV student loans and scholarships and/or Health Professions Student Loans, they must be accredited by an accrediting agency recognized by the USDE as a reliable authority on the quality of education provided by the institution or program (Schray, 2006).

The task of American accreditation agencies, whether national, regional, or specialized, is to identify and develop quality standards, determine whether institutions and programs meet these standards, and foster a process for continuous quality improvement. In the United States, accreditors may be recognized by the USDE and may also choose to be recognized by the Council for Higher Education Accreditation (CHEA), a nongovernmental agency (Schray, 2006).

According to the standards established by the USDE, every recognized accrediting organization must demonstrate that it has an accreditation process that effectively addresses the quality of institutions or programs in several areas, including successful student achievement; curricula; faculty; facilities, equipment, supplies; fiscal and administrative capacity; student support services; recruiting and admission practices; hard-copy and electronic communications; program specifics; student complaints; and compliance under Title IV of the Higher Education Act.

The process of accreditation of the institution by the accrediting organization usually involves institutional self-study, peer review, site visits, a status decision by the organization, and specified monitoring and oversight throughout the accreditation cycle. Three major issues stimulating reform in the higher education accreditation system in the United States are the accountability of the accreditation system, support for innovation in education delivery, and the consistency of accreditation standards and processes across different accrediting organizations, to allow for greater transparency across different accrediting institutions (Schray, 2006).

Specialized accreditation follows the same process; however, the accreditation standards are focused on the specific profession or area of study, and are developed with input from the profession and other stakeholders. Although accreditation status is voluntarily sought by veterinary medical educational programs, accreditation by an accrediting agency acceptable to the veterinary statutory body (VSB), which oversees the quality and competence of veterinarians in a particular country, is required for eligibility for licensure in the United States and Canada. The same cannot be said of accreditation systems of educational institutions in different regions of the world.

In the field of human medical education, there is wide variability in the prevalence of national accrediting bodies by region, ranging from 20% in Africa to 75% in Southeast Asia (WHO-WFME, 2005). This variability is expected to be wider in veterinary medical education. For example, in the United States and Canada, the AVMA COE is recognized as an accreditor of veterinary medical education programs by state and provincial VSBs; the Royal College of Veterinary Surgeons (RCVS) and its accrediting body has statutory authority to accredit veterinary medical educational programs in the United Kingdom; and the Australasian Veterinary Boards Council (AVBC) and its accrediting agency have statutory authority to accredit veterinary medical educational programs in Australia and New Zealand. The European Association of Establishments for Veterinary Education (EAEVE) and the Federation of Veterinarians of Europe (FVE), through the European System of Evaluation and Training (ESEVT), have a system of evaluation for veterinary medical educational programs in Europe. The decision-making body for this system, the European Committee of Veterinary Education (ECOVE), is an independent entity whose office operates under the umbrella of the EAEVE. This system does not have ties to a VSB. Other nations have implemented or are in the process of implementing systems to evaluate or accredit veterinary medical educational programs. Examples include the Accreditation and Recognition of Veterinary School Qualifications & Accreditations Committee of the Malaysian Veterinary Council, the Accreditation Board for Veterinary Education in Korea (ABOVE-K), and El Consejo Nacional de Educación de la Medicina Veterinaria y Zootecnia in Mexico (CONEVET).

A number of nations have not yet implemented any sort of evaluation or accreditation system. This is unfortunate, since accreditation enhances the improvement of educational processes and could lead to quality, state-of-the-art education throughout the world. In practice, even in world regions where accreditation systems exist, standards and processes vary in intent, procedural complexity, transparency, accountability, and consequences of the evaluation (Zarco, 2009; van Zanten *et al.*, 2008; ECFMG, 2010). It is for this reason that, in medical education at least, there is a move toward the evaluation and recognition of accrediting bodies by a single international agency using globally accepted criteria, in the aim that this would create a meaningful system of international accreditation (ECFMG, 2010). We are a long way from implementation of any sort of truly international accreditation in veterinary medicine.

History of Accreditation

The first European veterinary school was established in France in 1761. In the United States, 34 veterinary colleges were opened between 1854 and 1900. These early colleges struggled to survive due to inadequately trained faculty, a lack of committed students, poor admission standards, and unethical behavior, such that 19 of them closed (Banasiak, 2012). The lack of standardization of education between the early colleges and the inconsistent quality of the diplomas that were conferred played a role in the formation of the standing Committee on Intelligence and Education (CIE) within the United States Veterinary Medical Association (USVMA) in the late 1800s. The CIE would eventually evolve into the current COE (AVMA, 2014).

A major milestone in America's journey to a quality veterinary professional education system was the creation of the Bureau of Animal Industry (BAI) within the United States Department of Agriculture (USDA) at the beginning of the twentieth century. The federal bureau became a major employer of veterinarians, and only graduates of a bureau-acceptable veterinary school could sit for the civil service examination required for BAI employment (Banasiak, 2012). Whether or not a school was acceptable by BAI standards was determined by a committee, appointed by the Secretary of Agriculture and consisting of representatives of the BAI, the Association of Veterinary Faculties of North America that was formed in 1894, and the AVMA (the USVMA underwent a name change in 1898). A bureau-acceptable veterinary school had to comply with a series of prescriptive recommendations in order to remain on the acceptable list. The recommendations included stipulations about length of study, minimum number of instructional days in a year, minimum number of teaching/contact hours, the nature of the curriculum, and the textbooks to be used. The bureau even maintained a file on each student. However, the CIE became increasingly concerned that the bureau's rigid curriculum requirements and faculty standards also harbored a disregard for sound teaching principles (Banasiak, 2012).

In 1921, the AVMA adopted minimum standards of education called the Essentials of an Approved Veterinary College, which specified requirements such as minimum number of major departments and veterinary leadership and administration. These essentials were the beginnings of the modern COE standards of accreditation. An amendment to the AVMA Bylaws in 1928 officially terminated the CIE and created a new five-member Committee on Education. At least three members had to be faculty members representing different colleges. School acceptance took place through questionnaires; visits to the colleges by members of this group did not take place until the late 1940s. In 1946, the AVMA restructured the Committee on Education and replaced it with a nine-member Council on Education. Since then, the essentials have been revised and developed into the COE standards of accreditation (AVMA, 2014).

After World War II, veterinary colleges found it a burden to be accredited by both the USDA, then the largest accreditor, and the COE (Banasiak, personal communication). The United States Army also was compiling a list of accredited schools (Banasiak, personal communication). Efforts by the National Council on Accrediting (NCA) and the GI Bill of 1952 (the Veterans Readjustment Benefits Act of 1952) allowed the COE to be on a list of regional and specialized accrediting associations recognized by the military. In 1956, the NCA recognized the AVMA COE as its official accrediting association for veterinarians (UBSA 1967), but USDA relinquished its accrediting activities only after veterinary colleges and the Association of Deans of American Colleges of Veterinary Medicine recommended that it do so, in 1961 (Banasiak, personal communication).

The AVMA COE was included on the first list of nationally recognized accrediting agencies by the USDE in 1952. In addition to recognition by the USDE, the COE also earned the recognition of the CHEA, which it has maintained since 1949 (AVMA, 2015a). The CHEA is a nongovernmental organization that sets recognition standards that agencies must meet to be awarded recognition. CHEA recognition has

three purposes: the advancement of academic quality; demonstration of accountability by agencies; and assurance that agencies have standards that encourage institutions to review, plan, and implement change as needed (CHEA, 2010). The COE seeks renewal of recognition by the USDE every five years and by the CHEA every ten years. Recognition by the USDE and CHEA is voluntary.

In 1973, the COE first granted accreditation to a school outside of North America, the Faculty of Veterinary Medicine at the State University of Utrecht in the Netherlands. As of 2014, the COE has accredited 49 schools in total, 14 of which are located outside of the United States and Canada (AVMA, 2015b). Liaison and/or advisory relationships are also held by COE members with committees overseeing the education and activities of veterinary technology programs in North America, credentialing of graduates of foreign veterinary medical colleges, and licensing examinations (AVMA, 2015b).

Integration with University-Level Systems of Accreditation

All COE-accredited colleges of veterinary medicine must be a part of an institution of higher learning accredited by an organization recognized for that purpose by its country's government. In the United States, most institutions of higher learning voluntarily seek institutional accreditation by one of several regional or national accreditors. Institutional accreditation involves a comprehensive review of all institutional functions. It assures the educational community, the general public, and other organizations that an accredited institution has met high standards of quality and effectiveness. A veterinary college may be accredited only when it is a major academic administrative division of the parent institution and is afforded the same recognition, status, and autonomy as other professional colleges in that institution. For example, if a veterinary college seeking AVMA COE accreditation was affiliated with a university that also offered medical, dental, and nursing programs, then the deans of each of those programs should be subject to the same reporting and hierarchical structure as the dean of the veterinary medical program.

Goals of Accreditation

The goal of accreditation for the profession is to ensure that all students are offered a veterinary medical education that provides them with the knowledge, critical thinking, and clinical skills to be employed in the occupations that society values and that require veterinary medical training. To be eligible to take the North American Veterinary Licensing Examination (NAVLE), passing of which is required to practice veterinary medicine in the United States, students must graduate from an AVMA COE–accredited school or have passed the necessary licensing examinations for graduates of nonaccredited schools – Educational Commission for Foreign Veterinary Graduates (ECFVG) or Program for the Assessment of Veterinary Medical Equivalence (PAVE) (ICVA, 2015). Accreditation is not a tool to control market forces. For example, accreditation status is not used to control the number of accredited schools or the number of veterinary students trained in a given country or region. Accreditation is also not used to rank schools for quality. All schools are held to a defined set of standards and are judged only on whether or not they meet that standard, not by how much they may exceed the standard.

The goal of accreditation for a school is to ensure ongoing process improvement. The standards are evaluated and updated regularly to ensure that veterinary medical education is contemporary. Meeting accreditation standards at a given point in time is not a sinecure; schools are required to remain abreast of changes in society and in pedagogy that may alter the standards over time.

Current Mechanism of COE Accreditation

The reader is directed to the AVMA Center for Veterinary Education Accreditation (AVMA, 2016) for complete and continuously updated information regarding the processes of accreditation.

Membership of the COE

American members of the COE are chosen by the AVMA and by the Association of American Veterinary Medical Colleges (AAVMC). Members are selected to represent the profession and the public, and include representatives from academia and industry; different occupational sectors such as private practice (small animal, equine, food animal, mixed animal), basic science, preventive medicine, and nonprivate, nonacademic veterinary medicine; and research. Public members cannot be affiliated with a veterinarian or veterinary college. Canadian members of the COE are chosen by the Canadian Veterinary Medical Association and usually are appointed from that country's National Examining Board. All members of the COE sign confidentiality and conflict-of-interest agreements, which state that they will not divulge private information about specific schools, and will not participate in discussions or voting for institutions where they are or have been employed or with which they have substantial affiliations.

Accreditation Processes

All accreditation processes start with submission by the college of an in-depth report known as a self-study. The self-study follows a prescribed format and is a concise body of documentation by the school regarding how it meets the standards of accreditation. The COE provides review of materials submitted by colleges and provides site teams to visit the college. The goal of the site visit is to verify and supplement information presented in the self-study documents, and to address questions or concerns occasioned by reading of the self-study by members of the site team and the full Council.

Several types of site visits may take place, depending on the stage of development of the veterinary college:

- *Consultative site visit.* A consultative site visit is a nonbinding review of a developing school in North America or an established school elsewhere in the world, and is described in more detail later in this chapter.
- *Comprehensive site visit.* A comprehensive site visit is a 3–5-day on-site evaluation of the school and associated educational facilities. A team is made up of trained site team members who are not sitting members of the COE, with approval of that membership by the dean of the college that is being visited. Site teams for schools in the United States have one Canadian representative and site teams for Canadian schools have two representatives from the United States. Observers may be part of the team; these may include COE members, and other people requiring training in how site visits are conducted, or in place to ensure proper protocols are followed. A staff member also accompanies every team to provide logistical support and ensure that proper protocols are followed and that all documentation is completed. Observers and the staff member are nonvoting members of the team. There are a set number of required meetings between the site team and the college's administration, faculty, and staff to ensure complete understanding of the school's compliance with all standards (Table 22.1). The site team uses information gathered from the self-study, its tour of the facilities, and these meetings to complete a rubric (AVMA, n.d.).
- *Focused site visit.* Focused site visits are undertaken by small groups, usually including site team members who have previously visited the college, to evaluate specific standards of concern or new initiatives instituted by the college.

Accreditation Standards

There are 11 standards that must be met by any school striving to achieve or maintain accreditation. The following is a list of the standards, the rationale behind each standard, and specific items assessed to determine whether a school is meeting the standard.

Standard 1: Organization

The overall goal of this standard is to ensure a governance structure that will permit ongoing decision-making by knowledgeable individuals within the college and adequate support from the larger institution. Specific factors that are evaluated by the site team and Council include the following:

- Does the college have a well-developed mission statement and does it follow that mission statement and its associated values and purposes?
- Is the college part of an institution of higher learning that is accredited by an organization recognized by that country's government?
- Is the college afforded the same recognition, status, and autonomy as other professional colleges in that institution?
- Are the dean and officer(s) responsible for the professional, ethical, and academic affairs of the college veterinarians?
- Are there sufficient administrative staff to manage the affairs of the college?

Standard 2: Finances

The overall goal of this standard is to ensure that current finances and financial planning are adequate to ensure continuation of the program, with support for growth or change as deemed necessary by the college. Specific factors that are evaluated by the site team and Council include the following:

- Are current finances adequate to sustain the educational programs and mission of the college?
- What is the impact of non-DVM programs offered by the college, if applicable (undergraduate degree programs, veterinary technical programs, etc.)?
- Does instructional integrity take priority over the financial self-sufficiency of clinical services, field services, and teaching hospitals?

Standard 3: Physical Facilities and Equipment

The overall goal of this standard is to ensure adequate and safe facilities and equipment for

Table 22.1 Site team meetings.

MEETING	STANDARDS ADDRESSED	GOAL OF MEETING
Required meetings		
Dean and selected administrators	Organization, Finance	To confirm governance structure in the school/college, including effectiveness and flexibility; to clarify data in finance tables and discuss factors influencing financial viability of the school/college
Admissions Committee, admission officer, outcome officer(s)	Admissions, Outcomes Assessment	To clarify admissions processes as described in the standard
Curriculum Committee, outcome officer(s)	Curriculum, Outcomes Assessment	To clarify curriculum, verify processes for ongoing curricular review
DVM students – 2–3 representatives of each class, chosen by their peers	Students, Curriculum, Admissions, Organization, Physical Facilities and Equipment, Clinical Resources	To gather from the students their impressions/concerns regarding all aspects of their experience in veterinary school
Research Committee	Research	To document the adequacy of the research program and how DVM student learning is affected by the research program
Postgraduate students, interns, and residents – representatives who interact with DVM students, all clinical departments	Research, Students, Curriculum, Clinical Resources, Physical Facilities and Equipment	To determine how postgraduate students and house officers interact with DVM students
Faculty – 2–3 faculty members from each department or administrative units who are not administrators	Faculty, Physical Facilities and Equipment, Clinical Resources	To clarify faculty employment as described in the standard, and to gather impressions/concerns regarding the educational program
Confidential meetings with DVM students	All Standards	
Confidential meetings with faculty	All Standards	
Alumni – representatives reflecting career paths taken by students, president of alumni association, any alumni acting as adjunct faculty members	All Standards	To verify that career goals could be reached with the education provided by the school/college
Department heads	Faculty, Organization	To determine coordination between faculty and administration and impact on DVM students, faculty development process, adequacy of resources
Course leaders/instructors of record and relevant staff of laboratory-intensive courses (e.g., Anatomy, Microbiology)	Faculty, Organization, Curriculum, Students, Finances	To determine coordination between faculty and administration and impact on DVM students, faculty development process, coverage of the veterinary curriculum

(continued)

Table 22.1 (Continued)

MEETING	STANDARDS ADDRESSED	GOAL OF MEETING
Section chiefs (VTH)	Curriculum, Students, Faculty, Clinical Resources	To gather information from mid-level administrators about functionality of the DVM program as a whole
Outcomes officer(s)	Outcomes Assessment	How is information from outcomes transferred to the appropriate stakeholders – completing the loop
Optional meetings		
Technical staff in teaching hospital	Physical Facilities and Equipment, Faculty	To verify working conditions in the hospital, staff and faculty support of the DVM program, role of paraprofessionals in training and assessment of students
Library	Information Resources	To question the librarian and library staff about factors beyond those captured during the tour, to see demonstrations of specific technologies

the teaching, research, and service missions of the college. This includes on-campus facilities and any affiliated teaching facilities that are used by a large number of students or are required for any portion of a student's education. For colleges with a distributed model, where all clinical training takes place away from the college, this includes all distributed sites that are designated as primary instructional sites (core instructional sites). Specific factors that are evaluated by the site team and Council include the following:

- Are the classrooms, teaching laboratories, teaching hospital educational areas, ambulatory vehicles, and other teaching spaces adequate in size, clean, in good repair, and contemporary?
- Is there sufficient office space for administration, staff, and faculty?
- Is there an on-campus teaching hospital that is adequate in size, clean, in good repair, and contemporary? If there is no on-campus teaching hospital, do all core instructional sites meet these criteria?
- Are facilities for housing animals for teaching and research adequate in size, clean, and in good repair, such that they meet minimum welfare standards?

- Is there sufficient equipment for examination, diagnosis, and treatment of all animal species regularly managed by the college? Are pharmacy, diagnostic imaging, diagnostic support services, isolation facilities, intensive/critical care, and necropsy services and equipment available?
- Student and patient safety must be assured at all times – are there appropriate signs designating hazards and enforcing infection control and radiation safety standards?

Standard 4: Clinical Resources

The overall goal of this standard is to ensure adequate caseload or provision of animals in species regularly managed by the college or stressed in the curriculum, to guarantee adequate exposure of students throughout their training. Specific factors that are evaluated by the site team and Council include the following:

- Does the college provide an adequate number of normal and diseased animals of various domestic and exotic species for instruction throughout the curriculum? These may be client-owned animals, animals associated with an affiliate site, or animals specifically made available by the college for instruction.

- Are students provided with the necessary ancillary resources to permit them to manage clinical resources, including access to subject matter experts, technical staff, appropriate equipment and services, and reference resources?
- Is the medical record system comprehensive and searchable?

Standard 5: Information Resources

The overall goal of this standard is to ensure that students, staff, and faculty members have timely access to materials necessary for teaching and learning, research, and service. Specific factors that are evaluated by the site team and Council include the following:

- Do students, staff, and faculty have adequate access to materials and the personnel necessary to help them retrieve these materials?
- Do faculty members have access to the personnel and technology necessary for the creation and maintenance of instructional materials?

Standard 6: Students

The overall goal of this standard is to ensure that students have the necessary support mechanisms in place to help them succeed in the curriculum and beyond, and to safeguard their physical and mental health. Specific factors that are evaluated by the site team and Council include the following:

- Are the number of directly enrolled, transfer, and any additional clinical-year students consistent with the resources of the college?
- Are there internships, residencies, and advanced degree programs available that complement and strengthen the DVM program?
- Are student services within the college adequate?
- Is current information readily available for prospective and enrolled students, including admission requirements and procedures, tuition and fees, financial aid information, licensing requirements, and an accurate academic calendar?

- Is there a mechanism for students to comment anonymously on the standards of accreditation as applied at their college?

Standard 7: Admissions

The overall goal of this standard is to ensure that the admissions process is transparent and fair to all prospective students, and that admissions processes are driven by the mission of the college. Specific factors that are evaluated by the site team and Council include the following:

- Does the college have an Admissions Committee primarily made up of full-time faculty members trained in admissions that makes recommendations of students for enrollment based on the college's admissions policy?
- Do the college's trends in number of applicants, and offers made and accepted, demonstrate the sustainability of the program?
- Are the prerequisites appropriate?
- Does the committee consider factors other than academic achievement as part of its stated admissions process?
- Does the college strive to increase diversity in its admitted population?

Standard 8: Faculty

The overall goal of this standard is to ensure that the number and qualifications of faculty can sustain the program. Specific factors that are evaluated by the site team and Council include the following:

- Are there enough faculty members with the varying qualifications necessary to sustain the teaching, research, and service missions of the college?
- What professional development and promotion opportunities, and other benefits, exist for faculty members so as to ensure stability and continuity in the program?
- Does the college strive to increase diversity in its faculty population?

Standard 9: Curriculum

The overall goal of this standard is to ensure that students are exposed to appropriate content in varying ways, and that application of the content is assessed. Specific factors that are evaluated by the site team and Council include the following:

- Does the curriculum extend over four academic years, including at least one year of clinical training?
- Does the college have a Curriculum Committee primarily made up of full-time faculty members that guides oversight of the curriculum?
- Is the curriculum complete and flexible, with student exposure to all topics and disciplines, such that they graduate as entry-level veterinarians with knowledge of biomedical sciences, clinical sciences, and professional and clinical skills?
- Has the curriculum been reviewed as a whole within the last seven years, with revisions made as necessary?
- Is the grading/student promotion process fair and equitable?

Standard 10: Research

The overall goal of this standard is to ensure that students have opportunities to participate in research and understand how to incorporate research findings into clinical practice. Specific factors that are evaluated by the site team and Council include the following:

- Does the college have an active, substantial research program of high quality, with many faculty members having some research activity?
- What opportunities exist for students to participate in research, and to what extent?
- How are students trained to access and evaluate the primary literature?

Standard 11: Outcomes Assessment

The overall goal of this standard is to ensure that the college is assessing the outcomes of its processes (for example, admissions), students (for example, clinical competencies), and overall program (for example, benchmarking against other institutions), and that the college recognizes deficiencies, acts on them, and then reassesses. Specific factors that are evaluated by the site team and Council include the following:

- Does the college survey students at graduation, alumni, employers, and other stakeholders regarding their education and competencies permitting them to work as a veterinarian? What is the employment rate of graduates?
- Do all graduating students demonstrate the defined clinical competencies and, if not, how are students identified and remediated before graduating?
- How many students take and pass the NAVLE?
- Does the college evaluate the outcomes of its processes and the overall program and what is done with the collected data?

Accreditation Decisions

The site team does not make binding accreditation decisions, but instead provides documentation for consideration by the full Council. When evaluating a school on a comprehensive site visit, for each component of the rubric within each standard, the college is defined as having met the standard, having a minor deficiency, or having a major deficiency. For any designation of minor or major deficiency, the site team must provide within the report observations supporting that decision. The site team also may choose to make recommendations or suggestions for improvement. The site team report is sent to the dean of the college for factual corrections, and the amended document sent to the COE for consideration of the accreditation status of that college.

Accreditation classifications for established schools are accredited, accredited with minor deficiencies, probationary accreditation, and terminal accreditation (see Figure 22.1).

Accredited

Accredited is an accreditation status granted to a college that has no deficiencies in any of the standards. Accreditation is granted for a period of up to seven years.

Accredited with Minor Deficiencies

Accredited with minor deficiencies is an accreditation status granted to a college that has one

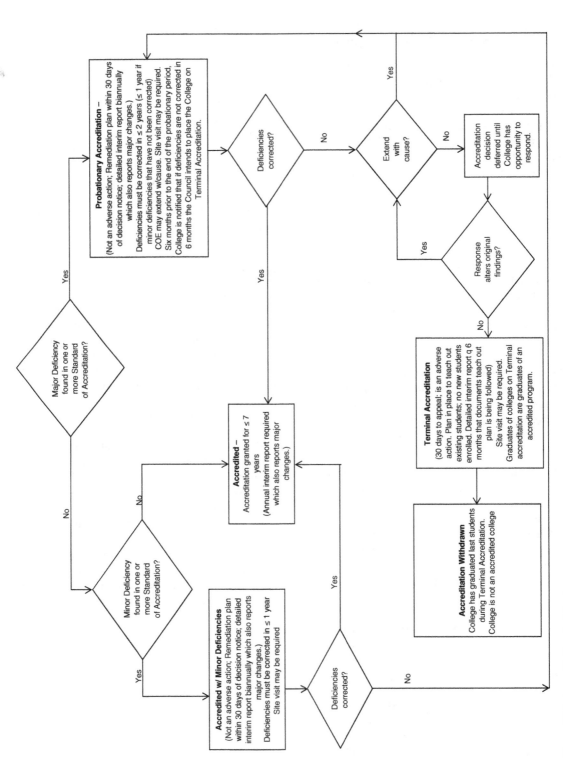

Figure 22.1 Accreditation decision tree.

or more minor deficiencies in one or more of the standards. Minor deficiencies are those that have minimal or no effect on student learning or safety, and that can be corrected by the college within one year. Minor deficiencies must be corrected within one year or the school must be moved to probationary accreditation for one year. The Council provides the school with specific reporting requirements to ensure steady progress on the correction of deficiencies. The Council may accept a variety of forms of evidence of correction of deficiencies, or may require a focused site visit.

Probationary Accreditation

Probationary accreditation is an accreditation status granted to a college that has one or more major deficiencies in one or more standards. Major deficiencies are those that have more than a minimal impact on student learning or safety. Major deficiencies must be corrected within two years. The Council provides the school with specific reporting requirements to ensure steady progress on the correction of deficiencies. The Council may accept a variety of forms of evidence of the correction of deficiencies, or may require a focused site visit. If a college does not correct a minor deficiency after a year on probationary accreditation, or does not correct a major deficiency within two years, it must be placed on terminal accreditation.

Terminal Accreditation

Terminal accreditation is an accreditation status assigned to a college that is unable to correct deficiencies within the specified time period. This is an adverse decision, and the Council and college will work through a specific set of legal proceedings to ensure that prospective and currently enrolled students are not at risk of graduation from a nonaccredited school, which would hinder their ability to become licensed to practice veterinary medicine in the United States.

Most established schools will be accredited or accredited with minor deficiencies. After having received an accreditation status, schools must supply the Council with regular documentation to demonstrate ongoing process improvement. Developing schools are discussed in the next section. Established schools are expected to correct any minor or major deficiencies within set timelines, as previously described. Every school must submit an interim report annually; the Council may require more frequent communications with developing schools or those in the midst of correcting deficiencies. Schools also are expected to provide the Council with information regarding any substantive change that could affect one or more of the standards, for example increasing class size.

Developing Schools

The COE does not provide any sort of recommendation for developing schools outside of North America. For new schools in North America, the COE will review documentation from the school and send a site team for initial review, to help the school determine for which standards the school has adequate resources or plans in place and to provide an unofficial appraisal. This is a consultative visit. Classifications assigned to developing schools are reasonable assurance and provisional accreditation.

A new school seeking the classification of reasonable assurance must send a formal letter of application to begin the process. A comprehensive site visit is conducted in a similar manner to that for accredited schools. After this comprehensive visit, if the college demonstrates reasonable resources and planning, the Council may grant it a letter of reasonable assurance. This is not an automatic decision; reasonable assurance is not a pre-accreditation action and does not confer an accreditation status on the college. The college must demonstrate ongoing progress toward the achievement of standards to maintain its letter of reasonable assurance, and must admit its first class within three years. On admission of the first class and provision of sufficient proof that it is making adequate progress in complying with the standards, the developing school is granted provisional accreditation. A school that is provisionally accredited must demonstrate completion of plans in place and respond to any concerns brought forward by the COE. A site team will visit the developing school as students enter and move through the program. A school may not be provisionally accredited for more than five years. If it cannot be granted accreditation, it is placed on terminal accreditation, as described earlier.

Established Schools Outside of the United States and Canada

Established schools are defined as those that have graduated enough classes to permit them to complete outcomes assessment. Established schools from any country can contact the COE and request consideration for accreditation. A consultative site visit is performed, with documentation from the school and a site visit with a small site team and one staff member. The school is provided with written documentation regarding any perceived deficiencies. If deficiencies are corrected, the college can request a comprehensive site visit. The site team sent for a comprehensive site visit cannot include those members who served on the consultative visit. The comprehensive visit and associated documentation and accreditation decisions are as already described.

Alternate Mechanisms of Accreditation

Accreditation in the United States is a peer-reviewed system in which a veterinary medical educational program is assessed by people who are knowledgeable in the field, to assure educational quality and a system of continuous quality improvement (ASPA, 2002). Accreditation and licensure are administered by separate bodies.

In some countries the higher educational system is overseen by a governmental agency, for example the ministry of education. The ministry in those countries may regulate many functions of the college, including number of students admitted; which students are admitted; the curriculum, including content and length; and the number of faculty, including the number of faculty of specific rank. The college may have input, but does not have full autonomy.

Accreditation agencies can have statutory authority that is granted by law, and have multiple duties.

For example, the RCVS is responsible under the Veterinary Surgeons Act of 1966 for maintaining the register of veterinarians eligible to practice in the United Kingdom, setting the standards for veterinary education, and the regulation of the professional conduct of veterinarians (RCVS, 2016a). The RCVS Education Committee is charged with setting the policy for veterinary education. Thirty-eight weeks of extramural studies (EMS) is a required part of the curriculum (RCVS, 2016b). EMS are practical experiences with practitioners that are broken into 12 weeks of preclinical (animal husbandry) experience and 26 weeks of clinical experiences. Day One Competencies that all graduates are expected to meet are defined in the accreditation criteria. In addition, as part of the professional development phase, new graduates must also complete year-one competencies within approximately one year of graduation (RCVS, 2016c). Year-one competencies cover the same areas as Day One Competencies, but the expectation is that at the end of this first year after graduation, the veterinarian "will be able to perform a range of common clinical procedures, or manage them without close supervision, in a reasonable period of time and with a high probability of a successful outcome" (RCVS, 2016c).

The AVBC also has multiple functions (AVBC, 2011). It has the authority to speak and act on behalf of the registering authorities in Australia and New Zealand. In addition to working with veterinary accreditation, the AVBC is involved in the assessment of foreign veterinary graduates, recognition criteria for qualifications for registration as a veterinarian, and regulation of veterinarians for both general and specialist registration. AVBC accreditation also requires EMS and the attainment of Day One Competencies. The accreditation process is managed by a committee of the AVBC, the Veterinary Schools Accreditation Advisory Committee (VSAAC). The accreditation criteria follow a strong outcomes-based approach, similar to the AVMA COE and the RCVS.

EAEVE is an association of veterinary medical colleges that have established minimum standards for veterinary medical education programs. EAEVE manages their accreditation process, which is accomplished via the ESEVT. EAEVE has joint responsibility for this process with the FVE. This system separates the approval process into two stages (EAEVE/FVE, 2012). In Stage One, the college is assessed to determine whether it conforms with Directive 2005/36:

> Directive 2005/36/EC establishes that the training of veterinarians ("or equivalent professional denomination") shall comprise a total of at least five years of full-time theoretical and practical study at a university or at a higher institute of education providing training recognised as being of an equivalent level, or under the supervision of a university, covering at least the study programme referred to in Annex V.4. of the Directive: Veterinarian, which lists the requirements for knowledge and skills (5.4.1.), the study programme for veterinarians as well as a clear description of extramural practical training. (European Parliament and Council of the European Union, 2005, Section 5, Article 38)

Colleges that conform with Directive 2005/36 are granted "Approval." In Stage Two, the college is assessed to determine whether it meets specific academic standards and provides appropriate learning opportunities. Colleges that meet Stage Two criteria are granted "Accreditation." All members of EAEVE must meet Stage One requirements; however, participation in a Stage Two assessment is voluntary (EAEVE/FVE, 2012). This system incorporates a number of ratios in the assessment process. Colleges must be in the listed range for the ratio to meet the criteria, for example number of support staff per faculty member (EAEVE/FVE, 2012). Approval or accreditation by EAEVE is not a prerequisite for licensure or registration. However, it should be remembered that accreditation processes are dynamic and subject to review and revision. The EAEVE routinely reviews their process for the evaluation of veterinary education establishments and posts the most recent Standard Operating Procedure on their website (EAEVE/ESEVT, 2016).

Schools outside of North America may pursue AVMA COE accreditation, as already described. Often, joint site visits are held with the COE and one of these other agencies. Accreditation decisions and voting are managed separately by the COE and these other agencies.

Future of COE Accreditation

Just as the veterinary profession has changed how medicine is practiced given the advent of new scientific discoveries, the process of accreditation and the standards of accreditation will change as new modalities for the delivery of education are developed, and as the needs of the profession and society change. Governments may have an influence by encouraging educational systems to look at educational models in which time in a classroom seat is disconnected from the completion of a class and credit granted (USDE, 2015).

If colleges of veterinary medicine adopt modalities like the Massive Open Online Course (MOOC), hybrid online education, competency-based education, and others, the COE will need to review these educational systems and determine whether the educational program can meet its expectations that graduates are firmly based in the fundamental principles, scientific knowledge, and physical and mental skills of veterinary medicine, and that they will be able to apply these fundamentals to solving veterinary medical problems. In addition, each veterinary medical program must continue to be in compliance with the standards of accreditation, which are regularly reviewed by the Council with extensive input from the colleges and the public.

Conclusion

Accreditation is not a one-time event, but rather is an underlying support system for ongoing quality improvement in veterinary medical education. Schools are strongly encouraged to participate as requested in evaluating and refining the standards of accreditation. Veterinarians from all aspects of the profession are strongly encouraged to volunteer for training as a site team visitor or as a member of the Council. For faculty members, participation in site visits and on the Council provides value for your place of employment as you develop expertise around the topic of accreditation, and is personally rewarding. For the profession, the more of us who participate the better, as our varied viewpoints and skills are what bring such great depth and validity to this process.

References

ASPA (2002) *About Accreditation: Resources, Documents and Definitions.* Association of Specialized and Professional Accreditors. http://www.aspa-usa.org/content/about-accreditation (accessed June 18, 2015).

AVBC (2011) *Veterinary School Accreditation.* Australasian Veterinary Boards Council. http://esvc000063.wic046u.server-web.com/school.htm (accessed November 20, 2016).

AVMA (n.d.) *The Standards of Accreditation Site Team Evaluation Rubric.* American Veterinary Medical Association. https://www.avma.org/ProfessionalDevelopment/Education/Accreditation/Colleges/Documents/coe_pp_appendix_i.pdf (accessed November 12, 2016).

AVMA (2014) *Accreditation Policies and Procedures of the AVMA Council on Education (COE).* American Veterinary Medical Association. https://www.avma.org/ProfessionalDevelopment/Education/Accreditation/Colleges/Pages/coe-pp.aspx (accessed June 17, 2015).

AVMA (2015a) *COE Recognition by the Council on Higher Education Accreditation.* American Veterinary Medical Association. https://www.avma.org/ProfessionalDevelopment/Education/Accreditation/Colleges/Pages/COE-Recognition-by-the-Council-for-Higher-Education-Accreditation.aspx (accessed June 17, 2015).

AVMA (2015b) *Accredited Veterinary Colleges.* American Veterinary Medical Association. https://www.avma.org/ProfessionalDevelopment/Education/Accreditation/Colleges/Pages/colleges-accredited.aspx (accessed June 17, 2015).

AVMA (2016) *AVMA Center for Veterinary Education Accreditation.* American Veterinary Medical Association. https://www.avma.org/professionaldevelopment/education/accreditation/pages/default.aspx (accessed November 12, 2016).

Banasiak, D. (2012) Rooted in knowledge, in *The AVMA: 150 Years of Education, Science, and Service*, American Veterinary Medical Association, Schaumburg, IL, pp. 161–178.

CHEA (2010) *Recognition of Accrediting Organizations: Policy and Procedures.* Council for Higher Education Accreditation. http://www.chea.org/pdf/Recognition_Policy-June_28_2010-FINAL.pdf (accessed June 17, 2015).

EAEVE/FVE (2012) *European System of Evaluation of Veterinary Training (ESEVT): Manual of Standard Operating Procedure.* European Association of Establishments for Veterinary Education/Federation of Veterinarians of Europe. http://www.eaeve.org/fileadmin/downloads/SOP/EAEVE_Budapest_SOPs_merged.pdf (accessed Nov 20, 2016).

EAEVE/ESEVT (2016) *Standard Operating Procedure (SOP).* European Association of Establishments for Veterinary Education/European System of Evaluation of Veterinary Training. http://www.eaeve.org/esevt/sop.html (accessed January 13, 2017).

ECFMG (2010) Requiring Medical School Accreditation for ECFMG Certification – Moving Accreditation Forward. Educational Commission for Foreign Medical Graduates. http://www.ecfmg.org/forms/rationale.pdf (accessed February 18, 2016).

European Parliament and Council of the European Union (2005) Directive 2005/36/EC of the European Parliament and of the Council of 7 September 2005 on the recognition of professional qualifications. *Official Journal of the European Union*, **L 255/22**, 1–121.

ICVA (2015) *North American Veterinary Licensing Examination (NAVLE®): Frequently Asked Questions*. National Board of Veterinary Medical Examiners. https://www.icva.net/navle-general-information/faqs/ (accessed Nov 12, 2016).

RCVS (2016a) *About*. Royal College of Veterinary Surgeons. http://www.rcvs.org.uk/about-us/ (accessed November 12, 2016).

RCVS (2016b) *Extra-Mural Studies (EMS)*. http://www.rcvs.org.uk/education/extra-mural-studies-ems/#what (accessed November 12, 2016).

RCVS (2016c) *Professional Development Phase (PDP)*. http://www.rcvs.org.uk/education/professional-development-phase-pdp/ (accessed November 12, 2016).

Schray, V. (2006) Assuring quality in higher education: Key issues and questions for changing accreditation in the United States. Issue paper #4. United States Department of Education. http://www2.ed.gov/about/bdscomm/list/hiedfuture/reports/schray.pdf (accessed February 18, 2016).

Simmons, D. (2004) Developing an accreditation system. *Journal of Veterinary Medical Education*, **31** (2), 89–91.

UBSA (1967) Organizations designated by the Commissioner of Education as nationally recognized accrediting agencies and associations. *United Business Schools Association Bulletin*, **67** (7), 4. http://cdm16804.contentdm.oclc.org/cdm/compoundobject/collection/ACICS01/id/1231/rec/6 (accessed June 17, 2015.

USDE (2015) *Competency-Based Learning or Personalized Learning*. United States Department of Education. http://www.ed.gov/oii-news/competency-based-learning-or-personalized-learning (accessed June 15, 2015).

van Zanten, M., Norcini, J.J., Boulet, J.R., and Simon, F. (2008) Overview of accreditation of undergraduate medical education programmes worldwide. *Medical Education*, **42**, 930–937.

WHO-WFME Task Force on Accreditation (2005) Accreditation of medical education institutions: Report of a technical meeting. Schaeffergarden, Copenhagen, Denmark, 4–6 October 2004. World Health Organization/World Federation for Medical Education, Geneva. http://www.who.int/hrh/documents/WFME_report.pdf (accessed February 18, 2016).

Zarco, L. (2009) Current approaches to veterinary school accreditation in Latin America. *Revue scientifique et technique*, **28** (2), 855–860.

Part VI

Teaching and Assessing Professional Competencies

23

Communication

Cindy L. Adams[1] and Suzanne M. Kurtz[2]

[1] *Department of Veterinary & Clinical Sciences, University of Calgary, Canada*
[2] *College of Veterinary Medicine, Washington State University, USA*

 Box 23.1: Key messages

- Communication is an essential clinical skill that must be taught with the same level of attention and rigor as other clinical skills.
- Communication can be taught and learned.
- Seven elements are necessary to learn skills and change behavior:
  - Systematic delineation and definition of the evidence-based skills to be learned.
  - Observation and assessment of learners performing the skills (live and/or on video, but for communication skills preferably with some video or at least audio recording of the interaction).
  - Well-intentioned, detailed, descriptive feedback (guided reflection, coaching, peer feedback, and self-assessment).
  - Practice and rehearsal of skills in various veterinary contexts.
  - Planned reiteration (a helical, reiterative teaching/learning model rather than a linear, once-and-done model; this includes applying the skills in increasingly complex situations or contexts over time).
  - Interactive small group or one-to-one experiential teaching/learning format.
  - Performance-based assessment strategies.
- There are evidence-based benefits to be gained from skilled communication.
- Thinking about communication education will systematically move the development of communication teaching forward.

Introduction

The overarching purpose of this chapter is to improve communication education in veterinary medicine, from the beginning of veterinary school and throughout a career. To accomplish this, we offer a practical guide to teaching communication effectively. We include reasons to invest in communication skills teaching programs, what we are trying to teach, and methods to develop learners' communication skills that enable learners to use these skills in practice and continue to develop them throughout their careers. We conclude by advocating for clinical communication programs and offering several suggestions to build a program that extends the impact of the dedicated communication course.

Veterinary Medical Education: A Practical Guide, First Edition. Edited by Jennifer L. Hodgson and Jacquelyn M. Pelzer.
© 2017 John Wiley & Sons, Inc. Published 2017 by John Wiley & Sons, Inc.

A Practical Guide for Teaching and Learning Clinical Communication

The first steps in teaching (and learning) communication effectively are to gain an evidence-based understanding of why we teach communication and to determine just what it is we are trying to teach. The reason we have added "and learning" is to underscore the fact that learners need this orientation and understanding as much as intructors do.

Why Bother?

An extensive body of research developed over the past 45 years in human medicine, and more recently in veterinary medicine, indicates that improving clinical communication in specific ways leads to the benefits summarized in Box 23.2.

These findings confirm that communication is an influential *clinical* skill in veterinary (and human) medicine that deserves to be taught and learned with the same rigor as medical technical knowledge, clinical reasoning, physical examination, and other procedural skills. The clinical outcomes that depend on communication are too central to leave the development of skilled communication to chance (Cake *et al.*, 2016). The research evidence is too strong to refute. For an in-depth review of the studies substantiating the benefits in Box 23.2, see Silverman *et al.*, (2013) in relation to human medicine and Adams and Kurtz (2017) for veterinary medicine.

In keeping with the evidence base, the broad learning goals of clinical communication are as follows:

- Ensure increased accuracy, efficiency, and supportiveness of client interaction.
- Enhance client *and* veterinarian satisfaction.
- Improve outcomes of veterinary care.
- Promote collaboration and partnership (relationship-centered care).
- Enhance coordination of care (between healthcare providers, patients, clients, families, and production animal workers).

The goal of communication education is not merely to improve knowledge and understanding of communication, but to improve clinical communication skills to a professional level of competence. Professional competence implies heightened awareness, greater ability to reflect and articulate with precision, heightened intentionality, and more consistent performance across all situations. Moreover, professional competence is evidence based. These goals of communication training remain the same across all levels of medical education. At more senior levels, deeper mastery of skills and development of attitudes or capacities is expected. Contexts and problems become more complex as learners advance, but the goals of training remain constant.

A second rationale for communication education is that the veterinary profession, recognizing the significance of the contribution that communication makes to clinical practice, is making communication a required part of the curriculum. Many key studies and reports emphasized the need for a focus on the development of veterinary students' "professional competencies." Subsequent studies indicated that many veterinary graduates were clinically competent, but lacked the crucial skills, knowledge, and attitudes essential for practice success (Brown and Silverman, 1999; Cron *et al.*, 2000; Chadderdon, King, and Lloyd, 2001; Lloyd and Walsh, 2002). These findings have played a significant role in terms of communication training in veterinary education.

Responding to these reports and recent research, professional organizations and veterinary medical education councils have acknowledged and taken on communication training as an essential component of the curriculum. For example, the American Veterinary Medical Association Council on Education (AVMA, 2012) lists client communication as an essential outcome of the Doctor of Veterinary Medicine (DVM) program, and states that graduating students must be able to demonstrate communication competence (AVMA, 2012). Veterinary educators in many countries have begun to include communication teaching

Box 23.2: Evidence-based benefits gained from skilled communication

Improving communication in specific ways leads to:

- More effective consultations for client(s), veterinarian(s), and patient(s):
  - Greater accuracy
  - Heightened efficiency
  - Enhanced supportiveness and trust
  - Relationships characterized by collaboration and partnership.
- Better coordination of care with clients and their families, with teams responsible for animal care, with veterinary team members

and colleagues, etc.
- Improved outcomes:
  - Greater satisfaction for everyone involved
  - Better understanding and recall
  - Improved adherence and follow-through
  - Greater patient safety and fewer clinician errors
  - Better outcomes for patients
  - Reduced numbers of conflicts, complaints, and malpractice claims.

Source: Silverman, Kurtz, and Draper, 2013; Adams and Kurtz, 2017.

within the veterinary curriculum (see, e.g., Heath, 1996; Radford *et al.*, 2006; Adams and Ladner, 2004; Adams and Kurtz, 2006; Kurtz, 2006; Shaw and Ihle, 2006; Mills, 2006; Gray *et al.*, 2006; Chun *et al.*, 2009; Baillie, Pierce, and May, 2010; Hecker, Adams, and Coe, 2012; Artemiou *et al.*, 2014; Everitt *et al.*, 2013; Hafen *et al.*, 2013; Hodgson, Pelzer, and Inzana, 2013; McArthur and Fitzgerald, 2013; McDermott *et al.*, 2015; Mossop *et al.*, 2015), and clients and veterinarians have recognized the importance of communication (Blach, 2009; Walsh, Klosterman, and Kass, 2009; Mellanby *et al.*, 2011).

Defining What We Are Trying to Teach

Given that communication is an essential clinical skill in veterinary medicine, how do we define effective clinical communication, and how do we decide what to teach?

A Skills-Based Approach
Whether enhancing our own clinical communication skills, assisting others, or designing communication education programs, how we think about communication significantly influences how we teach communication and what we do with it in practice. Consequently, it is helpful in defining what to teach and learn to distinguish between three types of clinical communication skills:

- *Content skills*: what you communicate, for example the substance of your questions and responses, the information you gather and give, the issues and treatments you discuss.
- *Process skills*: how you communicate, for example how you go about discovering the history or providing information, structure interactions, ask and respond to questions, relate to clients and patients, use nonverbal skills, involve clients in decision-making.
- *Perceptual skills*: what you are thinking and feeling, for example your internal decision-making, clinical-reasoning, and problem-solving skills; your attitudes, values, and personal capacities for compassion, mindfulness, integrity, respect, flexibility; your awareness of feelings and thoughts you have about the patient, the client, and the problems or other issues that may be concerning them; what you do with your own feelings and those of your clients; awareness of your self-concept and confidence and of your assumptions, biases, and distractions.

Content, process, and perceptual skills are highly interdependent – a weakness or strength in one set of skills translates into a weakness or strength in all. We must give attention to all three when trying to teach and learn effective clinical communication (Riccardi and Kurtz, 1983; Kurtz, Silverman, and Draper, 2005).

Three approaches to communication teaching and learning are prevalent: skills based, issues based, and attitude based. We deliberately encourage taking a predominantly skills-based approach rather than an issues-based approach. The skills-based approach gives primary emphasis to the development of learners' communication process skills, since these tend to be least emphasized in other parts of the curriculum, and secondary attention to content and perceptual skills, since they are taken up elsewhere. The issues-based approach organizes coursework and learning around issues such as end of life, ethics, cost discussions, informed consent, communicating treatment risks and benefits, communicating with children, cultural issues, etc. These issues are important, but the focus needs to be on the skills required to deal with these issues; once individuals understand and develop competence in applying the skills, communication issues and challenges can be much more readily tackled. There is no need to invent a new set of skills for each issue. Instead, we need to develop the learners' core communication skills, along with the awareness that some skills will need to be used with greater intention, intensity, and awareness. We need to deepen understanding of these core skills and enhance the level of competence with which we apply them. For a detailed example of how to apply the skills differentially to cultural issues, see Kurtz and Adams (2009).

The attitudes-based approach organizes teaching around learners' attitudes, and biases, by developing the values and capacities that influence communication. Skilled communication without the commensurate development of values quickly becomes manipulation. On the other hand, developing values and capacities without the skills to demonstrate them is also insufficient.

Only the skills-based approach provides the communication skills that enable learners to deal with issues and to put capacities, values, beliefs, and intentions into practice. The core skills that we describe represent the foundation for effective clinical communication in all circumstances.

What It Takes to Learn (and Teach) Skills, Change Behavior and Master Skills

Seven elements are necessary to change behavior and master any skill set:

- Systematic delineation and definition of the evidence-based skills to be learned.
- Observation and assessment of learners performing the skills (live and/or on video, but for communication skills preferably with some video or at least audio recording of the interaction).
- Well-intentioned, detailed, descriptive feedback (guided reflection, coaching, peer feedback, and self-assessment).
- Practice and rehearsal of skills in various veterinary contexts.
- Planned reiteration (a helical, reiterative teaching/learning model rather than a linear, once-and-done model; this includes applying the skills in increasingly complex situations or contexts over time).
- Interactive small group or one-to-one experiential teaching/learning format.
- Performance-based assessment strategies.

Finding or making opportunities to bring all seven elements into play is a primary challenge for anyone who wants to enhance clinical communication skills in veterinary medicine. This is true for learners at any level: individual veterinarians who want to improve their personal clinical communication skills or the skills of their practice group; coaches and preceptors, faculty members, or program directors involved in coursework or clinical rotations, residency training, or continuing education programs or acting as role models; veterinary hospital or other organizational administrators. How these challenges are met depends on what can be made possible in each of those contexts, both through course/program design and via the efforts of individual teachers. (For detailed explanations and review of research evidence regarding these elements, see Kurtz, Silverman, and Draper, 2005.)

Deciding How to Teach and Learn Clinical Communication: The Elements Elaborated

We use the essential elements listed on the previous page as a way to organize the discussion of how to structure and teach clinical communication.

Systematic Delineation and Definition of Communication Skills

Placing the delineation of specific skills at the top of the list of essential elements is not accidental. All the other components are dependent on that first basic element.

Specific Communication Process Skills Worth Teaching and Learning We know that knowledge about the clinical communication skills that learners are trying to enhance and the research behind those skills is useful and important. Yet, as with other clinical skills, knowledge does not translate directly into either competence (can you do it?) or performance (do you [choose to] do it in practice?). Nor does simply watching the experts. I can read a lot of books on tennis and watch a lot of excellent tennis and still improve my skills very little if I never really focus on developing them. Yet still, just what are the specific communication skills that enable everything else?

While several skills models and frameworks are available, one of the most comprehensive, applicable, and utilized in veterinary medicine is the Calgary–Cambridge Communication Process Guide and its companion Content Guide, known collectively as the Calgary–Cambridge Guides (Kurtz *et al.*, 2003; Kurtz, Silverman, and Draper, 2005; Silverman, Kurtz and Draper, 2013; Adams and Kurtz, 2017). Evolving since the 1980s, the Calgary–Cambridge Process Guide includes 58 highly evidence-based communication process skills, plus another 15 process and content skills related to common focuses of explanation and planning. Validated by a large body of research, the communication skills in the guides are applicable to routine

and complex medical situations, to an array of issues (finances, ethics, end of life) in veterinary medicine, and across all contexts (e.g., small and large animal practice). The guides were originally developed in faculties of medicine at the University of Calgary (Canada) and, in a later collaboration, Cambridge University (UK). First published in 1998 (Kurtz, Silverman, and Draper; Silverman, Kurtz, and Draper, 1998) the guides have continued to evolve in subsequent editions of these two companion books and are used world-wide in human medicine. Initially adapted for veterinary medicine in 2000, the use of the guides in veterinary contexts has also expanded (Adams, 2000; Adams and Ladner, 2004; Adams and Kurtz, 2006; Gray *et al.*, 2006; Latham and Morris, 2007; Hecker, Adams, and Coe, 2012).

Taken together, the skills in the guides represent the state of the evidence regarding the communication skills that make a difference to clinical practice outcomes. These are the skills that research and experience indicate are necessary in order to achieve the benefits and outcomes listed in Box 23.2. Corresponding directly to what transpires in veterinary consultations, Figure 23.1 depicts the organizational framework for the Calgary–Cambridge Process Guide. See total guide in Adams and Kurtz (2017).

The guides have three broad aims: to help learners and practitioners conceptualize and structure their communication learning and practice; to summarize the clinical communication literature in an accessible way; and to assist clinical teachers and communication program directors in their efforts to establish training programs for both learners and those facilitating the learning, whether working in veterinary schools, residency, or continuing education. The guides are the backbone of communication program design, teaching, learning, feedback, assessment, and coaching, whether in an educational setting or in practice. Providing a common foundation for communication teaching and learning at all levels, the Calgary–Cambridge Guides are applicable to all types of practice, and to everyone from

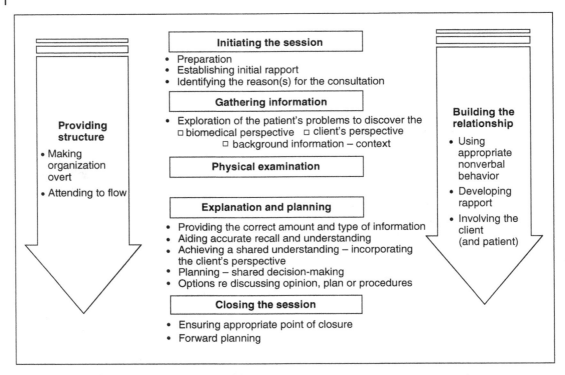

Figure 23.1 Expanded framework for the Calgary–Cambridge Process Guide. Source: Adapted from Kurtz *et al.*, 2003. Used with permission. For complete guide see Adams and Kurtz (2017), pp 29–33 and 259–263.

veterinary students to veterinarians who have years of experience.

First Principles of Effective Communication (and Teaching) Thinking in terms of first principles that characterize effective communication offers another useful resource for teaching and learning communication skills. The principles help us keep in mind what we are trying to do, which process skills to bring into play (Kurtz, 1989; Dance and Larson, 1972; Dance, 1967), and where the skills in the Calgary–Cambridge Guides are needed to put the principles into practice. Importantly, these same principles also characterize effective teaching.

Effective communication (or teaching):

- *Ensures interaction not just transmission.* Only giving information or telling someone what to do is insufficient; accuracy, efficiency, and relationship require two-way conversation, feedback, questions and responses from both client and clinician.

- *Reduces unnecessary uncertainty.* Uncertainty distracts attention and interferes with accuracy, efficiency, and relationship; for example, we can reduce uncertainty about the patient's problems and anticipated outcomes, the client's expectations for a visit, the clinician's expectations, the structure of the interview, how the team works, and so on.

- *Requires planning, thinking in terms of outcomes.* Effectiveness can only be determined in the context of the particular needs and outcomes toward which the clinician and the client are working and consideration of the patient's needs at any given moment. If I am angry and want to vent that anger, then I communicate in one way, but if I want to get at the misunderstanding that caused the anger, then to be effective I must communicate in an entirely different way.

- *Demonstrates dynamism.* This principle includes engaging with the patient/client, and being present, responsive, and flexible. Clinicians need to develop a repertoire of skills that allow different approaches with different individuals, or even with the same individual as circumstances change.

- *Follows a helical rather than a linear model.* Saying something once is not enough; repetition and feedback are essential. Each reiteration moves us up the spiral to a higher level of understanding. Similarly, the helix is an excellent learning/teaching model. Developing communication skills and maintaining competence require reiteration as skills are deepened and applied in different contexts.

These principles are a useful self-assessment tool for learners (and teachers). Ask yourself what you did to ensure that each of the principles was in play during a given consultation (or teaching session). The first principles of effective communication also serve as a useful reference point – whenever in doubt about what skills would be most effective, go back to first principles to help you decide.

Communication process skills are the primary focus of teaching and learning clinical communication. However, what about the content of the consultation?

Ideas for Linking Content with Communication Process Skills Although communication courses do not focus primarily on the medical content of the consultation, you cannot teach or learn process skills without keeping in mind what learners are trying to communicate about in veterinary contexts, as well as the interdependence between process and content skills. So content becomes a secondary focus of communication teaching and learning. A "content guide" that helps learners to structure what they are saying (or trying to say) is a useful resource to incorporate. One such guide forms the second part of the Calgary–Cambridge Guides. This content guide (see Table 23.1) works directly with the Calgary–Cambridge Process Guide. Because the two guides are closely aligned, they reinforce each other and encourage integration of content with process skills.

While the Calgary–Cambridge Content Guide offers a useful way to structure any given

veterinary consultation from start to finish, learners frequently require additional direction in order to collect pertinent details of history from the client regarding the patient. Recognizing this fact led to the development of four species-specific history-taking "pyramids" at the University of Calgary that learners there use from Year 1 to the end of veterinary school (see Wilson *et al.*, in Adams and Kurtz, 2017). Figure 23.2 offers an example of one of the pyramids.

Like the Calgary–Cambridge Guides, the pyramids are based on the premise that the best patient care can be delivered if learners (and ultimately veterinarians) can identify not just the chief complaint, but all of the patient's problems or issues as well as the client's perspectives. Developed using the same template, the other species-specific pyramids reflect pertinent content that needs to be collected relative to those species. For instance, with production animals, herd considerations versus individual animal considerations are needed. Included in the communication course, the pyramids then become a means for integrating aspects of communication with the rest of the veterinary curriculum. The pyramids help ensure consistency between what students learn in small-group simulations and what they do in real-life settings.

Ideas for Linking Perceptual Skills with Communication Process and Content Skills The communication course also offers opportunities to underscore the interdependent relationship between perceptual skills and communication process and content skills. For example, we use the straightforward clinical method map in Figure 23.3 (Bryan and Cary, 2010) to help learners conceptualize how their communication with any given client fits into the sequential pattern of the clinical method.

Asking students to identify points on the map where communication process and content skills affect what students are doing with clients and animals helps learners visualize just how frequently veterinarians rely on communication skills during clinical practice. Asking learners then to discuss the points on the map at which

Table 23.1 Calgary–Cambridge Content Guide – Veterinary Medicine.

Signalment

Patient and/or flock, herd problem list

Present history – exploration of patient/flock/herd problems

 Veterinary medical perspective

  Sequence of events

  Analysis of signs

  Relevant systems review

 Client's perspective

  Ideas and beliefs

  Concerns

  Expectations

  Effects on life (of animal and client)

  Feelings

Background information – context

 Past medical history

 Environment and lifestyle

 Current medications, adverse drug reactions, and allergies

 Genetic and familial background

 Behavioral/social history

 Review of systems

Physical examination

Differential diagnosis – hypotheses (veterinarian's and client's)

Veterinarian's plan of management

 Investigations

 Treatment alternatives

Explanation and planning with client

 What the client has been told

 Plan of action negotiated

Source: Adams and Kurtz, 2017, pp. 35–36. Adapted for veterinary medicine from Kurtz *et al.*, 2003, pp. 802–809.

communication process and content skills have an impact on their clinical reasoning and what that impact is – or to consider how what they are thinking at any given point affects how they are communicating with clients or patients – helps students to realize how these skills influence each other (Kurtz, 2016):

- *Clinical reasoning* consists of the thought processes in which you engage as you collect information and opinions from various sources (e.g., the patient, the client, and others; physical examination; diagnostic tests; veterinary staff and colleagues; the medical record) and synthesize that information with your knowledge and experience to generate hypotheses, differentials, diagnoses, and action/treatment plans. These perceptual skills occur at the intrapersonal level of communication.

- *Clinical communication skills and capacities* are what you employ to initiate interactions with those involved in the communication; develop relationships; gather information from others accurately and efficiently; structure your interactions so that all participants can engage in them at optimal levels; give explanations and participate in planning and decision-making; close interactions; and

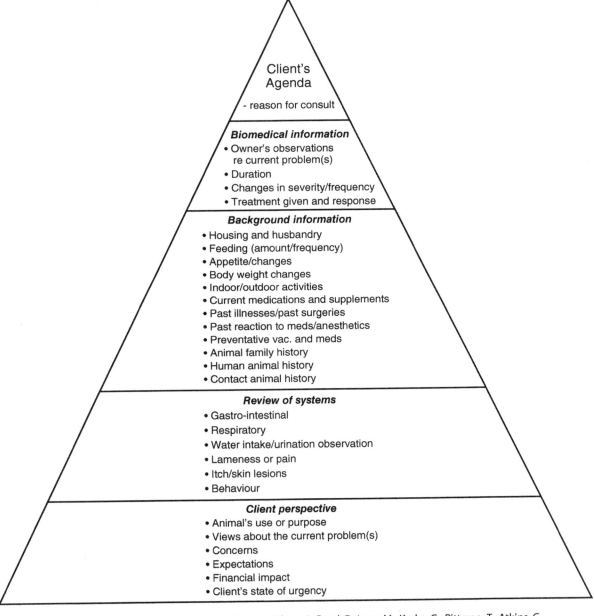

Client's Agenda
- reason for consult

Biomedical information
• Owner's observations
 re current problem(s)
• Duration
• Changes in severity/frequency
• Treatment given and response

Background information
• Housing and husbandry
• Feeding (amount/frequency)
• Appetite/changes
• Body weight changes
• Indoor/outdoor activities
• Current medications and supplements
• Past illnesses/past surgeries
• Past reaction to meds/anesthetics
• Preventative vac. and meds
• Animal family history
• Human animal history
• Contact animal history

Review of systems
• Gastro-intestinal
• Respiratory
• Water intake/urination observation
• Lameness or pain
• Itch/skin lesions
• Behaviour

Client perspective
• Animal's use or purpose
• Views about the current problem(s)
• Concerns
• Expectations
• Financial impact
• Client's state of urgency

Figure 23.2 Small animal historical investigation. Source: Wilson, J., Read, E., Levy, M., Krebs, G., Pittman, T., Atkins, G., Leguillette, R., Whitehead , A., Donszelmann, D., and Adams, C. (2012). Used with permission.

follow up appropriately. Communication content and process skills play major roles here, along with perceptual skills related to feelings, attitudes, values, assumptions, biases, intentions, and capacities.

• *Medical problem-solving* is what you get when you have well-developed clinical reasoning and clinical communication skills and capacities and are adept at integrating all of them.

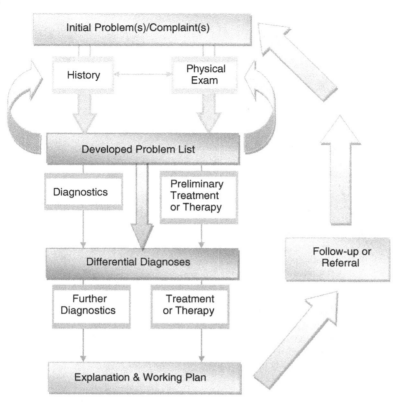

Figure 23.3 The clinical method map. Source: Bryan and Cary, 2010. In Adams and Kurtz, 2017. Used with permission.

For a more detailed description of how to use simulation and feedback with learners at any level to enhance clinical reasoning and other perceptual skills along with communication process and content skills, see Cary and Kurtz (2013).

Another idea for integrating perceptual skills has to do with the relationship between process skills and values or capacities such as mindfulness, compassion, integrity, and flexibility. These capacities and values have a significant impact on how learners (choose to) communicate in veterinary contexts. Conversely, communication process and content skills provide the means through which veterinarians – and veterinary students and teachers – demonstrate their capacities and values to clients. Incorporating feedback and discussion about each of these into small-group sessions and discussing how they influence each other contributes to the development of each of these skills, values, and capacities.

Observing Learner's Performance and Rehearsal of Skills

Because what we are really trying to do in communication training is to develop learners' understanding *and* their actual clinical communication skills, we have to be able to work experientially and individualize instruction. Although useful, neither large-class lectures nor demonstrations are sufficient. Small-group and one-to-one teaching are necessary, including the small learning groups that meet in simulation labs or during rounds, the one-to-one learning in clinics and large animal settings, and so on. Planning for the overall course as well as individual small-group sessions has to be orchestrated to give individual learners maximum opportunity to engage in observable consultations or other interactions, observe the performances of others, and participate in the feedback process in both instances. Members of the small group take responsibility for careful observation, well-intentioned feedback, and ongoing learning in the communication course. Expert facilitation that guides reflection and ensures systematic, comprehensive feedback is critical to maximize learning and participation for all. Program directors, individual faculty who facilitate learning, and the curriculum committee share the responsibility to make sure that all of this happens.

In order to ensure that each learner has multiple opportunities to engage, small learning groups ideally consist of five to six members plus an expert coach. (For convenience, we use the term "coach" throughout this chapter to refer to the experts who facilitate small-group or one-to-one learning rather than calling them facilitators, preceptors, small-group leaders, or small-group teachers, and so on.) In small-group settings, coaches are responsible for working with individual learners and coaching them through their consultations with real or simulated clients. At the same time, coaches are also working with the rest of the small group, inviting them to share their feedback when appropriate, and taking advantage of the dynamics of group process and the insights and ideas that emerge from all participants to promote both support for the individual and stimulation for the learning of all.

Finding, recruiting, training, and sustaining small-group coaches for the communication course is an ongoing challenge. In most communication courses, the majority of small-group coaches are faculty members and veterinarians recruited from nearby communities. Occasionally, experienced veterinary technicians, communication specialists, and others who are immersed in the veterinary profession also serve as coaches. Since formal communication training is still a relatively recent development in veterinary education, many (probably most) coaches have limited if any training regarding clinical communication or small-group teaching when they first take on coaching responsibilities. While "new" coaches generally require an orientation regarding expectations, how the course works, what is involved in assessment, and so on, all coaches benefit from regular

training sessions at various points during the year, for example at the beginning of each segment of the course and before each assessment. In our programs we also sit in as observers or participant observers with individual coaches during some small-group sessions, and then engage in coach-the-coach sessions with those individuals after the students have left. In other words, like student learning, coach training is organized around an ongoing helical model. Coaches are always in a position to learn more.

Lasting anywhere from an hour to two days and generally incorporating experiential learning techniques, these training sessions focus on questions and issues the coaches raise and on introducing or deepening understanding about ideas and methods to enhance coaching. For example, training often includes discussion of approaches that are working particularly well; updates about new community volunteer or simulated clients and the cases they bring; and ideas for enhancing coaching around cases with which coaches are already familiar, implementing the feedback process to maximize participation and learning, developing consistency across small groups regarding everything from attendance policies to the use of instruments like the Calgary–Cambridge Guides, making the most of cases that are included in the course, dealing with defensiveness or conflicted points of view, and so on. Training frequently also presents research evidence that validates both what and how coaches are teaching in the clinical communication course. During ongoing training, coaches experiment with ways to refine their coaching, deal with difficult situations, enhance interactions between learners, improve efficiency, and bring research findings into discussion. Bonvicini and Keller (2006) and Adams and Kurtz (2012) describe additional approaches to faculty development for communication teaching.

As with all clinical skills, there are two essential contexts for teaching and learning communication:

- The formal communication curriculum of dedicated courses, lectures, demonstrations, modules, workshops, and rounds that are explicitly designed for teaching and learning.

- The informal curriculum occurring in clinics, teaching hospitals, community veterinary practices, and other real-world veterinary settings where animal care is the primary focus. Here, "in-the-moment" teaching addresses the integration of communication and other clinical skills. Just as with the teaching of physical examination, procedural skills, and medical technical knowledge, teaching also occurs via intentional and unintentional modeling of communication skills, what veterinarians choose to focus on regarding that modeling, and, for communication, the "hidden" curriculum of how learners are treated and see their peers and mentors treating animals, clients, and others.

Effectively coaching communication skills in the "real world" requires excellent communication role models who are highly aware of how they are communicating, ongoing observation and feedback, and time to engage in feedback and coaching. The informal curriculum is very influential in veterinary clinical rotations, electives, and during intern and residency training. This aspect of the curriculum provides essential reinforcement and validation of the applicability of communication in the real world of practice. The coaching that happens in these settings has the potential to reach performance issues that other training cannot. Like the formal curriculum, informal curricula can have a profound effect on attitudes, values, and beliefs as well as communication skills and capacities, such as compassion for humans and animals and respect. For concrete ideas on effective coaching in the informal curriculum, see Adams and Kurtz (2012), Lane and Cornell (2013) and Smith and Lane (2015). For specific ideas on how to teach to the evidence in either context, see Adams and Kurtz (2017).

Using Appropriate Paradigms for Coaching Historically, three paradigms have influenced how we think about veterinary education, interact with learners, and actually teach: teacher-centered, learner-centered, and relationship-centered teaching. Veterinary education is moving away from teacher-centered education, where teachers hold control and essentially tell students what to think and do, toward a more learner-centered approach, employing teaching and learning strategies that are more interactive, participatory, and experiential.

This is similar to the shift in how we conceptualize veterinarian–client interactions. We have moved from a doctor-centered paradigm, in which the veterinarian holds the control, does most of the talking, and tells clients what to do with their animal(s), to a more client/patient-centered paradigm, which requires veterinarians to understand the client(s)' perspective as well as the patient(s)' problems or needs. In the client/patient-centered approach, veterinarians elicit and respond to the client(s)' thoughts, beliefs, expectations, concerns, and other feelings and expectations about their animal(s)' issues, care, and treatment.

Inspired by research in human and veterinary medicine, another shift is in progress, this time toward relationship-centered care (RCC). In veterinary medicine, RCC regards relationships – between veterinarians and clients, veterinarians and practice teams or colleagues, referring and referral veterinarians, and veterinarians' with their communities – as central to important outcomes, including satisfaction, retention of employees, adherence, and ultimately patient health. So, while the relationship between veterinarian and client remains central, veterinarians' relationships with themselves, colleagues, and communities are also important. Like the other two paradigms, RCC has parallels in teaching, and translates into relationship-centered education. One way to prepare learners for RCC is to model it in the form of relationship-centered education. Working in human medicine, Beach and Inui (2006) identified four principles on which RCC is built (we have substituted client and veterinarian to put RCC in the veterinary context):

- Relationships in veterinary medicine and education ought to include dimensions of personhood, with veterinarians and clients, teachers and students bringing their authentic and whole person to the encounter.

- Affect and emotion are important components of relationships in veterinary medicine and education, and support is provided through the emotional presence of the veterinarian or teacher; this challenges the notion of detached concern.
- All relationships occur in the context of reciprocal influence. While not precluding the primary importance of learners' goals, the client's goals for the patient and the patient's needs, this principle acknowledges that teachers also benefit from working with learners as do veterinarians when they serve clients and patients.
- RCC has a moral foundation – humans are morally committed to those with whom they are in relationships.

These shifting perspectives and attitudes toward communication in veterinary medicine are undoubtedly influenced not only by the changing environment in professional veterinary education, but also by societal changes regarding the role of animals in people's lives, and the recognition that other professions, most notably human medicine, are gaining insights and making evidence-based connections between communication and outcomes that have relevance for veterinary medicine and how we teach communication.

Importantly, these are not competing paradigms (Lussier and Richard, 2008). The question is not which is best, but which is most appropriate. In practice contexts, that depends on the nature of the animal's issues or problems, the client's preferences and needs, and the veterinarian's needs and preferences at any given time within a consultation. In teaching contexts, which paradigm is most appropriate depends on the nature of what you are trying to teach and students are trying to learn, as well as the group's needs and preferences at any given time, and the teachers' preferences and insights at that same time. All three paradigms are useful in large-group settings, but in small-group

and one-to-one teaching, learner-centered and relationship-centered teaching are essential.

Working with Simulated and Real Clients Simulated clients (SCs) have been a particularly useful part of communication training in veterinary medicine since the late 1990s and in human medicine since the early 1980s. They have been used at all levels in veterinary education, including veterinary schools, practice settings, major conferences, and so on. Where veterinary and medical schools are in reasonably close proximity, both have used the same bank of simulators. Simulated clients can be actors or people without acting experience who are trained to portray the clients in actual veterinary cases, including whatever medical or other information about their animal(s) the client in the case had; that client's personality, demeanor, perspectives, and issues; and the communication challenges that client presented. In other words, SCs are trained to reflect, to the degree possible and with appropriate protection of anonymity, the actual client that the simulation portrays.

Simulated clients require knowledge about the course and training regarding the cases and clients they will portray. Their training therefore includes:

- Information about the objectives of the communication course, specific skills, and learning objectives for the sessions of which they are a part, and methods used in the course.
- Discussion of difficulties that learners may experience in the context of working on communication skills in a simulated environment.
- Training to a particular role, understanding the case setting and description of the client, understanding and memorizing what they as the client know about their animal(s)' situation, rehearsing the case, and ongoing discussion of their role and the case with the SC director or coordinator.
- Direction on how to accurately portray the client's specific attitudes, beliefs, emotions, and behaviors regarding medical details and issues in the case.
- Direction on working with timeouts and rewinds.

- Direction and practice on how to give well-intentioned, specific feedback to learners.

Simulated clients offer many advantages over real clients. The first is safety. Working with SCs, learners can practice and learn communication skills and make errors with no consequences to any of the animals or people involved (including themselves and the veterinary practice). Animal models (when appropriate) and SCs reduce the pressure on students who are trying out and learning to master skills. Simulated clients make it possible for learners to stop and rewind or begin again at any point in the interaction, to rehearse skills over and over again, and to try out ideas that are generated in the small group. Because specific cases can be selected for inclusion in the course, the use of SCs ensures that every learner will be exposed to the same key cases and at appropriate times. With SCs it is also possible to focus on one aspect of the consultation rather than the entire interaction. When SCs are appropriately trained, another important advantage is their ability to provide feedback to learners from the client's perspective. This would generally be unavailable from real clients.

Periodically relying on real clients during the dedicated communication course is useful, including review of pre-recorded real consultations or live interviews with clients who are invited to participate in small-group teaching sessions for various reasons. Of course, learners also interact with real clients during rotations and electives in teaching hospitals and veterinary practices.

Developing Simulated Client Cases Simulations are much more realistic if they are based on real cases. When cases are developed locally, case content material (physical examination findings and results of diagnostic tests or procedures) and the client's perspective can be provided by veterinarians who saw these cases in real life. The original history of the case may be adapted to the goals of the course and the learners by increasing or decreasing its complexity. Teams consisting of faculty members, community veterinarians, program organizers, coaches,

simulated client trainers, and sometimes even the client work together to develop cases. For examination purposes, case development might also involve examiners or curriculum committee members.

When writing up cases, use of a template promotes consistent formatting and efficiency for authors. Varying in length from a paragraph to several pages depending on case complexity and intended use, write-ups include the animal(s)' medical history (presenting problems, history of those problems or concerns, progression of the case, past history, and background information) and the client's perspective (ideas, concerns, expectations, effect of the animal on life, feelings). Directions about the client's communication style and affect are also included, since these details are needed to train the SC effectively. Write-ups describe the context in which the case takes place (e.g., small animal exam room, barn, field) and invariably begin with a case scenario that learners see just before meeting with the client. Case scenarios briefly describe the setting, who the learner is about to meet, information already gathered, and the task for the interaction (e.g., your task is to meet with Mrs. Jamieson and Rocky, build a relationship, and take an initial history).

It is practical to develop organized case banks sorted according to year offered, species, communication issues, and how the case might be used in an integrative or assessment capacity. For cases that do integrate communication with other clinical skills, we include appropriate findings such as radiographs, results of laboratory tests, and so on. Whether learners are seeing no animals, animal models, or live animals in the case, you will need to think through how and when accurate findings are given to learners.

Using Video and Audio Recordings Video recordings and review are essential tools in communication education. Developing any skill is helped by self-observation, which is an opportunity that video recording uniquely provides. Learner–client interactions can be captured in small-group teaching and learning sessions and on rotations in large and small animal settings.

Wall-mounted, hand-held, or head-mounted cameras can be used to capture interactions as appropriate. Before making any recording of simulated or real interactions, it is necessary to obtain written, informed consent from all parties.

Video allows us to see ourselves as others see us. It equips us to reinforce our strengths and identify improvements we need to make in order to be more effective. Learners and coaches can rewind to look at something twice, or stop the video to discuss skills or find the words for an alternative approach. With video we can review the use and impact of specific skills or parts of the interaction. Video recordings can also be used in formative assessments, for example for "guided critical appraisal" assignments (Adams, Nestel, and Wolf, 2006), reflective journal writing assignments, and video review (Kurtz, Silverman, and Draper, 2005). In summative assessments that are performance based, video provides an accurate record of what actually transpired, thereby resolving disagreements about what individuals thought took place.

We sometimes use audio recordings too, for example when we are teaching and learning about telephone communication or when video is not an option. However, while audio is useful, video reveals more regarding nonverbal communication and interplay between the participants.

Differences between Teaching and Learning Communication and Other Clinical Skills

While the process of teaching and learning communication skills has much in common with what it takes to teach and learn other clinical skills, it is also substantively different. Communication is more complex than simpler procedural skills, because so many variables influence how we communicate. Communication is tightly bound to self-concept. Students are not invested in how they palpate a dog's liver before they learn to do it, but are already invested in how they communicate. Whether they are students or experienced veterinarians, learners can be heavily invested in their way of communicating. Perceiving that their communication "style"

defines them in some significant way, they may resist trying out new skills.

Competence in communication has no achievement ceiling. Even if we apply communication skills masterfully today, an unfamiliar situation or a variety of distractions can significantly reduce our effectiveness the following day. A final difference is that while faculty are acknowledged experts in the other clinical skills or subjects they teach, many communication coaches have had little to no formal training in this area. In light of these differences and the complexity that surrounds communication, learners and coaches must take particular care with how they engage in the feedback process.

Using Agenda-Led Outcome-Based Analysis: A Protocol for Feedback and Small-Group Facilitation

This leads us to a protocol for the feedback process called Agenda-Led Outcome-Based Analysis (ALOBA; Kurtz, Silverman, and Draper, 2005). This process was developed for giving and receiving feedback in the experiential learning environments preferred for teaching clinical communication. A relationship-centered approach, ALOBA maximizes the participation and learning of the entire group, reduces defensiveness, and personalizes teaching and learning. It transforms feedback from a mini-lecture or an evaluation of what was good and bad into a constructive analysis, discussion, and problem-solving session. The protocol is meant to be used flexibly. The steps involved in ALOBA resemble the tasks around which the Calgary–Cambridge Guides are organized, and the skills required to coach a small-group session are very similar to the veterinary–client communication skills in the guides.

The ALOBA process begins by setting the stage for the small-group session, including greeting the group, and in the early stages getting to know the group members, establishing rules of conduct with the group, and discussing expectations and goals. Next, the coach prepares the learner(s) for the consultation with a simulated or real client that provides the basis for discussion and feedback. Before the consultation begins, the coach asks what the learner wants to work on during the interaction (agenda led), followed by the sharing of thoughts, questions from the other group members, and possibly some refinement of the learner's goals.

Prior to the learner beginning the consultation, the coach divides up the sections of the Calgary–Cambridge Guides so that each small-group member takes primary responsibility for observation and feedback regarding one or two sections of the guides. Next, the learner begins the consultation. As observers take notes on the guides, the learner or coach might call a "timeout" to get ideas or help the learner shift their communication in a direction more in line with the learner's intended objectives. Returning to the consultation, a "rewind" to a slightly earlier section can then allow the learner to apply feedback and practice suggestions made during the timeout. Questions from the coach such as "What are you trying to achieve in this portion of the interview?" or "What would you like to see happen?" enable the learner to think through alternative ways to communicate with the client. Once the consultation is complete, the coach asks for the learner's perspective and insights about the interaction, before inviting other group members to offer feedback or ask questions about the case. The coach invites client feedback and offers insights at appropriate points. For everyone, descriptive comments ("Here's what I saw") take the place of evaluation ("That was good, that was not…"). The coach and group members are responsible for ensuring that feedback is well intentioned, specific, based on what could be observed rather than on assumptions about client's or learner's intent, and balanced between reinforcing what worked and other approaches that could be taken. Coaches encourage learners to try out alternative approaches with the simulated client.

The outcome-based portion of ALOBA occurs when individuals are trying to determine what skills or approaches would be most effective. The coach might ask the learner "What were you trying to achieve at that point?" or "What was the client in need of or trying to accomplish at that same point?" or "What did the animal need then, if anything?" In an effort to deepen the learners' skill development, the coach might ask "What is another approach that we can take to get closer to your goals and the outcomes the client was working on?" or "What would you like to do differently to meet your goal of building a solid relationship with your client?" Questions such as these that structure feedback around ALOBA help learners think through and apply their own ideas, rather than the coach telling them what to do. If we as coaches are doing the majority of the talking, we are likely in lecture mode. That said, there are times when we do need to provide more specific ideas about skills that may be worth trying, and times when we can discuss research or integrate process or perceptual skills with content to enhance learners' understanding of how these skills work together.

Developing Performance-Based Assessment Strategies

Another challenge of a comprehensive program is assessment of learners' communication skills. The best form of assessment is one that is not just a decision-making tool (pass/fail), but also a learning exercise that helps students to be "even better," thereby having an educational impact. Evaluation methods should mirror the way in which we teach communication, for instance by using the same model for the teaching and assessment instruments (such as the Calgary–Cambridge Guides) and the same methods (video recordings, simulated client interactions, and so on). Educational impact should be an important objective rather than assessment alone. Such evaluations require that we consider the content, format, and feedback process for the assessment.

An objective structured clinical examination (OSCE) fulfills all of these requirements (Hodges, 2006). For example, at the University of Calgary, the Year 1 OSCE assesses only communication skills. In later years' assessments, subsequent OSCEs integrate history taking, physical examination, diagnosis, explanation and planning, treatment recommendations decided on, and the completion of the medical record (including documentation of the client's perspective). Live large and small animals are incorporated into the OSCEs in Years 3 and 4. Multiple examination checklists are used to assess communication skills, pertinent history, procedural skills, and the medical record (e.g., accuracy and completeness). The parallel nature of assessment in the later years reflects the integration of the communication course into the larger curriculum. For a more detailed account of workplace-based assessment in a primary care setting, see Hecker, Norris, and Coe (2012).

We can assess more accurately and develop the learner's skills beyond what the learner demonstrated during the examination by reviewing video recordings of the consultation done for the examination. This video review process combines assessment, feedback, and a mini-tutorial. As part of capstone assessment exercises for two phases of the clinical communication program at Washington State University, pairs of students and an evaluator participate in video review. Using instruments based on the Calgary–Cambridge Guides, all three assess each learner's video, stopping it periodically for a mini-tutorial including consideration of alternative approaches. The coach incorporates written client feedback and each learner's self-assessment of content filled in immediately after interacting with the client. Learning is deepened by comparing and contrasting two learners' video-recorded interviews done with the same simulated client case. At the University of Calgary, video review with pairs of veterinary students and coach is used as part of the formative assessment of communication during the first three years of the program.

Ensuring Planned Reiteration and Ongoing Development of Skills

Skill development requires that the communication course – and even individual sessions within the course – follow a helical, reiterative teaching and learning model rather than a linear, once-and-done model. We have already described examples of planned reiteration,

including ways to make it possible for students to lead and observe multiple consultations, engage in feedback related to their own and others' performance, employ timeouts and rewinds to rehearse skills, try out alternative approaches, or see how other small-group members might do something differently.

Course design offers additional opportunities for ongoing reiteration and helical development. Course directors can selectively develop simulated cases or choose real cases that include a variety of species and situations, where learners can apply skills in routine and increasingly complex situations.

Designing assessment strategies such as those described that emphasize educational impact is another way to build in reiteration. In the next section we describe a major strategy for the reiteration and integration of communication with the rest of the veterinary curriculum and beyond.

Advocating for Clinical Communication Programs: Moving Beyond the Course

During the past decade, schools of veterinary medicine in a number of countries have begun to develop strong clinical communication courses. Despite this substantial progress and all of the ideas for course development detailed in this chapter, veterinary educators and researchers continue to identify common challenges and unresolved issues. How do we:

- ensure mastery and retention of evidence-based communication skills and capacities and transfer skills to practice?
- ensure that what is learned in the communication course is appropriately integrated into other parts of the curriculum and applied with increasing competence in actual clinical practice?
- assess clinical communication skills more effectively and efficiently?
- develop well-trained faculty for teaching/learning/assessment?

- find adequate time for all of this in an already overburdened veterinary curriculum?
- secure the status of communication as a bona fide clinical skill, important across all species and in all types of practice?
- incorporate large and small live animals and models into communication teaching?

The problems implicit in these questions stem partly from the fact that course organizers (and curriculum committees) tend to structure communication training into a single, self-contained course offered in the preclinical years and concluding with an evaluation of communication skills in isolation from other clinical skills. The development of isolated communication courses and evaluations is appropriate, and we are definitely not suggesting doing away with them. In fact, continuing to strengthen the design and teaching of the dedicated communication course is one important way to address these challenges. Learners' communication skills evolve in tandem with their increasing levels of knowledge, clinical sophistication, and maturity over the course of their veterinary education and beyond. As Latham and Morris (2007) found, final-year veterinary students who receive more comprehensive communication training do in fact have better communication skills at their disposal.

In order to resolve the persistent questions we have raised, we need to both strengthen and move beyond the self-contained course and examination. In other words, we need to build a clinical communication *program* that actively integrates communication with other parts of the veterinary curriculum, and translates communication skills developed during the course into actual veterinary practice.

Figure 23.4 illustrates one way to define what we mean by a clinical communication program (CCP), which is already being implemented at Washington State University (WSU) and also fits how the University of Calgary (U of C) conceptualizes its program. In both schools, developing a CCP around the five components shown in Figure 23.4 has proven to be a useful way to respond to the challenges of developing substantive communication training in veterinary

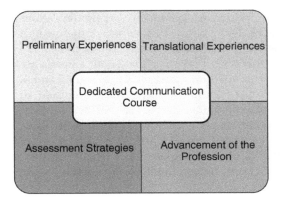

Figure 23.4 Structure of a clinical communication program. Source: Cary, J., DeBowes, R., Haley, D., Jensen, R., and Kurtz, S. 2013. Used with permission.

medicine. It has also been invaluable in helping us to describe what we are doing with respect to course organization, integration, and collaboration to administrators, curriculum committee, and external funders.

Dedicated Communication Course

The dedicated communication course is the centerpiece of the program. It includes some large-group lectures, but for the vast majority of the course learners meet in small groups with an expert facilitator/coach who is trained in communication and small-group methods. Incorporating well-chosen simulation cases, this separate course remains essential. It provides a venue (the clinical or communication skills lab) in which learners can observe and undertake learner–client consultations without being disruptive (e.g., observation rooms paired with consultation rooms separated by one-way glass in small animal settings, or a stall with enough space to accommodate the small group safely). Video and audio recordings can be made routinely. Repeated timeouts and rewinds are possible and can be encouraged to deal with difficulties or simply to consider and try out alternative ways of communicating without adverse consequences to the patient or anyone else. The number of hours you are able to secure for the dedicated course makes a considerable difference in how you divide up what you do with the other four program components.

Preliminary Experiences

Occurring before the dedicated course begins or concurrent with it, these formative experiences lay important foundations by introducing communication concepts, skills, and capacities in contexts outside the course, and by contributing to students' understanding of experiential learning, group dynamics, and how to work effectively with peers. For example, orientation, leadership, and team-building coursework is undertaken outside the communication course.

Translational Experiences

Providing follow-through after (or concurrent to) the dedicated course, translational experiences provide opportunities to apply, reinforce, and enhance communication skills and capacities even when there are time constraints, integrate them with other clinical skills, and to translate them into real-world contexts. Conversely, faculty who teach in other courses can be invited to contribute and help develop specific cases from their content area that lend themselves to simulation in the communication course. In this way, the communication course can reinforce, integrate, and extend the efforts of those other courses.

For example, the U of C communication course design team collaborates with a community organization to set up student-run clinics for low-income pet owners. The student–client consultations at the clinic are well supervised by a communication-trained veterinarian and/or coach. The WSU communication course design team collaborates with the organizer of the Field Investigation Unit course to review with pairs of students their audio-taped (and often transcribed) telephone conversations with dairy or beef producers who requested the services of the unit regarding the producers' actual problems. To guide the review and engage in the feedback process regarding the students' interactions with the producer, an adapted version of the Calgary–Cambridge Guides is used to guide the review.

Assessment Strategy

Rather than a single, stand-alone examination, the CCP develops an assessment strategy in which educational impact plays as significant a role as evaluation of student progress. Coach/examiner, peer and self-assessment, and simulated client feedback are all important elements of the strategy during the dedicated course. Capstone assessments and experiences or exercises are another part of the strategy, including video review and integrated clinical skills assessments that are scheduled either during the course or, better still, weeks or even months after the course ends.

Advancement of the Profession

Because communication is so central to the veterinary profession and yet is a relatively new addition to the curriculum, the CCP includes "outreach" to enhance clinical communication skills and capacities in veterinary medicine, promote more coherent clinical skills training, and advance the profession. For example, coach training for the dedicated course has impacts on both community veterinarians and veterinary school faculty, which ultimately affects what they do with clinical communication both within and beyond the course. Continuing education workshops on clinical communication at conferences for practicing veterinarians and technicians, or for veterinarians who have our students in their practices during rotations, raise participants' awareness of communication in veterinary medicine and their ability to model skilled communication (especially if these workshops incorporate the same simulation, video recording, and coaching methods that we use in the dedicated course).

Figure 23.4 helps us visualize communication programs more clearly. While it is essential to identify and capitalize on existing opportunities elsewhere in the curriculum, three other factors are even more important to developing coherent programs: building relationships with colleagues, collaborating with these colleagues over time for mutual benefit, and constructing a conceptual framework around which to build a coherent, systematic program that includes but extends beyond the dedicated course.

One of the reasons the U of C and WSU have been able to implement longitudinal communication programs is that we and our teams have been able to argue effectively that communication is an essential clinical skill, and that the communication program is a logical place for the necessary integration of clinical skills with each other and with learners' deepening knowledge base. In both veterinary schools, the success of the communication program has depended on the ability to pull so many threads together, and to build collaborative relationships with others in the faculty and with community practitioners and preceptors for mutual benefit. Examples of other longitudinal communication programs that have been implemented include those at the University of Sydney (Collins and Taylor, 2002) and Ontario Veterinary College (Stone, Conlon, and Cox, 2012) and several in the UK (Mossop *et al.*, 2015).

Our longitudinal programs are designed to ensure that learners develop substantive, evidence-based clinical communication skills and capacities during their DVM training, and also gain the tools and grounding needed to continue developing these skills and capacities to a professional level of competence throughout their careers. Without this kind of longitudinal planning, the benefits of the dedicated communication course would be compromised. Integrated longitudinal programs achieve a more effective, sustained increase in communication skills than stand-alone courses (van Dalen *et al.*, 2002).

Although communication skills teaching and learning is a core competency in veterinary medicine and is beginning to be required in veterinary curricula, there is a great deal of variation in what schools are offering. Communication education ranges from a few lectures embedded into ethics and practice management courses to full-blown programs that start in undergraduate training and continue through to intern and resident training. There are strong, evidence-based methods for teaching clinical communication, yet often these have not been taken up. The ability to implement effective communication training is compromised where human resources, time, funding, and commitment are inadequate.

Conclusion

This chapter provides numerous complementary ideas and strategies for enhancing veterinary education for the benefit of the profession and the animals and people it serves. Certainly, no one individual can put all of these ideas into practice in short order. Educational revolution takes commitment and perseverance.

The goal of this chapter has been to enhance clinical communication in veterinary medicine by improving communication education for learners at all levels. To that end, it provides compelling evidence-based rationales and proven methods for teaching and learning communication in veterinary medicine. We have organized the chapter around three important questions: Why bother? What are we trying to teach in the clinical communication curriculum? How do we teach and learn this subject – what are the most efficacious methods and approaches? The framework presented here offers several pragmatic ways to think systematically and move the development of communication courses and programs forward. You have to start with what you have, but no matter where you are now, there is much to do in this dynamic process. Producing truly effective communication courses and programs is not for the faint of heart, as this chapter has demonstrated, but the payoff is well worth the effort.

Acknowledgments

The authors wish to thank Jonathan Silverman and Juliet Draper; Julie Cary and Richard Debowes; Linda Ladner, Brian Gromoff, and Jack Wilson for their generous contributions to the development of these ideas and our communication programs in veterinary medicine.

For a more in-depth description and analysis of the theory and research evidence on which this chapter is grounded, see Kurtz, Silverman, and Draper (2005), Silverman *et al.* (2013), and

Adams and Kurtz (2017). The co-authors of these books have previously published some of the material in this chapter, in other articles and book chapters.

References

Adams, C.L., with Conlon, P.D., Power, B., and Tait, J. (2000) Art of Veterinary Medicine I, course syllabus. University of Guelph, Ontario Veterinary College, Guelph.

Adams, C.L., and Kurtz, S.M. (2006) Building on existing models from human medical education to develop a communication curriculum in veterinary medicine. *Journal of Veterinary Medical Education*, **33** (**1**), 28–37.

Adams, C.L., and Kurtz, S.M. (2012) Coaching and feedback: Enhancing communication teaching and learning in veterinary practice settings. *Journal of Veterinary Medical Education*, **39** (**3**), 217–228.

Adams, C.L., and Kurtz, S. (2017) *Skills for Communicating in Veterinary Medicine*, Otmoor Publishing, New York.

Adams, C.L., and Ladner, L.D. (2004) Implementing a simulated client program: Bridging the gap between theory and practice. *Journal of Veterinary Medical Education*, **31** (**2**), 138–145.

Adams, C.L., Nestel, D., and Wolf, P. (2006) Reflection: A critical proficiency essential to the effective development of a high competence in communication. *Journal of Veterinary Medical Education*, **33** (**1**), 58–64.

Artemiou, E., Adams C.L., Hecker, K.G., *et al.* (2014) Standardized clients as assessors in a veterinary communication OSCE: a reliability and validity study. *Veterinary Record*, **175** (**20**), 509.

AVMA (2012) COE Accreditation Policies and Procedures: Requirements: Standard 11, Outcomes Assessment. American Veterinary Medical Association. https://www.avma.org/ProfessionalDevelopment/Education/Accreditation/Colleges/Pages/coe-pp-requirements-of-accredited-college.aspx (accessed November 12, 2016).

Baillie, S., Pierce, S., and May, S.A. (2010) Fostering integrated learning and clinical professionalism using contextualized simulation in a small-group role-play. *Journal of Veterinary Medical Education*, **37** (**3**), 248–253.

Beach, M.C., and Inui, T. (2006) Relationship-centered care: A constructive reframing. *Journal of General Internal Medicine*, **21**, 53–58.

Blach, E.L. (2009) Customer service in equine veterinary medicine. *Veterinary Clinics of North America: Equine Practice*, **25** (**3**), 421–432.

Bonvicini, K., and Keller, V.F. (2006) Academic faculty development: The art and practice of effective communication in veterinary medicine. *Journal of Veterinary Medical Education*, **33** (**1**), 50–57.

Brown, J.P., and Silverman, J.D. (1999) The current and future market for veterinarians and veterinary medical services in the United States. *Journal of the American Veterinary Medical Association*, **215**, 161–183.

Bryan, J., and Cary, J. (2010) Clinical Method Map. Clinical Communication Program, course resources. Washington State University, College of Veterinary Medicine, Pullman, WA.

Cake, M.A., Bell, M.A., William, J.C. *et al.* (2016) Which professional (non-technical) competencies are most important to success of graduate veterinarians? A Best Evidence Medical Education (BEME) systematic review. BEME Guide No. 38. *Medical Teacher*, **38** (**6**), 1–4.

Cary, J., DeBowes, R., Haley, D., *et al.* (2013) Moving beyond the course: Advocating for clinical communication programs in veterinary medicine. Poster presented at the International Conference on Communication in Veterinary Medicine, St. Louis, MI, November 4–6.

Cary, J., Kurtz, S. (2013) Integrating clinical communication with clinical reasoning and the broader medical curriculum. *Patient Education and Counseling*, **92** (3), 361–365.

Chadderdon, L.M., King, L.J., and Lloyd, J.W. (2001) The skills, knowledge, aptitudes, and attitudes of successful veterinarians: A summary of presentations to the NCVEI subgroup (Brook Lodge, Augusta, Michigan, December 4–6, 2000). *Journal of Veterinary Medical Education*, **28**, 28–30.

Chun, R., Schaefer, S., Lotta, C.C., *et al.* (2009) Didactic and experiential training to teach communication skills: The University of Wisconsin-Madison School of Veterinary Medicine collaborative experience. *Journal of Veterinary Medical Education*, **36** (2), 196–201.

Collins, G.H., and Taylor, R.M. (2002) Attributes of Australasian veterinary graduates: Report of a workshop held at the Veterinary Conference Centre Faculty of Veterinary Science, University of Sydney, January 28–29, 2002. *Journal of Veterinary Medical Education*, **29** (2), 71–72.

Cron, W.L., Slocum, J.V., Goodnight, D.B., and Volk, J.O. (2000) Executive summary of the Brakke management and behaviour study. *Journal of the American Veterinary Medical Association*, **217**, 332–338.

Dance, F.E.X. (1967) Toward a theory of human communication, in *Human Communication Theory: Original Essays* (ed. F.E.X. Dance), Holt, Rinehart and Winston, New York, pp. 288–309.

Dance, F.E.X., and Larson, C.E. (1972) Speech Communication: Concepts and Behavior. Holt, Rinehart and Winston, New York.

Everitt, S., Pilnick, A., Waring, J., and Cobb, M. (2013) The structure of the small animal consultation. *Journal of Small Animal Practice*, **54** (9), 453–458.

Gray, C.A., Blaxter, A.C., Johnston, P.A., *et al.* (2006) Communication education in veterinary education in the United Kingdom and Ireland: The NUVACS project coupled to progressive individual school endeavors. *Journal of Veterinary Medical Education*, **33** (1), 85–92.

Hafen, M., Jr.,, Siqueira, D.A.A., Rush, B.R., and Nelson, S.C. (2013) Using authentic client interactions in communication skills training: Predictors of proficiency. *Journal of Veterinary Medical Education*, **40** (4), 318–326.

Heath, T. (1996) Teaching communication skills to veterinary students. *Journal of Veterinary Medical Education*, **23**, 2–7.

Hecker, K.G., Adams, C.L., and Coe, J.B. (2012) Assessment of first-year veterinary students' communication skills using an objective structured clinical examination: The importance of context. *Journal of Veterinary Medical Education*, **39** (3), 304–310.

Hecker, K.G., Norris, J., and Coe, J.B. (2012) Workplace-based assessment in a primary-care setting. *Journal of Veterinary Medical Education*, **39** (3), 229–240.

Hodges, B.D. (2006) The objective structured clinical examination: Three decades of development. *Journal of Veterinary Medical Education*, **33** (4), 571–577.

Hodgson, J.L., Pelzer, J.M., and Inzana, K.D. (2013) Beyond NAVMEC: Competency-based veterinary education and assessment of the professional competencies. *Journal of Veterinary Medical Education*, **40** (2), 102–118.

Kurtz, S.M. (1989) Curriculum structuring to enhance communication skills development, in *Communicating with Medical Patients* (eds M. Stewart and D. Roter), Sage, Newbury Park CA, pp. 153–166.

Kurtz, S. (2006) Teaching and learning communication in veterinary medicine. *Journal of Veterinary Medical Education*, **33** (1), 11–19.

Kurtz, S.M. (2016) Clinical communication education for surgeons, in *Communication in Surgical Practice* (eds S.J. White and J.A. Cartmill), Equinox Publishing, Sheffield, pp. 366–395.

Kurtz, S.M., and Adams, C.L. (2009) Cultural communication: Essential education in communication skills and cultural sensitivities for global public health in an evolving world. *Revue scientifique et technique*, **28** (2), 635–647.

Kurtz, S., Silverman, J., Benson, J., and Draper, J. (2003) Marrying content and process in clinical method teaching: Enhancing the Calgary–Cambridge Guides. *Academic Medicine*, **78** (8), 802–809.

Kurtz, S., Silverman, J., and Draper, J. (1998) *Teaching and Learning Communication in Medicine*, 1st ed, Radcliffe Medical Press, Oxford.

Kurtz, S., Silverman, J., and Draper, J. (2005) *Teaching and Learning Communication in Medicine*, 2nd edn, Radcliffe Publishing, Oxford.

Lane, I.F., and Cornell, K.K. (2013) Teaching tip: Making the most of hospital rounds. *Journal of Veterinary Medical Education*, **40** (**2**), 145–151.

Latham, C.E., and Morris, A. (2007) Effects of formal training in communication skills on the ability of veterinary students to communicate with clients. *Veterinary Record*, **160**, 181–186.

Lloyd, J.W., and Walsh, D.A. (2002) Template for a recommended curriculum in veterinary professional development and career success. *Journal of Veterinary Medical Education*, **29** (**2**), 84–93.

Lussier, M.T., and Richard, C. (2008) Because one shop doesn't fit all: A repertoire of doctor–patient relationships. *Canadian Family Physician*, **54** (**8**), 1089–99.

McArthur, M.L., and Fitzgerald, J.R. (2013) Companion animal veterinarians' use of clinical communication skills. *Australian Veterinary Journal*, **91** (**9**), 374–380.

McDermott, M.P., Tischler, V.A., Cobb, M.A., *et al.* (2015) Veterinary-client communication skills: Current state, relevance, and opportunities for improvement. *Journal of Veterinary Medical Education*, **42** (**4**), 305–314.

Mellanby, R.J., Rhind, S.M., Bell, C., *et al.* (2011) Perceptions of clients and veterinarians on what attributes constitute "a good vet". *Veterinary Record*, **168** (**23**), 616.

Mills, J.N. (2006) Development of veterinary communication skills at Murdoch University and in other Australian veterinary schools. *Journal of Veterinary Medical Education*, **33** (**1**), 93–99.

Mossop, L., Gray, C., Baxter, A., *et al.* (2015) Communication skills training: what the vet schools are doing. *Veterinary Record*, **176** (**5**), 114–117.

Radford, A., Stockley, P., Silverman, J., *et al.* (2006) Development, teaching, and evaluation of a consultation structure model for use in veterinary education. *Journal of Veterinary Medical Education*, **33** (**1**), 38–44.

Riccardi, V.M., and Kurtz, S.M. (1983) *Communication and Counselling in Health Care*, Charles C. Thomas, Springfield, IL.

Silverman, J., Kurtz, S., and Draper, J. (1998) *Skills for communicating with patients*, 1st ed., Radcliffe Medical Press, Oxford.

Silverman, J., Kurtz, S., and Draper, J. (2013) *Skills for communicating with patients*, 3rd ed., Radcliffe Publishing, London and New York.

Shaw, D.H., and Ihle, S.L. (2006) Communication skills training at the Atlantic Veterinary College, University of Prince Edward Island. *Journal of Veterinary Medical Education*, **33**, 100–104.

Smith, J.R., and Lane, I.F. (2015) Making the most of five minutes: The clinical teaching moment. *Journal of Veterinary Medical Education*, **42** (**3**), 271–280.

Stone, E.A., Conlon, P., and Cox, S. (2012) A new model for companion-animal primary health care education. *Journal of Veterinary Medical Education*, **39** (**3**), 210–216.

van Dalen, J., Kerkhofs, E., van Knippenberg-van den Berg, B.W., *et al.* (2002) Longitudinal and concentrated communication skills programmes: Two Dutch medical schools compared. *Advances in Health Sciences Education: Theory and Practice*, **7**, 29–40.

Walsh, D.A., Klosterman, E.S., and Kass, P.H. (2009) Approaches to veterinary education - tracking versus a final year broad clinical experience. Part two: Instilled values. *Revue Scientifique et Technique*, **28** (**2**), 811–822.

Wilson, J., Read, E., Levy, M., *et al.* (2012) Species specific history taking pyramid. Professional Skills course resources, University of Calgary Veterinary Medicine, Calgary.

24

Clinical Reasoning Skills

Jill Maddison

Royal Veterinary College, UK

 Box 24.1: Key messages

Problem-based inductive clinical reasoning:

- Provides a structured and teachable approach to clinical reasoning centred on three or four main steps:
  - Define and refine the problem.
  - Define and refine the system.
  - Define the location (where appropriate).
  - Define the lesion.
- Can be applied to any clinical sign.
- Provides the student with a framework on which to hang their growing knowledge, allowing them to recognize and retrieve the information they need more easily.

- Reinforces understanding of key pathophysiological principles.
- Reduces the need to remember long lists of differentials.
- Helps avoid diagnostic bias.
- Allows students to "see" the clinical reasoning strategies used by their teachers and mentors.
- Provides the student with memory triggers to ensure that an appropriate history is taken and a through clinical examination performed.
- Provides a clear rationale for choosing diagnostic tests or treatments that can be communicated to the owner.

Introduction

Veterinarians must make rapid decisions every day about diagnostic and treatment options for their patients. Clinical reasoning skills form the cornerstone of those decisions, as well as providing a sound knowledge base that is appropriate to the case. The latter also must include an understanding of important pathophysiological principles relevant to the patient's clinical problem. However, knowing the facts is not the same as knowing what to do. Knowledge is only useful if it can be accessed, formulated, and applied to the problem at hand. For example, a good understanding of the mechanics of an automobile engine is highly useful if the problem to be solved is a malfunctioning car, but not as useful when learning to drive.

Clinical Reasoning Education

It would seem self-evident that a competent clinician needs clinical reasoning and interpersonal skills, as well as knowledge and

Veterinary Medical Education: A Practical Guide, First Edition. Edited by Jennifer L. Hodgson and Jacquelyn M. Pelzer.
© 2017 John Wiley & Sons, Inc. Published 2017 by John Wiley & Sons, Inc.

understanding of diseases and their prevention or management. However, the emphasis of medical and veterinary education is usually more heavily weighted toward knowledge-building than the development of professional and communication skills. Over the past couple of decades, the attitudes of veterinary educators to the social science aspects of veterinary practice have shifted substantially. Teaching related to professional, interpersonal, and business skills has become an integral part of the veterinary curricula in many countries (Heath, 2006). Despite this, although clinical problem-solving is regarded as a core competency expected of a new graduate (AVMA, 2015), explicit teaching in clinical reasoning is not as well established. The reasons for this are multiple, and are perhaps primarily due to the belief that such skills will naturally develop as students acquire greater depth and breadth of knowledge, supplemented by exposure to clinical cases (May, 2013). Yet veterinary graduates report that they feel ill equipped in relation to clinical reasoning when they graduate (May, 2013).

The relative lack of formal training in reasoning may also be because the process by which clinicians reason clinically remains the subject of much debate. Many studies and reviews discuss clinical reasoning strategies, and the literature has been elegantly reviewed and critiqued by May (2013). However, there is a paucity of practical guidance about *how* to help students develop robust clinical reasoning skills. The general assumption seems to be that how experts "do it" is the gold standard, although how to get to that exalted state is rarely explained. If all clinicians eventually developed superb clinical reasoning skills with experience, then it perhaps would be reasonable not to worry too much about specifically educating undergraduate students in this area – the skills would come with time. However, diagnostic error is an important healthcare issue (Del Mar, Doust, and Glasziou, 2008), and stress and anxiety arising from difficult medical cases is reported by even experienced veterinarians. While the reasons for this are multifactorial and include issues such as financial constraints

and owner compliance, concern about the veterinarian's clinical reasoning abilities are also cited (Mant, 2014). Every clinical specialist is aware that poor clinical decision-making occurs in a proportion of cases referred to specialists by general practitioners. And, of course, clinical specialists remain at risk of making diagnostic errors themselves.

Comparing Medical and Veterinary Graduates

It is important to review studies in the literature on clinical reasoning development in medical students and novices with care when applying the results to veterinary student education. Graduates from medical school spend a considerable time after graduation in supervised clinical training programs before they are able to practice. Veterinary students, in contrast, are deemed fit to practice as soon as they graduate. Although they may seek further supervised clinical training in the form of internships (if they practice in countries where these are available), these are not a requirement to practice, and only a small proportion of those who plan to enter general practice will do so. Thus, a novice medical graduate will still be in a clinical training program, whereas a novice veterinary graduate will usually not be. The level of support and mentorship that a veterinary graduate may experience in their first year of practice varies enormously and may influence their whole career.

Another difference to note between medical and veterinary clinical education and practice is that a greater proportion of a graduating class in veterinary medicine will enter general practice than of a graduating medical class. Most veterinary graduates will never become clinical specialists, although they may well become expert general practitioners (May, 2013). The breadth of the skills required for a successful general veterinary practitioner is huge. The veterinary general practitioner must not only be an astute diagnostician (usually for more than one species), but also a surgeon, anesthetist, radiologist, pharmacist, and more. Access to specialist care is influenced by client finances as well as geographical location. Referral of difficult cases is an option in some countries but not others, in some geographical areas within a country, state, or city but not others, and, in almost every practice where referral services are accessible, for some clients but not others. Veterinarians in general practice therefore are constantly faced with the challenge of patients with problems that require complex knowledge and decision-making skills, who have owners with high expectations of a successful outcome for their animal. Even if referral to a specialist is an option, the choice of specialist requires sufficient clinical reasoning skills to recognize when referral is indicated and to which specialist.

Diagnostic Errors

The literature relating to problem-solving in human medicine is broadly driven by the desire to enhance clinical teaching and/or to understand the decision-making process in order to reduce diagnostic errors (Graber, Gordon, and Franklin, 2002; Graber, Franklin and Gordon, 2005; Berner and Graber, 2008; Graber, 2009; Norman and Eva, 2010; May, 2013; Mamede *et al.*, 2014). Diagnostic errors have been monitored and reported for a range of different specialties and clinical environments in humans. The estimate is that the rate of diagnostic error in clinical medicine is around 15%, thus affecting almost one in seven patients (Berner and Graber, 2008). The level of diagnostic error in veterinary medicine has not, to the author's knowledge, been estimated, but we would be foolish as a profession to believe that our diagnostic accuracy was any better than that of our medical colleagues.

Of most relevance to this chapter is that cognitive skill errors (processing biases) are reported to be a far more common reason for diagnostic error than errors caused by knowledge gaps (Graber, Franklin, and Gordon, 2005; Berner and Graber, 2008; Norman and Eva, 2010). Although experts may reach the correct diagnosis more often and more quickly than novices, no level of expertise confers zero risk of diagnostic errors.

Clinical Reasoning Models

As in many other situations where the science involved is more closely related to the social sciences than the physical sciences, there are no definitive or unequivocal results from many of the studies on clinical reasoning. Clinical reasoning is a complex process that varies enormously depending on the clinician's preferred thinking and learning styles (of which they are often unaware), their past experiences and expertise, the clinical problem itself, and the context in which that problem is encountered. It is not at all surprising that "measuring" reasoning strategies is difficult, and that study methods and results may be vigorously debated.

The current understanding (which has evolved considerably since the 1980s) is that the clinical reasoning strategies used by physicians can be broadly classified as Type 1 (nonanalytic) and Type 2 (analytic). A blended approach or triangulation of both types to cross-check clinical reasoning and diagnostic conclusions is advocated for successful diagnostic decision-making (Eva, 2004; Bowen, 2006; Graber, 2009; Coderre *et al.*, 2003; Vandeweerd *et al.*, 2012; May, 2013). Although some authors believe that the risk of bias and diagnostic error is higher with nonanalytic reasoning than analytic reasoning, improving and supplementing nonanalytic reasoning, rather than replacing it, is believed to reduce diagnostic error (Norman, Young, and Brooks, 2007).

Nonanalytic Clinical Reasoning

Nonanalytic reasoning occurs quickly and subconsciously, and primarily relies on the clinician accessing knowledge and patterns from past experiences that can be applied to the present case. It is often referred to as "pattern recognition," and relies on the clinician having developed a number of illness scripts for a particular presentation. Because of limited previous case exposure, pattern recognition is inherently weaker in novice medical students compared to more experienced clinicians. However, there is disagreement about whether this means that students should disregard nonanalytic methods in their clinical reasoning, or whether some use of intuition and pattern recognition improves diagnostic accuracy in novices (Norman and Brooks, 1997; Coderre *et al.*, 2003; Eva, 2004; Cockcroft, 2007; Norman, Young, and Brooks, 2007; Smith, 2008). Surprisingly, evidence from both nonclinical problem-solving studies (Pretz, 2008) and clinical studies (Norman and Eva, 2010) demonstrates that explicit, analytic thought may be most appropriate for experienced individuals, whereas holistic, intuitive problem-solving may be more effective for novices. Other educators have exactly the opposite view: "Given the amount of expertise required, this type of diagnostic reasoning strategy [pattern recognition] is generally unavailable to novice medical students" (Coderre *et al.*, 2003 p. 695).

Use of pattern recognition as the primary mode of clinical reasoning has positives and negatives. It works well for many common disorders and has the advantage of being quick and cost effective, provided that the diagnosis is correct. Use of pattern recognition as the major form of clinical reasoning is also effective if a disorder has a unique pattern of clinical signs; if there are only a few diagnostic possibilities that are simply remembered or can easily be ruled in or out by routine tests; and if the clinician has extensive experience (and thus a rich bank of illness scripts to recall), is well read and up to date, reviews all of the diagnoses made regularly and critically, *and* has an excellent memory.

However, nonanalytic reasoning based on pattern recognition can be flawed and unsatisfactory when the clinician is inexperienced (and therefore has access to few illness scripts) and/or only considers or recognizes a small number of salient factors in the case (incomplete problem presentation). Even if the clinician is experienced, use of pattern recognition as the primary clinical reasoning process can be problematic for uncommon diseases, for common diseases presenting atypically, when the patient is exhibiting multiple clinical signs that are not immediately recognizable as a specific disease and may or may not be related to one diagnosis,

or if the pattern of clinical signs is suggestive of certain disorders but not specific for them. In addition, for the experienced clinician, the success of pattern recognition relies on a correct diagnosis being reached for the pattern observed previously. This may not always be the case, especially in general practice, where the clinician must often form a provisional diagnosis and make treatment decisions in the absence of complete knowledge or data, without ever having the diagnosis confirmed (May, 2013). This will be reinforced by the presumption that the diagnosis was correct if the patient clinically improves with treatment.

Nonanalytic reasoning to solve diagnostic puzzles involves a wide variety of heuristics (subconscious rules of thumb or mental shortcuts to reduce the cognitive load and speed resolution of problems), which can be powerful clinical tools but also predispose to diagnostic bias. They tend to be viewed more favorably in some disciplines, for example emergency care, than others, such as internal medicine. Even experienced clinicians are vulnerable to bias in nonanalytic reasoning. Such bias is generally subconscious (although some authors suggest that an awareness of bias can help one avoid such errors). These biases have been clearly described (Croskerry, 2003; Berner and Graber, 2008; Norman and Eva, 2010; McCammon, 2015) and are outlined in Table 24.1. Often diagnostic error can involve a combination of biases. Physician overconfidence is believed to be a major factor contributing to diagnostic error and bias, even (or perhaps especially) among specialists (Berner and Graber, 2008).

Enhancing Nonanalytic Clinical Reasoning Skills in Veterinary Students

By nature of its automaticity, pattern recognition is not something that can be taught (or suppressed). A new case will inevitably trigger memories and suggest possible diagnoses if similar patients have been seen previously. Proponents of using (rather than ignoring) pattern recognition in clinical reasoning recognize that for this to be useful, a large bank of illness scripts is required. There may be different views

Table 24.1 Diagnostic biases in clinical medicine.

Bias	Description
Availability bias	A tendency to favor a diagnosis because of a case the clinician has seen recently.
Anchoring bias	Where a prior diagnosis is favored but is misleading. The clinician persists with the initial diagnosis and is unwilling to change their mind.
Framing bias	Features that do not fit with the favored diagnosis are ignored.
Confirmation bias	When information is selectively chosen to confirm, not refute, a hypothesis. The clinician only seeks or takes note of information that will confirm their diagnosis, and does not seek or ignores information that will challenge it.
Premature closure	Narrowing the choice of diagnostic hypotheses too early.

in the literature about whether or not students can effectively solve clinical problems using pattern recognition, but nevertheless there are practical strategies recommended to assist students in strengthening their nonanalytic reasoning skills.

Using pattern recognition responsibly has two requirements: the patterns need to be in place (as many correct illness scripts as possible); and there needs to be a learned process for acknowledging, then double-checking, the favored illness script. Strengthening students' pattern-recognition skills and development of illness scripts requires recognition of the typical presentation for a problem, as well as the variations and atypical presentations (Bowen, 2006). Formation of patterns used for illness scripts can only be constructed by each learner based on the patients they have seen (Fleming *et al.*, 2012) and the knowledge they have accumulated.

Educational strategies that are recommended to assist with the development of illness scripts are to ensure that students are exposed to patients with common problems, ideally with prototypical presentations, followed by similar

problems to provide them with an appreciation of atypical or subtle findings (Bowen, 2006). In other words, students must have adequate exposure to pedagogically useful cases. Teachers need to recognize that complex and elaborate cases may be suboptimal as teaching tools (Eva, 2004), unless efforts are made to "convert" them to useful teaching cases. Rare diseases that may make exciting problem-solving opportunities for postgraduate training scholars and clinical specialists, especially if they lead to publication, may not be particularly useful teaching cases unless there are relevant "teaching points" that can be utilized. These usually relate to logical and analytic decision-making rather than pattern recognition. In the author's experience, relatively complex (but not bizarre) medical cases *can* be powerful learning tools, provided that the clinical teacher clearly identifies the key learning features of the case, those learning points are transferable and core to good medical practice and clinical reasoning, and the teacher does not get bogged down in clinical minutiae of questionable relevance.

If a student is almost exclusively exposed during their clinical training to secondary- and tertiary-level referral cases, there is limited opportunity for them to build a bank of illness scripts relevant to general practice. It can be difficult for students to transfer clinical reasoning experienced in one context, for example a high-level specialist hospital, to another, such as first-opinion practice (Del Mar, Doust, and Glasziou, 2008). One unfortunate consequence is that the new graduate, exposed in their first year of general practice to a barrage of clinical situations that they have rarely encountered, may dismiss as irrelevant the "academic" learning in their clinical student years, and place a much higher value on their practical, extramural work-based placements in general practice. As a result, the rich learning resource provided by the intellectual academic rigor and expertise in clinical teaching hospitals may be wasted.

Analytic Clinical Reasoning

In cases where nonanalytic reasoning is not helpful, analytic reasoning is required. An analytic approach to clinical reasoning is also needed to double-check presumptive diagnoses based on pattern recognition – the clinical reasoning safety net.

In contrast to nonanalytic reasoning, analytic reasoning is reflective and systematic, permitting hypothesis formation and abstract reasoning (May, 2013). Analytic reasoning is less prone to bias than nonanalytic reasoning (May, 2013), but is limited by working memory capacity, unless strategies are developed to provide the clinician with a logical, methodical, and memorable process through which to problem-solve any case presentation. The most pertinent question, though, is how to do it? There is almost a complete lack of guidance in the literature on how to teach analytic reasoning. Audétat *et al.* (2011) do, however, provide a very practical overview of clinical reasoning difficulties that students may experience, why they may occur, and remediation strategies to help overcome them.

Analytic reasoning can be deductive, inductive, or abductive. Deductive reasoning (also referred to as hypothetico-deductive) is guided by generated hypotheses that the clinician then tests. This is the basis of the "rule out" approach – that is, "I will use diagnostic tests to rule out differentials until I am left with the most correct one." The intellectual process used in deductive reasoning, where there are many potential diagnoses, has been described (Cockcroft, 2007) and makes interesting, if exhausting, reading. It appears to be a very useful basis for the development of computer programs to generate differential diagnoses taking into account the clinical data provided, all possible diagnoses, and the ranking of probabilities of disease (probabilistic reasoning based on Baye's theorem). However, as an accessible method of clinical reasoning the method can be "time-consuming and laborious" (Cockcroft, 2007). It is certainly not feasible in the short time available during a first-opinion consultation, especially for a novice clinician who cannot formulate a relatively short and accessible list of alternative hypotheses.

Inductive reasoning makes broad generalizations from specific observations. From these observations, patterns and regularities are detected, then tentative hypotheses formulated, leading to general conclusions or theories. Inductive reasoning, by taking a more exploratory, "diagnosis open" approach, avoids eliminating the appropriate hypothesis too early, but is overwhelming without specific advice on how to do it. Coderre *et al.* (2003) describe scheme-inductive diagnostic reasoning. In this approach there is an organized structure for the learning and use of decision trees. The clinician seeks information from the patient that will distinguish between categories of conditions. It is very similar to the "small worlds" hypothesis proposed by Kushniruk, Patel, and Marley (1998), where expert clinicians select relatively small sets of plausible diagnostic hypotheses (small worlds) and focus on the most relevant medical findings that distinguish them. Neither author, however, provides any real guidance about *how* to develop this decision-making approach or create these "small worlds." It is on this aspect that we will focus in the problem-based clinical reasoning approach covered later in the chapter.

The third form of reasoning described is abductive reasoning. This usually starts with an incomplete set of observations and proceeds to the most likely possible explanation for the group of observations. It is based on making and testing hypotheses using the best information available. It often entails taking an educated guess after observing a phenomenon for which there is no clear explanation. We recognize, and should make students aware, that this reasoning process occurs, and that it will be used more often in general practice than specialist practice. Abductive reasoning is descriptive, but by its nature cannot be explicitly taught.

Enhancing Analytic Clinical Reasoning Skills in Veterinary Students

As discussed, the literature on clinical reasoning provides an insight into how clinicians think, even if not all studies agree, but very little about how to specifically teach and develop students' clinical reasoning skills. Vandeweerd *et al.* (2012) concluded from their study of clinical reasoning strategies used by Belgian veterinarians that students should be made aware of the reality of the decision-making strategies that clinicians use, but this does not mean that they should not be taught a rational decision-making model: "Teaching must not only train students to behave as current practitioners do, but to behave more as veterinarians ideally should." (Vandeweerd *et al.* 2012 p. 147) Of particular importance in clinical education is the recognition that no two clinical students can ever have exactly the same clinical experiences – they will see different cases, reflect on different aspects of their experience, and as a result gain different insights. It is for this reason that students need to be guided to multiple strategies to enable them to work through clinical problems (Eva, 2004).

Teaching a clinical reasoning structure explicitly can be challenging. Experienced clinical teachers may use both nonanalytic reasoning and analytic reasoning to solve clinical cases. They often do this very quickly. Their clinical reasoning process may be opaque for students, as it is based on the clinician's accumulated experience and wisdom, which are vastly different from those of the students, as well as on subconscious analytic checking of their clinical instincts. This is one reason why some experts may not necessarily be good teachers (May, 2013). Of course, the teacher may provide a rich learning experience by articulating, for example, that they discarded several differentials because the clinical signs did not fit expectations, outline the key features of the case that led them to the diagnosis, and discuss any atypical features of relevance. They almost certainly have developed clinical reasoning strategies that include what were originally analytic processes, but have now become part of their nonanalytic reasoning. Yet the failure to remember what it was like "not to know" can be an impediment to explicitly teaching and enhancing students' critical reasoning skills. Practitioners not accustomed to working in a collegial or scholarly environment may not be skilled in articulating their clinical reasoning process, even when it is well constructed and analytic.

The aim of the clinical reasoning approach described in the remainder of this chapter is to help veterinary students and practicing clinicians, particularly those involved in clinical teaching, develop and articulate a structured and pathophysiologically sound approach to the diagnosis of common clinical presentations. It has been most extensively described for clinical signs in dogs and cats (Maddison, Volk, and Church, 2015), but the principles are applicable to other clinical disciplines. The method aims to avoid the student having to remember long lists of differentials (as is often the result when other methods of analytic reasoning have been taught), and allows them to place their knowledge (which is often scaffolded by body system in the typical veterinary curriculum) into an appropriate problem-solving context.

The method is similar in some aspects to clinical algorithms, which can be found in some textbooks (e.g., Ettinger and Feldman, 2010) and have been suggested by Safi, Hemmati, and Shirazi-Beheshtiha (2012), who used the approach to the vomiting dog as an example. These algorithms can be very helpful in guiding decision-making for specific clinical problems. Their potential drawback is that the key decision points are usually clinical sign specific, and thus not transferable to atypical or complex clinical scenarios or other clinical signs. The principles of the problem-based inductive reasoning approach described in this chapter can be applied to virtually any clinical problem or combination of problems in a clinical scenario. It explicitly articulates key clinical reasoning steps that an expert diagnostician almost always will use, even if subconsciously, so that the student can "see" the clinical reasoning brain of their mentors and teachers at work. An additional benefit is that the key questions reinforce fundamental pathophysiological principles and understanding.

The Minimum Database

Before specifically discussing strategies to develop a problem-based inductive clinical reasoning approach, it is appropriate to include just a few words about the other fall-back that the clinician may use when nonanalytic reasoning is not available, helpful, or needs to be supplemented. That is the use of the minimum database – or colloquially, "I'll do bloods."

Routine diagnostic tests such as hematology, serum biochemistry panel, and urinalysis can be enormously useful and often essential in progressing understanding of a patient's clinical condition. However, relying on a minimum database to give more information about the patient before the clinical reasoning brain is engaged may be reasonable for disorders of some body systems, but totally unhelpful for others. Serious, even life-threatening disorders of the gastrointestinal tract, neuromuscular system, pancreas (especially in cats), and heart rarely cause significant diagnostic changes in the routine hematological and biochemical parameters measured in general practice. In addition, diagnostic tests are rarely 100% sensitive and 100% specific. Using blood testing to "screen" for diagnoses therefore can be misleading, as the positive and negative predictive value of any test is very much influenced by the prevalence of a disorder in the population.

Abnormal or even normal results in an unwell patient can create confusion rather than clarity if they are not critically reviewed as an integral part of the clinical assessment of all data relevant to the patient and related to the presenting problem(s). There is a tendency for physicians (and clients, which further biases the clinician) to overestimate the information that is gained from laboratory and imaging results (Del Mar, Doust, and Glasziou, 2008). This risk is exacerbated if the fundamentals – a comprehensive history and a thorough clinical examination – are bypassed in favor of tests. Overreliance on empirical testing to steer the clinician in the right clinical direction can also be problematic when the results do not clearly confirm a diagnosis. The clinician can waste much time and the client's money searching without much direction for clues to the patient's problem – formally referred to as "information gathering" (Del Mar, Doust, and Glasziou, 2008), less formally as a "fishing expedition." And, of course, the financial implications of nondiscriminatory testing can be considerable. Many clients are unable or unwilling to pay for comprehensive testing. And in many parts of the world where small animal practice is emerging, access to clinical pathology is currently very limited.

Many veterinary students spend considerable time during their undergraduate course in referral specialist hospital settings. Here they are exposed to the model of clinical practice where comprehensive and sophisticated diagnostic testing is integral to the management of patients, because the focus of the specialist is almost exclusively on reaching an accurate diagnosis and instituting rational therapy as soon as possible (May, 2015). This is not to say that the learning experience for students from such cases cannot be deep and rich. However, it is easy for the student to form the belief that such a level of testing is essential for all cases. They then may enter general practice and find to their horror that they are faced with many cases where the problems are ill defined, access to comprehensive diagnostics is much more limited, and owners' expectations may be more focused on resolution than a specific diagnosis (May, 2015). If students' clinical reasoning skills are weak, then their ability to influence clients to follow recommended diagnostic and treatment paths is impaired, there is further disillusionment with the value of their clinical education, and they face higher stress levels when they encounter any complex or chronically unresolved clinical case.

Problem-Based Inductive Clinical Reasoning

In problem-based inductive clinical reasoning, each significant clinicopathological problem is assessed before being related to the patient's other problems. Using this approach, the pathophysiological basis and key questions for the most specific clinical signs the patient is exhibiting are considered before a pattern is sought. This ensures that the clinician's mind remains more open to other diagnostic possibilities than what might seem to be initially the most obvious, and thus helps prevent pattern-based diagnostic bias.

The Problem List

An aspect of clinical reasoning that can be overlooked is the importance of clinical presentation and problem formulation. Problem formulation means structuring the elements of the clinical presentation into a recognizable form. This involves realizing what in the patient's data is important, giving it a recognizable shape, and formulating a structure of concepts linked by relations (Auclair, 2007). In problem-based inductive clinical reasoning, the formation of a prioritized problem list and ensuring that the problem or problems have been appropriately defined are the key steps.

The initial step in problem-based inductive reasoning is to clarify and articulate the clinical problems with which the patient has presented. This is best achieved by constructing a problem list. Constructing a problem list (either mentally, orally, or in written form) helps make the clinical signs explicit to the clinician's current level of understanding, transforms vague presenting information to specific problems, and helps the clinician determine which are the key clinical problems ("hard findings") and which the "background noise" ("soft findings"). Most importantly, it helps prevent the clinician overlooking less obvious but nevertheless crucial clinical signs and becoming overwhelmed with information. Problems do need to be prioritized and those that are most specific/diagnostically useful will act as "diagnostic hooks." This concept is described in more detail elsewhere (Maddison, Volk, and Church, 2015).

The Problem-Based Approach

Once the problem list has been formulated, it can be used as the lynchpin for the problem-based approach. It is important to clarify at this point that this approach means different things to different people. Some regard the problem-based approach as meaning: "Write a problem list, then list every differential diagnosis possible for every problem." Not a feasible task unless you have an amazing factual memory and endless time! Others view the problem-based approach as meaning: "Write a problem list, then list your differential diagnoses." This is in essence a form of pattern recognition, but at least a problem list is formed.

Problem-based inductive clinical reasoning is a more accurate definition of the clinical reasoning approach outlined here than is "problem-based approach." This approach provides steps to bridge the gap between the problem list and the list of differential diagnoses via a structured format. The approach to specific presenting problems is described in more detail in Maddison, Volk, and Church (2015).

The specific problems identified should be investigated by the rigorous use of key steps, which are highlighted in Box 24.2.

The answers to these questions or the pursuit of the answers will determine the appropriate questions to ask in the history. They may alert the clinician to pay particular attention to aspects of the physical examination, and/or they may indicate the most appropriate diagnostic test(s) to use to find the answers, as well as prepare the clinician intellectually to assess the results of the tests chosen.

Box 24.2: Focus on the key questions in problem-based clinical reasoning

- What is the problem? Define and refine the problem.
- What system is involved and how is it involved? Define and refine the system.
- Where within the system is the problem located? Define the location.
- What is the lesion? Define the lesion.

Define the Problem

When considering the important clinical signs that the patient is exhibiting, it is essential to try to define the problem as accurately as possible. "A problem well defined is a problem half solved" is a good maxim from which to work. The first question to ask is "Is there another clinical sign with which this problem could be confused?" This is a vital step, and failure to define the problem correctly has often derailed a clinical investigation that might otherwise have been relatively straightforward. Examples are shown in Box 24.3.

Refine the Problem

Some problems require further refinement to clarify the best diagnostic approach. Examples are shown in Box 24.4.

Box 24.3: Examples of defining the problem

- The owner reports that the dog is vomiting. Is the animal really vomiting or regurgitating – or perhaps even gagging or coughing?
- The owner says that the dog is having fits – is it having seizures, episodes of syncope or vestibular attacks, or other strange episodes?
- The owner says that the dog has red urine – is it blood, hemoglobin, myoglobin, or another pigment such as beet?

Box 24.4: Examples of refining the problem

- Weight loss – is this because of inappetence or despite a normal appetite?
- Collapse – with or without loss of consciousness?

The range of diagnoses to consider, diagnostic tools used, and potential treatment or management options for clinical problems that may be perceived by the owner to be the same and present similarly to the veterinarian can be very different. Or the owner might perceive the presenting signs to be attributable to one problem, but in fact the signs indicate another problem to the veterinarian.

Define and Refine the System

Once the problem is defined, the next step is usually to consider the body system that is malfunctioning. For every clinical sign there is a system (or systems) that *must* be involved; that is, that "creates" the clinical sign. However, the really important question is "How is it involved?" The key specific questions here are "What systems could be involved in causing this clinical sign?" and "Is it a primary – that is, structural – problem of a body system or a secondary – that is, functional – problem whereby the system involved in creating the particular clinical sign is secondarily affected in the pathophysiological process?" Examples are shown in Box 24.5.

The range of diagnoses to consider, diagnostic tools used, and potential treatment or management options for primary, structural problems of a body system are often very different from those relevant to secondary, functional problems of that system. Investigation of primary, structural problems often involves imaging the system in some manner (radiology, ultrasound, advanced trans-sectional imaging, endoscopy, surgical exploration) and/or biopsy. Routine hematology, serum biochemistry panel, and urinalysis are often of little value in confirming the diagnosis. For secondary, functional disorders, on the other hand, hematology and serum biochemistry are often critical in progressing our understanding and reaching a diagnosis.

An alternative, although closely related, question for some problems is "Is the problem local or systemic?" or "Is the clinical sign or lesion asymmetric (more apparent in one region) or

Box 24.5: Examples of defining and refining the system

The body system that is always involved when a patient vomits is the gastrointestinal (GI) system. However, it may be directly involved due to primary pathology of the gut, such as parasites, inflammation, neoplasia, or a foreign body. This is defined as primary (structural) GI disease. Or vomiting may be occurring due to the dysfunction of nongastrointestinal organs such as the liver, kidney, adrenal glands, and/or pancreas, which activate the vomiting center in the brain. This is defined as secondary (functional) GI disease.

The body system that is always involved when a patient has generalized weakness is one or more components of the neuromuscular system (central nervous system, peripheral nervous system, neuromuscular junction, or muscles). However, it may be directly involved due to primary (structural) neuromuscular pathology (e.g., inflammation, toxins, neoplasia, infection). Or the neuromuscular system may be malfunctioning due to the effect of pathology in other organs causing metabolic derangements that impair neuromuscular function, such as hypoglycemia, anemia, hypoxia, and electrolyte disturbances. This is defined as secondary (functional) neuromuscular disease.

Other examples:

- Chronic cough – primary respiratory system or secondarily affected by cardiac disease?
- Jaundice – due to prehepatic (hemolysis) or hepatic/posthepatic disorder?
- Cardiac arrhythmia – due to primary (structural) cardiac disease, e.g., dilated cardiomyopathy, or extracardiac disease, e.g., gastric dilation and volvulus, splenic disease?
- Polyuria/polydipsia – due to primary polydipsia or primary polyuria? If primary polyuria, is this due to structural renal disease or extrarenal dysfunction, e.g., diabetes mellitus, hypercalcemia, hypoadrenocorticism?

 Box 24.6: Examples of local versus systemic disease

- Epistaxis – due to local nasal disease or systemic disease, e.g., coagulopathy, hyperviscosity?
- Melena – GI bleeding due to local disease (ulceration, which in turn may be due to primary or secondary GI disease) or systemic disease, e.g., coagulopathy?

- Seizures – due to local and/or asymmetric structural brain disease, e.g., neoplasia, infection/inflammation, or systemic disease, e.g., electrolyte disturbances, hypoglycemia, or intoxication.

symmetric (affecting the system diffusely)?" Examples are given in Box 24.6.

There are often clues from the history and/or clinical examination that help the clinician define and refine the body system involved; or they may not be able to answer this question until further diagnostic tests are done. Nevertheless, just asking the question ensures that the clinician remembers that body systems can malfunction due to structural causes – direct pathology of that system – or functional problems, where pathophysiological processes not originating in the body system can have an impact on its function.

If the clinician does nothing else when assessing a case before seeking the diagnostic "pattern," they should ask, for each of the specific problems, "What system could be involved and how – primarily (structural) or secondarily (functional)?" This simple question can immediately open their mind to diagnostic possibilities that they may never have contemplated if they were just focusing on the "obvious pattern." The consequences of failing to define the problem and/or system can be serious and are outlined in Box 24.7.

Define the Location within the Body System

Having determined that vomiting is due to primary gastrointestinal disease, where in the gastrointestinal tract is the lesion located? In this example, by asking this question the clinician will select the most appropriate method to either answer the question or move on to the next step. For example, if they believe

that the history and physical examination and other ancillary data indicate a lower small intestinal lesion, endoscopy will not be an appropriate method of visualizing the area or obtaining biopsies. On the other hand, if all information obtained suggests a gastric lesion, endoscopy, if available, may be the most appropriate diagnostic tool. Examples are given in Box 24.8.

Define the Lesion

Once the location of a problem within a body system is determined, usually the next key question is "What is it?" The clinician now needs to identify the pathology. It can be helpful to remember the types of pathology that can occur in broad terms – for instance, degeneration, anomaly, metabolic, neoplasia, nutritional, infection, inflammation, idiopathic ("genetic"), trauma, toxic, vascular (DAMNIT-V). The type of pathology present is most likely to depend on the body system or organ involved, the signalment of the patient (species, breed, age,

---

Box 24.7: Focus on failure to define and refine the problem and/or system

- Can delay reaching a correct diagnosis and implementing appropriate treatment
- May prolong the disease and therefore the patient's suffering
- May endanger the life of the patient

- May unnecessarily increase the costs to the client
- May frustrate the veterinarian and/or client
- May potentially impair the relationship between veterinarian and client

---

Box 24.8: Examples of defining the location

- Vomiting due to primary GI disease – stomach, small intestine, or large intestine?
- Vomiting due to secondary GI disease – liver, kidney, adrenals, pancreas, endogenous toxicity from infection/inflammation, electrolyte disturbances?

- Hind limb weakness has been determined to be due to neurological dysfunction – is the lesion in the central nervous system (and where), peripheral nerves, or brain?
- Hematuria – blood from urethra, prostate, bladder, or kidneys?

Box 24.9: Examples of defining the lesion

- Gastric lesion – tumor, foreign body, or ulcer?
- Spinal cord lesion visible on magnetic resonance imaging – inflammation, infection, or a neoplasm?
- Hematuria due to lower urinary tract disease – infection, calculi, or neoplasia?
- Large bowel diarrhoea – parasites, infection, ulceration, stricture, neoplasia, diet related, inflammation?

sex, etc.), the clinical onset and course of the clinical signs, pain involvement (for neurological problems), the geographical location of the patient, and what disorders are common in that population. Since the lesion is now accurately localized and characterized, the list of differential diagnoses will be short.

This assessment can be influenced by whether the patient is in a general clinic or a specialist hospital. Common things occur commonly. This does not mean that uncommon diagnoses should not be considered (and they will, of course, be more common in specialist referral hospitals). However, in general practice at least, common disorders usually receive diagnostic priority at the beginning of a clinical investigation. Examples are given in Box 24.9.

Teaching Clinical Reasoning

As discussed earlier in the chapter, use of blended nonanalytic and analytic reasoning is the method by which most successful diagnoses are made. It is important to reiterate that pattern recognition for many cases is appropriate and justified, depending on the clinician's level of experience, knowledge, and skill base as well as mindset. However, clinical teachers need to be cognizant that pattern recognition is a process of thinking that does not require explicit teaching – it happens naturally – whereas developing a robust, structured inductive approach *does* require explicit articulation and practice of the steps involved. If the student is not overtly guided to develop the key steps and is not able to practice on relatively simple clinical cases, when they are faced with complex cases they will not be able to apply problem-based principles and as such will flounder if pattern recognition fails. The aim is for the student to progress from conscious competence to subconscious/unconscious competence in a problem-based approach to common clinical signs. It is also important to be aware that reasonable knowledge of anatomy and physiology and a detailed knowledge of pathophysiology are required in order to learn and apply problem-based inductive clinical reasoning. The veterinary curriculum needs to include suitable training prior to, or in conjunction with, the introduction of this form of clinical reasoning. Without knowledge and understanding of pathophysiology, the process can only be learned in theory and cannot be practiced.

When teaching problem-based inductive reasoning, a case-based approach is essential to support theoretical concepts. Some key features of educationally rich cases that are useful to consider as teaching cases are outlined in Table 24.2.

As with all skills, it takes time to develop the knowledge base and mental discipline required for successful problem-based inductive clinical reasoning. However, once the approach is embedded (and indeed, ideally becomes part of the clinician's nonanalytic reasoning), it can save time by assisting the clinician in quickly eliminating extraneous information and focusing on the particular information that is important for the patient and client. It will provide a firm base for the future and, most importantly, will not "go out of date" no matter how many new diseases/disorders are discovered. It is "future proof."

Table 24.2 Characteristics of useful cases for teaching problem-based reasoning.

Characteristic	Learning objective addressed
Clinical signs are suggestive of a diagnosis (thus may result in pattern recognition for the student), but there are several plausible alternatives with very different clinical outcomes if they are not recognized.	Application and pitfalls of pattern recognition.
Clinical signs preclude pattern recognition, but the diagnosis can be reached by application of problem-solving principles through rigorous application of key questions relating to defining/refining the problem and system for the specific problems.	Enhance recognition of the value of a problem-based approach.
Problem definition is key to a successful diagnostic approach – failure to define the problem correctly results in a poor clinical outcome.	Importance of complete and accurate initial problem list. Importance of defining the problem before progressing.
Cases with multiple clinical signs – some of which are specific and key, others are "background noise."	Formulation of a structured and prioritized problem list. Prioritization of problems by diagnostic utility.
Clinical signs have different chronology (acute vs. chronic). Acute and chronic signs may be due to the same disorder, due to different but related disorders (e.g., one a risk factor for the other), or due to two unrelated disorders.	Pathophysiological interpretation of problem list – use of chronology to group problems. Helps build competence in assessing cases with potentially more than one diagnosis.
System definition is key to successful diagnostic approach – failure to seek to define and refine the system correctly results in poor clinical outcome.	Importance of defining and refining the system in relation to primary (structural) vs. secondary (functional) or local vs. systemic.
Clinical signs indicate disease in multiple body systems.	Pathophysiological interpretation of problem list – recognition of comorbidities.
Clinical signs suggest a very large number of possible diagnoses, including those that are quite plausible but not as familiar, e.g., hypercalcemia is a cause of polydipsia/polyuria.	Help to reinforce the value of problem-based reasoning, as pattern recognition not possible. Increase knowledge base in relation to potential differential diagnoses.
There are other learning issues to discuss as well as clinical reasoning, e.g., interpretation of clinical pathology results, choice of diagnostic imaging modalities, interpretation of diagnostic imaging results, management decisions.	Learning of ancillary diagnostic skills that support problem-based reasoning.

References

Auclair, F. (2007) Problem formulation by medical students: An observation study. *BMC Medical Education*, **7**, 16. doi:10.1186/1472-6920-7-16

Audétat, M.-C., Béïque, C., Caire Fon, N., et al. (2011) *Clinical reasoning Difficulties: A Guide to Educational Diagnosis and Remediation.*

http://healthsci.queensu.ca/assets/ohse/
Remediation_Guide.GRILLE_ang_final1er_
sept11.pdf (accessed September 18, 2015).

AVMA (2015) *COE Accreditation Policies and Procedures: Requirements.* American Veterinary Medical Association. https://www.avma.org/ProfessionalDevelopment/Education/Accreditation/Colleges/Pages/coe-pp-requirements-of-accredited-college.aspx (accessed September 18, 2015).

Berner, E., and Graber, M.L. (2008) Overconfidence as a cause of diagnostic error in medicine. *American Journal of Medicine,* **121**, S2–S23.

Bowen, J.D (2006) Educational strategies to promote clinical diagnostic reasoning. *New England Journal of Medicine,* **355**, 2217–2225.

Cockcroft, P.D. (2007) Clinical reasoning and decision analysis. *Veterinary Clinics: Small Animal Practice,* **37**, 499–520.

Coderre, S., Mandin, H., Harasym, P.H., and Fick, G.H. (2003) Diagnostic reasoning strategies and diagnostic success. *Medical Education,* **37**, 695–703.

Croskerry, P. (2003) The importance of cognitive errors in diagnosis and strategies to minimize them. *Academic Medicine,* **78**, 775–780.

Del Mar, C., Doust, J., and Glasziou, P. (2008) *Clinical Thinking: Evidence, Communication and Decision Making.* Blackwell, Oxford.

Ettinger S.J. and Feldman, E.C. (2010) *Textbook of Veterinary Internal Medicine.* Saunders, Missouri.

Eva, K.W. (2004) What every teacher needs to know about clinical reasoning. *Medical Education,* **39**, 98–106.

Fleming, A., Cutrer, W., Reimschisel, T., and Gigante, J. (2012) You too can teach clinical reasoning! *Pediatrics,* **130**, 795–797.

Graber, M.L. (2009) Educational strategies to reduce diagnostic error: Can you teach this stuff? *Advances in Health Science Education,* **14**, 63–69.

Graber, M., Gordon, R. and Franklin, N. (2002) Reducing diagnostic error in medicine: what's the goal? *Acad Med,* **77**, 981–992.

Graber, M., Franklin, N., and Gordon, R. (2005) Diagnostic error in internal medicine. *Archives of Internal Medicine,* **165**, 1493–1499.

Heath, T. (2006) The more things change, the more they should stay the same. *Journal of Veterinary Medical Education,* **33**, 149–154.

Kushniruk, A.W., Patel, V.L., and Marley, A.A.J. (1998) Small worlds and medical expertise: Implications for medical cognition and knowledge engineering. *International Journal of Medical Informatics,* **49**, 255–271.

Maddison, J.E., Volk, V.A., and Church, D.B. (2015) *Clinical Reasoning in Small Animal Practice.* Wiley Blackwell, Oxford.

Malmede, S., van Gog, T., van den Berg, K., *et al.* (2014) Why do doctors make mistakes? A study of the role of salient distracting clinical features. *Academic Medicine,* **89**, 1–7.

Mant, N. (2014) *What frustrations do veterinarians experience in practice and how might their attendance on a "Logical Approach to Clinical Problem Solving" course affect these frustrations?* BVetMed final-year student research project, Royal Veterinary College.

May, S.A. (2013) Clinical reasoning and case-based decision making: The fundamental challenge to veterinary educators. *Journal of Veterinary Medical Education,* **40**, 200–209.

May, S.A. (2015) Towards a scholarship of primary health care. *The Veterinary Record* **176**, 677–682.

McCammon, C. (2015) How to avoid the mistakes that everyone makes. *Emergency Medicine,* **47**, 58–63. http://www.mdedge.com/emed-journal/article/97331/how-avoid-mistakes-everyone-makes (accessed September 18, 2015).

Norman, G.R and Brooks, L.R. (1997) The non-analytical basis of clinical reasoning. *Advances in Health Science Education* **2**, 173–184

Norman, G.R., and Eva, K.W. (2010) Diagnostic error and clinical reasoning. *Medical Education,* **44**, 94–100.

Norman, G., Young, M., and Brooks, L. (2007) Non-analytical models of clinical reasoning: The role of experience. *Medical Education,* **41**, 1140–1145.

Pretz, J.E. (2008) Intuition vs analysis: Strategy and experience in complex everyday problem solving. *Memory and Cognition*, **36**, 554–566.

Safi, S., Hemmati, P., and Shirazi-Beheshtiha, S. (2012) Developing a clinical presentation curriculum in veterinary education: A cognitive perspective. *Comparative Clinical Pathology*, **21**, 1521–1526.

Smith, C.S. (2008) A developmental approach to evaluating competence in clinical reasoning.

Journal of Veterinary Medical Education, **35**, 375–381.

Vandeweerd, J.-M., Vandeweerd, S., Gustin, C., *et al.* (2012) Understanding veterinary practitioners' decision-making process: Implications for veterinary medical education. *Journal of Veterinary Medical Education*, **39**, 142–151.

25

Professionalism

India Lane[1] and Liz Mossop[2]

[1] *College of Veterinary Medicine, University of Tennessee, USA*
[2] *School of Veterinary Medicine and Science, University of Nottingham, UK*

Box 25.1: Key messages

- Recognition of the nontechnical skills required of veterinarians has increased attention to defining and teaching veterinary professionalism.
- Definitions from other health professions provide useful starting points. Key elements include excellence, dignity, humanism, trust, integrity, altruism, and accountability.
- Educators must consider the concept of professional identity formation when designing a professionalism curriculum.
- The influence of the hidden curriculum on students must also be considered, including role models, rituals, and routines within the institution.

- Relevant educational theory includes experiential learning and situated learning; early clinical experiences are rich experiences for development and assessment of professionalism.
- Delivery methods include interactive presentations, case studies, simulated client encounters, and reflective exercises.
- Assessment methods are chosen based on a reasonable expectation of validity and reliability for assessing professional behaviors and feasibility of implementation.

Introduction

Professionalism has been a hot topic in medical education for over a decade. The current emphasis on professionalism has rapidly proceeded through a trajectory that included significant consternation over the meaning of the word, a proliferation of educational efforts, and serious challenges to the inclusion of professionalism in formal curricula. For physicians, changes in societal demands and new models of care delivery have led to an extensive discourse around medical professionalism. Increased primacy for patient autonomy, informed consent, and patient confidentiality are examples of societal pressures influencing professional expectations in human medicine. For veterinarians, economic realities spurred exploration of the nontechnical skills, knowledge, aptitudes, and attitudes (SKAs) that aid practice

Veterinary Medical Education: A Practical Guide, First Edition. Edited by Jennifer L. Hodgson and Jacquelyn M. Pelzer.
© 2017 John Wiley & Sons, Inc. Published 2017 by John Wiley & Sons, Inc.

and career success. Two major assessments of market forces and veterinarian incomes in the late 1990s, known as the KPMG and Brakke studies, illuminated the importance of personal characteristics, communication skills, and savvy business practices in veterinary success (Cron *et al.*, 2000; Brown and Silverman, 1999). Recommendations arising from these studies essentially became a call for a new notion of professionalism in veterinary practice. Additional strategic initiatives, including the North American Veterinary Medical Education Consortium Roadmap (NAVMEC, 2011), later included communication; collaboration; management of self, teams, and systems; leadership; and adaptability as core competencies for future veterinary graduates. The veterinary community responded with numerous educational and professional development opportunities, from revised admissions practices, ceremonies, orientation sessions, and workshops to new courses, curricula, and continuing education strategies (Lloyd and King, 2004).

Despite these efforts, professionalism remains an ill-defined competency or competency domain, and still may be neglected in the veterinary curriculum (Mossop, 2012). In veterinary medicine and other health professions, educators have struggled with whether professionalism can be defined, taught, and assessed. The emergent veterinary literature has focused more heavily on concrete skills, such as communication and business skills, and wellness, but includes limited contributions tackling the concept of professionalism.

Medicine's contemporary "professionalism movement" first called for a useful definition of terms, especially to distinguish professionalism from content areas such as jurisprudence, ethics, and communication (Hafferty and Levinson, 2008). Although related, legal regulations and professional skills such as interviewing, physical examination, and general communication training should be distinct from the professionalism curriculum. Ethics, long a standard component of veterinary curricula, also does not quite capture the essence of professionalism, although ethical dilemmas often underlie professional dilemmas. Educational perspectives in ethics, animal welfare, and communication skills are found elsewhere in this text.

Redefining professionalism was followed by attention to teaching and assessing professionalism across the continuum of undergraduate, clinical, and graduate medical education. A plethora of programs hoped to institutionalize a shared commitment to appropriate conduct. In the aftermath, though, counterpoints arose, where students and others recognized the limitations of professionalism as taught. Evidence grew that empathy and idealism declined, rather than blossomed, during medical training (Hilton and Slotnick, 2005; Patenaude, Niyonsenga, and Fafard, 2003). Students struggled with an idealistic depiction of professionalism in the classroom and a different reality outside it. By recognizing the challenges of professional lives, the reality that professional lapses occur, and the imperfect relationships within healthcare systems, professionalism has become a dynamic and evolving concept and is expected to change just as state-of-the-art medicine changes.

What is Professionalism?

Attempts to define professionalism suffer from the inherent difficulty of defining an ethos that crosses so many intangible and interrelated lines. Birden *et al.* (2014) listed no fewer than 70 definitional papers published between 1999 and 2007. Drawing on the dictionary definition and literature from multiple professions, Cruess, Johnston, and Cruess (2004) developed an expanded definition of "profession" that can be used to introduce students to the service orientation and accountability that bound organized veterinary medicine:

> An occupation whose core element is work based upon the mastery of a complex body of knowledge and skills. It is a vocation in which knowledge of some department of science or learning or the practice of an art founded upon it is used in the service of

others. Its members are governed by codes of ethics and profess a commitment to competence, integrity and morality, altruism, and the promotion of the public good within their domain. These commitments form the basis of a social contract between a profession and society, which in return grants the profession a monopoly over the use of its knowledge base, the right to considerable autonomy in practice and the privilege of self-regulation. Professions and their members are accountable to those served and to society. (Cruess, Johnston, and Cruess, 2004, p. 74)

Additionally, veterinary students are usually quickly introduced to a form of professional statement or oath, in which we publicly *profess* to meet core obligations.

Definitions of professionalism have been suggested for physicians. Most are expansive, with lists of principles, attributes, or competencies (see Box 25.2). The many elements that bleed into professionalism are illustrated by Stern's conceptualization of professionalism as a portico with the "pillars" of excellence, humanism, accountability, and altruism sitting atop a "base" of ethics, jurisprudence, communication, and competence (Arnold and Stern, 2006). Two other frequently cited definitions (the American Board of Internal Medicine Physician's Charter and the Royal College of Canadian Physicians and Surgeons CANMeds Role of the Professional) are framed as *commitments*. The CANMeds model is updated every 10 years.

Both Hafferty (2006) and Birden *et al.* (2014) offer meta-analyses of the definitional literature. Hafferty distills five thematic conclusions, including three common threads — altruism, civic engagement, and self-reflection/mindfulness. He also points out the many ways in which these themes and definitions appear and notes how context influences meaning. Birden makes similar conclusions about context, including geographical region, medical specialty, and personal interpretation. Indeed, Mossop (2012) recognized the importance of

context and the limitations of simply adapting a definition created for physicians to veterinary medicine. The unique and foremost responsibility of veterinary professionals to the welfare of the animal creates a complex professional web, including relationships among veterinarians, animal caretakers, and practice employers. Mossop's proposed definition emphasizes these diverse responsibilities and the attributes employed in meeting them (see Box 25.2).

Eloquent articulations of professionalism can also be complemented by effective personalized sayings, phrases, or mottos for individuals, institutions, or veterinary practices. Veterinary schools often have a professionalism statement or a list of professional values. Detailed codes of conduct, while useful, frequently are too specific to reflect the essence of professionalism. More simply, one or two powerful words can easily be diffused through the daily language of an organization or college. A respected mentor who led several large campuses during his professional career used the single word "dignity" to promote the culture that he expected.

Professionalism as Identity

Those who struggle with defining professionalism can be troubled by the naivety of thinking that such a concept can be reduced to discrete behaviors, attributes, or values. A renewed call has urged medical educators to embrace the development of professionalism as the development of *professional identity*. Indeed, professional identity has been the end goal of educational efforts all along. Using a definition of identity as "a representation of self, achieved in stages over time during which the characteristics, values, and norms of the medical profession are internalized, resulting in an individual thinking, acting, and feeling like a physician" (Cruess *et al.*, 2014, p. 1447), one can imagine a curriculum tailored to emphasize self-awareness, the relationship of actions and behaviors to core attitudes, and the continual development of identity through a professional lifetime.

Box 25.2: What's the meaning of medical and veterinary professionalism – some definitions

American Board of Internal Medicine, "A Physician's Charter" (ABIM, 2002)

Fundamental Principles
- Primacy of patient welfare.
- Patient autonomy.
- Social justice.

Commitments
- Professional competence, including lifelong learning and competence of profession as a whole.
- Honesty, including informed patient consent, reporting, and analyzing medical errors.
- Patient confidentiality.
- Appropriate relations.
- Improving quality of care.
- Improving access to care.
- Just distribution of finite resources.
- Scientific knowledge.
- Managing conflicts of interest.
- Professional responsibilities.

CanMEDs Physician Competency Framework, "Role of the Professional" (CanMEDS, 2015)

Definition:

As Professionals, physicians are committed to the health and well-being of individual patients and society through ethical practice, high personal standards of behavior, accountability to the profession and society, physician-led regulation, and maintenance of personal health.

[Professionals honor] commitments to:
- patients, profession and society through ethical practice;
- society by recognizing and responding to societal expectations in health care;

- the profession by adhering to standards and participating in physician-led regulation; and
- physician health and well-being.

Behaviors That Demonstrate Medical Professionalism (Swick, 2000)

- Subordination of their own interests to the interests of others.
- Adherence to high ethical and moral standards.
- Responsiveness to societal needs.
- Consideration of the societal contract with the communities they serve.
- Demonstration of core humanistic values (honesty, integrity, caring, compassion, altruism, empathy, respect, trustworthiness).
- Accountability.
- Commitment to excellence.
- Commitment to scholarship and advancement.
- Ability to deal with high levels of complexity and uncertainty.
- Reflection on actions and decisions.

Proposed Definition of Veterinary Professionalism (Mossop, 2013)

To demonstrate professionalism, veterinary surgeons should at all times consider their responsibilities to, and the expectations of, their clients, the animals under their care, society and the veterinary practice that provides their employment. The ability to balance these demands and therefore demonstrate professionalism is helped by the following attributes: efficiency, technical competence, honesty, altruism, communication skills, personal values, autonomy, decision-making, manners, empathy, confidence and acknowledgment of limitations. (p. 224)

Professional identity formation does not replace, but builds on, the foundational knowledge, abilities, and attitudes that we attempt to make explicit in professionalism curricula. The lens of professionalism as identity does shift the emphasis from "doing" professional things to "being" professional, a subtle but effective gradation that influences how professionalism is taught and assessed (Cruess, Cruess, and Steinert, 2015). Using this lens for professionalism education, a higher purpose is kept in the forefront, the charge to "raise the ceiling so that everyone can reach their highest potential" (Gunderman and Brown, 2013, p. 1183).

Why Bother Teaching Professionalism?

History and wordsmithed definitions will not capture students' passion, nor will a checklist of competencies required for accreditation. A compelling "why" is necessary for students to embrace professionalism content. The lead arguments highlight the impact of poor behavior or communication. Unprofessional physician behavior has been linked to compromised treatment, poor patient outcomes, dysfunctional healthcare teams, and malpractice suits (Johnson, 2009; Bahaziq and Crosby, 2011). Attention to student behavior is imperative as well: physicians disciplined by state medical boards were more likely than control-matched physicians to have been cited for professional breaches during medical school (especially failure to demonstrate responsibility or failure to respond to feedback; Papadakis *et al.*, 2005). While these important consequences grab attention, starting from a negative orientation may set a punitive or preachy tone. Reframing the positive reasons why professionalism is important, with extensive student input, may be more effective and collaborative in gaining buy-in. "Reasons to be professional" usually include meeting client expectations and fostering client satisfaction, preserving the positive public perceptions of veterinarians, and abiding universal norms of morality and decency (e.g., the "golden rule"; Lane, 2006). Professionalism is indeed a core competency, albeit one frequently

taken for granted. Notions of professionalism, including "practice with integrity" and "have a good attitude," were included among the top three most frequently used skills cited by small animal practitioners (Greenfield, Johnson, and Schaeffer, 2004). Five of six themes emerging from diverse groups of exemplars to define veterinary "success" were nontechnical SKAs grounded in a professional work environment: personal fulfillment, pride, and fun in work; a helping orientation; a balanced lifestyle; respect and professional recognition; and personal goal achievement (Lewis and Klausner, 2003).

Above all, professionalism connotes the manner in which we serve the public. Hafferty (2006) includes professionalism in the "three social movements in medicine today: evidence-based medicine; patient safety; and professionalism (p 194)," and relates all three to quality of care. A recent review by Mueller (2015) recaps the positive impact of professionalism on patients and medical practice. Professionalism of the physician improves clinical outcomes by increasing confidence and trust, motivating patients to follow the doctor's recommendations. A practice culture that prizes high-quality medicine, teamwork, and patient care generates better outcomes as well (Mueller, 2015) and has economic benefits. Veterinary income has been correlated with nontechnical skills (Cron *et al.*, 2000). In a limited veterinary market, nontechnical SKAs can distinguish an exemplary veterinarian from competitors (Lloyd, 2006). Unprofessional behavior has negative impacts on practice reputation and referrals.

Further, contemporary professionalism education emphasizes self-awareness, self-management, and reflection, all skills that foster adaptability and ongoing personal growth. Professionals who have the ability and the opportunity to shape their working environment and respond constructively to professional challenges may be more likely to avoid burnout.

All of these are compelling reasons to include professionalism explicitly in the curricula for veterinarians in training. Of course, the primary reason to embrace professionalism is to preserve the health of the profession. A commitment to the manner in which we meet professional obligations should be just as strong as our commitments to quality medical care and rigorous biomedical research.

Professionalism in the Curriculum

The steps in creating a professionalism curriculum are no different than for curriculum development in general (see Part One, Chapter 1: Curriculum Design, Review, and Reform). The most important decisions surround the content to be included and how it will be framed in theoretical and structural terms. The anticipated goals and outcomes must be articulated so that the content, delivery, and assessment of students and the program follow purposefully. Outcomes can be described as competencies or behaviors, including knowledge of a cognitive foundation. Professionalism can also be considered a competency domain or thread that weaves throughout the curriculum. Within this framework, professionalism is a curricular theme that appears in all courses or blocks, presented in a manner relevant to the setting.

Regardless of the approach, the curricular goals must be intentional and clearly communicated to students and faculty. If the content appears haphazard, it may feel like multiple, orphaned topics have been thrown together into a professionalism or "doctoring" course. Organizing such a course so that it appears in the schedule prominently, alongside "regular" courses, can also raise credibility and status (Hafferty, Gaufberg, and O'Donnell, 2015). Common topics that form or complement a professionalism curriculum are listed in Table 25.1, and Box 25.3 considers who should deliver the curriculum.

Structurally, professionalism curricula usually balance formal and informal approaches so that delivery of a cognitive base and experiential and reflective work are included (Cruess and Cruess, 2009; Inui *et al.*, 2009). Ideally, content flows from the early preclinical curriculum to clinical and postgraduate scenarios in a fashion that builds an individual's "capacity to personalize professionalism" (Cruess and Cruess, 2009, p. 78). Modules or vignettes that can be revisited at various points in the educational continuum can be useful for this

Table 25.1 Suggested content for professionalism curricula.

Frequent core curricular topics	Contemporary issues to consider
AVMA Principles, Veterinarian's Oath	Corporate veterinary medicine
Practice Acts or equivalent	Industry relationships and conflicts of interest
Professional values and behaviors	Professional and personal use of images
Evidence-based practice and continuing education	Social media, blogs, and internet presence
Confidentiality	Professional use of smartphones
Leadership	Referrals and consultations with veterinary specialists
Integrity and responsibility	Giving and receiving feedback
Teamwork and conflict management	Veterinarian or veterinary student impairment
Cultural competence	Veterinary students/veterinarians on reality TV
Informed consent	Managing change
Euthanasia/resuscitation	Appropriate humor
Self-awareness and self-management	
Reflection	
The veterinary team–patient–client relationship	
Coping/adaptability	
Professionalism in the classroom and student groups	
Emotional intelligence	

Box 25.3: Reflections on who should deliver the formal professional curriculum

Although veterinary programs often have limited personnel to draw from, the following points illustrate the varied perspectives on who should "teach" professionalism:

- *Ethicists*: The existing ethics curriculum, with its obvious overlap in content, has been expanded to include the formal teaching of professionalism in many schools. However, ethicists may not be well suited to include the clinically relevant and practical aspects of professionalism (Roberts *et al.*, 2004). Additionally, some ethicists argue that professionalism

should not be considered a "division" of ethics and detract from the importance of the ethics curriculum (Dudzinski, 2004).
- *Anatomists*: Anatomy courses are early in the curriculum and provoke the first considerations of professionalism (respect for cadavers, teamwork, communication; Swartz, 2006; Pawlina, 2006; Swick, 2006).
- *Clinicians*: Professionalism issues often require a problem-solving approach, which is frequently effectively delivered by clinicians (d'Oronzio, 2004).

Box 25.4: Examples of professionalism sessions for the veterinary curriuclum (Mossop and Cobb, 2013)

Throughout the curriculum:

- "What makes a good veterinarian?" facilitated discussions.
- Case studies in empathy for reflection and small-group discussion.

Early in curriculum:

- Cognitive base of professionalism, including example disciplinary cases.
- Honor code exercise: students work in small groups to write their own code.

- Early clinical experience, including opportunities to observe veterinary professionals and debrief in facilitated discussions.
- Critical incident reporting, in writing or in confidential small-group discussions.

Later in curriculum:

- Communication and professionalism: scenarios with simulated clients and debriefing/feedback.
- "What would you do?" case studies or games.

purpose. A sample longitudinal curriculum for veterinary students is posed by Mossop and Cobb (2013; see Box 25.4), who emphasize early immersion in clinical practice or the community. These opportunities create space for students to reflect on the behavior of role models and to shape their own professional identity. Mossop and Cobb (2013) also highlight the guidance needed to help students *learn how to learn* in this new educational landscape. The contrast between material requiring rumination, empathy, and nuance and the rest of

the curriculum, or a busy practice, is strong (Piemonte, 2015).

Additional steps in curriculum planning include planning ahead for individual and programmatic assessments, and methods for updating or adjusting the curriculum. Finally, the curriculum must be dynamic and flexible. Educators must be on the alert for and proactively address contemporary issues that challenge or reshape our notions of professionalism (Table 25.1). Recent examples include industry influences on veterinary students, appropriate use of social media, and the ubiquitous photographs that are easily taken with smartphones (Coe *et al.*, 2011). Digital professionalism is now a distinct field of study (Ross *et al.*, 2013; Ellaway *et al.*, 2015).

Student Feedback and the Hidden Curriculum

When designing a professionalism curriculum, much can be learned from the experiences of others, including students. Medical students pointedly reveal the limitations of a formal course or curriculum in professionalism. Leo and Eagen (2008), nearing graduation, wrote: "How can medical students, who are hopefully the proponents of professionalism, be so hostile towards the subject?" (p. 509) They suggest that students quickly tire of the subject due to a primary orientation on unprofessional behaviors versus professional ones; a double standard and "do as I say, not as I do" view of faculty and staff behavior; and a perceived personal affront – professionalism curricula seem to suggest that one might not be a good person, much less a good doctor. Furthermore, curricular content was perceived to project positive behaviors as unachievable, abstract ideals, whereas unprofessional behaviors were common, realistic, and worthy of a scolding. The most disturbing aspect of the curriculum for these students was the disconnect between what was taught and what was observed; a laundry list of unprofessional faculty behaviors was noted (Leo and Eagen, 2008). Other medical students have chimed in on the apparent double standard (Brainard and Brislen, 2007). Students who stood up for principles appeared more likely to be punished for rocking the boat than applauded. The latter authors write: "Students are genuinely confused as to what constitutes professional behavior (p. 1010)."

Despite this disappointing pushback, Levinson *et al.* (2014) point out the value of struggling with definitions of professionalism and with professionalism education: "In short, the arrival of medicine's modern-day professionalism movement helped both to uncover, but also to create and label, the very tensions between professionalism-as-an-ideal and professionalism-in-practice." (p. 44) It is important that students have the ability to recognize lapses in professionalism and to use these observations to reflect on what is and is not professional behavior. With this insight, conversations about professionalism can emphasize: "We are generally good people; what are the stressors and situations that challenge us?"

Additionally, students resent the time devoted to professionalism and, by default, "taken away" from scientific courses. Resentment may be particularly strong when the content feels patronizing (Leo and Eagen, 2008; Hafferty, Gaufberg, and O'Donnell, 2015; Stockley and Forbes, 2014). Students are offended by content that feels like common sense, a kindergarten lesson, or a sermon. Faculty may also resent the time devoted to professionalism and other nontechnical competencies – curricular time has long been symbolic of relative importance and power among academic disciplines or departments (Lane, 2007).

Hafferty, Gaufberg, and O'Donnell (2015) suggest that these student reactions result from the *hidden curriculum*; they describe early medical students as "hypersensitive readers of the environment (p133)." The set of unseen influences known as the hidden curriculum contribute as much, if not more, than any formal curriculum to the process of professional identity formation of veterinary students (Figure 25.1). The hidden curriculum is difficult to define precisely, but the definition of Karnieli-Miller *et al.* (2010)

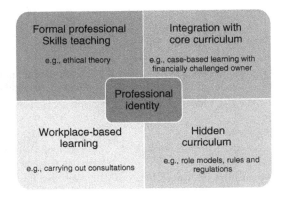

Figure 25.1 The elements that contribute to professional identity formation in veterinary students.

is useful: "the physical and workforce organizational infrastructure in the academic health center that influences learning process and the socialization to professional norms and rituals." Important components of this are the people, rituals, regulations, and language that students encounter on a daily basis, in both the academic environment and the clinical environment. Role models are one of the strongest influences on the hidden curriculum (Cruess, Cruess, and Steinert, 2008); faculty must be aware of this aspect of student learning and consider their professional behaviors accordingly. Students must also be introduced to the powerful influence of the hidden curriculum early in a professionalism curriculum. Students who are aware of the influence of role models and language can be encouraged to identify and reflect on both positive and negative incidents, hopefully encouraging them to mirror appropriate rather than inappropriate behaviors.

Fortunately, students tend to recognize the value of nontechnical content increasingly as they progress through the overall curriculum. Heath, Lanyon, and Lynch-Blosse (1996) found that Australian veterinary students' attitudes toward the importance of communication skills, self-management, and understanding of others in the curriculum increased from the first to the fifth year of training and beyond. The importance of professional skills as compared to other technical skills also increased in fourth-year students and graduates of a Canadian veterinary college (Tinga *et al.*, 2001).

Third-year students in another veterinary college felt confident that they would "turn on" professionalism when it mattered (Lane, 2006). Not surprisingly, professionalism curricula in residency training programs tend to be highly effective and well received, given the immersion of residents in clinical work (Deptula and Chun, 2013). Although reassuring, this reality presents significant dilemmas regarding what to include in formal curricula and when to include it.

Educational Theory Relevant to the Teaching of Professionalism

As with any curricular component or approach, it is important to consider relevant educational theory when developing a curriculum of professionalism. There are several useful theories that help faculty consider how to deliver this teaching, and all have reflective practice as a core component.

Situated Learning

The concept of situated learning (Lave and Wenger, 1991) is often used as an overarching framework for professionalism curricula (Cruess and Cruess, 2006). This framework acknowledges classroom learning as a fairly ineffective contribution to the development of professionalism as a standalone element. Cognitive foundations must be brought together with contextualized experience to make professionalism authentic and recognizable to students (Table 25.2). Situated learning is the notion of

Table 25.2 Key components of situated learning.

Cognitive apprenticeship	The traditional apprenticeship model is expanded where teachers make task elements explicit and ensure that relevance is explained to the learner
Collaborative learning	Learning takes place with others, encouraging group problem-solving, often in an interprofessional context
Reflection	Reflection on action and considering future actions are essential
A chance to practice skills	Repetition of tasks allows development of automation and the ability to perform tasks in a range of situations
Articulation of learning skills	The overt description of task elements and the way in which problems have been solved is important to developing experts

Source: McLellan, 1996.

putting knowledge acquisition in a real-life context, ensuring the development of the novice to an expert with a professional identity and a core set of common values (Maudsley and Strivens, 2000). By nature, situated learning is a social learning process, requiring interaction and collaboration with others. Students go through a phase of "legitimate peripheral participation," being allowed to learn from the skills and behaviors of others, before developing these things themselves and becoming firmly embedded in the workplace and entrusted to carry out appropriate tasks. The key components of situated learning as described by McLellan (1996) are outlined in Table 25.2. The experience-based learning model of clinical students learning in the workplace draws much from situated learning, and has "supported participation" at its core, leading to both emotional and practical learning (Dornan *et al.*, 2007).

Experiential Learning and Reflection

The concept of experiential learning is well recognized in clinical curricula, and is of great importance when developing a curriculum of professionalism. The classic experiential learning cycle (Kolb and Fry, 1975) explains how experience contributes to learning in four cyclical steps: concrete experience, reflective observation, abstract conceptualization, and active experimentation (see Figure 6.1 in Part Two, Chapter 6: Collaborative Learning).

A prominent way in which students will learn professionalism is by participating in tasks and reflecting on their performance; ample opportunities for workplace-based experience form a key component of ensuring that this occurs, alongside teaching students to engage in reflective practice. Simulation can also be used to deliver experiential learning, and this can be an effective way to improve readiness for the workplace and a smooth transition (Kneebone *et al.*, 2002).

It is important to ensure that students reflect *on action* as well as the more spontaneous reflection *in action* (Schön, 1983), and this can be facilitated by the use of reflective diaries or portfolios, in which students describe their thoughts and actions and their impact on others. Formal reflection should also ensure that students plan learning goals, which is important as they develop their professional identity. Reflective practice is also generally included as a component of professionalism, and so it is not only a part of students' learning, but something that they must be able to do effectively in order to progress to being an expert with the ability to think critically and solve problems (Lachman and Pawlina, 2006).

Delivery Methods

The relevant educational theories inform delivery methods: methods for highlighting professionalism are by necessity experiential and interactive. The nature of the material to be delivered also compels there to be a variety of methods employed in a variety of settings (Table 25.3). Intensive sessions during orientation or inter-semester periods can provide some space for exploration, but may suffer from a lack of context and experience (Walton *et al.*, 2013). The separation also may place the professionalism symbolically outside of the "regular" curriculum. Didactic presentations should be limited, but are sometimes necessary for foundational material. Lectures or large-group discussions can be enhanced by using student response systems (clickers) to unveil diverse or consensus student opinions (Mueller, 2015). Formal courses also employ small groups for discussion of case studies or critical reflections. Periodic faculty-led case presentations and guest speakers can be effective too (Byszewski *et al.*, 2012). The use of critical incident reporting and reflection has been described to formalize debriefing of real-life observations (Branch, 2005). Students discuss behaviors and situations that they have encountered in small groups, and consider professionalism issues. These conversations also serve to uncover the hidden curriculum and make it an identifiable component of their professional development. Simulation, role play, and interviews with veterinary team members, clients, producers, or public health officials are other commonly used methods (Ramani and Orlander, 2013; MacPherson *et al.*, 2014).

Table 25.3 Curricular activities for professionalism education.

Activity	Advantages	Disadvantages	Potential assessment
Ceremony or orientation	Introduces necessary basic knowledge Symbolism can be powerful	Usually prior to context Empty gesture if not followed up in practice Can empower students excessively	Not usually done; quiz could cover basic points or reflective writing
Intensive workshops or bootcamps	Particularly useful for house officers Provides space for reflection and dialog	Time and labor intensive	OSCE or performance-based assessment
Didactic cognitive foundation course	Provide cognitive base in consistent message Offers opportunity to build	Students may resent time commitment May not be in experiential context	Multiple options: exam, OSCE, portfolio
Personal mission statements or projected obituary exercises	Student directed and personal	Lack of relevance for early curriculum Students may not engage	Portfolio
Medical humanities Literature, poetry, art, music	Ability to see another's point of view Create meaning independently	Brief exposures may not be effective Students may not engage	Reflective writing
Role modeling (e.g., mentoring program)	Situational and resource independent Most effective for learners, especially with debriefing opportunities	Role-modeled behaviors are positive and negative Message can confuse students	Reflective writing
Case studies	Can cover many different types of scenarios Delivered to small groups or in online fora	Often feel open-ended for students May not be realistic	Reflection or discussion
Scenario-based videos	Capture situations or interactions for review in multiple settings	May not appear realistic or authentic Can be expensive to produce	Reflection or discussion
Peer group discussions	Student directed authentic and relevant to student experience	Schedule coordination may be difficult Peer training required for consistency	Reflective writing or group report
Owner or veterinarian interviews, panels, or testimonials	Authenticity Most effective with small groups of students	Labor intensive to coordinate Outcome of sessions may be unclear	Participation Reflective writing
Virtual scenarios/patients	Allows individual exploration and safe practice in making decisions	Authenticity can be challenging in online delivery	Direct observation
Simulation	Provides safe space for practice and simulates actual workplace	Can be labor intensive or expensive	Performance-based assessment

(Continued)

Table 25.3 (Continued)

Activity	Advantages	Disadvantages	Potential assessment
Early clinical experience	Allows situated learning and context Fosters the socialization process	Experiences are likely to be inconsistent	Reflection or journal review
Journals or narrative reflections	Personal interaction with content Skill-building for reflection in practice	Time consuming for students require practice and feedback	
Community service or service learning experiences	Authentic experiences Develop multiple skills	Labor intensive to facilitate Hidden curriculum difficult to control	Direct observation Narrative or reflective report
Critical incident discussions	Use real-life content, foster reflective practice	Facilitators must foster safe and confidential disclosure and reflection	

Note: OSCE = objective structured clinical examinations.

The importance of role modeling as an educational method cannot be overemphasized. Role modeling tends to be a preferred opportunity for learners of all levels (Riley and Kumar, 2012; Morihara, Jackson, and Chun, 2013; Byszewski *et al.*, 2012). Faculty and staff should be aware that students are continually watching for clues as to how to act. In the clinical environment, students are expected to absorb constant messages from observing and participating in client interactions, diagnostic and treatment decisions, and veterinary team operations. The professionalism component can be made more explicit by educators, however. Attention to positive and negative expressions of professionalism can be regularly added to discussions of medical or surgical details. Activities can also be designed to raise awareness of language, communication, teamwork, respect, and responsibility (Lane and Cornell, 2013). Debriefing of critical incidents is useful as well. Again, educators must be prepared to elicit observations and discussion from students, rather than simply relaying their own experience or perspective.

Preparing Content and Using Examples

Content used for teaching and assessing professionalism must be current, authentic, and relevant. Content organization requires a challenging balancing act to hit the mark for context and relevance at each point in the curriculum, avoiding redundancy to maintain student interest. As illuminated by medical student pushback, content must avoid the appearance of simply trying to teach morality. By focusing on the impact of professional actions and decisions, rather than the moral grounds for decisions (as important as that seems), messages may find better reception. Additionally, the circumstances that make *just doing the right thing* more challenging in practice can be emphasized, especially when peer behavior or role-model behavior alters the context (Levinson *et al.*, 2014; Huddle, 2005). Attention to professional lapses must be balanced with sufficient examples of positive behavior. Elementary points about professional dress, classroom etiquette, and respect for others may be best addressed separately, or left up to the students themselves to explore (Leo and Eagen, 2008).

Listening to student input or client input is particularly useful when forming content and illustrative examples. In one medical school, students in internal medicine and pediatrics clerkships wrote case observations identifying ethical or professional issues, and redacted versions were used to facilitate seminar discussion. Based on qualitative analysis of hundreds of student reports, the most frequent issues included (in decreasing order) inadequate communication, end-of-life or quality-of-life treatment concerns, discord between doctor's and patient's wishes, disrespect to patient or family, resuscitation decisions, and lapses in patient confidentiality. Student roles and reactions were also themes in the observations (Kaldjian *et al.*, 2012). Public views of professionalism can inform content too: the most prized elements of medical professionalism include doctors' genuine (attentive, empathetic, compassionate) interactions with patients and colleagues, confidentiality, fairness, accessibility, and accountability (Chandratilake *et al.*, 2010).

Other examples can be pulled from news articles, videos, television shows, or other narratives. Literature and art are particularly rich media for expanding a learner's ability to see through others' eyes (Marchalik, 2015; Stone and Weisert, 2004). A young academic physician who teaches literature in medicine poignantly relates how this is usually learned – the hard way:

> As interns we learned that recognising the depth of another's suffering is a skill earned the hard way – by repeatedly bearing witness to it – because we were seldom taught to imagine the world from another's point of view in the classroom. (Marchalik, 2015, p. 2346)

He reminds us how storytelling is a compelling educational strategy, provided that learners are allowed to explore personal thoughts and feelings in a safe environment.

Organizational Professionalism and the Learning Environment

The success of a professionalism curriculum also depends on the professionalism and support of the institution. While a few dedicated individuals often carry professionalism efforts in veterinary schools, visible institutional support can make these efforts truly successful. Institutional support is usually found in mission and values statements, participation by top leaders, and commitment of resources.

In the health professions, organizational professionalism can go further than the student curriculum. Stern and Papadakis (2006) plead for a systemic environment of professionalism in academic medical centers and professional organizations, where all personnel are trained to role model professional behavior and administrative decisions prioritize the delivery of compassionate and professional healthcare. Levinson *et al.* (2014) summarize *institutional professionalism* as a pie chart of prevention, education, intervention, and reward, spanning all units and levels of the school and hospital. Rewards and scholarships are popular and meaningful ways to visibly recognize exemplary professional behavior (Byszewski *et al.*, 2012; Hammer, 2000).

Leadership by experienced and respected faculty, particularly those whose responsibilities and credibility cross departmental lines, is key to successful curricular planning and implementation. Extensive faculty engagement and input into curriculum development, including attention to the hidden curriculum, will both enable planners to understand faculty perspectives and improve buy-in for a significant investment of curricular time (Cruess and Cruess, 2009).

Faculty Development and Professionalism of Educators

Faculty development in how to teach, how to assess, and how to role model professionalism is critical. Although veterinary faculty agree that nontechnical skills are important for veterinary graduates, they are less likely to feel that it is their responsibility to foster these skills (Lane and Bogue, 2010). Individual faculty probably were not exposed to professionalism education in their own training, and may never have articulated a personal meaning of professionalism for themselves (Cruess and Cruess, 2009). When considering a curricular element of professionalism teaching, faculty development is an essential component, so that this teaching is not undermined by the overt behavior of teachers

Box 25.5: Quick Tip – faculty and staff development

Faculty and staff members may not be comfortable or well equipped enough to assess professionalism in learners. Fortunately, the adage "we miss more by not seeing than not knowing" applies here, as it does in medical diagnosis. Observing, noticing, and articulating positive and negative professional behaviors simply require attentiveness, some help with examples, and practice.

and clinicians (Steinert *et al.*, 2005). While behaviors that clearly disrupt patient care, the laboratory, or the department are probably clear to faculty and staff, the professionalism expected of an educator may surprise them. Medical students pointed to unprofessional behavior in the preclinical environment: lectures canceled, delayed meeting start times, unanswered phone calls or e-mails, weak or late evaluations, breaches of confidentiality, and frequent, disruptive turnover of faculty and administrators (Brainard and Brislen, 2007). During professionalism week activities in one veterinary college, faculty, house officers, and staff met together for dialogue about recently adopted professionalism guidelines. Pointedly, behaviors such as simply saying "hello" in the morning and paying attention during rounds and seminars were suggested to improve faculty professionalism (Lane, 2006).

The behavior and commitment of faculty participating in formal professionalism activities is also important. Faculty members who put little effort into facilitating small-group activities or discussions can diminish their perceived value (Stockley and Forbes, 2014). Fundamental training for faculty and staff emphasizes recognition of professional behavior, observational skills, descriptive skills, and feedback skills. Providing significant, intensive, and longitudinal development opportunities so that faculty and staff take the same journey as we envision for our students takes time, commitment, and resources; however, simple conversations can still raise awareness and open dialog for college-wide progress.

Assessment of Professionalism

The importance of professionalism in the curriculum must be supported by appropriate evaluation. Veterinary colleges also have an obligation to affirm the achievement of professionalism in graduates to their institution, accreditors, the profession, and the public. In general, features of good assessment practice include defined outcomes and expected performance, appropriate methods, and reasonable reliability, validity, and feasibility (see Chapter 20). Students should also have opportunities for practice and formative feedback prior to summative or high-stakes assessments. Assessment of professionalism is challenging, especially if behaviors reflecting professional values are not defined. Faculty must work together to compose a collective vision of "what professionalism looks like." Added concerns for evaluating professionalism include the following (Stern, 2006):

- Frequent formative feedback and longitudinal development are required to change attitude or behavior and to allow for occasional lapses; early assessments should primarily be oriented toward improvement.
- Direct measures are most reliable for assessing behaviors, but are labor and time intensive.
- Assessments always have an element of subjectivity.
- Professionalism can be expressed in many different ways.
- Professional dilemmas rarely have only one correct resolution.

- Observed behavior (positive or negative) does not necessarily reflect underlying attitudes, intentions, or values.
- Raters may perceive learner behaviors in different ways.
- Assessment of professionalism feels quite personal to both rater and learner and must be handled sensitively.

In order to meet some of these challenges, the assessment program is usually carefully planned and multipronged; the plan and methods should evolve as the meaning of professionalism evolves. Like the teaching methods, assessment methods should be as authentic and experiential as possible, leading to a heavy emphasis on direct measures. Embedding assessments and direct observations across multiple points in the curriculum helps spread the workload and encourage continual development.

Ideally, students have a clear path to final goals and outcomes from the outset of the curriculum. Key indicators should be aggregated for programmatic review and reporting purposes. Many methods have been described to assess professionalism (Amin, Seng, and End, 2006; Mossop and Cobb, 2013; Levinson et al., 2014) and can be adapted for specific needs (Table 25.4). A few commonly used methods are highlighted in what follows.

Self-Assessment and Portfolio

Portfolios are increasingly used in health professions education as a method for students to demonstrate their development and reflect on their strengths and weaknesses (Hall et al., 2012; Mossop and Senior, 2008). A portfolio consists of a collection of evidence and accompanying narrative reflection, all linked to competencies outlined by the learner's curriculum. Electronic formats are becoming increasingly popular and several bespoke e-portfolios are available to educators, including open-source options. Educators can utilize the portfolio to assess student progress formatively or summatively and to rate students on their written reflective

skills. To elicit insight into professional identity development, learners must be directed specifically to reflect on elements of professionalism during learning experiences, for example in summaries of clinical cases encountered in school or the workplace. Using portfolios as capstone, summative assessments certainly helps drive student engagement with the tool (Driessen et al., 2005).

Portfolios are appealing for professionalism assessment because they complement and reduce the time commitment of direct observation. Portfolio documentation and reflective work also promote lifelong learning skills, which will benefit learners throughout their professional career (Friedman et al., 2001). However, portfolios are considered indirect measures of professionalism, because student behavior is not being directly observed, a concern that limits the validity of the method. Implementation is also challenging; adequate support is critical to ensure that students understand the requirements and format or technical platform. Faculty development is also vital for successful implementation (Driessen et al., 2005). Finally, portfolio design for assessing professionalism should be developed in a student-centered manner. If the portfolio largely comprises templates provided by instructors or administrators, self-assessment and self-discovery are diminished. Well-designed portfolio initiatives encourage students to engage in reflective practice and develop essential professional skills; these vital elements are undermined if there is little freedom for exploration and creativity (Driessen et al., 2005).

Performance-Based Observation and Checklists

Teaching and assessment of skills often involve breaking those skills down into their component steps or parts. Learners are then assessed based on their demonstration of each step, along with a global, overall rating or score. Behaviors reflecting professionalism can also be listed in this manner for a course, small-group exercise, practical examination,

Table 25.4 Methods for assessing professionalism.

Method of assessment	Brief description	Best applications	Advantages	Disadvantages
Participant self-reports	Survey or inventory	Pre- and post-assessments of attitudes	Easy to implement and collect	Reliance on self-assessment
Written examinations	Usually multiple-choice format	Assessment of basic knowledge and principles of professionalism	Can measure knowledge base Can be adapted to provide limited test of decision-making	Disconnected from practice, therefore limited validity
Objective structured clinical examination (OSCE)	Usually a timed and focused assessment delivered in a series of stations Scored with a rubric or checklist	Clinical-level interactions such as interviews, delivering bad news, deflecting anger and conflict	Reliable checklists are possible for consistency	Labor intensive Relies on well-trained assessors Disconnected from real-life practice, therefore limited validity
Journals or narrative reflections	Students asked to record experiences relating to professionalism	Formative feedback in experiences	Ideal for capturing individual progress Models and enhances reflective skills	Labor intensive to implement and assess Reflection is challenging to assess, therefore reliability limited Validity also questionable
Portfolio	Student collects evidence, usually including evaluations, narratives, projects, etc.	Longitudinal assessment for and demonstration of performance across curriculum, course, or experience	Provides varied evidence for periodic formative assessment	Labor intensive to implement and assess Reflection is challenging to assess, therefore limited reliability Validity also questionable
Unannounced standardized clients (SCs)	Trained actor visits with prepared scenario	Clinical setting	Provides consistent case and reliability Validity good with well-trained SCs	Labor intensive and challenging to implement
Peer assessment	Anonymous structured feedback by comments or rubrics	Clinical setting Small groups As supplement to faculty	Peers are most attuned to performance in time and context of other students Know each other best Mimics future regulation of colleagues and feedback to other professionals	Potential for bias, self-interest or reluctance to criticize Poor reliability

(Continued)

Table 25.4 (Continued)

Method of assessment	Brief description	Best applications	Advantages	Disadvantages
Whole-case observation	Videotaped client interactions or direct observation of client interaction or other case management (e.g., anesthesia or radiology)	Clinical setting	Takes advantage of regular caseload and practice context	Time intensive for assessor Reliability low unless multiple encounters are observed
Professionalism Mini-evaluation exercises	Short checklist for on-the-spot direct observation	Daily, frequent, formative assessment of student performance with patients/clients	Feasible for clinical use Reliable with 4–6 assessments	Requires trained assessors
Clerkship/clinical rotation end-of-course ratings	Scales or rubrics		Clarifies expected levels of performance Can include detailed and global ratings	Often in-house and lack validation and assessor training Reliability low
360° assessments (multisource feedback)	Incorporates feedback and impressions from multiple sources: peers, supervisors, staff, clients	Clinical students or house officers; also useful for faculty and staff evaluation	Combines multiple perspectives for valid input, good reliability with reasonable number of respondents	Challenging to implement – recruitment of respondents needs care Potential bias
Client feedback	Usually a post-visit survey	Clinical setting	High levels of validity High educational impact	Quality of feedback variable Poor reliability between clients
Review complaints or lapses	Log of complaints or reported incidents	Clinical setting	Feasible and important for organizational improvement	Poor reliability depending on reporting methods; Overemphasizes negative behaviors

Sources: Mossop and Cobb, 2013; Levinson *et al.*, 2014; Amin, Seng, and End, 2006.

or clinical rotation (see Figure 25.2). Checklists are easy to create and distribute and add consistency to evaluations. However, they may "over-anatomize" a complex and nebulous ethos and fail to capture the essence of professionalism (Hafferty, Gaufberg, and O'Donnell, 2015). Too much reliance on checklists may diminish the countless ways in which learners can find their own flavor and identity, as well as restrict the lens through which evaluators see professionalism.

Rubrics

Rubrics differ from checklists in that components (or dimensions) of performance are described, but levels of performance are delineated from unsatisfactory to exemplary (see Table 25.5). Two to five levels of performance are defined; the minimally acceptable level is set somewhere along the scale.

Rubrics can be applied to many types of learning activities, from essay questions and journals to participation scores, presentations, clinical

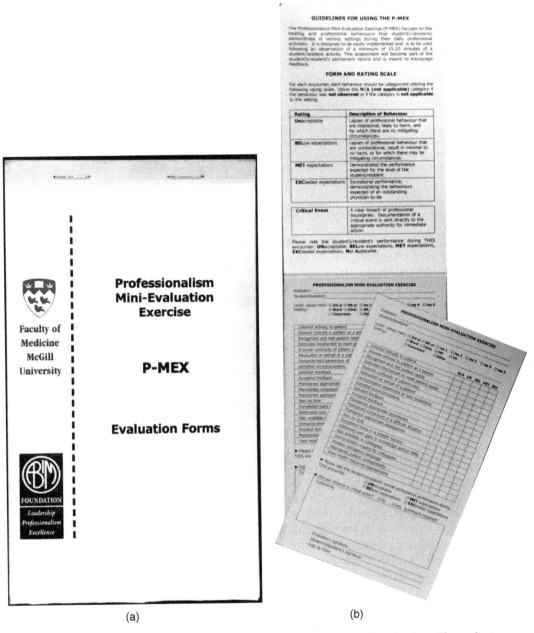

Figure 25.2 Example mini-evaluation of a patient or client encounter. (a) Booklet developed for evaluators. (b) Evaluation page that is immediately provided to learner. Source: Courtesy of the American Board of Internal Medicine and McGill University.

Table 25.5 Sample rubric descriptors for professionalism in a clinical environment.

	Exemplary Performance	Good Performance	Satisfactory Performance	Unacceptable Performance
Overall Professionalism				
	Demonstrates high level of maturity, is always prepared and dependable, interacts respectfully with clinicians, staff, classmates and clients; appears eager to learn and participate	Demonstrates good level of maturity, is usually prepared and dependable, interacts respectfully with clinicians, staff, classmates and clients; appears eager to learn and participate	Demonstrates acceptable level of maturity, preparedness and dependability; generally interacts respectfully with others or has minor areas for improvement in professional behavior (must comment)	Does not display appropriate professionalism; is unenthusiastic about learning and participation; demonstrates gaps in professional behavior based on UTCVM guidelines (must comment)

Source: University of Tennessee College of Veterinary Medicine (UTCVM). Used with permission.

performance, and medical record-keeping. Rubrics communicate the expectations for performance, increase consistency among raters, and save time for evaluators. Although rubrics are not as restrictive as checklists, the descriptors are still limited in scope.

Clinical Performance Ratings

Clinical performance ratings are familiar to veterinary faculty and either utilize a rubric or a simple anchored scale (e.g., 1 = unsatisfactory, 5 = outstanding). Without additional narrative feedback, these ratings give students little insight into their strengths or guidance for how to improve. Performance ratings are highly subject to error, including some errors related to rater ability and many more related to subjectivity and bias. Common errors in the use of a rating scale include lack of discrimination (giving an individual learner similar ratings on all items), inappropriate use of extremes, and centralizing tendencies (giving all learners similar ratings). Validity is also compromised when evaluators put minimal effort into rating learners, make assessments based on limited evidence, or let fatigue, cowardice, or bias affect results (Royal and Hecker, 2015). In the domain of professionalism, such errors are magnified. Raters should be trained to interpret

the anchors, use the rubric or scale properly, and add qualitative feedback.

Multisource Feedback, Including Peer Assessment

Feedback by multiple methods and in multiple contexts (time and setting) offers an integrated assessment of ability (Levinson *et al.*, 2014). Data sources include performance ratings as already described, as well as input from staff, clients, and peers. Online systems facilitate collection and distribution. Peer assessment creates an opportunity for learners to practice giving feedback, another essential professional skill (Cohen, 1999). Peer assessment is usually aggregated and shared with the student anonymously. In small-group and clinical team settings, however, an established team can grow to exchange constructive face-to-face feedback. When peer and multisource assessment is implemented across the institution (including staff and faculty), constructive feedback becomes the organizational norm.

Conclusion

Professionalism is an important, but challenging concept to thread through veterinary curricula. Effective programs utilize a working definition or set of principles to engage discussion and practice, with the lofty end goal of each graduate reaching a personalized professional identity. Early experiential opportunities and effective role models are keys to successful delivery; frequent, direct observation with individualized

feedback provides the ideal assessment. Significant faculty, staff and student input is critical in order to maintain relevant content as the expression of professionalism and the challenges to professional behavior change over time.

References

ABIM (2011) *A Physician's Charter*. American Board of Internal Medicine. http://abimfoundation.org/what-we-do/medical-professionalism-and-the-physician-charter/physician-charter (accessed November 13, 2016).

Amin, Z., Seng, C.Y., and End, K.H. (2006) *Practical Guide to Medical Student Assessment*, World Scientific, Hackensack, N.J.

Arnold, L., and Stern, D.T. (2006) What is medical professionalism? in *Measuring Medical Professsionalism* (ed. D.T. Stern), Oxford University Press, New York, pp. 15–37.

Bahaziq, W., and Crosby, E. (2011) Physician professional behaviour affects outcomes: A framework for teaching professionalism during anesthesia residency. *Canadian Journal of Anaesthesiology*, **58**, 1039–1050.

Birden, H., Glass, N., Wilson, I., *et al.* (2014) Defining professionalism in medical education: A systematic review. *Medical Teacher*, **36**, 47–61.

Brainard, A.H., and Brislen, H.C. (2007) Viewpoint: Learning professionalism: A view from the trenches. *Academic Medicine*, **82**, 1010–1014.

Branch, W.T., Jr. (2005) Use of critical incident reports in medical education. *A perspective. Journal of General Internal Medicine*, **20**, 1063–1067.

Brown, J., and Silverman, J. (1999) The current and future market for veterinarians and veterinary medical services in the United States. *Journal of the American Veterinary Medical Association*, **215**, 161–183.

Byszewski, A., Hendelman, W., Mcguinty, C., and Moineau, G. (2012) Wanted: Role models – medical students' perceptions of professionalism. *BMC Medical Education*, **12**, 115–123.

CanMEDS (2015) Physician Competency Framework. Royal College of Physicians and Surgeons of Canada. http://canmeds.royalcollege.ca/en/framework (accessed November 13, 2016).

Chandratilake, M., McAleer, S., Gibson, J., and Roff, S. (2010) Medical professionalism: What does the public think? *Clinical Medicine*, **10**, 364–369.

Coe, J.B., Weijs, C.A., Muise, A., *et al.* (2011) Teaching veterinary professionalism in the face(book) of change. *Journal of Veterinary Medical Education*, **38**, 353–359.

Cohen, J.J. (1999) Measuring professionalism: Listening to our students. *Academic Medicine*, **74**, 1010.

Cron, W., Slocum, J., Goodnight, D., and Volk, J. (2000) Executive summary of the Brakke management and behavior study. *Journal of the American Veterinary Medical Association*, **217**, 332–338.

Cruess, R.L., and Cruess, S.R. (2006) Teaching professionalism: General principles. *Medical Teacher*, **28**, 205–208.

Cruess, R.L., and Cruess, S.R. (2009) Principles for designing a program for the teaching and learning of professionalism at the undergraduate level, in *Teaching Medical Professionalism* (eds R.L. Cruess, S.R. Cruess, and Y. Steinert), Cambridge University Press, Cambridge, pp. 73–92.

Cruess, R.L., Cruess, S.R., Boudreau, J.D., *et al.* (2014) Reframing medical education to support professional identity formation. *Academic Medicine*, **89**, 1446–1451.

Cruess, R.L., Cruess, S.R., and Steinert, Y. (2015) Amending Miller's pyramid to include professional identity formation. *Academic Medicine*, **91**, 180–185.

Cruess, S.R., Cruess, R.L., and Steinert, Y. (2008) Role modelling – making the most of a powerful teaching strategy. *BMJ*, **336**, 718–721.

Cruess, S.R., Johnston, S., and Cruess, R.L. (2004) "Profession": A working definition for medical educators. *Teaching and Learning Medicine*, **16**, 74–76.

Deptula, P., and Chun, M.B.J. (2013) A literature review of professionalism in surgical education: Suggested components for development of a curriculum. *Journal of Surgical Education*, **70**, 408–422.

Dornan, T., Boshuizen, H., King, N., and Scherpbier, A. (2007) Experience-based learning: A model linking the processes and outcomes of medical students' workplace learning. *Medical Education*, **41**, 84–91.

D'Oronzio, J.C. (2004) Avoiding fallacies of misplaced concreteness in medical professionalism. *American Journal of Bioethics*, **4**, 31–33.

Driessen, E.W., Van Tartwijk, J., Overeem, K., et al. (2005) Conditions for successful reflective use of portfolios in undergraduate medical education. *Medical Education*, **39**, 1230–1235.

Dudzinski, D.M. (2004) Integrity in the relationship between medical ethics and professionalism. *American Journal of Bioethics*, **4**, 26–27.

Ellaway, R.H., Coral, J., Topps, D., and Topps, M. (2015) Exploring digital professionalism. *Medical Teacher*, **37**, 844–849.

Friedman, B.D., Davis, M., Harden, R., et al. (2001) AMEE medical education guide no. 24: Portfolios as a method of student assessment. *Medical Teacher*, **23**, 535–551.

Greenfield, C., Johnson, A., and Schaeffer, D. (2004) Frequency of various procedures, skills, and areas of knowledge among veterinarians in private small animal exclusive or predominant practice and proficiency expected of new graduates. *Journal of the American Veterinary Medical Association*, **224**, 1780–1787.

Gunderman, R.B., and Brown, B.P. (2013) Teaching professionalism through case studies. *Academic Radiology*, **20**, 1183–1185.

Hafferty, F.W. (2006) Definitions of professionalism: A search for meaning and identity. *Clinical Orthopaedics and Related Research*, **449**, 193–204.

Hafferty, F.W., Gaufberg, E.H., and O'Donnell, J.F. (2015) The role of the hidden curriculum in "on doctoring" courses. *AMA Journal of Ethics*, **17**, 130–139.

Hafferty, F.W., and Levinson, D. (2008) Moving beyond nostalgia and motives: Towards a complexity science view of medical professionalism. *Perspectives in Biology and Medicine*, **51**, 599–615.

Hall, P., Byszewski, A., Sutherland, S., and Stodel, E. (2012) Developing a sustainable electronic portfolio (ePortfolio) program that fosters reflective practice and incorporates CanMEDS competencies into the undergraduate medical curriculum. *Academic Medicine*, **87**, 744–751.

Hammer, D.P. (2000) Professional attitudes and behaviors: The "A's and B's" of Professionalism. *American Journal of Pharmaceutical Education*, **64**, 455–464.

Heath, T.J., Lanyon, A., and Lynch-Blosse, M. (1996) A longitudinal study of veterinary students and recent graduates 3. Perceptions of veterinary education. *Australian Veterinary Journal*, **74**, 301–304.

Hilton, S., and Slotnick, H. (2005) Protoprofessionalism: How professional occurs across the continuum of medical education. *Medical Education*, **39**, 58–65.

Huddle, T.S. (2005) Teaching professionalism: Is medical morality a competency? *Academic Medicine*, **80**, 885–888.

Inui, T.S., Cottingham, A.H., Frankel, R.M., et al. (2009) Supporting teaching and learning of professionalism – changing the educational environment and students' "navigational skills," in *Teaching Medical Professionalism* (eds R.L. Cruess, S.R. Cruess, and Y. Steinert), Cambridge University Press, Cambridge, pp. 108–123.

Johnson, C. (2009) Bad blood: Doctor–nurse behavior problems impact patient care. *Physician Executive*, **35**, 6–11.

Kaldjian, L.C., Rosenbaum, M.E., Shinkunas, L.A., et al. (2012) Through students' eyes: Ethical and professional issues identified by third-year medical students during clerkships. *Journal of Medical Ethics*, **38**, 130–132.

Karnieli-Miller, O., Vu, R., Holtman, M.C., *et al.* (2010) Medical students' professionalism narratives: A window on the informal and hidden curriculum. *Academic Medicine*, **85**, 124–133.

Kneebone, R., Kidd, J., Nestel, D., *et al.* (2002) An innovative model for teaching and learning clinical procedures. *Medical Education*, **36**, 628–634.

Kolb, D.A., and Fry, R. (1975) Toward a theory of experiential learning, in *Theories of Group Process* (ed. C. Cooper), John Wiley & Sons Ltd, Chichester, pp. 33–57.

Lachman, N., and Pawlina, W. (2006) Integrating professionalism in early medical education: The theory and application of reflective practice in the anatomy curriculum. *Clinical Anatomy*, **19**, 456–460.

Lane, I.F. , Strand, E., Sims, M., and Hendrix, D. (2006) A college-wide approach to promote professional behavior in a college of veterinary medicine. *International Association of Medical Science Educators 10ᵗʰ Annual Meeting*. San Juan, Puerto Rico.

Lane, I.F. (2007) Change in higher education: Understanding and responding to individual and organizational resistance. *Journal of Veterinary Medical Education*, **34**, 85–92.

Lane, I.F., and Bogue, E.G. (2010) Perceptions of veterinary faculty members regarding their responsibility and preparation to teach non-technical competencies. *Journal of Veterinary Medical Education*, **37**, 238–247.

Lane, I.F., and Cornell, K.K. (2013) Teaching tip: Making the most of hospital rounds. *Journal of Veterinary Medical Education*, **40**, 145–151.

Lave, J., and Wenger, E. (1991) *Situated Learning*, Cambridge University Press, Cambridge.

Leo, T., and Eagen, K. (2008) Professionalism education: The medical student response. *Perspectives in Biology and Medicine*, **51**, 508–516.

Levinson, W., Ginsburg, S., Hafferty, F.W., and Lucy, C.R. (2014) *Understanding Medical Professionalism*, McGraw-Hill Education, New York.

Lewis, R., and Klausner, J. (2003) Nontechnical competencies underlying career success as a veterinarian. *Journal of the American Veterinary Medical Association*, **222**, 1690–1696.

Lloyd, J. (2006) Current economic trends affecting the veterinary medical profession. *Veterinary Clinics of North America: Small Animal Practice*, **36**, 267–279.

Lloyd, J., and King, L. (2004) What are veterinary schools and colleges doing to improve the nontechnical skills, knowledge, aptitudes and attitudes of veterinary students? *Journal of the American Veterinary Medical Association*, **224**, 1923–1924.

MacPherson, A., Lawrie, I., Collins, S., and Forman, L. (2014) Teaching the difficult-to-teach topics. *BMJ Supportive and Palliative Care*, **4**, 87–91.

Marchalik, D. (2015) Saving the professionalism course. *Lancet*, **385**, 2346–2347.

Maudsley, G., and Strivens, J. (2000) Promoting professional knowledge, experiential learning and critical thinking for medical students. *Medical Education*, **34**, 535–544.

McLellan, H. (1996) *Situated Learning Perspectives*, Educational Technology Publications, Englewood Cliffs, N.J.

Morihara, S.K., Jackson, D.S., and Chun, M.B. (2013) Making the professionalism curriculum for undergraduate medical education more relevant. *Medical Teacher*, **35**, 908–914.

Mossop, L.H. (2012) Is it time to define veterinary professionalism? *Journal of Veterinary Medical Education*, **38**, 93–100.

Mossop, L.H., and Cobb, K. (2013) Teaching and assessing veterinary professionalism. *Journal of Veterinary Medical Education*, **40**, 223–232.

Mossop, L.H., and Senior, A. (2008) I'll show you mine if you show me yours! Portfolio design in two UK veterinary schools. *Journal of Veterinary Medical Education*, **35**, 599–606.

Mueller, P.S. (2015) Teaching and assessing professionalism in medical learners and practicing physicians. *Rambam Maimonides Medical Journal*, **6**, e0011.

NAVMEC (2011) *Roadmap for Veterinary Medical Education in the 21st Century: Responsive, Collaborative, Flexible.* North American Veterinary Medical Education Consortium. http://www.aavmc.org/data/files/navmec/navmec_roadmapreport_web_single.pdf (accessed January 14, 2016).

Papadakis, M.A., Teherani, A., Banach, M.A., *et al.* (2005) Disciplinary action by medical boards and prior behavior in medical school. *New England Journal of Medicine*, **353**, 2673–2682.

Patenaude, J., Niyonsenga, T., and Fafard, D. (2003) Changes in students' moral development during medical school: A cohort study. *Journal of the Canadian Medical Association*, **168**, 840–844.

Pawlina, W. (2006) Professionalism and anatomy: How do these two terms define our role? *Clinical Anatomy*, **19**, 391–392.

Piemonte, N.M. (2015) Last laughs: Gallows humor and medical education. *Journal of Medical Humanities*, **36**, 375–390.

Ramani, S., and Orlander, J.D. (2013) Human dimensions in bedside teaching: Focus group discussions of teachers and learners. *Teaching and Learning Medicine*, **25**, 312–318.

Riley, S., and Kumar, N. (2012) Teaching medical professionalism. *Clinical Medicine*, **12**, 9–11.

Roberts, L.W., Green Hammond, K.A., Geppert, C.M., and Warner, T.D. (2004) The positive role of professionalism and ethics training in medical education: A comparison of medical student and resident perspectives. *Academic Psychiatry*, **28**, 170–182.

Ross, S., Lai, K., Walton, J.M., *et al.* (2013) "I have the right to a private life": Medical students' views about professionalism in a digital world. *Medical Teacher*, **35**, 826–831.

Royal, K.D., and Hecker, K.G. (2016) Rater errors in clinical performance ratings. *Journal of Veterinary Medical Education*, **43**, 5–8.

Schön, D.A. (1983) *The Reflective Practitioner: How Professionals Think in Action*, Basic Books, New York.

Steinert, Y., Cruess, S., Cruess, R., and Snell, L. (2005) Faculty development for teaching and evaluating professionalism: From programme design to curriculum change. *Medical Education*, **39**, 127–136.

Stern, D.T. (2006) A framework for measuring professionalism, in *Measuring Medical Professionalism* (ed. D.T. Stern), Oxford University Press, Oxford, pp. 3–13.

Stern, D.T., and Papadakis, M. (2006) The developing physician – becoming a professional. *New England Journal of Medicine*, **355**, 1794–1799.

Stockley, A.J., and Forbes, K. (2014) Medical professionalism in the formal curriculum: 5th year medical students' experiences. *BMC Medical Education*, **14**, 259.

Stone, E.A., and Weisert, H.A. (2004) Introducing a course in veterinary medicine and literature into a veterinary curriculum. *Journal of the American Veterinary Medical Association*, **224**, 1249–1253.

Swartz, W.J. (2006) Using gross anatomy to teach and assess professionalism in the first year of medical school. *Clinical Anatomy*, **19**, 437–441.

Swick, H. (2000) Toward a normative definition of medical professionalism. *Academic Medicine*, **75**, 612–616.

Swick, H.M. (2006) Medical professionalism and the clinical anatomist. *Clinical Anatomy*, **19**, 393–402.

Tinga, C., Adams, C.L., Bonnett, B.N., and Ribble, C.S. (2001) Survey of veterinary technical and professional skills in students and recent graduates of a veterinary college. *Journal of the American Veterinary Medical Association*, **219**, 924–931.

Walton, M., Jeffery, H., Van Staalduinen, S., *et al.* (2013) When should students learn about ethics, professionalism and patient safety? *Clinical Teacher*, **10**, 224–229.

26

Working in Professional Teams

Tierney Kinnison[1,2], David Guile[1] and Stephen A. May[2]

[1] Institute of Education, University College London, UK
[2] Royal Veterinary College, UK

 Box 26.1: Key messages

- Veterinarians no longer work in isolation. During a typical day, they are likely to work with several groups within their practice: veterinary nurses/technicians, receptionists, and practice managers, as well as other groups outside the practice.
- Initiatives designed specifically to address the competency of working within professional teams are rare within veterinary curricula.
- Two examples of simple but effective face-to-face interventions are described: Talking Walls and an emergency-case role play.
- Not all schools and universities will be able to offer face-to-face initiatives. Online tools are described that address logistical challenges.

- In order to reinforce the importance of working in teams, this competency should be assessed. Methods of assessment could include attendance, project work, behavioral marker team rating scores, surveys, and workplace multi-source feedback.
- Teaching and assessing working in professional teams within the veterinary field is rare. Research is required to evaluate how to design contextual interventions that have positive outcomes for student learning identifiable through assessment.

Introduction

We begin this chapter with a brief consideration of semantics. In Part Two, Chapter 7, John Tegzes gave an excellent account of teaching interprofessionalism. The interprofessional education (IPE) that he described primarily involved looking outward to veterinary students learning with members of the human healthcare team, such as doctors, nurses, dentists, and pharmacists. This type of learning can have far-reaching benefits through the consideration of humans, animals, and the environment as an interconnected ecosystem. It is therefore a style of One Health IPE. This chapter, however, looks inward and takes a more focused look at the veterinary team. It considers the professions and occupations that work together within typical veterinary practices across the globe on a more day-to-day basis. Indeed, the title

Veterinary Medical Education: A Practical Guide, First Edition. Edited by Jennifer L. Hodgson and Jacquelyn M. Pelzer.
© 2017 John Wiley & Sons, Inc. Published 2017 by John Wiley & Sons, Inc.

of this chapter could have been very similar to John Tegzes's and included the term interprofessional; its subject is interprofessional working, but at a different level. In the United Kingdom, where our research has so far been based, veterinarians have been recognized as a profession since the Royal College of Veterinary Surgeons (RCVS) was set up in 1844. Far more recently, in February 2015, a new Royal Charter came into effect that acknowledges veterinary nurses as a profession in their own right, and ensures their coherent regulation alongside veterinarians. Therefore, we have called our previous research regarding the relationship between veterinarians and veterinary nurses interprofessional. This chapter is instead termed working in professional teams. The important point is that, in the modern day, members of the veterinary profession will work alongside members of the veterinary nursing profession (in countries including the United Kingdom) and veterinary technicians (for example in the United States), as well as those in other occupations such as practice managers, receptionists, and animal physiotherapists, and animal charities. They must work as a team, whether we call it an interprofessional, multiprofessional, uniprofessional, or simply a professional team.

Published research on the topic of the veterinary team, whether it is regarding working in practice or educational strategies, is sparse. This chapter will therefore, in addition, make use of research from the medical field, which currently is ahead of veterinary research. We hope, as the importance of veterinary teamwork is increasingly appreciated, to encourage those in our field to help us catch up.

The chapter will first consider the rationale for teaching students about working in veterinary professional teams. It will then outline in detail an example of designing, running, and evaluating two educational interventions designed for veterinary and veterinary nurse students, with reflection on where to go next. Finally, the issue of assessing teamwork will be discussed.

Rationale for Teaching Students How to Work in Professional Teams

The veterinary profession has evolved enormously over the course of its existence. Initially, the first veterinary schools in the world focused almost exclusively on the horse as the type species (Mitsuda, 2007), with some attention paid to cows and sheep in terms of their use as food animals. The students were all male, would graduate within a few years, and would set up practice on their own. They would charge for their services, but would perhaps also accept payment in kind, as in the portrayal of British veterinary surgeon James Herriot, who inspired a generation of veterinarians. Today this scene is an increasing rarity. Veterinary practices are becoming larger businesses, which these days are more likely to see a multitude of pet cats and dogs rather than any other species. They frequently employ a large group of veterinarians (including specialists) who carry out disease diagnosis and create treatment plans, along with veterinary nurses/veterinary technicians and assistants who cover all aspects of patient care. Practice managers, human resources managers, and finance managers have the expertise to deal with running the business side. Receptionists provide a front-of-house role and are the first point of contact for clients. Outside of the practice itself, veterinarians may work alongside other animal-related groups such as charities, farriers, farmers, equine dentists, and drug company representatives, as well as other nonmedical groups, for example accountants, web designers, and law enforcement officers, to name but a few (Root Kustritz, Molgaard, and Tegzes, 2013).

All of these groups, especially the in-practice groups, have developed their working roles alongside veterinarians, whose roles also continue to change. Creating a team with complementary knowledge, skills, and attributes is desirable for service efficiency and effectiveness. The availability of different ideas and perspectives can enable a team to solve problems in

written about them. Give them a red pen to make amendments, additions, and deletions.

- Bring each subgroup back together to discuss the charts. Ensure that there is an atmosphere of sharing and encourage explanation of thoughts to overcome stereotypes and misconceptions.
- Bring the whole group together to explore the results and to extend the session to consider other groups with which they will both work.

Emergency-Case Role Play

The second intervention aimed to enhance the appreciation of communication skills between members of the veterinary team while allowing practical teamwork skills to be practiced. Communication is now an integral part of veterinary curricula (Mossop *et al.*, 2015), but, as with physicians in healthcare (Stone 2010), it focuses on veterinarians communicating with clients and often neglects communication within the team, or between the team and clients. This intervention is a basic simulation using a model of a dog requiring cardiopulmonary cerebral resuscitation (CPCR). CPCR is an emergency situation that could happen at any time and requires effective teamwork from any and all available staff. During the evaluation of the intervention, pairs of students (one veterinary student and one veterinary nurse student) undertook the scenario separately. Since the evaluation it has become apparent that this is unfeasible given logistical issues such as time and group size. Therefore, the session is now run as a group session in which pairs of students conduct the role play in front of their peers. The role play is run several times with suggested improvements incorporated.

At the beginning of the role play, a facilitator describes the patient's clinical situation. The patient has "crashed" (no spontaneous ventilation or circulation) and the students are told to resuscitate the patient as if in a real-life situation. The facilitator observes clinical as well as interpersonal aspects of the task, such as how long it took for any action to occur, leadership, and the effectiveness of communication. During the intervention evaluation, the students were

provided with feedback as a pair. In the new format, peers also volunteer feedback to the pair, both during and after the role play.

Evaluating Teamwork Interventions

Freeth *et al.* (2005) developed a typology of interprofessional education outcomes based on Kirkpatrick's original four-level evaluation pyramid. The levels are:

1) Reaction
2a) Modification of attitudes/perceptions
2b) Acquisition of knowledge/skills
3) Behavioral change
4a) Change in organizational practice
4b) Benefits to patients/clients, families, and communities.

Freeth *et al.* (2005) claim that their levels, like Kirkpatrick's, are not hierarchical. As the levels are not hierarchical and each has its own value, it is desirable to conduct evaluations that cover all levels. However, the majority of publications that focus on evaluation concentrate on the first levels in terms of asking students about the value and feasibility of the initiative, while longitudinal demonstrations of behavior change are rare (Olson and Bialocerkowski, 2014).

Our initial evaluation was part of this trend and was aimed at Levels 1 (reaction) and 2a (modification of attitudes and perceptions). This was achieved through a questionnaire regarding the individual interventions alongside an adapted version of the Readiness for Interprofessional Learning Scale (RIPLS), developed by Parsell and Bligh (1999). Suggesting that there are attitudinal, organizational, and structural challenges to implementing IPE, but that attitudes are the hardest to change, we wanted to create a questionnaire that could assess readiness for interprofessional learning.

Thannhauser, Russell-Mayhew, and Scott (2010) conducted a review of instruments designed to measure aspects of interprofessional collaboration and education, and included instruments that could involve a range of roles and situations, rather than being specific to one interaction or team. The inclusion criteria reduced the hundreds of abstracts found to eight formal measures. The majority of these questionnaires, however, were only ever used once or twice and had limited assessments of validity. Only two instruments were considered to be accessible and psychometrically validated. These were RIPLS and the Interdisciplinary Education Perception Scale (IEPS), originally developed by Luecht *et al.* (1990). While the IEPS was designed specifically to be a pre- and post-intervention assessment of changing attitudes, the RIPLS is an assessment of readiness for interprofessional learning that can be used once or repeatedly, and according to the literature has been validated across disciplines, stages of education, and countries (e.g., Reid *et al.*, 2006; McFadyen *et al.*, 2005; Lauffs *et al.*, 2008). However, there is a continuing debate over the precise makeup of the scale items, and indeed the validity of the scale as a whole, due to low internal consistency of subscales, which has promoted the recent suggestion of utilizing individual scales for different competencies (Mahler *et al.*, 2015). Back in 2010 when we undertook this pilot to gauge the veterinary professions' changing opinions of team interventions, the RIPLS was chosen as the instrument to adapt and use. The adaptation primarily consisted of the term "healthcare students" being replaced by "veterinary and veterinary nursing students" or "students from the other veterinary professions" where appropriate. The "healthcare team" became the "veterinary team." The scale is split into three subscales – Teamwork and Collaboration, Professional Identity, and Client and Patient Centeredness – with a total of 23 items rated on a five-point Likert scale from strongly disagree to strongly agree. Demographic questions relating to gender, age, area, time of qualification, route to qualification, and current employment were also included. The scale was then sent to two veterinary nurses and two veterinarians involved in education at the RVC who are knowledgeable regarding the design of questionnaires. Comments were sought regarding clarity of instructions, accuracy of items, and layout. All appropriate edits were included.

Student participants completed the questionnaires in the following timeframe:

- Immediately pre intervention: RIPLS 1.
- Immediately post intervention: RIPLS 2 and intervention-specific questionnaire.
- Follow-up, 4–5 months post intervention: RIPLS 3.

Box 26.2 reports the project's data analysis regarding the 39 participants. Attitudes toward team collaboration learning significantly improved immediately after the intervention across all three subscales. However, in the follow-up, the scores had reverted to pre-intervention levels, although they remained significantly better for the subscale Teamwork and Collaboration. This implies that although the interventions had a positive effect on the students' attitudes, encouraging them to appreciate learning with their future colleagues, this was not maintained once they returned to their normal student lives.

It is suggested that teamwork initiatives should be horizontally and vertically integrated throughout the curriculum to maintain the positive views, and that training staff with regard to the teamwork concept will reduce any hidden curriculum relating to power and status that may prevent positive attitudes to teamwork. There was no significant difference between members of the professions in their RIPLS scores, except for veterinary students having a higher professional identity score prior to the intervention, which indicates a view of isolation and feelings of hierarchical professional superiority that are potentially detrimental to teamwork. The interventions reduced this view.

The intervention questionnaire demonstrated that half of the students (from both professions) were apprehensive about learning with students from another profession prior to the intervention, while the other half were not. However, 38 of the 39 participants agreed or strongly agreed that the intervention was enjoyable, suggesting that any fears were unfounded. Positive feedback was provided by all participants in free-text sections. Two examples are shown in Box 26.3.

Box 26.2: Where's the Evidence?

Within our first peer-reviewed paper regarding veterinary team interprofessional education, we assessed changes in students' attitudes toward IPE. The analysis we used was as follows:

> Statistical analysis to measure the attitudinal change to readiness for interprofessional learning was conducted in SPSS, Friedman's tests compared the results over the three intervals of time, and Wilcoxen tests with a Bonferroni correction were used to compare pairs within significant results. Mann–Whitney U tests were used for comparison between the results of veterinary and veterinary nursing students and the two interventions. Descriptive statistics were carried out in SPSS to summarize the quantitative sections of the resource-specific questionnaire, and the main themes were explored within the open-ended responses. (Kinnison *et al.*, 2011, p. 313)

Attitudes initially improved, but not all were maintained several months after the intervention, as described in this chapter.

Box 26.3: Student reflections

"Able to see things from the other profession's point of view. Able to leave uni, qualify and help future students with concerns raised today. Work differently in a team." (Talking Walls, veterinary nurse student)

"Really enjoyed it despite feeling nervous. Was a good example of a teamwork situation and the 'pressure' of the role play made it more realistic and easier to interact with someone I don't know." (Emergency-case role play, veterinary student)

Suggestions for improvements reflected the need for vertical integration into the curriculum, with the majority of comments concerning integrating the session into the curriculum with additional scenarios, activities, and people.

Online Veterinary Team Tools

While the support from students and staff was apparent for our interventions, the logistical challenges of making this style of teaching available to all students became all the more apparent. Another interprofessional, and this time intercollegiate, project was started to develop an online tool to introduce the concepts of interprofessional/team working within veterinary practices to students of all stages of study, colleges, and disciplines, at any time. It is acknowledged that this type of online tool – which does not have synchronous or asynchronous interactions with other people, and instead relies on quizzes and tasks whereby feedback is generated from the program – challenges the concept of interprofessional education and by association professional team education. However, it overcomes many challenges and is therefore a useful adjunct to face-to-face initiatives.

The tool was initially based on the previous project, although input was also received from veterinary nurses in practice and university, a specialist small animal chartered physiotherapist, and two students, one veterinary and one veterinary nursing, who had a special interest in veterinary teamwork. It was created using Xerte, a toolkit that allows those without computer programming skills to develop online tools. This "Introduction to Interprofessional Education" is freely available (Kinnison, Mossop, and Baillie, 2014). Students from all veterinary-related courses, such as veterinary medicine, veterinary nursing, veterinary technology, physiotherapy, animal behavior, and veterinary practice management, are invited to use the tool.

Most recently we have created a short, 10-minute e-lecture that introduces the concept of veterinary-specific teamwork to veterinary students. After introducing teamwork issues, it makes practical suggestions for students when considering teamwork during their studies, both within and outside of university. This e-lecture is freely available from Kinnison (2016) as part of the VET Talks project, which was created by the International Veterinary Students' Association's Standing Committee on Veterinary Education (SCoVE) and Wikivet. We again encourage you as veterinary educators to make it available to your students.

What is Next?

Small steps have been made in integrating professional team competencies into some veterinary curricula. Similar interventions, driven by a particular individual's interest, have also been seen in other universities, although publications regarding their use and evaluation are missing. The context of educational activities is key to their success, and anecdotally veterinary students need to see the clinical relevance of a topic prior to accepting its worth. We suggest that it is prime time to take a step back in order to consider the real-life working and learning within veterinary practices, and to use this to guide future team-based pedagogical interventions in an evidence-based manner.

The lead author has undertaken a PhD, completed in 2016, with this aim. It used a unique methodological structure involving both quantitative and qualitative research within an overarching case study. A quantitative questionnaire using social network analysis (SNA) comprised the first part of the project. It identified common patterns of interprofessional working and learning within a range of veterinary practices in the United Kingdom (Kinnison, May, and Guile, 2015; Kinnison, Guile, and May, 2015a). The results of the SNA enabled two practices to be chosen for further study. Embedded case studies were carried out in each practice and consisted of one week of general observations, one week of shadowing focus individuals (veterinarians, veterinary nurses, managers, and receptionists), and one week of interviews. Field notes, transcripts, and artifacts were collected. The data from all three weeks at both practices was triangulated with the SNA data to produce a concept of interprofessional working and learning in practice (Kinnison, Guile, and May, 2016). An interesting outcome related to the identification of potential or actual errors caused by mistakes within interprofessional communication (Kinnison, Guile, and May, 2015b) reiterates the need for teaching interprofessional skills to students of all professions within the veterinary team.

The United Kingdom is fortunate to be among the leaders in veterinary team development in terms of the professionalization of veterinary nurses and the rise of other occupations. Much of this research is highly relevant to other countries where veterinarians will work alongside other groups, perhaps with an even more distinct hierarchical formation. It is likely that veterinary teams across the globe will continue to develop and will face similar confusion over roles, jostles for jurisdiction, differences in professional perspectives, and the need for trust and respect. It is hoped that these primarily UK examples will assist other countries in recognizing the need for professional team competencies to be taught to veterinary students. Yet if we are to teach these competencies, how are we to assess them?

Assessing the Professional Competency of Working in Teams

The first question regarding assessment suggested by Della Freeth in her interprofessional chapter in the medical equivalent of this book (Freeth, 2013) was whether we should assess the competencies that are the target of interprofessional education. She proposed that immersion in the topic may be more important, and that there are challenges such as being able to produce defined summative criteria and dealing with the requirements of all professions and departments. It has been noted that if the assessment for the professional cohorts in the same intervention differs, this may cause certain professions to be reluctant to take part (Hammick *et al.*, 2007). The choice of how to assess team-based skills therefore influences how the intervention will be perceived by the participants, and the facilitators, and the degree to which it will succeed. Freeth (2013) goes on to suggest that having no assessment may lead to limited perceived value and subsequent issues such as absenteeism. Assessment in the form of attendance, knowledge tests, essays, reflective journals, and group presentations was proposed. Some of these have already been introduced in Chapter 7, and in addition, interprofessional Objective Structured Clinical Examinations (OSCEs) were explored and considered to be very useful for assessing interprofessional skills, behaviour and attitudes; although they are challenging to implement. Active engagement was suggested to facilitate peer and self-assessment. Assessment is often quoted as driving learning, as an external motivator, and while we hope that our students have an intrinsic motivation to learn about working in teams, providing constructively aligned assessment can only promote the culture of valuing this type of learning and working (Freeth, 2013). Formal assessment that is relevant to practice also increases students' own awareness of team-based skills, which may otherwise go unnoticed (Stone, 2010), at least until they begin to practice.

As outlined earlier, there is little formal teaching of the professional competency of working in teams within current veterinary curricula. Although we evaluated the interventions during our project in terms of the self-assessment of attitude change, we did not go so far as to measure objectively whether or not learning had taken place in terms of knowledge, skills, attitudes, or behavioral change. Evaluating IPE is strongly linked to assessing professional competencies, as both seek to identify changes in students' abilities and perceptions. The two aspects should therefore be developed together.

Despite the lack of formal veterinary IPE, there is evidence of assessment of teamwork within veterinary curricula. During intramural rotations at the RVC, students are assessed in three categories: Professional Activity, Practical Skills, and Clinical Reasoning and Application of Knowledge. In each category the student will either pass or fail, and students receiving one or more "Fail" in any rotation will also be considered to have failed the rotation. All rotations must be passed before a student can proceed to take finals examinations. Example activities in Professional Activity include interaction with staff and other students in the clinical environment; communication skills on all levels, including written and oral communication; and ability to work within a team. Therefore, demonstrating satisfactory teamwork is required to qualify as a veterinary surgeon. It is, however, mixed with skills of punctuality and neatness, for example, and it is suggested that more focused assessment of teamwork specifically would be beneficial to highlight its importance.

Therefore, as we develop formal teamwork initiatives, we must also consider objective assessment in more detail than at present. Historically there has been an individualist notion within healthcare, with a focus on the autonomous force of a physician with regard to their education and assessment of skills and knowledge, and subsequently regarding errors and adverse events (Lingard, 2009; Gawande, 2007). It is important to consider an individual's abilities in granting them a professional award; however, the working lives of doctors, and now veterinarians, are not an isolated existence.

As discussed extensively in this chapter, veterinarians work alongside members of several professions and occupations on a day-to-day basis, and the outcomes of the work done in a veterinary practice do not rely on the veterinarian alone, but on an effective and efficient team. It has been suggested that individual competence does not automatically result in an effective team with collective competence. A team with high collective competence has (in addition to individual knowledge, skills, and attitudes) elements of communication and collaboration that lead to distributed cognition and shared mental representations (Lingard, 2009). Therefore, although individuals can be assessed during group work regarding elements such as communication – for instance by NOTTS, Non-Technical Skills for Surgeons (Yule *et al.*, 2006) – it is more realistic for the team to be assessed (e.g., Cooper *et al.*, 2010). This requires an educational change. It is mirrored in an example of training of nontechnical skills for anesthetists called CARMA (Crisis Avoidance and Resource Management for Anaesthetists). Once trialed, CARMA was adapted to include other professions, due to the most difficult interactions being identified as interprofessional, and subsequently the course is just called CARMa (Crisis Avoidance and Resource Management; Flin and Maran, 2004).

One way for teamwork to be assessed, although primarily for qualified practitioners, is through a team-rating score. CARMa was, for example, based on ANTS (Anaesthetists' Non-Technical Skills), which involves teamwork skills but is again an example of a profession-specific tool. Due to the context-specific nature of scores, there are a multitude of examples of team-rating scores in the healthcare literature. In addition to NOTTS (of surgeons during surgery) and ANTS (of anesthetists during surgery), OTAS (Observational Teamwork Assessment for Surgery) involves observations of each professional sub-team (surgeons, nurses, anesthetists) separately during surgery, but focuses on interprofessional behavioral constructs: communication, coordination, cooperation, leadership, and situational awareness (Hull *et al.*, 2011).

TEAM (Team Emergency Assessment Measure) is a true rating of teamwork performance in a medical emergency setting (Cooper *et al.*, 2010). It includes three categories (leadership, teamwork, and task management), with specific observations of events including "the team worked together to complete tasks in a timely manner" and "the team monitored and reassessed the situation." Team-rating scores tend to consist of categories, elements, and examples of good behaviors and poor behaviors, which form a behavioral marker system used during observations. They can be developed through methods such as literature reviews, interviews, cognitive task analysis, surveys, observations (Yule *et al.*, 2006), expert reviews (Cooper *et al.*, 2010), and incident analysis (Flin and Maran, 2004). The tools themselves are assessed through means including expert consensus (content validity), correlation analysis, and interobserver agreement (reliability; Hull *et al.*, 2011). Such team-based scales have also been used in education; for example, a scale was developed at an Australian dental school and was suggested to be useful in evaluating interprofessional or intraprofessional team-based processes (Storrs *et al.*, 2015).

A review of surveys to measure teamwork in healthcare (which are easy to apply in comparison to observations of behaviors) showed similar results, with a multitude of examples, but a lack of consistency in the conception of teamwork and a lack of fulfillment of psychometric criteria (Valentine, Nembhard, and Edmondson, 2011).

Multisource feedback (MSF, or 360° assessment) in the workplace is interprofessional by nature, since members of other professional groups may provide feedback on an individual's work, offering unique insights. In a systematic review of MSF for physicians, in order to achieve high reliability, validity, and feasibility, 25 patients with eight medical colleagues and eight coworkers (nurses, psychologists, pharmacists, and allied health professionals) were required (Donnon *et al.*, 2014). Different professional groups have been demonstrated to provide reliable ratings of student physicians using an interprofessional collaborator assessment rubric (ICAR) within MSF, quelling any thoughts that nurses and allied health professionals are not able to evaluate student physicians appropriately (Hayward *et al.*, 2014). Although going back to assessing an individual, the domains evaluated in MSF include elements of teamwork, for example communication, interpersonal relationships, and management/leadership. The student's ability to act on the feedback and improve their work is imperative, although research has shown that there are varying levels of success, dependent on the usefulness of the assessor's free-text comments (Vivekananda-Schmidt *et al.*, 2013). Within the veterinary field, MSF was the only method identified for assessing teamwork in a Best Evidence Veterinary Medical Education (BEVME) systematic review, which produced a Guide to Assessment Methods, although MSF can be included in global rating scores used with other methods (Baillie, Warman, and Rhind, 2014). Clearly, the inclusion of teamwork competencies in teaching and assessment is new, but its importance is increasing quickly.

Conclusion

Professional teamwork is here to stay. It has arisen due to the benefit it offers of providing a better and more efficient service than any one individual profession could strive for. However, it requires a change of focus, from the individual and their knowledge and faults, to the team and their collective/distributed knowledge. For veterinary practice teams to work well, it is suggested that these groups should learn with, from, and about each other throughout their education and their subsequent careers. We would like to promote the development and evaluation of university-based pedagogical initiatives that target the professional competency of working within teams. Through the evaluation of these interventions, which should aim to span the levels of outcomes (from reaction, through student acquisition of knowledge, and on to benefits to patients and clients), ways of assessing students' progression in these competencies, as part of a team, should also be considered.

Acknowledgments

The authors would like to acknowledge the research grants that have allowed the work detailed here to be undertaken: Veterinary interprofessional education interventions development and evaluation – VETNET Lifelong Learning Network (2009/2010); online IPE tool – funding through the National Teaching Fellowship Award (Sarah Baillie) and the Royal Veterinary College, with access to Xerte and support provided through the University of Nottingham; PhD – Bloomsbury Colleges PhD studentship, undertaken by Tierney Kinnison 2012–2016.

References

Adler, P.S., Kwon, S.-W., and Heckscher, C. (2008) Perspective – Professional work: The emergence of collaborative community. *Organization Science*, **19** (2), 359–376. doi:10.1287/orsc.1070.0293

Alvarez, G., and Coiera, E. (2006) Interdisciplinary communication: An uncharted source of medical error? *Journal of Critical Care*, **21** (3), 236–242. doi:10.1016/j.jcrc.2006.02.004

Baillie, S., Warman, S., and Rhind, S. (2014) *A Guide to Assessment in Veterinary Medicine*. http://www.bris.ac.uk/vetscience/media/docs/guide-to-assessment.pdf (accessed November 17, 2015).

Cooper, S., Cant, R., Porter, J., *et al.* (2010) Rating medical emergency teamwork performance: Development of the Team Emergency Assessment Measure (TEAM). *Resuscitation*,

81 (4), 446–452.
doi:10.1016/j.resuscitation.2009.11.027

Donnon, T., Al Ansari, A., Al Alawi, S., and Violato, C. (2014) The reliability, validity, and feasibility of multisource feedback physician assessment: A systematic review. *Academic Medicine*, **89 (3)**, 511–516.

Flin, R., and Maran, N. (2004) Identifying and training non-technical skills for teams in acute medicine. *Quality and Safety in Health Care*, **13** (Suppl 1), i80–i84.

Freeth, D. (2013) Interprofessional education. In *Understanding Medical Education: Evidence, Theory and Practice* (ed. T. Swanwick), Wiley-Blackwell, Chichester, p. 520.

Freeth, D., Hammick, M., Reeves, S., *et al.* (2005) *Effective Interprofessional Education: Development, Delivery and Evaluation.* Blackwell, Oxford.

Gawande, A. (2007) *Better*. Profile, London.

Hall, L.W., and Zierler, B.K. (2015) Interprofessional education and practice guide no. 1: Developing faculty to effectively facilitate interprofessional education. *Journal of Interprofessional Care*, **29 (1)**, 3–7. doi:10.3109/13561820.2014.937483

Hammick, M., Freeth, D., Koppel, I., *et al.* (2007) A best evidence systematic review of interprofessional education: BEME guide no. 9. *Medical Teacher*, **29 (8)**, 735–751. doi:10.1080/01421590701682576

Hayward, M.F., Curran, R., Curtis, B., *et al.* (2014) Reliability of the Interprofessional Collaborator Assessment Rubric (ICAR) in Multi Source Feedback (MSF) with post-graduate medical residents. *BMC Medical Education*, **14 (1)**, 1–9. doi:10.1186/s12909-014-0279-9

Horsburgh, M., Lamdin, R., and Williamson, E. (2001) Multiprofessional learning: The attitudes of medical, nursing and pharmacy students to shared learning. *Medical Education*, **35 (9)**, 876–883.

Hull, L., Arora, S., Kassab, E., *et al.* (2011) Observational teamwork assessment for surgery: Content validation and tool refinement. *Journal of the American College of Surgeons*, **212 (2)**, 234–243.e1–5. doi:10.1016/j.jamcollsurg.2010.11.001

Kinnison, T. (2016) *VET Talks – Veterinary Interprofessional Teamwork.* https://www.youtube.com/ watch?v=NGp_XCidQ-0 (accessed November 30, 2016).

Kinnison, T., Guile, D., and May, S.A. (2015a) Veterinary team interactions part two: The personal effect. *Veterinary Record*, **177**, 541.

Kinnison, T., Guile, D., and May, S.A. (2015b) Errors in veterinary practice: Preliminary lessons for building better veterinary teams. *Veterinary Record*, **177**, 492.

Kinnison, T., Guile, D., and May, S.A. (2016) The case of veterinary interprofessional practice: From One Health to a world of its own. *Journal of Interprofessional Education and Practice*, **4**, 51–57.

Kinnison, T., Lumbis, R., Orpet, H., *et al.* (2011) Piloting interprofessional education interventions with veterinary and veterinary nursing students. *Journal of Veterinary Medical Education*, **38 (3)**, 311–318. doi:10.3138/jvme.38.3.311

Kinnison, T., Lumbis, R., Orpet, H., *et al.* (2012) How to run Talking Walls: An interprofesional education resource. *Veterinary Nurse*, **3 (1)**, 4–11.

Kinnison, T., May, S.A., and Guile, D. (2014) Inter-professional practice: From veterinarian to the veterinary team. *Journal of Veterinary Medical Education*, **41 (2)**, 172–178. doi:10.3138/jvme.0713-095R2

Kinnison, T., May, S.A., and Guile, D. (2015) Veterinary team interactions part one: The practice effect. *Veterinary Record*, **177 (16)**, 419.

Kinnison, T., Mossop, L., and Baillie, S. (2014) *An Introduction to Interprofessional Education – Learning about, from and with the Veterinary Team.* Royal Veterinary College/University of Nottingham/University of Bristol. http://www.nottingham.ac.uk/ toolkits/play_5724 (accessed November 17, 2016).

Lauffs, M., Ponzer, S., Saboonchi, F., *et al.* (2008) Cross-cultural adaptation of the Swedish version of Readiness for Interprofessional Learning Scale (RIPLS). *Medical Education*,

42 (**4**), 405–411.
doi:10.1111/j.1365-2923.2008.03017.x

Lingard, L. (2009) What we see and don't see when we look at "competence": Notes on a god term. *Advances in Health Sciences Education*, **14** (**5**), 625–628.

Lingard, L., Espin, S., Whyte, S., *et al.* (2004) Communication failures in the operating room: An observational classification of recurrent types and effects. *Quality and Safety in Health Care*, **13** (**5**), 330–334. doi:10.1136/qshc.2003.008425

LIVE (n.d.) *Interprofessional Education*. Lifelong Independent Veterinary Education. http://www.live.ac.uk/our-work/ interprofessional-education (accessed November 17, 2016).

Luecht, R. *et al.* (1990) Assessing professional perceptions: Design and validation of an Interdisciplinary Education Perception Scale. *Journal of Allied Health*, **19** (**2**), 181–191.

Mahler, C., Berger, S., and Reeves, S. (2015) The Readiness for Interprofessional Learning Scale (RIPLS): A problematic evaluative scale for the interprofessional field. *Journal of Interprofessional Care*, **29** (**4**), 289–291. doi:10.3109/13561820.2015.1059652

McFadyen, A.K. *et al.* (2005) The Readiness for Interprofessional Learning Scale: A possible more stable sub-scale model for the original version of RIPLS. *Journal of Interprofessional Care*, **19** (**6**), 595–603. doi:10.1080/13561820500430157

Mitsuda, T. (2007) The equestrian influence and the foundation of veterinary schools in Europe, c. 1760–1790. *eSharp*, **10**, 1–20.

Mossop, L., Gray, C., Blaxter, A., *et al.* (2015) Communication skills training: What the vet schools are doing. *Veterinary Record*, **176**, 114–117.

Olson, R., and Bialocerkowski, A. (2014) Interprofessional education in allied health: A systematic review. *Medical Education*, **48** (**3**), 236–246.

Parsell, G., and Bligh, J. (1999) The development of a questionnaire to assess the readiness of health care students for interprofessional learning (RIPLS). *Medical Education*, **33** (**2**), 95–100.

Parsell, G., Gibbs, T., and Bligh, J. (1998) Three visual techniques to enhance interprofessional learning. *Postgraduate Medical Journal*, **74**, 387–390.

Patterson, K., Grenny, J., Maxfield, D., *et al.* (2001) *Crucial Conversations: Tools for Talking When Stakes Are High*, McGraw-Hill, New York.

Reid, R., Bruce, D., Allstaff, K., and McLemon, D. (2006) Validating the Readiness for Interprofessional Learning Scale (RIPLS) in the postgraduate context: Are health care professionals ready for IPL? *Medical Education*, **40** (**5**), 415–422. doi:10.1111/j.1365-2929.2006.02442.x

Rhind, S.M., Baillie, S., Kinnison, T., *et al.* (2011) The transition into veterinary practice: Opinions of recent graduates and final year students. *BMC Medical Education*, **11** (**1**), 64. doi:10.1186/1472-6920-11-64

Root Kustritz, M.V., Molgaard, L.K., and Tegzes, J.H. (2013) Frequency of interactions between veterinarians and other professionals to guide interprofessional education. *Journal of Veterinary Medical Education*, **40** (**4**), 370–377. doi:10.3138/jvme.0413-065R1

Stone, J. (2010) Moving interprofessional learning forward through formal assessment. *Medical Education*, **44** (**4**), 396–403.

Storrs, M.J., Alexander, H., Sun, J., *et al.* (2015) Measuring team-based interprofessional education outcomes in clinical dentistry: Psychometric evaluation of a new scale at an Australian dental school. *Journal of Dental Education*, **79**, 249–258.

Thannhauser, J., Russell-Mayhew, S., and Scott, C. (2010) Measures of interprofessional education and collaboration. *Journal of Interprofessional Care*, **24** (**4**), 336–349. doi:10.3109/13561820903442903

Valentine, M.A, Nembhard, I.M., and Edmondson, A.C. (2011) Measuring teamwork in health care settings: A review of survey instruments. *Medical Care*, **53** (**4**), e16–e30. doi:10.1097/MLR.0b013e31827feef6

Vivekananda-Schmidt, P., MacKillop, L., Crossley, J., and Wade, W. (2013) Do assessor comments on a multi-source feedback instrument provide learner-centred feedback? *Medical Education*, **47** (**11**), 1080–1088.

Xyrichis, A., and Lowton, K. (2008) What fosters or prevents interprofessional teamworking in primary and community care? A literature review. *International Journal of Nursing Studies*, **45** (**1**), 140–153. doi:10.1016/j.ijnurstu.2007.01.015

Yule, S., Flin, R., Paterson-Brown, S., *et al.* (2006) Development of a rating system for surgeons' non-technical skills. *Medical Education*, **40** (**11**), 1098–1104.

How to Become a Self-Directed Learner

Readiness to Learn

Students entering veterinary education will differ in the way they learn, which depends largely on characteristics such as intelligence, personality, and former learning experiences, but also on their – often implicit – beliefs about knowledge and knowing (personal epistemology; Hofer and Pintrich, 2002). Such beliefs drive behaviors. It makes all the difference to learning whether (see Box 27.3) an individual believes that knowledge is something received from others; that problems are solvable and answers can be right or wrong; or, at the other end of the spectrum, that knowledge is constructed on what one already knows, and develops through experience and reflection on experiences (Hofer and Pintrich, 2002). Students engaging in SDL should be aware of their own epistemological beliefs, and how these beliefs influence their learning. For example, when participants in a group discussion have a relativist understanding, where "all opinions are equally right" (Kuhn, 1999, p. 23), group discussion will not become a valuable learning experience or an opportunity for knowledge-sharing (Weinberg, 2015).

Since not all students entering a course will be familiar with the concepts of SDL and reflective practice, these concepts require explicit explanation regarding their meaning, the competencies required, and how they can be learned. Various skills and attitudes toward learning are required for successful SDL, for example the abilities to:

- diagnose their own learning needs realistically;
- take the initiative in making use of resources (i.e., teachers and peers as resources for diagnosing learning needs or as facilitators or helpers, as well as learning materials appropriate to different learning objectives);
- translate learning needs into learning objectives (Knowles, 1975).

However, most of all students require an adequate self-concept as a nondependent and self-directed person.

Learning Objectives

Learning objectives are motivating, especially for learners with a goal-oriented learning orientation (Teunissen and Bok, 2013). Learning objectives direct learning activities; achieving objectives is perceived as a successful (learning) experience that raises self-efficacy. Once learners have diagnosed their learning needs and translated these into learning objectives, they formalize them by making a personal development plan. In formal training, the preparation of development plans is often a joint process between student and mentor.

Engaging in the Learning Process

Students need to understand themselves as learners in order to understand their needs as

---

 Box 27.3: Focus on epistemology

Epistemological beliefs influence knowledge-sharing at work and learning at school, and may have the following dimensions (Hofer and Pintrich, 2002):

- Whether knowledge is certain – absolute *to* tentative
- How knowledge is structured – simple *to* complex

- What is the best source of knowledge – handed down by authorities *to* derived by reason
- Whether knowledge is under your own control – you are born with a certain ability to learn *to* your ability to learn can be changed
- With what speed knowledge is acquired – quickly or not at all *to* gradually

self-directed learners. These needs concern, for example, the instructional methods they prefer for gathering and processing information. Do they prefer active or reflective learning, verbal or visual explanations? They need to understand their own learning preferences because SDL requires a deep approach to learning. Understanding themselves as learners means that they know what learning resources they need. As women now dominate student enrollment in veterinary education all over the world, it is relevant to examine the consequences for teaching, learning, mentoring, professional development, and leadership. Male and female students might have different ways of knowing and learning. Research focusing on women's development and ways of knowing reveals that women prefer a less authoritarian and more person-centered learning environment, and supports the adoption of student-centered approaches to teaching and learning in veterinary education (Taylor and Robinson, 2009).

Evaluating Learning

Evaluating learning should not be confused with assessment only, although summative assessments can be valuable for evaluation of the acquisition of knowledge (i.e., exams, case reports, or essays) or mastering specific skills (i.e., objective structured clinical examinations). Evaluating learning in an SDL context involves evaluation of progress, for example by seeking feedback of peers, colleagues, or faculty members and subsequently reflecting on the feedback gathered. Self-reflection includes examining assumptions, beliefs, and emotions regarding learning and learning objectives. It is one of the most important and at the same time most difficult aspects of SDL.

Reflective Practice

The aforementioned strategies for the development of SDL call for curricula that allow for authentic learning experiences, such as longer clinical placements or extramural education, where students integrate theory into real-life practice and learn teamwork competencies

through socialization. Here, in the workplace, they will have authentic practice experiences on which to reflect and become reflective practitioners.

Reflective practice is an increasingly important aspect of CPD. Reflective skills and reflective practice seem to be essential for continuing personal and professional development in young veterinarians (Mastenbroek et al., 2015). Reflective practice enables individuals to look back on, learn, and improve their own practice. Since the obligation to keep their knowledge and skills up to a professional standard is part of the implicit social contract that health professionals have with society, it needs no further explanation that helping students be prepared for reflective practice must be part of the veterinary curriculum.

Reflection-on-Action

Schön (1983) argues that it is impossible for professionals to possess all the knowledge and skills required to solve problems in each and every complex situation they face every day. Despite this, professionals have to act and while acting use reflection. Schön (1983) called this type of reflection reflection-*in*-action, in contrast to reflection-*on*-action, which is reflection in which professionals engage after they have solved the problem and look back on their decisions.

Many descriptions of reflective practice exist, and often they are intermingled with terms such as reflection, reflective thinking, and critical reflection (Brookfield, 2009). Differences between these concepts are related to the focus of the reflection: whether reflection should be on your own behavior, on assumptions guiding your behavior, or on power structures at play in the workplace, which affect how the work is being done. In this chapter, we will look at reflective practice as deep approaches to learning and meaning-making in the workplace or during authentic learning situations within the curriculum.

Reflection-on-action helps to make subsequent meaning of complex situations and enables professionals to learn from experience.

Box 27.4: Focus on benefits to, and limitations of, reflective practice

Davies (2012) identified the benefits as well as the limitations to reflective practice in her review of the literature on behalf of general practitioners.

The benefits are:

- Increased learning from an experience or situation
- Promotion of deep learning
- Identification of personal and professional strengths and areas for improvement
- Identification of educational needs
- Acquisition of new knowledge and skills
- Further understanding of own beliefs, attitudes, and values
- Encouragement of self-motivation and self-directed learning

- Could act as a source of feedback
- Possible improvements in personal and clinical confidence

The limitations are:

- Some practitioners may not understand the reflective process, may feel uncomfortable challenging and evaluating own practice, and may have some confusion as to which situations/experiences to reflect on
- Reflective practice could be time consuming and may not be adequate to resolve clinical problems

The inclination to and ability for reflection appear to vary across individuals and across contexts in which individuals practice (see Box 27.4). Nevertheless, the ability for reflective practice seems to be amenable to development provided that the learning environment is encouraging, for example by supervisors' behaviour. Curricular interventions (see Box 27.5), aimed at promoting reflection and reflective practice, are now being incorporated in veterinary undergraduate curricula, even though the evidence to support and inform these interventions and innovations is limited.

How to Support Learning of Lifelong Learning Competencies in (Veterinary) Medicine

The main methods for preparing students for LLL are the use of portfolios, mentoring, and learning from consulting the research literature. As reflection is an essential skill in the process of SDL, and as we know that this is a competency that has to be developed through training, it is important to guide educators in structuring the development process.

Box 27.5: Examples of curricular interventions aimed at promoting reflective practice

Individual reflective writing assignments

- Learning journals in which students reflect on the learning processes they experienced
- Daily blog writing concerning critical incidents or meaningful events
- Mission statements to help them make professional identity formation explicit

Assignments for groups

- Critical incident technique where students reflect with peers on critical incidents that occurred in their workplace
- Peer-group meetings with the aim of making sense of experiences in relation to self, to others, and to contextual conditions, and planning how to act or to respond in such situations in the future

Source: Smith, 2011.

Learning with Portfolios

To support the learning of reflective practice and SDL, portfolios are frequently used. A portfolio serves as an outline for independent study, a letter of intent, and a tool to aid in the evaluation of achievement. Knowles (1975) describes how, in the design of a learning portfolio that serves in the achievement of SDL skills (he used the term "learning contract"), one should include learning objectives, learning resources, and strategies to be used, evidence of accomplishment, and criteria and means of validating evidence. To be effective:

- The design of the portfolio should be tailored to the intended purpose.
- Portfolios should best be introduced in curricula where learning in authentic situations is a key feature.
- Conditions must be met that facilitate successful introduction of portfolios, such as teacher and student support and commitment by educational leaders (van Tartwijk *et al.*, 2007).

Portfolios in veterinary education may have a focus primarily on formative assessment or on summative assessment (Mossop, 2008). A learning portfolio that contributes to LLL competencies should include reflective writing in action, on action, and for action, which makes the design complex. And even with a well-designed learning portfolio, an active and committed teacher (mentor) is indispensable (Driessen *et al.*, 2005).

Mentoring

A mentor is a more experienced adult who helps a less experienced individual learn to navigate the world of work through career-related and psychosocial support (Kram, 1985). In veterinary medicine, professionals have recognized the importance of mentoring students, since the recruitment and retention of students appear to be difficult (Niehoff, Chenoweth, and Rutti, 2005). In a study on mentoring within the veterinary world, mentors' behaviors aimed at career development and socioemotional support appeared to be positively related to the perceived effectiveness of the relationship. Mentors developed trusting relationships with their protégés by encouraging and reinforcing them, accepting them as competent professionals, helping them attain desired positions, and providing appropriate challenges (Niehoff, Chenoweth, and Rutti, 2005). Mentors may also function as role models. When reflective practice or SDL is supported by portfolios, several studies show that stimulating and guiding reflection on portfolio issues through mentoring was even more important than the portfolio use itself (Bok *et al.*, 2013; Mann, Gordon, and MacLeod, 2009; Driessen *et al.*, 2005).

Learning from Evidence-Based Practice

Practicing evidence-based veterinary medicine is an opportunity for veterinarians to keep their knowledge up to date, because in the literature they will find recent knowledge from their domain. Therefore, they have to (learn to) search for and judge the literature during their studies (Cockcroft and Holmes, 2004). As an example, to enhance veterinary technology students' research capabilities, a teaching program has been described where students worked in self-selected dyads to author a scientific case report, based on authentic cases from their clinical practice. This approach was reported to be an enjoyable and valuable learning experience, and not only contributed to writing and presentation skills, but helped students to become more fully formed professionals (Clarke *et al.*, 2013).

Learning in Social Interaction: Learning Communities

In veterinary practice much of the learning takes place in social interaction: veterinary professionals learn during their interactions with patient owners, during dyads with students on extramural placements and in learning groups, within their own practice, or with professionals from other practices (May and Kinnison, 2015; Scholz, Trede, and Raidal, 2014). Nevertheless, studies about (lifelong) learning of veterinarians rarely pay attention to communities, disregarding the collaborative nature of their work (Scholz, Trede, and Raidal, 2014; de Groot *et al.*, 2012). Learning groups may have different goals and different names. A broad division could be made between groups where discussion has their personal and professional development, management, and communication in mind (Mastenbroek *et al.*, 2015), and groups where discussions are primarily set up to keep their veterinary knowledge up to date and to solve problems in the veterinary domain that occurred in their clinical practice (de Groot *et al.*, 2012). The latter are often called learning communities or communities of practice.

The concept of communities of practice, introduced by Etienne Wenger (1998), has transformed from a model about a master with apprentices, to a model focusing on the interaction between individuals, toward a knowledge management concept (Cox, 2005). We consider the second the most attractive kind of learning communities for veterinarians: small groups to share and create knowledge about their profession collaboratively. Participants in these communities should be active in their learning process and engage in collective inquiry.

Critically Reflective Dialogs in Communities

Learning in communities is potentially valuable, but it has to be ensured that learning in communities does not only socialize people into existing practices, but helps them innovate and observe their work in a critically reflective manner (de Groot *et al.*, 2012). Essential behaviors in such learning communities are asking for feedback, challenging groupthink, critical opinion-sharing, research utilization, and openness about mistakes (de Groot *et al.*, 2012). In order to become valuable contributions to LLL, communities need organizational support (Jang and Ko, 2014), and they require a moderator who asks reflective questions and enables members to critically reflect on their learning process (see Box 27.6). And finally, the groups should be heterogeneous but not too heterogeneous (van Knippenberg, de Dreu, and Homan, 2004). When the background of participants is too diverse, they lack common ground for an in-depth discussion, while when it is too similar, there is a risk of confirmation bias and groupthink.

Communities for Professionalism

Learning in communities within curricula as well as in veterinary practice is used to build and share subject-specific knowledge and to contribute to professionalism. An example of the latter is the development of personal or professional skills such as communication, collaboration, and management (Mossop, 2013). In models for reflection, a moderator may help clarify a question from a group member who brings up a problem, and assist in collective reflection on the solutions that came to the fore in the group (see Box 27.7). Taking part in communities for professionalism in turn contributes to reflective behavior through sharing of experiences, and the corresponding feelings and thoughts, allowing for a different perspective on a personal situation (Mastenbroek *et al.*, 2015).

How to Prepare Students for Learning in Social Interaction

To help students acquire LLL competencies during their studies, they have to develop the ability for critically reflective dialog in group discussions (see Box 27.6). Students develop this ability during education that pays attention to questions such as "How can we deal with the ambiguity of not knowing?" and "How can we ask for and give feedback?" (Bleakley and Bligh, 2008). And, self-evidently, students have to be allowed to work in groups often and get feedback on their behavior in such groups regularly (Koskinen, 2010).

How to Support the Development of Lifelong Learning Competencies

A common misconception with concepts such as SDL is that teachers do not have a role to

Box 27.6: Focus on critically reflective dialogues

Discussions within learning communities need to be critically reflective, which asks for the following behaviors:

Openness about mistakes

Members talk about a mistake at their own workplace, or ask questions about presumed mistakes of others. They show concern. They evaluate what went wrong, and give some indications about the effect the mistake had, or will have, on their future behavior or knowledge. Community members interact about possible explanations and discuss alternatives.

Research utilization

Members mention research findings, and indicate that these influenced their thinking and understanding. Research findings can come from different sources: literature, experts, continuing education meetings or pharmaceutical companies.

Challenging groupthink

A member doubts whether the conclusion reached is valid by challenging the consensus or the lack of alternative options. Consensus can be about the content ("That is just the way it is") or

the group process (the way the discussion has developed thus far)

Feedback asking and giving

A member mentions something they have done, and reflects on what happened and what thoughts they had about the effect on their future behavior. These evaluative remarks show that a participant wants to know what others think about (their thoughts on) their behavior. Others interact on the issue at hand.

Experimentation

Members talk about thought experiments, and formulate hypotheses to explore, generate, and imagine alternatives. The purpose of their explorations is to understand the issue at hand better. They discuss the thought experiment collectively. The hypothetical situation can have its origins in their own practice, but it is not just a real-life situation that they remember and share with others.

Critical opinion sharing

Members present information, ideas, and opinions in a manner that makes joint evaluation possible, which requires being explicit about reasons.

play. This is not true: they need to perform a different role, which may be quite challenging. Teachers need to encourage and guide students to become self-directed learners through setting the climate for collaborative and supportive learning, where educators and students are mutually respectful. Teachers should explain their own role and stimulate the establishment of fruitful relationships between students for the enhancement of collaborative learning.

In addition, teachers need to provide adequate student mentorship. Teachers should be

role models with regard to LLL and have a solid understanding of the necessary competencies and its associated skills. For teachers, as for students and their mentors, epistemological beliefs are highly relevant to the way they teach. Their capacity for nurturing autonomy in students has shown to be related to such beliefs (Roth and Weinstock, 2013).

Faculty Development

To equip students with the skills and competencies to continue their own LLL, teachers

Box 27.7: How to be a moderator in a learning community

The main role of the moderator in a learning community is to support and inspire the communication processes for knowledge construction. Moderators need to be well informed about the clinical case and also its objectives. Moderators may fulfill their role in different ways: as more of a chairperson or more as someone who creates the conditions for fruitful discussions (Heron, 1999). They may display the following kinds of behavior:

- Goal-oriented planning
- Helping to articulate reasons for doing things, meaning raising the consciousness of the whole group
- Making emotions negotiable
- Structuring, similar to the role of a chairperson
- Assisting in creating an inspiring climate

This boils down to several essential activities of moderators (Lane, 2008; Sargeant, 2010):

- Posing higher-order and reflective questions to promote discussion and activate reasoning processes
- Asking group members to explain phenomena or define terms
- Keeping members on track by reminding them of their learning goals
- Role modeling positive interactions
- Identifying, in a constructive manner, differences in opinion between members
- Making power structures in the group explicit.
- Seeking, when relevant, to reach a consensus
- Encouraging, acknowledging, or reinforcing participants' contributions
- Setting a climate for learning by encouraging people to explore
- Presenting follow-up topics for discussion (*ad hoc*) and summarizing discussions
- Refraining from "teaching" the group

have to broaden their skill set and abandon the idea of knowledge transfer (Boerboom *et al.*, 2009). In addition, they should become more knowledgeable about learning theories. In a survey in the United States, veterinary teachers expressed an interest in knowledge about learning theories (Haden *et al.*, 2010). In 2006, Steinert and Mann already identified that faculty development programs in general ask for a longitudinal setup with peer coaching, mentorship, learning communities, and SDL. How and whether evidence about faculty development from the medical education research literature has been translated into veterinary initiatives and what specific context-specific challenges have been met along the way is as yet unknown (Bell, 2013).

In preparing teachers to help students in the acquisition of LLL competencies, they have to experience such learning processes themselves, individually and in social interaction. Through such experiential learning processes, teachers will probably learn that their own role modeling is more relevant for students than (the development of) valid and time-consuming assessment practices. Nevertheless, even though assessment of LLL competencies is hard, it is not impossible.

Assessment of Lifelong Learning Competencies

For assessment to become useful as a means of enhancing LLL competencies, the most important lesson is, as described by Candy, Crebert, and O'Leary (2004, p. 150), to "be weaned away from any tendency toward over-reliance on the opinions of others." Veterinary education should be designed in such a manner that professionals in practice are able to self-assess their performance as well as their learning processes. Such assessment practices ask for a focus on longitudinal assessment where students have to show evidence of their progress, for involvement of learners in the manner and the frequency with which they will be assessed, for peer and self-assessment, and for evaluation not only of the teaching but also of the assessments. Assessment in such educational formats is based on good reasoning, not on right or wrong answers (Ramaekers, 2011). To become effective lifelong learners, veterinary students have to have control over and feel responsible for their learning experiences and outcomes, during the curriculum and afterward.

An example of an assessment format that fits such an approach is peer feedback. Peer feedback may be helpful for the person who receives feedback as well as for the person who gives feedback, because it activates reflection on their own work (Nicol, Thomson, and Breslin, 2014). Peer-assisted learning may contribute to the acquisition of LLL competencies because it has a focus on reflecting on your own and other's work, and not waiting for the teacher's opinions. As an attractive side effect, it may save faculty time (Strand, Johnson, and Thompson, 2013). When peer feedback is used later on, when veterinarians work in practice, its introduction is probably not an easy task; for medical general practitioners the use of peer assessment in the context of a formal revalidation process has been difficult (Curnock *et al.*, 2012).

How to Enhance and Maintain Lifelong Learning in Veterinary Practice

Preparation for LLL in veterinary school is essential to equip individuals for active behaviors that influence their development. Once working in veterinary practice, being motivated to perform these active behaviors is crucial for LLL. Motivation for LLL alters over time, and is affected by personal factors and (social) experiences in the (work) environment.

Personal

Personal factors are not only learning skills, but also beliefs about learning and knowledge (Bath and Smith, 2009). The most important

beliefs are perceptions about knowledge and self-efficacy. For instance, when professionals during their career come to see the veterinary knowledge base as stable, their motivation for participation in learning activities will become low. Professional bodies could help sustain perceptions that are supportive for learning by focusing less on the transfer of core knowledge, which adds to the tendency for lifelong learning to evolve into lifelong assessment, and instead speak more about the dynamic nature of veterinary knowledge. When professional bodies desire "to empower learners by exercising more control over them" (Ecclestone, 1999), this will not help veterinary professionals to remain self-directed learners, because internal motivations are more powerful than external motivations (Knowles, 1975).

Likewise, self-efficacy is believed to undergo change across a lifetime and is influenced by life transitions. Employers may help to cross these transitions smoothly by alignment of the provision of support with employees' needs, and tailoring the level of autonomy provided with what the employee can cope with. Gender differences in the need for support and autonomy imply that this alignment must be established by dialog (Mastenbroek *et al.*, 2013). In other domains, studies about transitions and phases of change in a lifetime have been done, but no such work is available for veterinarians.

Workplace

Characteristics of the workplace, such as the level of autonomy, can help or hinder the further development of LLL competencies (Mastenbroek *et al.*, 2014). Even though workplaces in turn are influenced by larger developments in society, such as economic trends, we will restrict ourselves to the level of organizations. Work can provide the social environment that prevents decline or supports an increase in motivation for learning, like the provision of a safe learning environment where making mistakes is allowed. The aforementioned critically reflective learning communities can help. In Box 27.8 a conceivable format for organizing meetings in such learning

Box 27.8: How to run a learning community

A conceivable format for organizing a meeting in learning communities is the following:

- Agree on who will be the moderator and (re)confirm agreements about the way in which this group wants to discuss and work (5 minutes)
- Make an inventory of participants' learning issues for this meeting and choose what issue(s) will be discussed. (Time depends on group size, but no longer than 15 minutes)
- Problem owner (presenter) tells (part of) a problematic event from their own practice. Relate only what actually happened, not how you interpreted the events (5 minutes)

In learning communities focusing on discussing case reports:

- Each of the participants asks questions to come to grips with the problem (10 minutes)
- The moderator may ask whether other participants have experienced the same kind of problem, how they dealt with the problem, and why that approach was chosen (10 minutes)
- Is sufficient knowledge available within the group to solve this problem, in particular to reach an evidence-based – and feasible – solution?
- If not, what can be done to find sufficient knowledge? Agree on follow-up
- Reflection on the process: What went well? What is open to improvement? To begin with, the moderator gives feedback; in time, the learning community could use an observer from their group
- In learning communities focusing on competencies for professional development:
- Participants ask open questions for clarification. Be alert to closed questions, or hidden suggestions or solutions
- When participants have enough information and understanding of the situation and the presenter's dilemma, both the presenter and other participants reflect on the approach that was chosen and the possible alternatives that they can see or would explore. The presenter notes down the options
- The presenter reacts to the given advice, indicating what is appealing and what is not
- The presenter decides on what might be a first step to take

communities is outlined. Potentially, participation in such communities will affect perceptions about the knowledge base in the veterinary field. Professional bodies could support LLL through facilitating knowledge networks and, since one of the factors that hinders LLL is a lack of time, professional bodies could also contribute by means of easy access to the literature.

Challenges in Facilitating the Development of Lifelong Learning Competencies

To address reflective practice and SDL, and the assessment thereof, within the curriculum is not simple (Tummons, 2011). For educators who have acquired didactic skills within knowledge-heavy and assessment-driven curricula (May, 2008), shifting to a curriculum aimed at developing LLL competencies is a tremendous change. Such changes ask for faculty development, for design of curricula that leave room for authentic learning experiences, and for close alignment of developments within the curricula with the work of professionals. The latter is necessary because implementing authentic learning designs poses a challenge when students see differences between the ideals promoted in the curriculum and behavior observed in the workplace. In addition, such new formats may be resource intensive and require innovative logistics, such as have been described for problem-based learning within veterinary medicine (Hyams and Raidal, 2013).

Finally, even though different levels of reflection have been demonstrated in practice, higher levels of reflection are less frequently identified and appear to be more difficult to achieve. This resembles what has been found in different domains for higher-level learning competencies in general, where it has been said that even with the most optimal curriculum, many students will not attain these higher-level learning competencies (Kegan, 2009; Hofer and Pintrich, 2002).

Conclusion

For veterinarians to be effective lifelong learners, they have to start in veterinary school by taking responsibility for their own learning processes and outcomes. Veterinary schools may support these processes and prevent "growing pains" by offering opportunities for self-directed learning and reflective practice.

References

Bath, D.M. and Smith, C.D. (2009), "The relationship between epistemological beliefs and the propensity for lifelong learning", *Studies in Continuing Education*, **31**, **2**, 173-189.

Bell, C.E. (2013) Faculty development in veterinary education: Are we doing enough (or publishing enough about it), and do we value it? *Journal of Veterinary Medical Education*, **40** (**2**), 96–101.

Billett, S. (2010), "The perils of confusing lifelong learning with lifelong education", *International Journal of Lifelong Education*, **29**, **4**, 401-413.

Bleakley, A., and Bligh, J. (2008) Students learning from patients: Let's get real in medical education. *Advances in Health Sciences Education*, **13** (**1**), 89–107.

Boerboom, T.B.B., Dolmans, D.H.J.M., Muijtjens, A.M.M., *et al.* (2009) Does a faculty development programme improve teachers' perceived competence in different teacher roles? *Medical Teacher*, **31** (**11**), 1030–1031.

Bok, H.G., Teunissen, P.W., Favier, R.P., *et al.* (2013) Programmatic assessment of competency-based workplace learning: When theory meets practice. *BMC Medical Education*, **13** (**1**), 123.

Brookfield, S. (2009) The concept of critical reflection: Promises and contradictions. *European Journal of Social Work*, **12** (**3**), 293–304.

Candy, P., Crebert, G., and O'Leary, J. (1994) *Developing Lifelong Learners through Undergraduate Education*. Commissioned Report No. 28, National Board of Employment Education and Training. Australian Government Publishing Service, Canberra.

Caple, I.W. (2005) Continuing professional development for veterinarians. *Australian Veterinary Journal*, **83** (**4**), 200–202.

Clarke, P., Schull, D., Coleman, G., *et al.* (2013) Enhancing professional writing skills of veterinary technology students: Linking assessment and clinical practice in a communications course. *Assessment and Evaluation in Higher Education*, **38** (**3**), 273–287.

Cockcroft, P., and Holmes, M.A. (2004) Evidence-based veterinary medicine: 2. Identifying information needs and finding the evidence. *In Practice*, **26** (**2**), 96–102.

Cox, A. (2005) What are communities of practice? A comparative review of four seminal works. *Journal of Information Science*, **31** (**6**), 527–540.

Curnock, E., Bowie, P., Pope, L., and McKay, J. (2012) Barriers and attitudes influencing non-engagement in a peer feedback model to inform evidence for GP appraisal. *BMC Medical Education*, **12** (**1**), 12.

Dale, V.H.M., Pierce, S.E., and May, S.A. (2010) The importance of cultivating a preference for complexity in veterinarians for effective lifelong learning. *Journal of Veterinary Medical Education*, 37 (**2**), 165–171.

Dale, V.H.M., Pierce, S.E., and May, S.A. (2013) Motivating factors and perceived barriers to participating in continuing professional development: A national survey of veterinary surgeons. *Veterinary Record*, 173 (**10**), 247.

Davies, S. (2012) Embracing reflective practice. *Education for Primary Care*, 23 (**1**), 9–12.

de Groot, E., Endedijk, M., Jaarsma, D., *et al.* (2013) Development of critically reflective dialogues in communities of health professionals. *Advances in Health Sciences Education*, 18 (**4**), 627–643.

de Groot, E., Endedijk, M.D., Jaarsma, A.D.C., *et al.* (2014) Critically reflective dialogues in learning communities of professionals. *Studies in Continuing Education*, 36 (**1**), 15–37.

de Groot, E., Jaarsma, D., Endedijk, M., *et al.* (2012) Critically reflective work behavior of health care professionals. *Journal of Continuing Education in the Health Professions*, 32 (**1**), 48–57.

Driessen, E.W., van Tartwijk, J., Overeem, K., *et al.* (2005) Conditions for successful reflective use of portfolios in undergraduate medical education. *Medical Education*, 39 (**12**), 1230–1235.

Ecclestone, K. (1999), "Care or control?: Defining learners' needs for lifelong learning", *British Journal of Educational Studies*, 47, **4**, 332-347.

Haden, N.K., Chaddock, M., Hoffsis, G.F., *et al.* (2010) Preparing faculty for the future: AAVMC members' perceptions of professional development needs. *Journal of Veterinary Medical Education*, 37 (**3**), 220–232.

Heron, J. (1999) *The Complete Facilitator's Handbook*, Kogan Page, London.

Hofer, B.K., and Pintrich, P.R. (2002) *Personal Epistomology: The Psychology of Beliefs about Knowledge and Knowing*, Lawrence Erlbaum, Mahwah, NJ.

Hyams, J.H., and Raidal, S.L. (2013) Problem-based learning: Facilitating multiple small teams in a large group setting. *Journal of Veterinary Medical Education*, 40 (**3**), 282–287.

Jaarsma, A.D.C., Dolmans, D.H.J.M., Scherpbier, A.J.J.A. & Van Beukelen, P. 2009, "Educational approaches aimed at preparing students for professional veterinary practice", *OIE Revue Scientifique et Technique*, 28, **2**, 823-830.

Jang, H., and Ko, I. (2014) The factors influencing CoP activities and their impact on relationship commitment and individual performance. *Journal of Knowledge Management*, 18 (**1**), 75–91.

Kegan, R. (2009) *Immunity to Change: How to Overcome It and Unlock the Potential in Yourself and Your Organization*, Harvard Business School Press, Boston, MA.

Khosa, D.K., Volet, S.E., and Bolton, J.R. (2010) An instructional intervention to encourage effective deep collaborative learning in undergraduate veterinary students. *Journal of Veterinary Medical Education*, 37 (**4**), 369–376.

Koper, R., Giesbers, B., vanRosmalen, P., Sloep, P., vanBruggen, J., Tattersall, C., Vogten, H. & Brouns, F. 2005, "A design model for lifelong learning networks", *Interactive Learning Environments*, 13, **1-2**, 71-92.

Koskinen, H.I. (2010) Social interactions between veterinary medical students and their teachers in an ambulatory clinic setting in Finland. *Journal of Veterinary Medical Education*, 37 (**2**), 159–164.

Kram, K.E. (1985) *Mentoring at Work: Developmental Relationships in Organizational Life*, Scott Foresman, Glenview, IL.

Kuhn, D. 1999, "A developmental model of critical thinking", *Educational Researcher*, 28, **2**, 16-46.

Laal, M., and Salamati, P. (2012) Lifelong learning: Why do we need it? *Procedia – Social and Behavioral Sciences*, 31, 399–403.

Lane, E.A. (2008) Problem-based learning in veterinary education. *Journal of Veterinary Medical Education*, 35 (**4**), 631–636.

Larkin, M. (2010) Long road ahead to change veterinary education. *Journal of the American Veterinary Medical Association*, 237 (**5**), 474–478.

Lee, D.E. (2003) The case for continuing education in veterinary colleges. *Journal of Veterinary Medical Education*, 30 (**1**), 62–63.

Loyens, S.M.M., Magda, J., and Rikers, R.M.J.P. (2008) Self-directed learning in problem-based learning and its relationships with self-regulated learning. *Educational Psychology Review*, **20** (**4**), 411–427.

Mann, K., Gordon, J., and MacLeod, A. (2009) Reflection and reflective practice in health professions education: A systematic review. *Advances in Health Sciences Education*, **14** (**4**), 595–621.

Mastenbroek, N.J.J.M., Jaarsma, A.D.C., Demerouti, E., *et al.* (2013) Burnout and engagement, and its predictors in young veterinary professionals: The influence of gender. *Veterinary Record*, **174** (**6**), 144.

Mastenbroek, N.J.J.M., Jaarsma, A.D.C., Scherpbier, A.J.J.A., *et al.* (2014) The role of personal resources in explaining well-being and performance: A study among young veterinary professionals. *European Journal of Work and Organizational Psychology*, **23** (**2**), 190–202.

Mastenbroek, N.J.J.M., Van Beukelen, P., Demerouti, E., *et al.* (2015) Effects of a 1 year development programme for recently graduated veterinary professionals on personal and job resources: A combined quantitative and qualitative approach. *BMC Veterinary Research*, **11**, 311.

May, S.A. (2008) Modern veterinary graduates are outstanding, but can they get better? *Journal of Veterinary Medical Education*, **35** (**4**), 573–580.

May, S.J. (2012) Learning doesn't stop at university. *Veterinary Record*, **171**, i.

May, S.A., and Kinnison, T. (2015) Continuing professional development: Learning that leads to change in individual and collective clinical practice. *Veterinary Record*, **177** (**1**), 13.

McArdle, K., and Coutts, N. (2010) Taking teachers' continuous professional development (CPD) beyond reflection: Adding shared sense-making and collaborative engagement for professional renewal. *Studies in Continuing Education*, **32** (**3**), 201–215.

Moore, D.A., Klingborg, D.J., Brenner, J.S. and Gotz, A.A.(2000), "Motivations for and barriers to engaging in continuing veterinary medical education", *Journal of the American Veterinary Medical Association*, **217**, 7, 1001-1005.

Mossop, L.H., and Cobb, K. (2013) Teaching and assessing veterinary professionalism. *Journal of Veterinary Medical Education*, **40** (**3**), 223–232.

Mossop, L.H., and Senior, A. (2008) I'll show you mine if you show me yours! Portfolio design in two UK veterinary schools. *Journal of Veterinary Medical Education*, **35** (**4**), 599–606.

Nicol, D., Thomson, A., and Breslin, C. (2014) Rethinking feedback practices in higher education: A peer review perspective. *Assessment and Evaluation in Higher Education*, **39** (**1**), 102–122.

Niehoff, B.P., Chenoweth, P., and Rutti, R. (2005) Mentoring within the veterinary medical profession: Veterinarians' experiences as proteges in mentoring relationships. *Journal of Veterinary Medical Education*, **32** (**2**), 264–271.

Numan, A. (1827) Redevoering over de vee-artsenijkunde en de inrigting van derzelver onderwijs, overeenkomstig met het belang der maatschappy. *Veeartsenijkundig Magazijn*, **1** (**1–77**), 56.

Ramaekers, S. (2011) On the development of competence in solving clinical problems. PhD thesis, Utrecht University.

Roth, G., and Weinstock, M. (2013) Teachers' epistemological beliefs as an antecedent of autonomy-supportive teaching. *Motivation and Emotion*, **37** (**3**), 402–412.

Sargeant, J., Hill, T. and Breau, L. (2010), "Development and testing of a scale to assess interprofessional education (IPE) facilitation skills", *Journal of Continuing Education in the Health Professions*, **30**, 2, 126-131.

Scholz, E., Trede, F., and Raidal, S.L. (2013) Workplace learning in veterinary education: A sociocultural perspective. *Journal of Veterinary Medical Education*, **40** (**4**), 355–362.

Schön, D.A. (1983) *The Reflective Practitioner: How Professionals Think in Action*, Basic Books, New York.

Sfard, A. (1998) On two metaphors for learning and the dangers of choosing just one. *Educational Researcher*, **27** (**2**), 4–13.

Smith, E. (2011) Teaching critical reflection. *Teaching in Higher Education*, **16** (**2**), 211–223.

Steinert, Y., and Mann, K.V. (2006) Faculty development: Principles and practices. *Journal of Veterinary Medical Education*, **33** (**3**), 317–324.

Strand, E.B., Johnson, B., and Thompson, J. (2013) Peer-assisted communication training: Veterinary students as simulated clients and communication skills trainers. *Journal of Veterinary Medical Education*, **40** (**3**), 233–241.

van Tartwijk, J., Driessen, E., van der Vleuten, C., and Stokking, K. (2007) Factors influencing the successful introduction of portfolios. *Quality in Higher Education*, **13** (**1**), 69–79.

Taylor, K.A., and Robinson, D.C. (2009) Unleashing the potential: Women's development and ways of knowing as a perspective for veterinary medical education. *Journal of Veterinary Medical Education*, **36** (**1**), 135–144.

Teunissen, P.W., and Bok, H.G.J. (2013) Believing is seeing: How people's beliefs influence goals, emotions and behaviour. *Medical Education*, **47** (**11**), 1064–1072.

Tummons, J. (2011) "It sort of feels uncomfortable": Problematising the assessment of reflective practice. *Studies in Higher Education*, **36** (**4**), 471–483.

van Knippenberg, D., de Dreu, C.K.W., and Homan, A.C. (2004) Work group diversity and group performance: An integrative model and research agenda. *Journal of Applied Psychology*, **89** (**6**), 1008–1022.

Weinberg, F.J. (2015) Epistemological beliefs and knowledge sharing in work teams: A new model and research questions. *Learning Organization*, **22** (**1**), 40–57.

Wenger, E. (1998) *Communities of Practice: Learning, Meaning, and Identity*, Cambridge University Press, Cambridge.

28

Ethics and Animal Welfare

Joy M. Verrinder and Clive J.C. Phillips

Centre for Animal Welfare and Ethics, School of Veterinary Science, University of Queensland, Australia

---

 Box 28.1: Key messages

- The welfare of animals is the fundamental responsibility of all veterinarians.
- Animal welfare and ethics teaching is an essential component of any course for veterinarians.
- Teaching of the concepts of animal welfare should not be sacrificed in order to justify current animal management systems that compromise welfare for the sake of the financial profitability of the enterprise.
- Animal welfare science informs animal ethics, but they are two separate disciplines.

- Animal ethics education involves the scientific development of the four components of moral behavior: moral sensitivity, moral judgment, moral motivation, and moral character.
- A universal principles approach to ethics teaching utilizing ethical frameworks as complementary rather than competitive tools enables veterinarians to show ethical leadership in preventing and addressing animal ethics issues.

Introduction

Veterinary educators teaching animal welfare and, more rarely, animal ethics (how humans should behave toward animals) find themselves in an invidious position when determining what to teach. On the one hand, the future veterinarians will on graduating, by virtue of their detailed knowledge of animal form and function, always be regarded as one of the primary sources of information about the welfare of animals. To take on this responsibility effectively and with a good conscience, students need to be aware of, sensitive to, and capable of managing the many welfare issues with which they will be confronted. On the other hand, there will be pressures on veterinarians, in particular financial ones, to act in ways that support their clients and are not necessarily in the animals' best interests. Many of the animals that they treat are involved in an economic enterprise, for food production in particular, and the managers of these enterprises will often be required to take the course of action that maximizes profit, which may preclude expensive veterinary treatment. Similarly, the welfare of many companion animals may be compromised by both owners' treatment requirements not matching those

Veterinary Medical Education: A Practical Guide, First Edition. Edited by Jennifer L. Hodgson and Jacquelyn M. Pelzer.
© 2017 John Wiley & Sons, Inc. Published 2017 by John Wiley & Sons, Inc.

recommended by veterinarians and a surplus of animals in the community. Such dilemmas facing the veterinary student on graduation potentially lead to a disregard for the animals' interests and consequent moral distress. Moral distress occurs "when one knows the right thing to do, but institutional or other constraints make it difficult to pursue the desired course of action" (Raines, 2000, p. 30). A UK study found that veterinary practitioners experience stressful ethical dilemmas regularly, with most reporting one or two ethical dilemmas weekly, and one-third of practitioners reporting three to five per week in relation to animal ethics issues (Batchelor and McKeegan, 2012). One way in which veterinary schools deal with this is to desensitize veterinary students to the animals' interests. This is pursued by some staff in veterinary faculties because they perceive that it is necessary for students to cope with working in the animal industries and engaging in practices on animals that do not take full account of the animals' interests, for example tail docking in dogs or cattle. Staff may be defensive about breeding animals specifically for surgery practice for students, or about using apparently unwanted animals for this purpose.

However, the animal welfare and/or ethics instructor is responsible for ensuring that all students graduate with sufficient knowledge, understanding, and skills of animal welfare and ethics (AWE) to equip them to deal with welfare issues, not minimize or avoid them. Animal ethics in this respect should not be confused with professional ethics, the former requiring us to consider how we should treat animals, the latter usually concerned with how we should act in accordance with the veterinary profession's codes of conduct. To teach AWE, instructors need to be aware of the major animal welfare concerns in the most important animal industries, which include issues where it is expensive to provide adequately for the animals' welfare, for example provision of pain relief to farm livestock when invasive procedures are conducted. The availability of adequate space is another major cause for

concern, and so too are modifications to the animal to make it suit an economic production system, either by mutilating the body or by breeding for better performance, be it greater productivity, in the case of animals for food; greater appeal to the public, in the case of animals for companionship; or faster racing skills, in sport animals. Animal welfare and ethics educators can address these problems in two ways: they can attempt to describe all the major issues for all the industries, or they can attempt to draw out principles relating to the most common animal welfare problems, such as would emerge from an assessment of animal welfare in a dairy herd. Through these carefully chosen examples, they can analyze the problems that exist and how they can be addressed. The latter approach is advocated, since it teaches students to be proactive rather than just passively learn facts.

Veterinarians' Responsibilities for Animal Welfare

Veterinarians are seen as educators in animal welfare because of their expertise in animal-related topics, using their skills to teach their clients and the broader community about welfare issues. They are increasingly frequently becoming involved in public policy debates and in establishing appropriate regulatory frameworks to manage AWE to the satisfaction of the public. The One Welfare movement recognizes that human and animal welfare are closely linked (Dolby and Litster, 2015). Veterinarians can also take a preemptive role in developing local competitiveness between animal producers to enhance welfare (Pritchard *et al.*, 2012), or in analyzing new initiatives to identify possible ethical issues before they become entrenched in practice (Vergés, 2010), thereby preventing considerable disruption and intransigence.

Veterinarians have responsibilities to their clients, animal consumers, and the public more generally, but their fundamental responsibility lies in maintaining animals in a good welfare state. Veterinarians may be faced with the ethical dilemma of whether to treat animals in a system that they believe cannot possibly provide good welfare, for example chickens in battery cages, or whether to allow someone else to do this. Their responsibility for animals' welfare is shared with stockpeople, animal transporters, animal breeders, and a range of people with more limited roles in the provision of specific aspects of the animals' life. The primacy of the animal welfare responsibilities of veterinarians is recognized in some countries by an oath sworn at graduation in which they promise to uphold the welfare of animals within their charge (WSAVA, 2015). As such, developing skills in animal welfare and ethical behavior toward animals may be seen as the ultimate objective of veterinary training, although secondary goals of improving public health, supporting a viable rural environment, and fostering good human–animal interactions must be acknowledged.

Veterinarians operate largely in a clinical setting, and animal welfare education is the fundamental goal of clinical skills training, which is currently being supported by the opening of clinical skills laboratories in many veterinary schools worldwide (Rösch *et al.*, 2014). These are stocked with models and equipment for students to learn and practice key skills for treating animals, while maintaining a distance from the live animal for ethical reasons. Although some students fear that such opportunities could replace live animal practice, most students welcome the chance to improve their skills in tasks such as suturing, rectal examination, surgery, injection, ultrasound, obstetrics, blood sampling, X-ray, bandaging, and intubation (Rösch *et al.*, 2014). Overuse of animals in veterinary colleges is a reality that should be regularly monitored by ethics committees. Development of skills through use of alternatives to live animals in teaching clinical examination and surgical practice are now an important part of animal welfare training (Capilé *et al.*, 2015). Thus, veterinary educators have a responsibility for animal welfare and ethical practice in both veterinary training and practice.

Why Veterinarians Must Study Animal Welfare and Ethics

The first reason that veterinarians must study AWE is that all sentient beings have needs and interests in survival and wellbeing, a fact that grounds ethics in science (Harris, 2010). The development of veterinary medicine was originally based on the need to consider the physical welfare of animals in order to maximize their usefulness to humans (Bones and Yeates, 2012). This personal interest approach has become increasingly questioned. Through keeping animals as companions and through scientific studies, animals have been found to have a wide range of similar emotions to humans (Panksepp, 1998), including moral emotions such as empathy, which have an evolutionary basis through various animal species (de Waal, 2009). Furthermore, we are more and more recognizing that animals have capacities that humans do not (Ford, 1999). We no longer question whether animals deserve moral consideration (Sapontzis, 1987; Wise, 2002), and discussion is growing over how they should be treated (Rollin, 2006b). Thus, veterinarians need to be at the forefront of knowledge and research into animals' capabilities and to develop the skills for moral action. A universal principles approach (see Box 28.3) is ethically necessary, and tolerance of a multitude of other, less inclusive approaches is unreasonable.

The second reason for studying AWE is community expectation, or the new social ethic (Rollin, 2006a) regarding animals. Public concern for animal welfare is burgeoning as the animal industries intensify and production volumes increase in many countries. In conjunction with greater trade in other commodities, the long-distance trade in live animals is growing rapidly. The traditional curriculum for veterinarians, focused on basic and clinical sciences, animal handling and husbandry, diagnostics and surgery, is changing to incorporate areas of competence that will address the public concern for AWE.

The third reason is that veterinarians and veterinary students are indicating that they need it. In the UK study that identified regular exposure to moral distress in veterinary practice, 78% of respondents felt that they were not given enough (or in many cases any) ethics tuition during their training (Batchelor and McKeegan, 2012). In a study of Australian first- and fifth-year veterinary students (Verrinder and Phillips, 2014b), 96% agreed that they should be involved in the wider social issues of animal protection, 94% that the veterinary profession should be involved in addressing animal ethics issues, but only 33% considered that the veterinary profession was sufficiently involved. Also, 71% were morally motivated to put animals' interests over the interests of their owners/carers, although those in the fifth year were less strongly in agreement than first-year students.

What Is Happening in Animal Welfare and Ethics Teaching in Veterinary Science?

There is regional variation in the extent of the transition from the traditional curriculum to one that develops competencies in animal welfare and ethics. A European study identified a greater emphasis on such training in the northwest of the continent, in particular involving more interactive teaching (Illmann *et al.*, 2014). These courses are better held before the extramural placements, so that students are better able to detect welfare problems on farms (Kerr, Mullan, and Main, 2013). There is also a growing focus on animal welfare assessment and animal law. Most students agree that AWE courses enable them to identify and deal with ethical dilemmas more effectively (Abood and Siegford, 2012). The Royal College of Veterinary Surgeons' Day One Competences 2014 include understanding the ethical and legal responsibilities of the veterinary surgeon in relation to patients, clients, society, and the environment; the ethical framework within which veterinary surgeons should work; and ethical theories that inform decision-making in

professional and animal welfare-related ethics (RCVS, 2016). Veterinary medical education is increasingly providing training in nontechnical competence (Dolby and Litster, 2015), but the various aspects of animal welfare are not universally addressed in veterinary teaching. Graduating veterinarians are almost all good at understanding and treating the physical welfare issues, including infectious disease treatment and prevention, but psychological welfare issues are less well understood (Koch, 2009). However, a comprehensive understanding of all aspects of AWE gives students confidence in tackling animal welfare issues (Wu *et al.*, 2015). Veterinary students have shown more concerned attitudes for animals used for profit or regarded as pests following animal welfare courses (Hazel, Signal, and Taylor, 2011).

Ethics teaching in veterinary courses is relatively new, but is growing internationally, albeit with considerable variation in what is taught, and how, and little consistency in ethics competencies (Magalhães-Sant'Ana *et al.*, 2009, 2010; Morton, 2010). In many disciplines, including veterinary science, professional ethics teaching aims to develop ethical behavior toward people. However, the extent to which veterinary courses develop ethical behavior toward *animals* is unknown, despite this being central to the veterinary role. A major obstacle to the achievement of leadership in the veterinary profession addressing animal ethics issues is the reliance on a range of existing cultural perspectives on how animals should be treated (descriptive ethics), rather than universal principles (normative ethics). Consequently, students may finish veterinary school with a view that ethical decisions are based on personal choice, and that ethics is about tolerance of a range of conflicting perspectives. This provides little possibility for ethical direction and confidence in ethical decision-making. As well, "morality requires by definition the investment of knowledge in action" (Blasi, 1983, p. 205). Therefore, we advocate a more scientific approach to ethics teaching that includes the development of ethical behavior toward animals.

A Scientific Approach to Teaching Ethics

Ethical behavior has been identified as having four components – moral sensitivity, moral judgment, moral motivation, and moral character (see Box 28.2) – all of which can be developed through education (Rest, 1994). (The terms "ethical" and "moral" are often used interchangeably, as they are in this chapter.)

Ethics programs often emphasize just one of these components, moral judgment development to address ethical dilemmas. A number of moral judgment tests in relation to human ethics issues have been devised, including the frequently used Defining Issues Test (DIT; Rest *et al.*, 1999), a quantitative measure to determine the extent to which students use three moral reasoning schemas (Box 28.3). The DIT involves students choosing their preferred action, and then rating twelve considerations based on which are important when making a decision on a specific human ethics issue (such as stealing to feed one's family during a famine) and ranking the four that are most important. These rankings are used to quantify to what extent students rely on PI, MN, and UP reasoning (see Box 28.3). Education has been identified as one of the main predictors of moral judgment growth, particularly liberal arts programs. However, professional education programs do not appear to promote moral judgment unless the program includes a well-validated

---

Box 28.2: What's the meaning? The four components of moral behavior

Based on the literature on morality, including cognitive development and social learning, as well as behavioristic, psychoanalytic, and social psychological approaches, cognitive psychologist James Rest identified a Four Component Model (FCM) as a theory of what determines moral behavior:

- *Moral sensitivity*: interpreting the situation through awareness of how our actions affect others
- *Moral judgment*: determining which action is morally justifiable

- *Moral motivation*: prioritizing moral values relative to other values
- *Moral character*: having courage and persistence, overcoming distractions, and implementing skills

Rest proposed that these components constitute a logical analysis of what it takes to behave morally, and moral failure can occur because of deficiencies in any component.

Source: Rest, 1994.

Box 28.3: What is the Defining Issues Test (DIT)?

The DIT condenses Kohlberg's six hierarchical stages of moral judgment into three hierarchical schemas (Rest *et al.*, 1999):

- *Schema 1 Personal Interest (PI)*: recognition of authority and reciprocal relationships that result in reward or punishment for the person

- *Schema 2 Maintaining Norms (MN)*: abiding by existing rules and regulations set by governments or professional groups
- *Schema 3 Post-conventional, referred to here as Universal Principles (UP)*: emphasizing moral ideals that are constructive, applicable to all and not self-serving at the expense of others

ethics curriculum (Bebeau and Monson, 2008). Assessed by Rest's DIT based on human ethics issues, veterinary practitioners have shown a large variation in moral reasoning abilities, no different from that of the general public despite having a professional degree, and these abilities did not improve with experience (Batchelor, Creed, and McKeegan, 2015). However, until recently there has been no measure of moral reasoning in relation to the animal ethics issues faced by veterinarians.

In 2012, we developed a Veterinary Defining Issues Test (VetDIT; Verrinder and Phillips, 2014a) with three animal ethics scenarios involving companion, farm, and research animal ethics issues common to veterinary practice. Results of this test suggest that veterinary students of both animal- and nonanimal-related professions prioritize UP reasoning more, and PI reasoning less, on animal than on human ethics issues, and that MN reasoning is prioritized equally on animal and human issues (Verrinder, Ostini, and Phillips, 2016a).

Although moral judgment is a critical foundation for moral behavior because it produces moral meaning for an intended action (Bredemeier and Shields, 1994), the strength of association between moral judgment and action is low (Thoma, 1994). Thus, development of the other three components of moral behavior is also essential. Without the ability to recognize and interpret issues ethically (ethical sensitivity), it is unlikely that a person will engage in moral decision-making. Practice-specific tests have been created to assess ethical sensitivity in other professions, such as dentistry (Bebeau, Rest, and Yamoor, 1985) and life sciences (Clarkeburn, Downie, and Matthew, 2002). Recently, an ethical sensitivity measure for veterinarians using a written response and video-recorded role play demonstrated that students had increased capacity to identify elements of ethical sensitivity after instruction (Verrinder, Ostini and Phillips, 2016b). Moral motivation and moral character have been measured in other professions, but not so far in veterinary education. Table 28.1 provides samples of research on the four components of moral behavior.

Veterinary Students' Ethical Motivations

Australian veterinary students have indicated that their two main motivations for choosing to study veterinary science are "enjoyment in working with animals" and "wanting to help sick and injured animals." "Wanting to improve the way animals are treated" was the third most common motivation for more than one-third of students (Verrinder and Phillips, 2014b). Their past experience with animals, especially pets, is a major driver of this interest (Furnham and Pinder, 1990; Driscoll, 1992; Furnham and Heyes, 1993; Serpell, 2005). However, students' interest in AWE differs during their course. In English veterinary students, Paul and Podberscek (2000) observed less empathy toward animals in male students in the later years of their course, and this was confirmed for all students, not just males, in an Australian study (Pollard-Williams, Doyle, and Freire, 2014). Aligned with this evidence, Ling *et al.* (2016) found that as Asian veterinary students progressed through their course, there was greater acceptance of killing young, dependent animals and reduced concern about transporting animals from a developed to a developing country. There was also greater rejection of using animals that died naturally for products, which probably reflects a more advanced understanding of the risks of acquiring zoonoses. Such differences in ethical sensitivity and motivation suggest the need for a greater emphasis on animal welfare and ethics teaching and assessment.

Teaching Animal Welfare and Ethics

Animal welfare and ethics should initially be taught as a stand-alone course in the first year. Although it may be integrated into other relevant teaching, in particular animal behavior or husbandry, the latter often focuses on farm animals, and it is important that animal welfare teaching addresses all types of animals, including companion, zoo, wild, and sport animals. There is also a danger if animal welfare is subsumed within a husbandry course that the major AWE concerns will be seen to have to acquiesce to the demands of modern husbandry systems

Table 28.1 Research on the components of moral behavior.

Component of moral behavior	Publication type	Synopsis
Moral sensitivity	Paper presented at the Annual Meeting of the Association for Moral Education, Cambridge, MA	Review of 37 studies in which 23 measures to assess **ethical sensitivity** were described in dentistry, medicine, nursing, counseling, business, science, and school settings. Identified several well-validated measures showing that sensitivity can be influenced by educational interventions, and in some cases females demonstrated small but significantly higher levels of ethical sensitivity (You and Bebeau, 2005).
Ethical sensitivity	Journal article (submitted)	Reports results of animal ethics sensitivity tools in which third-year veterinary students increased ethical sensitivity scores in a written test following instruction (Verrinder, Ostini, and Phillips, 2016b).
Moral judgment	Journal article	Reviews 33 **moral judgment** studies (6600 respondents) in medicine, dentistry, law, and veterinary medicine, confirming that professional school education programs do not promote moral judgment development unless the program includes a well-validated ethics curriculum. Reviews effects of ethics teaching interventions and identifies significant benefits in law, nursing, and dentistry studies (Bebeau, 2002).
Moral judgment	Journal article	A longitudinal DIT study concluded that to facilitate moral development, opportunities for students to consider issues of fairness from less egocentric perspectives that serve the public good are required (Mayhew, Seifert, and Pascarella, 2010).
Moral judgment	Journal article	Results of three professional responsibility courses for law students showed small, moderate, and large gains in principled reasoning, as measured by the DIT (Hartwell, 2004).
Moral judgment	Journal article	Results of three variations of ethics course design and two comparison groups over a five-year period showed gains in principled reasoning scores equivalent to four to six years of formal education by teaching formal logic, development theory and stage typology, philosophical methods of ethical analysis, and application of methods to social issues. Peer discussion of moral issues was found to be less effective, as were general courses in the humanities and the political/social sciences (Penn, 1990).
Moral judgment	Journal article	A three-hour interactive workshop increased students' principled reasoning as determined by the VetDIT, whereas the same content presented in a lecture format did not. Growth in Universal Principles reasoning on animal ethics issues, similar to that achieved by Penn (1990) and McNeel (1994) using the DIT human ethics issues, suggests that direct teaching of moral development theory, and practice using principled reasoning, are effective (Verrinder and Phillips, 2016a).
Moral motivation	Book chapter	The Professional Role Orientation Inventory differentiates beginning and advanced students' role concept and is sensitive to the effects of instruction. Students at higher stages of professional moral identity (about 37% of students) were more likely to incorporate issues of access to care, serving medical assistance patients, and volunteering to help those in need as key expectations of self (Bebeau and Monson, 2008).
Moral action	Book chapter	In dental ethics education, students take on the role of a professional and analyze their responsibilities in complex situations, developing action plans and dialogs that are critiqued for professional effectiveness. This practice builds confidence in taking action (Bebeau, 1994).

Notes: DIT = Defining Issues Test; VetDIT = Veterinary Defining Issues Test.

for financial sustainability through high stocking rates, close confinement, limited pain relief, and so on. If AWE is taught as a separate course, it allows students opportunities to focus on the animals' welfare state without these constraints.

In the middle stages of the course, students' learning about animal husbandry, welfare, and ethics should be brought together into a systems-oriented course, which will include considerations of animal management economics. Student-centered learning is appropriate for an integrated course of this nature, with debates, workshops, and discussion, guided by an ethical approach. An ethical approach applies complementary universal ethical frameworks and principles to enable students to make the most fitting ethical decisions. Ideally, all teachers in the faculty will use the same ethical approach for a unified moral climate. This may require working with faculty to ensure a common understanding of this universal approach to using ethics concepts and frameworks.

Key Animal Welfare Concepts and Measures

It is important that veterinary students understand key concepts such as the five freedoms and other broader concepts of welfare, including the five domains (Mellor and Beausoleil, 2015) and animals' needs and capabilities (Nussbaum, 2001). Veterinary students also need to know the principles of and some methods of measuring animal welfare, especially those principles based on behavior, physiology, and animal production and product quality. It is particularly important that students understand the connections between good animal welfare and animal output. There are several online packages to assist in the teaching of AWE in veterinary schools, most notably the Concepts in Animal Welfare course produced by World Animal Protection (WSPA, 2003). Students should also be aware of the development and use of the Welfare Quality® Protocol (e.g., Gieseke *et al.*,

2014). Veterinary students should understand the complexity of the human–animal bond, as well as the diverse ways in which animals interact with humans, both advantageous and disadvantageous. They must recognize the correct way to move animals, using low-stress animal management techniques.

Animal Welfare Legislation

Animal welfare law is a rapidly developing subject, which forms the focus for whole courses in some veterinary schools (Whittaker, 2014). Such courses tend to be broad and multidisciplinary, including not just law but philosophy, economics, and animal welfare science. Regulatory frameworks can be described for the major animal groups; that is, companion, farm, wild (native and introduced), and animals in research and teaching. Given that veterinary students may practice outside their home countries, some international law comparisons should be included. The growing role of international organizations, in particular the World Organisation for Animal Health (OIE) and the World Trade Organization, should be acknowledged, as well as the role that the OIE plays in setting standards internationally.

Animal Ethics Concepts

Understanding the differences between animal welfare, animal ethics, and professional ethics, and between different approaches to animal ethics, is important (see Box 28.4). Based on moral philosophy and moral psychology, we take a normative approach to ethics teaching founded on universal principles and the complementarity of the main ethics frameworks; that is, deontological, utilitarian, virtue, and care ethics. The aim is to develop the capacity for ethical behavior toward both nonhuman and human animals.

Learning Methods

In the past 30 years, a large amount of material has become available on animal welfare,

Box 28.4: What's the meaning? Animal welfare and ethics definitions

Students are assisted in their understanding of the complexity of animal welfare and ethics if they are provided with clear definitions of discipline-specific terms:

- *Animal welfare*: an animal's physical and psychological state with respect to the quality and quantity of its experiences in the environment
- *Animal welfare science*: the intellectual and practical activities involved in systematically developing understanding of animals' needs and interests based on their physical and psychological states in relation to their environment
- *Animal ethics*: how humans should behave toward animals
- *Animal ethics as a scientific discipline*: the intellectual and practical activities to develop systematically the four components of moral behavior – that is, moral sensitivity, moral judgment, moral motivation, and moral character – to prevent and address animal ethics issues
- *Professional ethics*: often seen as the ethics of role – that is, the personal, organizational, and corporate standards of behavior expected of professionals – usually outlined in a code of practice. In its broadest sense, professional ethics involves a commitment to the public good and a strong emphasis on community service

- *Descriptive animal ethics*: values or rules of conduct that society historically and/or currently applies to the treatment of animals
- *Normative animal ethics*: standards based on universal principles and frameworks that guide human conduct on how we should behave toward animals
- *Relativist approach to ethics*: ethics seen as relative to one's personal background and/or one's culture or society
- *Pluralist approach to ethics*: accepting the existence of different ethical views within society and the right to choose one's own ethical view as long as one tolerates others' ethical views
- *Social consensus ethic or "common morality"*: what should be done is determined by the prevailing views of the society in which you live
- *Universal principles approach to ethics*: what should be done is based on principles that are sharable, fully reciprocal, and not self-serving at the expense of others. It includes respect for all sentient beings' survival and wellbeing, justice as fairness, and integrity
- *Ethical intelligence*: the ability to solve problems and create solutions that are fair and supportive of the life and wellbeing of sentient creatures affected by the situation or action

with differing levels of usefulness to veterinary students. This is in common with many other subjects and relates principally to the availability of information on the World Wide Web, but in animal welfare it is also connected to a rapid increase in research and development activity (Phillips, 2009, p. 139). Extension activities such as the European Union's Animal Welfare Science Hub (www.animalwelfarehub.com), the Animal Welfare Standards project led by the University of Queensland (www.animalwelfarestandards.org), and the animal welfare and ethics teaching project led by the University of Sydney (onewelfare.cve.edu.au) are just three examples of recent projects that have generated significant resources, and that are freely available for veterinary students to improve their understanding of animal welfare and ethics issues.

Box 28.5: Focus on the ten ethical sensitivity elements

These elements should be identified and expressed in response to a particular situation or action, for instance the use of excessive force to make animals move.

1) Physical responses of animals and people
2) Emotional responses of animals and people
3) Own thoughts (perceptions, appraisal, interpretation) of the situation
4) Own feelings in relation to the observed responses of animals and people

5) Why this is an ethical issue
6) All stakeholders' perspectives, including animals'
7) Empathy
8) Moral conflicts within and between stakeholders
9) Conflicts between legal, organizational, and ethical responsibilities
10) Alternative actions and their possible impacts on stakeholders

Hence, the role of the teacher has changed from one of providing a limited amount of information to students to one of helping to synthesize and recommend appropriate material, as well as enthusing students in their studies. With more information being available, students have to be far more selective than previously. Student-centered learning, using workshops, debates, seminars, and projects, is rapidly replacing didactic teaching.

Animal Ethics Learning Methods

Developing Ethical Sensitivity

Animal ethics sensitivity tools have been developed that include:

- An Animal Ethics Sensitivity Test (AEST) (see box 28.5) consisting of 10 ethical sensitivity questions for analysis of a situation.
- Videos demonstrating both ethically sensitive and insensitive ways to address an ethical issue, with a checklist for video analysis.
- A written and video assessment with a scoring manual.

The AEST aims to develop awareness, understanding, and articulation of the various elements of ethical sensitivity, so that students can raise ethical issues with stakeholders in a real situation. As it was not possible to use verbal dialog between professional and patient,

as used in the Dental Ethical Sensitivity Test and the Racial Ethical Sensitivity Test, the AEST uses short video clips representative of common animal ethics concerns in Australian farming. While the ethical issues seem already evident, this may not be the case for those inured to seeing such issues.

We identified 10 key elements of ethical sensitivity from previous research (Jordan, 2007) and adapted these to include animals (Box 28.5).

The learning process for using the AEST to develop ethical sensitivity includes the following steps:

- Prior to any discussion of ethical sensitivity, students complete a written response to the ethical sensitivity questions using stimulus videos or presentation of animals in a situation that adversely affects their wellbeing, e.g., sea transport of sheep for live export.
- Students' responses to the AEST questions are analyzed and areas needing development identified.
- Students become familiar with the Four Component Model of moral behavior, with an emphasis on ethical sensitivity and its relevance to animal ethics issues, through a lecture and/or focused reading and team-based learning.

- Because veterinary students know less about emotions in animals than about their physical characteristics (Verrinder and Phillips, 2014b), and emotions are often not accepted within scientific study (Smith and Kleinman, 1989), readings and videos may be necessary on the scientific research on emotions in animals, and on recognizing the importance of emotions in relation to ethics and cognition.
- Students analyze two videos of ethically insensitive and sensitive behavior using a checklist of key elements,
- Students form groups of three, and choose one of three provided videos of animal ethics issues, e.g., a lame dairy cow, cattle being herded with an electric prod, and flystrike in sheep.
- Each student researches the situation represented in their video, and in class independently identifies the 10 ethical sensitivity elements listed in Box 28.5. These responses can be used for summative assessment.
- Each student adapts their written responses to produce a script for a role-play video of a veterinarian raising the issue with a relevant stakeholder, e.g., farmer, manager, stockperson.
- In groups of three (rotating in roles as veterinarian, relevant stakeholder, and camera operator), each student produces a brief three-minute video of the role play using their mobile phone.
- Students are assessed on the post-test written response and the video. Research on inter-rater reliability shows that achieving rater consistency on written responses is easier than on video responses, which may require some specialized training (Verrinder, Ostini, and Phillips, 2016b). Nevertheless, the experience of applying ethical sensitivity is essential, and developing expertise in role-play video assessment is a good means of doing this. These videos can also be useful instructional tools for students in other year levels or universities, provided that student permission and human ethics approval have been obtained.

Developing Moral Judgment

To develop students' knowledge and skills of moral judgment and principled reasoning, a three-hour interactive workshop (Table 28.2) has been effective (Verrinder and Phillips, 2015). We also devised a template (Table 28.3) of Preston's Ethic of Response ethical decision-making model (Preston, 2001) to make it easier for students to compare alternative actions and determine the most fitting and ethically justifiable action. We used the following scenario as a basis for students completing the Ethic of Response template.

Breeding modification in confinement agriculture

In large-scale commercial egg production housing systems, laying hens often engage in feather pecking, which leads to damage to plumage, flesh wounds, and, in the worst cases, a risk of cannibalism. A common way of reducing these effects is removing the tips of the beaks of day old chickens. Another possible approach involves breeding congenitally blind hens. Research with blind adult hens at commercial stocking densities indicated these hens were physically and socially less active, with less feather pecking, less comb damage, and higher egg output, than sighted birds, whilst maintaining similar body weight. In another study, blind chickens up to six weeks old sat and preened more, did less environmental pecking, showed reduced behavioural synchrony and group aggregation, and lower body weight, and exhibited a number of abnormal behaviours, suggesting they may be more stressed, and likely to miss positive experiences of moving easily, social interaction, and finding food. A veterinarian, Dr Vivardi, is asked to provide professional advice regarding whether a proposed development plan, to breed congenitally blind chickens to assess welfare and productivity on a commercial scale, should proceed.

Using the universal ethical frameworks as complementary rather than competitive overcomes the confusion of relativism and pluralism

Table 28.2 Moral judgment and ethical decision-making workshop (3 hours).

Activity	Purpose	Resource	Time allowance (mins)
Complete Animal Ethics Issues Questionnaire	Reflection on ethical sensitivity, motivation, action	Animal Ethics Issues questionnaire	10
Human continuum	Taking a position on an ethical issue, considering others' positions, identifying the wide range of views and comparing with own view, possibly modifying their own position, raising question of how do we decide which position(s) are ethical	Suitable room for students to stand side by side in a semicircle from strongly agree to strongly disagree on an animal ethics issue Students take a position, discuss with others with similar positions, listen to the range of positions, possibly change positions	10
Explanation of Kohlberg's theory of moral development and the value of principled reasoning	Understanding how we develop morally and how we can identify an ethical position	Powerpoint™ presentation	10
Modelling use of Preston's Ethic of Response Template	Observing how to apply a comprehensive ethical decision-making model to an animal ethics issue	Powerpoint™ presentation of the template's step-by-step completion	10
In groups of three, Hot Potato activity (quick recording and passing of worksheets to add new ideas to facts, stakeholders, actions)	Focusing on the issue and identifying a wide range of ideas	Worksheet for brainstorming facts, stakeholders, possible actions	5
Completing Preston's Ethic of Response on a new issue (same for each group)	Using the main ethical frameworks (utilitarian, deontological, and virtue ethics) and universal principles of respect for life and wellbeing, justice as fairness, and integrity to come to a fitting ethical decision	Blank template for each group Completed model template and justification paragraph for each student	20
Each group reports their decision and justification back to whole group	Justifying ethical decisions using universal ethical frameworks and principles		10
Ethical decision-making survey	Evaluating ethical decision-making strategies used in workshop	Survey sheet for each student	10
Defining Issues Test – post-test	Reflect on own moral schema – what is important when making a decision on an ethical issue?	DIT for each student	20
Individual assessment	Application and justification for ethical decisions	Assessment sheet with new scenario to record justification Blank template for each student	30

Table 28.3 Ethic of Response Template (ERT) based on Preston's Ethic of Response ethical decision-making model
Sample scenario: Breeding modification for blind hens √ = Benefits; X = Harms.

STAKEHOLDERS	Action: Keep beak trimming		Action: Breed blind hens		Action: Move to less intensive production e.g. low-density free range *and* educate consumers to pay more	
	Respect life	Respect wellbeing	Respect life	Respect wellbeing	Respect life	Respect wellbeing
1 Hens	x Large numbers have short lives	x Painful trimming x Hens still frustrated	x Large numbers have short lives	x Lose one of their major senses/capacity for quality of life √ Less feather pecking	√ Fewer having short lives	√ Increased quality of life
2 Farmers/producers		√ Maintains production levels x Increasing pressure from consumers/general public/welfare groups		√ Easier to manage hens x Possibly greater repercussions from general public and concerns re industry future		x Lower production √ Increasing demand for free range
3 Consumers		√ Continued cheap eggs x Some do not like it and moving to keep own chickens		√ Increased supply of cheap eggs x More consumer backlash due to hens' permanent loss of sight capacity		x More expensive eggs √ Greater satisfaction with product and own integrity
4 Egg industry		√ Maintain production levels x Consumer/public concerns		√ Increased production levels x Possible decreased demand due to public concerns x Expense of research/time for trials		x Lower quantity of eggs produced √ Higher-value product √ Increased community satisfaction with egg industry
5 Researchers		x Less work		√ More work in this area x Loss of integrity		x Less work with genetic manipulation √ More time for less destructive research, e.g., better systems for hens' interests

	Option 1	Option 2	Option 3
6 General public	x Generally concerned about animal welfare	x Increasing concern about manipulation of animals' capacities	√ Less concern about animal welfare issues
7 Animal welfare groups	x More work to do to prevent beak trimming x Upset due to animal welfare concerns	x Extremely concerned about manipulation of animals' capacities x increased work to prevent this	√ Less concern about hens' wellbeing
8 Retailers	√ Plentiful eggs to sell x Some consumers unhappy	√ Plentiful eggs to sell x Probably more consumers unhappy due to more serious impact on hens	x Fewer cheap eggs to sell √ Increased satisfaction regarding product quality
9 Vet	x Concerned about pain to chickens and ongoing feeding issues if done badly x Loss of professional integrity to prevent harm to animals	x Concerned about permanent loss to hens' capacities; unknown further impacts on the species x Loss of personal and professional integrity – to heal not harm animals	√ Less worry about hens' wellbeing √ Increased integrity
UTILITARIAN ETHICS Rating 1–5 (1= Greatest benefits)	5	4	2
JUSTICE AS FAIRNESS Rating 1–5 (1= Fairest for least advantaged)	5	5	3
VIRTUE ETHICS/INTEGRITY Rating 1–5 (1=most virtuous, consistent)	4	5	3

Note: Students choose the most fitting action based on the three ratings and justify their choice using ethics language and reasoning from the template.

that is often associated with ethics and helps students come to a consensus. Students then construct a written justification for their decision using ethics language from the template, for example respect for life and wellbeing, fairness, and integrity.

Taking Animal Welfare and Ethics Assessment Seriously

Animal Welfare Assessment

An animal welfare assessment is made using scientific criteria and should be both reliable and repeatable. Students should know at what point in a continuum of animal welfare, from very good to very bad, animals are positioned. They should recognize the importance of knowledge of normal and abnormal behavior; key physiological indicators, such as cortisol, animal production, reproduction, and longevity parameters; and animals' mental states. Dichotomization of an animal's welfare state as simply good or bad should be discouraged in favor of an understanding of the need for a holistic approach.

Animal Ethics Assessment

In a review of medical ethics education, Eckles *et al.* (2005) identify a lack of systematic analysis of the measurable elements of ethical skills and the best means for assessing them, and suggest that educators should consider whether the ethics skills taught should be distilled into a competency. In veterinary education there has been a similar lack of analysis of measurable elements. However, the AEST provides the potential to develop and measure ethical sensitivity (Verrinder, Ostini, and Phillips, 2016b). The VetDIT provides a learning and formative measurement tool for moral judgment (Verrinder and Phillips, 2014a; 2015). The Ethic of Response template provides a summative moral judgment tool, to assess students' ability to use ethical frameworks and principles to identify, choose, and justify a chosen action as the most fitting decision (Verrinder and Phillips, 2015).

While there could be a range of ethical actions to address any particular issue, there will be some actions that are clearly more ethical than others based on respect for sentient beings' need for survival and wellbeing, fairness, and integrity. In this sense, moral judgment and actions can be assessed scientifically. As Harris (2010, p. 4) notes: "There are facts to be understood about how thoughts and intentions arise in the brain, there are facts to be learned about how these mental states translate into behaviour, there are further facts to be known about how these behaviours influence the world and the experience of other conscious beings."

Animal ethics is by nature comparative and highly complex, based on gathering and understanding as much as we can about our own thinking and motivations to act, as well as the needs and interests of all those sentient beings affected by our actions, and choosing those actions that are going to most benefit the least advantaged currently and into the future. Just because issues such as the shape of the Earth or climate change have been difficult to prove does not mean that they are not provable: "As with all matters of fact, differences of opinion on moral questions merely reveal the incompleteness of our knowledge, they do not oblige us to respect a diversity of views indefinitely" (Harris, 2010, p. 10).

Since these tools are fairly new and need to be extensively validated, teachers interested in using them are invited to contact us to obtain the latest versions and to contribute to their development. Further teaching strategies and tools for developing moral motivation and moral action in relation to animal ethics issues are needed. The development of these attributes in other professions provides a useful guide (see Table 28.1).

Conclusion

The chapter presents the justification for animal welfare and ethics education for veterinarians and the need for separate courses as well as integration in the veterinary program.

A scientific approach to animal welfare assessments and to the development of moral behavior is recommended. Tools to develop and measure competence in components of moral behavior in relation to animals are outlined.

References

Abood, S.K., and Siegford, J.M. (2012) Student perceptions of an animal-welfare and ethics course taught early in the veterinary curriculum. *Journal of Veterinary Medical Education*, **39**, 136–141.

Batchelor, C.E.M., Creed, A., and McKeegan, D.E.F. (2015) A preliminary investigation into the moral reasoning abilities of UK veterinarians. *Veterinary Record*, **177**, 124–129.

Batchelor, C.E., and McKeegan, D.E. (2012) Survey of the frequency and perceived stressfulness of ethical dilemmas encountered in UK veterinary practice. *Veterinary Record*, **170**, 19–22.

Bebeau, M.J. (1994) Influencing the moral dimensions of dental practice, in *Moral Development in the Professions: Psychology and Applied Ethics* (eds J. Rest and D. Narvaez), Lawrence Erlbaum, Hillsdale, NJ, pp. 121–146.

Bebeau, M.J. (2002) The Defining Issues Test and the Four Component Model: Contributions to professional education. *Journal of Moral Education*, **31**, 271–295.

Bebeau, M.J., and Monson, V.E. (2008) Guided by theory, grounded in evidence: A way forward for professional ethics education, in *Handbook of Moral and Character Education* (eds L.P. Nucci and D. Narvaez), Routledge, New York, pp. 557–582.

Bebeau, M.J., Rest, J., and Yamoor, M.A. (1985) Measuring dental students' ethical sensitivity. *Journal of Dental Education*, **49**, 225–235.

Blasi, A. (1983) Moral cognition and moral action: A theoretical perspective. *Developmental Review*, **3**, 178–210.

Bones, V.C., and Yeates, J.W. (2012) The emergence of veterinary oaths: Social, historical, and ethical considerations. *Journal of Animal Ethics*, **2**, 20–42.

Bredemeier, B., and Shields, D. (1994) Applied ethics and moral reasoning in sport, in *Moral Development in the Professions: Psychology and Applied Ethics* (eds J. Rest and D. Narvaez), Lawrence Erlbaum, Hillsdale, NJ, pp. 173–188.

Capilé, K.V., Campos, G.M.B., Stedile, R., and Oliveira, S.T. (2015) Canine prostate palpation simulator as a teaching tool in veterinary education. *Journal of Veterinary Medical Education*, **42**, 146–150.

Clarkeburn, H., Downie, J.R., and Matthew, B. (2002) Impact of an ethics programme in a life sciences curriculum. *Teaching in Higher Education*, **7**, 65–79.

de Waal, F. (2009) *The Age of Empathy*, Harmony Books, New York.

Dolby, N., and Litster, A. (2015) Understanding veterinarians as educators: An exploratory study. *Teaching in Higher Education*, **20**, 272–284.

Driscoll, J.W. (1992) Attitudes toward animal use. *Anthrozoos*, **5**, 32–39.

Eckles, R.E., Meslin, E.M., Gaffney, M., and Helft, P.R. (2005) Medical ethics education: Where are we? Where should we be going? A review. *Academic Medicine*, **80**, 1143.

Ford, B.J. (1999) *Sensitive Souls: Senses and Communication in Plants, Animals and Microbes*, Little, Brown, London.

Furnham, A., and Heyes, C. (1993) Psychology students' beliefs about animals and animal experimentation. *Personality and Individual Differences*, **15**, 1–10.

Furnham, A., and Pinder, A. (1990) Young people's attitudes to experimentation on animals. *Psychologist*, **10**, 444.

Gieseke, D., Lambertz, C., Traulsen, I., *et al.* (2014) Assessment of animal welfare in dairy cattle farming: Evaluation of the Welfare Quality (R) Protocol. *Zuchtungskunde*, **86**, 58–70.

Harris, S. (2010) *The Moral Landscape: How Science Can Determine Human Values*, Bantam, London.

Hartwell, S. (2004) Moral growth or moral angst? A clinical approach. *Clinical Law Review*, **11**, 115.

Hazel, S.J., Signal, T.D., and Taylor, N. (2011) Can teaching veterinary and animal-science students about animal welfare affect their attitude toward animals and human-related empathy? *Journal of Veterinary Medical Education*, **38**, 74–83.

Illmann, G., Keeling, L., Melisova, M., *et al.* (2014) Mapping farm animal welfare education at university level in Europe. *Animal Welfare*, **23**, 401–410.

Jordan, J. (2007) Taking the First Step Toward a Moral Action: A Review of Moral Sensitivity Measurement Across Domains. *The Journal of Genetic Psychology*, **168** (3), 323–359.

Kerr, A.J., Mullan, S.M., and Main, D.C.J. (2013) A new educational resource to improve veterinary students' animal welfare learning experience. *Journal of Veterinary Medical Education*, **40**, 342–348.

Koch, V.W. (2009) American veterinarians' animal welfare limitations. *Journal of Veterinary Behavior: Clinical Applications and Research*, **4**, 198–202.

Ling, R.Z., Zulkifli, I., Lampang, P.N., *et al.* (2016) Attitudes of students from south-east and east Asian countries to slaughter and transport of livestock. *Animal Welfare*, **25**, 377–387.

Magalhães-Sant'ana, M., Baptista, C., Olsson, I., *et al.* (2009) Teaching animal ethics to veterinary students in Europe: Examining aims and methods, in *Ethical Futures: Bioscience and Food Horizons: EurSafe 2009, Nottingham, United Kingdom, 2–4 July 2009* (eds K. Millar, P. Hobson West, and B. Nerlich), Wageningen Academic Publishers, Wageningen, p. 197.

Magalhães-Sant'ana, M., Olsson, I.A.S., Sandoe, P., and Millar, K. (2010) How ethics is taught by European veterinary faculties: A review of published literature and web resources, in *Global Food Security: Ethical and Legal Challenges* (eds C.M.R. Casabona, L.E. San Epifanio, and A.E. Cirión), Wageningen Academic Publishers, Wageningen, pp. 441–446.

Mayhew, M.J., Seifert, T.A., and Pascarella, E.T. (2010) A multi-institutional assessment of moral reasoning development among first-year students. *Review of Higher Education*, **33**, 357–390.

McNeel, S. (1994) College teaching and student moral development, in *Moral Development in the Professions* (eds J. Rest and D. Narvaez), Lawrence Erlbaum, Hillsdale, NJ, pp. 27–50.

Mellor, D., and Beausoleil, N. (2015) Extending the "Five Domains" model for animal welfare assessment to incorporate positive welfare states. *Animal Welfare*, **24**, 241–253.

Morton, D.B. (2010) A commentary on the animal welfare symposium, with possible actions. *Journal of Veterinary Medical Education*, **37**, 107–113.

Nussbaum, M.C. (2001) *Upheavals of Thought: The Intelligence of Emotions*, Cambridge University Press, Cambridge.

Panksepp, J. (1998) *Affective Neuroscience: The Foundations of Human and Animal Emotions*, Oxford University Press, New York.

Paul, E.S., and Podberscek, A.L. (2000) Veterinary education and students' attitudes towards animal welfare. *Veterinary Record*, **146**, 269–272.

Penn, W.Y.J. (1990) Teaching ethics: A direct approach. *Journal of Moral Education*, **19**, 124–138.

Phillips, C.JC. (2009) *The Welfare of Animals: The Silent Majority*, Springer, New York.

Pollard-Williams, S., Doyle, R.E., and Freire, R. (2014) The influence of workplace learning on attitudes toward animal welfare in veterinary students. *Journal of Veterinary Medical Education*, **41**, 253–257.

Preston, N. (2001) *Understanding Ethics*, 2nd edn, Federation Press, Sydney.

Pritchard, J.C., van Dijk, L., Ali, M., and Pradhan, S.K. (2012) Non-economic incentives to improve animal welfare: Positive competition as a driver for change among owners of draught and pack animals in India. *Animal Welfare*, **21**, 25–32.

group cultures, for example a lecture about African Americans followed by a lecture on individuals of Jewish descent. Such approaches can never be exhaustive and at best provide learners with overconfidence in their competence, based on static knowledge that is at risk of relying on stereotypes and not universally applicable information.

So, while this chapter advocates cultural competence content in teaching and curricula, we assert that veterinary medical faculty, students, and practitioners must strive to practice cultural humility. A cultural humility framework allows learners to focus on personal development and inwardly focused skills and behaviors. It moves the focus from the specifics of different cultures to the individual student, and through this humility framework provides a much better set of skills – the ability to embrace continued personal growth and self-reflection as an intrinsic quality of the veterinarian.

Cultural Competence and Humility Learning Models

The historical traditions of medicine, specifically western medicine, create a framework for how we understand the practice of appropriate and efficacious medical care for humans and animals. The framework tends to be narrowly defined and places an emphasis on the practitioner rather than the patient or client. Often

characterized as a nontechnical part of the practice of medicine, cultural competence is frequently seen as an "alternative to the epistemology of science" (Kirmayer, 2012, p. 156), and thus as a less important, at best, or unimportant, at worst, component of practice.

In reality, cultural competence and humility represent an increasingly important set of technical skills directly linked to health outcomes. Ever more pluralistic communities will demand and rely on culturally engaging, relevant, and responsive medical care. Teaching cultural competence and humility requires a framework that identifies competencies on which faculty must focus to practice and teach. Based on work by Seeleman, Suurmond, and Stronks (2009), the essential competencies framework is offered for veterinary medicine in Box 29.3.

Numerous models devoted to explaining the development of cultural competence suggest that it is best conceptualized as a continuum. Wells (2000) describes three developmental stages spread across two learning models. Cognitive learning phase outcomes include cultural incompetence, cultural knowledge, and cultural awareness; while cultural sensitivity, cultural competence, and cultural proficiency are affective phase learning outcomes (Wells, 2000, p. 192).

Veterinary students may achieve these learning outcomes in a variety of ways. In the classroom setting, teaching methodologies may focus on the use of lectures, case-based

---

Box 29.3: How to develop a framework for competencies

- Knowledge of how various forms of social privilege and disadvantage affect the relationship between the practitioner and the client
- Awareness of how culture shapes individual behavior and thinking
- Awareness of the social context in which specific ethnic groups live
- Awareness of one's own prejudices and tendency to stereotype

- Ability to transfer information in a way the client can understand and to know when external help with communication is needed
- Ability to adapt to new situations flexibly and creatively

Source: Seeleman, Suurmond, and Stronks, 2009.

learning, and online modules, coupled with reflective writing and student peer engagement. Faculty must also model these competencies for students in the clinical learning environment. As students are learning various clinical skills, there is an informal kind of teaching that occurs when students observe faculty behavior, including interactions with clients. This behavior models how veterinarians behave, how they are expected to practice, and whether skills like cultural competence and humility are valued in the practice of medicine. Arguably, the behaviors found in the "institutional curriculum" are a reflection of the college's values as well.

Institutional or Hidden Curriculum

The institutional or "hidden curriculum," a term coined in the 1980s, refers to the "subtle, less officially recognized" (Hafferty and Franks, 1994, p. 861) lessons taught in the academic environment. These are the informal lessons on how to be a professional, and more specifically how to be a veterinarian, taught from the modeled behavior of administrators, faculty, and staff. The hidden curriculum is an important part of student learning; it supports the formal curriculum and the reinforcement of appropriate professional behaviors (Keengwe, 2010). Discordant role modeling by members of the college community can have a deep impact on students; a hidden curriculum showing students how to be a "doctor" can inadvertently increase cultural insensitivity and the reconsideration of student career paths, among other outcomes (Murray-Garcia and Garcia, 2008). Further dissonant institutional curricula may also spurn more openly hostile campus climates that have a chilling effect on student learning in general.

Institutions have a responsibility to require training on diversity for faculty and staff in and around the college of veterinary medicine (Nazar *et al.*, 2015). Academic leaders should facilitate institutional investment in diversity as a core value, and the maintenance of consistent educational and clinical environments that demonstrate the importance of this value (Nazar *et al.*, 2015). Administrative leaders should ensure that the institutional climate and its hidden curriculum do not serve to undermine the other, more formal learning experiences of veterinary students, described in what follows.

Teaching Cultural Competence and Humility

The increased cultural competence that we seek within veterinary medical education should be manifested as a lifelong quest for increased cultural humility, evidenced by how veterinary practitioners ultimately affect the communities in which they live and practice. Specifically, we seek to provide an education that will guide and support the veterinarian who wishes to move beyond the role of professional healer to the role of social change agent, within and perhaps even beyond the field of veterinary medicine. Can this be done? Is effective multicultural education in the veterinary medical curriculum even feasible, given an already full and rigorous curriculum?

We submit that not only is it possible, it is critical. Wear (2003) argues, and we agree, that medical education has been getting it wrong for years, first by limiting the curricular approach to additional content, rather than infusion into existing courses, and second by expecting one-time visits to or participation in free clinics, and/or pop-up lectures, to produce a sustained cultural humility. We should not expect increased cultural competence to emerge miraculously from intermittent participation (whether voluntary or required) in a series of disconnected events, lectures, and activities. Teaching cultural competence and humility is a process requiring multiple educational experiences across the veterinary medical curriculum. The institutional goal should be to ensure that the curriculum provides numerous opportunities for learning through required and elective coursework, clinical simulation, and online learning, as well as other educational methodologies (Lipson and Desantis, 2007).

Preclinical Courses

The goal of a preclinical medical student curriculum focused on cultural competence and cultural humility should be to help students in their "individual diversity development" (Chavez, Guido-DiBrito, and Mallory, 2003). This involves engaging in work on personal development, including, but not limited to, lessons in social privilege, bias, epidemiological data on various demographic groups, and critical race and gender theories. Preclinical coursework must emphasize students' ability to become more self-aware of personal values, to become interpersonally sensitive, and to develop a willingness to learn from their clients. Further, students should learn to "value and [choose] to validate those who are other, as well as otherness within [themselves]" (Chaves, Guido-DiBrito, and Mallory, 2003, p. 457).

These courses may utilize a variety of approaches. While standard didactic lectures can be used to teach basic diversity and cultural concepts, they are also often employed to cover general cultural themes and customs of various social groups. While such content can be enormously helpful, it should sequentially follow material that focuses on enhancing student personal identity development with respect to diversity. Again, the goal of this coursework is specific to the development of the individual student. In addition to lectures, workshop or seminar courses offer opportunities for a high amount of student engagement with the material. Small groups using faculty as facilitators can be especially useful in teaching cultural competence and humility content. Students need many opportunities to engage with their colleagues as they wrestle with this content and its relationship to the practice of veterinary medicine.

Veterinary administrators and faculty may find that this type of coursework focused on personal identity development may be better suited to the preveterinary curriculum and/or to being taught and facilitated by faculty with expertise in these scholarly areas. In the case of the former, the authors would strongly urge

college faculty then to require evidence of such coursework in the prerequisites for admission into the professional veterinary medical program. In the case of the latter, we recommend offerings that are co-facilitated by expert faculty from the appropriate disciplines, who may be found in colleges outside of the college of veterinary medicine. It is critical to note that student cognitive development is the essential precursor to curricular content that facilitates effective behavioral change in practice. Either evidence of this curricular content is required for admission, or it is integrated as required course components in the Doctor of Veterinary Medicine (DVM) program.

Online Learning

The use of online learning technologies is certainly not new, but little has been published on its applicability to teaching cultural competence or cultivating cultural humility among health professions students (Wiecha *et al.*, 2010). That said, online learning technologies can be an important component of the teaching of elements of the veterinary medical curriculum, and student responses to online learning are very favorable (Pasin and Giroux, 2011). As professional students, veterinary students are more likely to be able to maximize the potential of online learning environments and to participate more fully in self-directed learning (Hung *et al.*, 2010). It is very likely, however, that online learning modules, particularly those addressing diversity and inclusion content, will be part of a blended learning environment that involves both online and face-to-face components. Although veterinary students have the skills to support self-regulated learning, there is a need for face-to-face engagement to underscore the importance of interpersonal relationships, as well as to provide students with the opportunity to verify and validate what they have learned in the online components (Paechter and Maier, 2010).

Online learning modules that create virtual worlds, such as the game *Second Life*, have been shown to be effective at creating safe environments for students to explore content related to diversity and inclusion (Games and Bauman, 2011). Virtual worlds in games provide students with the opportunity to try on different identities and make decisions based on those identities (Games and Bauman, 2011). This safe practice improves students' ability to approach sensitive cross-cultural issues with clients (Mack, 2013). Mack (2013) writes that the use of online gaming to facilitate the achievement of cultural competence or humility can require more time than other learning methodologies; students need time to work through scenarios fully, possibly repeating them several times, and there is a continued need for face-to-face meetings and other reflective assignments to facilitate the related learning.

Experiential Learning

Moving students from the confines of the classroom to the field is an important component of developing competence and the appropriate level of humility in multicultural settings. Experiential learning, or for these purposes a clinical externship, provides students with the opportunity to apply directly knowledge gathered in both the formal and informal curricula. While most of the rotations in the final year of the professional DVM curriculum are devoted to developing and refining Day One clinical skills, which include client communication, these rotations are rarely nuanced enough deliberately to provide students with the opportunity to practice navigating cross-cultural engagements.

Numerous factors will influence students' ability to leverage cultural learning opportunities in clinics; some students will express a natural motivation to seek out these experiences, while others will do so in order to conform behaviorally to the outcomes prescribed in the curriculum (Ng, van Dyne, and Ang, 2009). Clinical experiences enable faculty to utilize learning models that assist veterinary students in moving from simply experiencing a diverse interaction with clients and colleagues to achieving learning outcomes in cultural competence and humility.

Due to client pool limitations, faculty may find challenges in cultivating intentionally diverse learning situations for veterinary students. As faculty and administrators assist students in developing their clinical experience schedules, it is critical for students to be reminded that experiences should provide the opportunity to achieve learning objectives related to diversity, cultural competence, and cultural humility. Helping students find opportunities to engage with a wider clientele outside of the college or even the country may be necessary in achieving these goals. Additionally, novel approaches like virtual gaming, *Sims* for example, provide faculty with effective opportunities for targeted, project-based learning in these areas (Jarmon *et al.*, 2009).

The hinge point in experiential learning is the need for student reflection before and after experiences. Regular journaling and reflection papers are essential to facilitate student learning; they are not merely assessment tools, although their use as such will be discussed shortly. Reflective assignments assist students in developing a greater sense of self and understanding of the experimental situation; such assignments are also necessary for developing the competencies that lead to positive client relationships (Sandars, 2009). They are time consuming for both faculty and student; however, they are an important teaching tool in programs seeking to develop culturally competent and culturally humble health professionals.

As with any curriculum element, it is important that the professional curriculum in its entirety be evaluated for learning outcomes that help students improve their cultural sensitivity and humility toward a heterogeneous client base. Students must also be aware that the goal is not to master all or even individual cultures or subcultures, but to understand that culture plays an integral role in the client's life and influences their decision-making on what to do for the patient. The professional curriculum should provide opportunities to build the knowledge necessary to avoid bias, prejudice, and stereotypes, and this will aid in the reduction of health disparities (Tervalon and Murray-Garcia, 1998).

Assessment

Educational interventions centered on the practice and delivery of veterinary healthcare in various cultural settings are expected to benefit students in terms of increased cultural knowledge, appreciation, and competence. In order to assess the effectiveness of such interventions, intercultural competence is typically measured before and after multicultural training or an experience such as a study abroad program. Measuring cultural competence, specifically for those involved in medical fields, is not a simple or uniform task. In 2007, Kumas-Tan *et al.* revealed several problematic hidden assumptions in the top 10 widely used cultural assessment tools in approximately 20 years' worth of literature on this topic. These assumptions are listed in Box 29.4.

These instruments are far from ideal, because assessment of cultural competence based on the assumptions in Box 29.4 results in the development of professionals who are not sufficiently competent, but dangerously overconfident in their skills (Kumas-Tan *et al.*, 2007). As noted earlier in this chapter, multiple analyses have reached the following conclusions:

- The pursuit of cultural competence is represented by a lifelong pursuit of *cultural humility*, rather than by the acquisition and mastery of a finite body of cultural knowledge (Tervalon and Murray-Garcia, 1998).

- Traditional cultural competence pedagogy in medical education was incorrectly focused on individual biases and attitudes, and should be refocused on *insurgent multiculturalism* – an understanding of how institutionalized structures, organizations, and policies in western societies continually support and maintain imbalances of power and privilege (Giroux 2000).

- When insurgent multiculturalism is tied to professional development focusing on duty, respect, and altruism, the doctor–client relationship is improved through a reduction in the relational power imbalance (Wear, 2003).

Because the process of teaching cultural competence and cultural humility requires a high level of introspection and reflection of faculty and students, surely the next difficult decision to be made is the appropriate assessment tool that one should employ. Given the plethora of cultural competence assessment tools currently in use, how are and *should* we be measuring success? Many of these tools have been developed using the same basic experimental design as that outlined in detail by Matsumoto and Hwang (2013).

In a 2014 study, Leung, Ang, and Tan reported that there are over 30 cultural competence models with more than 300 related personal characteristics. It is important to note that not all of these tests have been subjected to reliability and validity studies. The personal

---

Box 29.4: Quick tips about cultural competence

- Culture is solely a matter of race and ethnicity.
- Culture is possessed by the Other; the Other is or has the problem. Dominant groups are assumed to have no culture.
- Cultural incompetence is due to the practitioner's lack of familiarity with the Other.
- Cultural incompetence is due to the practitioner's discriminatory attitudes toward the Other.

- Cross-cultural healthcare is solely about Caucasian practitioners working with patients from racial and ethnic minority groups.
- Cultural competence is about self-confidence and about the level of comfort with others.

Source: Kumas-Tan *et al.*, 2007.

characteristics represented throughout the various models can be generally grouped into three categories or domains: cultural traits, cultural attitudes and worldview, and cultural capabilities. Cultural competence models can be specific to these three domains or can be mixed, including aspects (or constructs) from multiple domains (Javidan and Teagarden, 2011).

The Intercultural Development Inventory or IDI is a culture-general assessment tool based on the Developmental Model of Intercultural Sensitivity (DMIS), which conceptually relies solely on an intercultural worldview domain. The DMIS was originally described by Milton Bennett (1986, 1993) and later revised by Milton Hammer (2011, 2012). Intercultural development using this model is described in terms of orientations and mindsets.

At one end of the DMIS continuum are monocultural mindsets (Denial and Polarization orientations), then a transitional orientation called Minimization, and finally at the other end of the continuum the intercultural mindsets of Acceptance and Adaptation. In Denial and Polarization, individuals believe that "one's own culture is central to all reality" (Bennett, 1993, p. 30), whereas individuals in Acceptance and Adaptation are capable of shifting perspective and changing behavior based on cultural context, and in response to changing cultural conditions.

The IDI measures cultural competence by determining where individuals or groups fall along the continuum as defined by the DMIS. This assessment tool is presently in its third iteration (v3), and is widely used throughout academia and industry to measure cultural competence. It also assesses Cultural Disengagement, defined as an individual or group level of disconnection from a primary cultural community. The IDI has been shown to be a method that is both valid and reliable regarding the measurement of orientation toward cultural difference, as described in the DMIS model (Hammer, Bennett, and Wiseman, 2003).

The IDI is currently used to assess increased cultural competence (as defined by positive movement along the DMIS continuum) by comparing pre- and post-test values for a number of activities, including student participation in curricular and/or co-curricular activities (Altshuler, Sussman, and Kachur, 2003), study abroad (Engle and Engle, 2004), and professional advancement opportunities (Box 29.5).

In adult education, the theory of transformative learning explains that we interpret our individual experiences based on "meaning perspectives," which are expectations framed within cultural assumptions and presuppositions (Mezirow, 1991). A 1994 study showed that acquiring cultural competence is based on a transformative learning process, manifested in the individual learner as an evolving cultural identity, a change in values, an increase in self-confidence, and a change in perspective (Taylor, 1994). More recent research suggests

---

Box 29.5: How to use the Intercultural Development Inventory (IDI) for assessment

The IDI is best used to measure mindset change, so it is most effectively utilized as a pre-and post-event assessment tool. It can be used in numerous ways across a veterinary college, for example:

- Course assessment
- Evaluation of curricular design related to diversity, cultural competence, and cultural humility. For example, at the Center of Excellence for

Diversity and Inclusion in Veterinary Medicine, pre- and post-IDI results are being used to evaluate the effectiveness of the curricular design for the certificate program being administered to faculty, students, and practitioners

- Assessment of cultural competence related to international programming
- Assessment of student-led diversity programming within the college

Box 29.6: How to create reflective writing prompts

Reflective assignments should be framed with prompts that encourage students to answer "what, so what, and now what." The prompts ask students to reflect on the specific exercise, ponder its relevance to the participant and the surrounding community, and finally consider how the experience might shape future behaviors.

Source: Northwest Service Academy, n.d.

that experiential learning activities such as reflective writing (journaling) and facilitated discussion are crucial for participants to reap the full benefits of participation in cultural activities, courses, and presentations (Jordi, 2011; Williams, 2009; Engle and Engle, 2004). Several studies indicate that reflective writing and/or facilitated discussion are key to improving cultural competence in medical students (Kripalani *et al.*, 2006; DasGupta and Charon, 2004; Yamada *et al.*, 2003), pharmacy students (Westberg, Bumgardner, and Lind, 2005), public health students (Kratzke and Bertolo, 2013), and dental students (Isaac *et al.*, 2015). Therefore, we submit that any program designed to increase cultural competence within a veterinary medical program should include reflective writing and facilitated discussion to realize maximum impact for individual students.

A common thread throughout the various teaching methodologies is the critical need for student reflection. The exercise of reflecting on lectures, online modules, and experiential learning can take various forms, including but not limited to writing, speaking, reading, and listening (Northwest Service Academy, (n.d.). The goal of assigning reflection activities is to foster personal identity development and a sense of awareness, which ultimately results in a desire and obligation to assess socially relevant issues in the practice of veterinary medicine (Kumagai and Lypson, 2009; Box 29.6).

Conclusion

Veterinary medical education is uniquely positioned to lead the way in providing cultural competence and humility training to its students, due in large part to the ability to learn from the years of experience and data produced by adjustments to human healthcare education. Allowing ourselves to learn from the efforts expended in the institutions of our human health counterparts can, if we let it, provide a springboard for the development of effective and resonant education for our veterinary medical students. Without the uniform history of curricula addressing these competencies, the major need is to create new programming, not to change what exists. With this comes a profound responsibility to understand the history of the approaches that have been employed in other professions.

References

Altshuler, L., Sussman, N.M., and Kachur, E. (2003) Assessing changes in intercultural sensitivity among physician trainees using the intercultural development inventory. *International Journal of Intercultural Relations*, 27 (4), 387–401.

Bennett, M.J. (1986) A developmental approach to training for intercultural sensitivity. *International Journal of Intercultural Relations*, 10 (2), 179–196.

Bennett, M. (1993) Towards ethnorelativism: A developmental model of intercultural sensitivity, in *Education for the Intercultural Experience* (ed. R.M. Paige), Intercultural Press, Yarmouth, ME, pp. 109–135.

Blanchet Garneau, A., and Pepin, J. (2015) A constructivist theoretical proposition of cultural competence development in nursing. *Nursing Education Today*, **35** (**11**), 1062–1068.

Brach, C., and Fraser, I. (2000) Can cultural competency reduce racial and ethnic disparities? A review and conceptual model. *Medical Care Research and Review*, **1**, 181–217.

Campinha-Bacote, J. (2001) Delivering patient-centered care in the midst of a cultural conflict: The role of cultural competence. *Online Journal of Issues in Nursing*, **16** (**2**), 5. doi:10.3912/OJIN.Vol16No02Man05

Chavez, A.F., Guido-DiBrito, F., and Mallory, S.L. (2003) Learning to value the "other": A framework of individual diversity development. *Journal of College Student Development*, **44** (**4**), 453–469.

Cross, T., Dennis, K., and Isaacs, M. (1989) *Towards a Culturally Competent System of Care, Vol.* **1**. Georgetown University Child Development Center, CASSP Technical Assistance Center, Washington, DC.

DasGupta, S., and Charon, R. (2004) Personal illness narratives: Using reflective writing to teach empathy. *Academic Medicine*, **79** (**4**), 351–356.

Engle, L., and Engle, J. (2004) Assessing language acquisition and intercultural sensitivity development in relation to study abroad program design. *Frontiers*, **10**, 219–236.

Games, A.I., and Bauman, E.B. (2011) Virtual worlds: An environment for cultural sensitivity education in the health sciences. *International Journal of Web Based Communities*, **7** (**2**), 189–205.

Giroux, H.A. (2000) *Stealing Innocence: Youth, Corporate Power, and the Politics of Culture*. St. Martin's Press, New York.

Hafferty, F.W., and Franks, R. (1994) The hidden curriculum, ethics teaching, and the structure of medical education. *Academic Medicine*, **69** (**11**), 861–871.

Hammer, M.R. (2011) Additional cross-cultural validity testing of the Intercultural Development Inventory. *International Journal of Intercultural Relations*, **35** (**4**), 474–487.

Hammer, M. (2012) The Intercultural Development Inventory: A new frontier in assessment and development of intercultural competence, in *Student Learning Abroad* (eds M. Vande Berg, R.M. Paige, and K.H. Lou), Stylus, Sterling, VA, pp. 115–136.

Hammer, M.R., Bennett, M.J., and Wiseman, R. (2003) Measuring intercultural sensitivity: The Intercultural Development Inventory. *International Journal of Intercultural Relations*, **27** (**4**), 421–443.

Hung, M.L., Chou, C., Chen, C.H., and Own, Z.Y. (2010) Learner readiness for online learning: Scale development and student perceptions. *Computers and Education*, **55** (**3**), 1080–1090.

Isaac, C., Behar-Horenstein, L., Lee, B., and Catalanotto, F. (2015) Impact of reflective writing assignments on dental students' views of cultural competence and diversity. *Journal of Dental Education*, **79** (**3**), 312–321.

Isaacs, M., and Benjamin, M. (1991) *Towards a Culturally Competent System of Care, Vol. II: Programs Which Utilize Culturally Competent Principles*, Georgetown University Child Development Center, CASSP Technical Assistance Center, Washington, DC.

Jarmon, L., Traphagan, T., Mayrath, M., and Trivedi, A. (2009) Virtual world teaching, experiential learning, and assessment: An interdisciplinary communication course in Second Life. *Computers and Education*, **53** (**1**), 169.

Javidan, M., and Teagarden, M.B. (2011) Conceptualizing and measuring global mindset. *Advances in Global Leadership*, **6**, 13–39.

Jordi, R. (2011) Reframing the concept of reflection: Consciousness, experiential learning, and reflective learning practices. *Adult Education Quarterly*, **61** (**2**), 181–197.

Keengwe, J. (2010) Fostering cross cultural competence in preservice teachers through multicultural education experiences. *Early Childhood Education Journal*, **38** (**3**), 197–204.

Kirmayer, L. (2012) Rethinking cultural competence. *Transcultural Psychiatry*, **49** (**2**), 149–164.

Kratzke, C., and Bertolo, M. (2013) Enhancing students' cultural competence using cross-cultural experiential learning. *Journal of Cultural Diversity*, **20** (**3**), 107–111.

Kripalani, S., Bussey-Jones, J., Katz, M.G., and Geano, I. (2006) A prescription for cultural competence in medical education. *Journal of General Internal Medicine*, **21** (**10**), 1116–1120.

Kumagai, A.K., and Lypson, M.L. (2009) Beyond cultural competence: Critical consciousness, social justice, and multicultural education. *Academic Medicine*, **84** (**6**), 782–787.

Kumas-Tan, Z., Beagan, B., Loppie, C., *et al.* (2007) Measures of cultural competence: Examining hidden assumptions. *Academic Medicine*, **82** (**6**), 548–557.

LCME (2015) *Functions and Structure of a Medical School*. Liaison Committee on Medical Education. https://med.virginia.edu/instructional-support /wp-content/uploads/sites/216/2015/12/2015 _16_functions_and_structure_march_2014.pdf (accessed November 30, 2016).

Leung, K., Ang, S., and Tan, M.L. (2014) Intercultural competence. *Annual Review of Organizational Psychology and Organizational Behavior*, **1** (**1**), 489–519.

Lipson, J.G., and DeSantis, L.A. (2007) Current approaches to integrating elements of cultural competence in nursing education. *Journal of Transcultural Nursing*, **18** (1 Supplement), 21S–27S.

Mack, A. (2013) *Using the virtual world of Second Life to teach cultural competence for health science professional students*. MS thesis. University of Louisville.

Matsumoto, D., and Hwang, H.C. (2013) Assessing cross-cultural competence: A review of available tests. *Journal of Cross-Cultural Psychology*, **44** (**6**), 849–873.

Mezirow, J. (1991) *Transformative Dimensions of Adult Learning*, Jossey-Bass, San Francisco, CA.

Murray-Garcia, J.L., and Garcia, J. (2008) The institutional context of multicultural education: What is your institutional curriculum? *Academic Medicine*, **83** (**7**), 646–652.

Nazar, M., Kendall, K., Day, L., and Nazar, H. (2015) Decolonising medical curricula through diversity education: Lessons from students. *Medical Teacher*, **37** (**4**), 385–393.

Ng, K., van Dyne, L., and Ang, S. (2009) From experience to experiential learning: Cultural intelligence as a learning capability for global leader development. *Academy of Management Learning and Education*, **8** (**4**), 511–526.

Northwest Service Academy (n.d.) *Service Reflection Toolkit*. http://www.dartmouth.edu/~tucker/docs/ service/reflection_tools.pdf (accessed July 21, 2015).

Paechter, M., and Maier, B. (2010) Online or face-to-face? Students' experiences and preferences in e-learning. *The Internet and Higher Education*, **13** (**4**), 209–297.

Pasin, F., and Giroux, H. (2011) The impact of a simulation game on operations management education. *Computers and Education*, **57** (**1**), 1240–1254.

Saha, S., Beach, M.C., and Cooper, L. (2008) Patient centeredness, cultural competence and healthcare quality. *Journal of the National Medical Association*, **100** (**11**), 1275.

Sandars, J. (2009) The use of reflection in medical education: AMEE guide no. 44. *Medical Teacher*, **31** (**8**), 685–695.

Seeleman, C., Suurmond, J., and Stronks, K. (2009) Cultural competence: A conceptual framework for teaching and learning. *Medical Education*, **43** (**3**), 229–237.

Sue, D.W. (2010) Microaggressions: More than just race. *Psychology Today*, November 17. https://www.psychologytoday.com/blog/ microaggressions-in-everyday-life/201011/ microaggressions-more-just-race (accessed July 7, 2015).

Sue, D.W., Capodilupo, C.M., Torino, G.C., *et al.* (2007) Racial microaggressions in everyday life: Implications for clinical practice. *American Psychologist*, **62** (**4**), 271–286.

Taylor, E.W. (1994) Intercultural competency: A transformative learning process. *Adult Education Quarterly*, **44** (**3**), 154–174.

Tervalon, M., and Murray-Garcia, J. (1998) Cultural humility versus cultural competence: A critical distinction in defining physician training outcomes in multicultural education.

Journal of Health Care for the Poor and Underserved, **9** (**2**), 117–125.

Thompson, D. (2013) The 33 whitest jobs in America. *The Atlantic*, November 5. http://www.theatlantic.com/business/archive/2013/11/the-33-whitest-jobs-in-america/281180/ (accessed July 23, 2015).

Waters, A., and Asbill, L. (2013) Reflections on cultural humility. *CYF News*, August. http://www.apa.org/pi/families/resources/newsletter/2013/08/cultural-humility.aspx (accessed July 7, 2015).

Watt, S.K. (2007) Difficult dialogues, privilege and social justice: Uses of the privileged identity exploration (PIE) model in student affairs practice. *College Student Affairs Journal*, **26** (**2**), 114–126.

Wear, D. (2003) Insurgent multiculturalism: Rethinking how and why we teach culture in medical education. *Academic Medicine*, **78** (**6**), 549–554.

Wells, M.I. (2000) Beyond cultural competence: A model for individual and institutional cultural development. *Journal of Community Health Nursing*, **17** (**4**), 189–199.

Westberg, S.M., Bumgardner, M.A., and Lind, P.R. (2005) Enhancing cultural competency in a college of pharmacy curriculum. *American Journal of Pharmaceutical Education*, **69**, AA1.

Wiecha, J., Heyden, R., Sternthal, E., and Merialdi, M. (2010) Learning in a virtual world: Experience with using Second Life for medical education. *Journal of Medical Internet Research*, **12** (**1**), e1.

Williams, T.R. (2009) The reflective model of intercultural competency: A multidimensional, qualitative approach to study abroad assessment. *Frontiers*, **18**, 289–306.

Williamson, M., and Harrison, L. (2010) Providing culturally appropriate care: A literature review. *International Journal of Nursing Studies*, **47** (**6**), 761–769.

Yamada, S., Maskarinec, G.G., Greene, G.A., and Bauman, K.A. (2003) Family narratives, culture, and patient-centered medicine. *Family Medicine*, **35** (**1**), 69–79.

30

Business and Practice Management Skills

Gary J. (Joey) Burt

College of Veterinary Medicine, Mississippi State University, USA

 Box 30.1: Key messages

- Recognize the need for teaching business skills in veterinary medicine.
- Identify the business skills that should be taught in the veterinary curriculum and demonstrate how to teach them.

- Determine who should teach business skills to veterinary students.
- Discern when the business skills should be taught within the veterinary curriculum.
- Define and delineate assessment methods for the teaching/learning of business skills.

Introduction

Business skills are defined as those skills necessary to market and manage the business around which one's technical skills are used. In veterinary medicine, this division occurs between the teaching and developing of medical reasoning and surgical skills versus the instruction of techniques devoted to the art of using these skills to their greatest potential. Traditionally, countless hours of veterinary curricula are devoted to formally teaching the medical skills, while little emphasis is placed on educating these future doctors in the art of practicing their chosen profession. Since the latter part of the twentieth century this has begun to change, however.

The teaching of business skills, knowledge, aptitudes, and attitudes (SKAs) in veterinary education has been deemed a core competency by organizations in North America and world-

wide (AVMA, 2014; Australia Learning and Teaching Council, 2009; NAVMEC, 2011; OIE, 2013). Practitioners are also demanding that the new graduates they hire possess business acumen. In one study of practicing veterinarians in California (Walsh, Osburn, and Schumacher, 2002), when asked what further expectations of new graduates they had, the overwhelming response was "improved knowledge of veterinary business practice." Similarly, in a survey of employers of graduates of the Iowa State University College of Veterinary Medicine (Danielson *et al.*, 2012), it was found that nontechnical veterinary skills such as business skills were important for predicting employer satisfaction. Although these vital skills are deemed a core competency, many times the challenge for an educator comes with where and when within the curricula to teach them. The ever-expanding veterinary medical knowledge

Veterinary Medical Education: A Practical Guide, First Edition. Edited by Jennifer L. Hodgson and Jacquelyn M. Pelzer.
© 2017 John Wiley & Sons, Inc. Published 2017 by John Wiley & Sons, Inc.

base makes available class time increasingly more limited. Likewise, inserting topics dealing with business early into a student's academic career may prove futile while they scramble to learn anatomy, physiology, or other seemingly overwhelming topics that they may view as more important. Yet others may argue that insertion of earlier instruction may mitigate some of the accumulation of student debt (Harris, 2012). Another variable is how veterinary curricula are structured (i.e., number of clinical years, distributive model, etc.). Thus, no single method of instruction seems to be a "one size fits all."

What Business Skills Should Be Taught, Who Should Teach Them, and Why?

Agreement about subject matter when teaching business SKAs is only slightly more straightforward. All veterinary educators would agree that underlying all of the business skills should be a strong foundation in communication skills, for without an ability to communicate effectively, much of the business knowledge and many of the applications of business skills would be difficult if not impossible. Volumes have been written on the teaching of communication skills, and a summary of that information can be found elsewhere within this textbook. Another area of agreement is that a student's understanding of these business skills is best accomplished by instilling their use in the student's personal finances and money management. With the average veterinarian completing four and a half years of undergraduate education prior to attending veterinary school, and many students pursuing additional training with internships (one year) and residencies (two to four years) (AVMA, 2015a), the burden of student educational debt is high. Providing this knowledge as early as possible would seem to allow an individual the most opportunity to make educated decisions, apply concepts, and potentially reduce their overall debt load. In fact, the Association of American Veterinary Medical

Colleges' Student Debt Initiative Report (Harris, 2012) states that by helping "students develop personal financial paths to graduation (i.e. improving their financial literacy) the students made better financial decisions while in school, had less anxiety and were better able to focus on their academic goals." Students should be counseled at the time of application to veterinary school on the real costs of the education and ways in which they can make smart choices in their decision-making processes.

The variances in curricular structure and the appropriate timing of relevant delivery dictate that business skill teaching is distributed throughout the learning process. Examples of methods used for teaching business skills and when they are taught are discussed in more detail in this chapter. As with clinical medicine, teaching of business skills should be performed by those who have education and experience. Students express appreciation of faculty members with private clinical experience who not only provide factual information, but also bring first-hand, "real-world" knowledge to the discussion. With veterinary business skills covering a wide range of topics, specific experts within each of the diverse areas may be utilized. For example, while a general practitioner may have lots of experience with face-to-face client interactions, someone formally trained in communications may provide a different and more effective perspective.

Personal Finance and Budgeting

Early within the educational process, students should receive instruction on preparing a personal budget. While this may be the most basic of the business skills, personal observation of informal first-year Doctor of Veterinary Medicine (DVM) student surveys reveals a surprising number of students admitting to not keeping a written budget for their personal finances and, by extension, not making informed, well-thought-out decisions with regard to their personal finances and spending. Many students enter veterinary school with four or more years of accumulated educational debt. Learning the basics of budgeting can provide these students with the knowledge necessary to manage their finances effectively, and subsequently mitigate the damages of excessive student loan debt. Ideally, this instruction should occur in the first semester of their veterinary education or earlier.

Numerous online templates on budgeting specifically designed for veterinary college students are available and easily utilized (AVMA, 2015b; University of Minnesota College of Veterinary Medicine, 2015; AAHA, 2015). Utilization of the template in a year-one, first-semester course to encourage early student use begins with projection of the template in class. This projected image of a monthly budget is then completed by the instructor, with student input to ensure participant understanding, thoroughness, and appropriate categorizing. This instruction should concentrate on the benefits of budgeting, such as controlling money by being intentional with spending; deliberately saving and managing income; setting monetary goals and planning for the expected and the unexpected; and determining what adjustments can be made with spending or saving habits to have the most positive effect on your debt (see Box 30.2). At this time the concept of marginal decision-making should be explained. Marginal decision-making is the incremental process of deciding cost versus benefit instead of an all-or-nothing decision. An example of this decision-making would be choosing to prepare lunch at home versus purchasing a prepared meal at a restaurant. Discussing the differences between needs and wants is also warranted at this time. By definition, a need is something necessary for a person's survival, whereas a want is something that is desirable but not necessary. Assessment of student understanding is accomplished by requiring students to complete a similar monthly budget exercise for their personal finances on their own and submit it for review. This review deals primarily with assuring that they understand the various expenses and income, along with ensuring that

the student's expectations are realistic. Feedback is provided where applicable. The goal of these exercises is for students to realize that budgeting reflects long-term money management and replaces their day-to-day financial decision-making. Even the overall organizational skills learned from budgeting can, and should, be applied to other life skills.

One of the first financial concepts that students must master is an understanding of the time value of money. While the processes and calculations of this concept do not necessarily require mastering, understanding the concept is a must (Drake and Fabozzi, 2009). In its simplest form, the time value of money states that money today (present value) is worth more and has more purchasing power than the same amount in the future (future value). With most veterinary students beginning a career path, time is on their side when it comes to financial decisions. Their comprehension of the time value of money should extend to its application to such behaviors as saving for retirement, as well as appreciation of its application to compounding of interest and debt management. This is a foundation on which they can build their future personal financial affluence and their business success.

Legal and Ethical Decision-Making

Again, beginning early in the educational process students must be exposed to moral philosophy. Ethics can be defined as an inner feeling of what is wrong versus what is right (Chadwick and Schroeder, 2002). So, can ethics be taught? Almost 2500 years ago, Socrates declared that ethics consists of knowing what one ought to do and, as such, this knowledge could be taught. While ethics is an individual's definition of wrong versus right, the profession's code of conduct can be taught and discussed. This standard should be assessed prior to veterinary school during the application process, and questionable candidates denied entry to the profession. Once in veterinary school, ethics

Box 30.2: How to set up a budget template

Budget template

Monthly income

Item	Amount
Salary	
Spouse's salary (if applicable)	
Dividends	
Interest	
Investments	
Reimbursements	
Other	
Total	

Monthly expenses

Item	Amount
Bills	
Groceries	
Mortgage	
Credit cards	

Item	Amount
Gas	
IRA (retirement plan)	
Laundry	
Car loan	
Utilities	
Clothing	
Daycare (if applicable)	
Medical/dental	
Household repairs	
Savings	
Property taxes	
Other	
Total	

Income vs. expenses

Item	Amount
Monthly income	
Monthly expenses	
Difference	

must not only be discussed but also modeled (Self, Baldwin, and Wolinsky, 2009). This may begin with a student code of conduct and introduction to the Principles of Veterinary Medical Ethics of the American Veterinary Medical Association (AVMA, 2015). Likewise, defining the veterinarian–client–patient relationship is important for these analyses. Additionally, instruction in basic veterinary and business law should occur. Real-life scenario case discussions (see Box 30.3) have proven a valuable and informative manner in which the differences between legal and ethical violations can be discussed (Wilson, Rollin, and Garbe, 2008).

One of the biggest fears facing new graduates is making a medical error. Fundamentally understanding the difference between committing a medical error versus negligently practicing veterinary medicine helps bolster confidence. Examples of issues that new graduates may face that would place them in a moral or ethical dilemma include cosmetic surgery (e.g., declaws, tail dock, ear crops), convenience euthanasia, and correction of congenital deformities in intact animals, to name just a few. Some of the legal and ethical issues that may be encountered include employment contract "noncompete clause" reasonableness, hospitalization of patients overnight without staff on premises, workplace safety (e.g., radiation exposure monitoring, anesthetic gas scavenging, use of chemical restraint), and individualized sterile surgical pack use. Further, it should be noted that instilling a sense of values is not counterintuitive to the teaching of business where material gain is sought.

Box 30.3: Example of a Case Study with Legal and Ethical Considerations

The neighbor's dog

Instruction of legal and ethical decision-making can be accomplished with real-life scenario presentations and discussion.

Scenario

One of your best clients presents a 4-year-old neutered male Labrador Retriever dog who has been hit by a car. They indicate that this dog belongs to their neighbor, whom they have tried to contact to no avail. Your quick assessment determines that the dog has a broken rear leg (femur) and exhibits moderate signs of shock.

Instructor questions
- *What are your ethical responsibilities?*

The Principles of Veterinary Medical Ethics of the American Veterinary Medical Association Supporting Annotations and the Veterinarian's Oath instruct a practitioner "to first consider the needs of the patient: to prevent and relieve disease, suffering, or disability while minimizing pain or fear." Therefore, minimally the veterinarian should administer emergency treatment to correct the signs of shock, provide stabilization of the fracture, and appropriately control the patient's pain.

- *What legal responsibilities does the veterinarian have?*

Unless a veterinarian–client–patient relationship exists, these duties may not apply to patient medical care or treatment beyond the ethical responsibilities. The veterinarian should continue to attempt to contact the owner or patient's regular attending veterinarian.

Scenario continued

After numerous attempts to contact the owner by telephone, you discover that they are out of the country on vacation and have placed the care of the dog with a neighborhood kid. The teenager is contacted and she indicates that the dog's regular veterinarian is Dr. Smith, a colleague who practices across town.

Instructor questions continued
- *Have the ethical implications changed in light of this new information?*

Generally, the ethical implications have stayed the same. One expected change would be that the patient's regular veterinarian should be contacted and the care transferred to them if mutually agreed.

- *Legally, who is financially responsible for the incurred charges?*

Depending on the laws where the presentation and subsequent treatment occurred, the neighbors who presented the dog may be liable. Ultimately, most legal minds would agree that the rightful owners are responsible for charges incurred. However, ethically we are reminded to discuss and inform all treatment with an owner, including proposed therapies, expected outcomes, and their associated costs, prior to rendering this medicine. It is with these two conflicting guidelines that most veterinarians would seek payment from the owner but, if rebuffed, they would not legally seek remuneration.

These types of scenarios and follow-up discussion can be successfully used to provoke thoughts and questions from students.

Communication and Interpersonal Interactions, Team Building, and Leadership Development

The next phase of business instruction naturally fits within the clinical education portion of the curriculum. As previously stated, communication skills are necessary for business success. During clinical instruction that involves student interaction with doctors, technicians, staff, fellow students, and clients, the students hone their skills at various levels and across the three types of communication – written, verbal, and nonverbal. It is just this type of varied communication that is needed to emphasize the important concepts when conveying their knowledge to the caregiver. Studies have shown that client relationships built out of effective communication between veterinarians and clients lead to comprehension of a pet's healthcare needs, better compliance, improved patient outcomes, and increased clinical revenue (Shaw, Adams, and Bonnett, 2004). The inverse – that is, poor communication with clients – leads to deficient care for the involved patient and dissatisfied clients. In this age of social media, the ramifications of having these disgruntled customers are magnified enormously, as will be discussed shortly (Tassava, 2014).

Not to be overlooked, the skill of *active listening* to clients has been shown to be one of the most sought-after communication skills and one of the most effective key skills for a practice's success (Opperman and Grosdidier, 2014). Recording students in real-life client interactions during their primary care rotation is an excellent means of assessing verbal and nonverbal communication. The recordings are reviewed by clinical faculty, with direction and feedback provided to students allowing refinement of these skills. Student self-assessment of these video recordings is shown to be more critical and, subsequently, very influential in changing their communication methods. Another method that can be used for assessing written communication skills is with the assignment of a client education handout. This is a written description of a disease process or husbandry practice provided in a format that is easy for the client to read and understand. It should be assessed for thoroughness, clarity, and practical usefulness for an owner. Other encompassing forms of assessment can be derived from the discharge instructions and communication logs within the medical record. Assessment can be surmised from recommendations followed and feedback on owner comprehension during follow-up visits.

One of the biggest challenges currently facing business owners is how to manage communication in the electronic age. Social media, e-mail, and web pages have allowed us to communicate vast amounts of information to an infinite number of people. The challenge lies with differentiating factual information from opinions or perceptions. Historically, the largest and most effective single marketing tool for veterinary practices has been client word-of-mouth recommendation (Molhoek and Endenburg, 2009; DVM360.com staff, 2014). Social media has allowed the number of potential clients that can be reached to explode. Likewise, dissatisfied clients can now release their feelings on a blog that has the potential to influence a multitude without the opportunity for rebuttal. Veterinarians will continue to find managing these communication portals a challenge.

While we have stressed the importance of communication with clients, perhaps equally important is learning the team-building and leadership skills necessary to work productively within healthcare teams and accomplish their collective goals. This frequently entails new graduates leading the case management effort, a task that many are unfamiliar with undertaking. An additional skill that has been identified as a fundamental key to the success of a practice and to the professional wellbeing of a business owner is delegation (Opperman and Grosdidier, 2014). Many veterinarians find it difficult to relinquish some of the "power" associated with business ownership, but, once they do, they find the benefits to be financially and personally rewarding. Delegation of any duty that is not directly associated with the practice of veterinary medicine can allow the veterinarian to focus their time and effort on that for which they were extensively trained and for which revenue is generated. The two primary areas that lend themselves to delegation are practice management and technical staff utilization. It has been shown that practices employing veterinary managers earn as much as 13% more than those without managers (Richardson and Osborne, 2006), and effective use of technical support staff also increases practice revenue (National Research

Council of the National Academies, 2015). Not only do earnings increase, job satisfaction for veterinarian owners also improves, leading to less professional "burnout." The effective utilization of veterinary technicians in practice revenue generation continues to be lacking (Liss, 2012; Veterinary Business Advisors, 2013).

Faculty modeling of team building and leadership development within the clinical setting may be one method to encourage support staff use and allow collaborative learning. Faculty members who leverage their staff (delegate) while dealing with clinical cases are viewed as more efficient, have more time to spend interacting with students, and are appreciated by the associated staff team members. Placing students in the role of "doctor" during their clinical education facilitates learning the skills necessary to be a team leader and promotes delegation of duties for efficient case workups (Bridges *et al.*, 2011). When professional students are instructed to utilize technical staff, they quickly learn the associated value of efficient time usage.

Another method used to teach the arts of delegation and team building involves scenario-based discussions. As an example, take a simple clinical procedure like a fecal flotation. Point out that while the leader (veterinarian) *could* perform all the steps needed to complete the task, it can be achieved in a much more time-efficient manner when multiple team members are involved. For instance, the owner can retrieve the sample at home and bring it with the pet. Discuss how much this frees the technician to do other productive procedures. A technician should set up the test sample and read the results. Discuss how this frees the veterinarian to do things such as case assessment, diagnostic test interpretation, and therapeutic treatment plan assignment. Isn't each member doing what he or she is trained and capable of? Are the results or outcome different? Do you think job satisfaction is greater than if the most qualified person performed all the tasks? Simple discussions such as this can be an eye-opening experience for students.

Goal Setting/Strategy

As students approach the end of their veterinary education, skills such as résumé construction, cover letter writing, interviewing techniques, and contract negotiation become imminently important. A combination of lecture, student project assignment exercises, role playing, and group discussions assists students with enhancing these essential skills.

Creating the professional résumé is an essential task that must be refined over time (Wilson, 2010). Whether submitting a curriculum vitae or résumé, students should begin this process early in their clinical studies and add the educational experiences they encounter. A résumé is a general and concise overview of personal experiences and skills and how they relate to the particular position that one is aiming to obtain. In contrast, a curriculum vitae (CV) is a detailed summary of one's life accomplishments. As a general rule, CVs are required when furthering one's academic career and résumés are utilized to acquire a professional position (job). Polishing how students present these experiences and the skills learned from them is critical. Critique of the résumé should be mindful of the tremendous power that each word possesses and the image that this document portrays.

Numerous marketing studies have shown that the writer has a brief amount of time to entice the reader to engage in further exploration of a document. What is commonly known as the "3-30-3 Rule" simply states that a writer has 3 seconds to capture the reader's attention, 30 seconds to engage the reader, and then 3 minutes to get the message across. While no single "perfect" professional résumé template exists, the following example demonstrates many of the key points necessary to garner the reader's attention. First, the overall look of the résumé should be appealing from across the desk. Next, the applicant's name should be easy to read. Contact information should be clear and concise. Educational degrees need to be readily discernable. Work experience and additional educational experiences should showcase the applicant's skills and knowledge.

Demonstration of involvement is seen with activities, volunteerism, and awards. Lastly, a brief list of references can provide the reader with a sampling of professional networking. A reference list with complete contact information can be separately presented at the interview. Every opportunity to place a supervisor's name on the résumé should be taken, as the veterinary profession is a relatively small community and name recognition can set the applicant apart. An example of a résumé template can be found at http://cvm.msstate.edu/resume-ex.pdf.

Mock interviews where students assume the role of applicant and an instructor takes the role of employer are excellent tools for teaching interview skills. The role-play activity can be recorded for review and discussion or performed in front of the class. The latter allows for group discussion and assessment of what could have be done better or differently. It should be noted that all participants must be made to feel comfortable and understand the reasons for taking part in such an open fashion. Likewise, the intensity of the encounter can be modulated by the instructor based on the individual's ability to handle the questioning. Role play can be a valuable instrument in preparing students for their job interviews.

It is also at the end of the professional curriculum that professional and personal goal setting should be reintroduced. Initial introduction of goal setting and strategy formulation should be discussed early in the curriculum, perhaps in the first year together with budgeting. For many students their single lifelong goal has been attaining a DVM degree. Now they must think about how they want to apply their new degree to a lifetime professional career. Likewise, many are at the age where significant personal life events will begin to occur, such as choosing a life partner, beginning a family, and so on. While it may seem intuitive to some, the goal-setting process improves the learning and motivation of students as they assume the responsibility and ownership of learning their set goals (Zimmerman, 1990). Turkay (2014) has said that "Although setting goals improves performance robustly across various settings, it is nevertheless a skill: one must learn how to effectively set goals." An individual's achievement of their goals has been shown to correlate directly with their commitment to that goal (Klinger, 1977). Instruction in goal setting can be best accomplished by helping students manage their goals with organization and prioritization. Another effective means of goal-setting instruction is through instructor modeling by setting challenging goals, working diligently to accomplish those goals, and constantly planning the next step. From observation of this modeling, students have shown more commitment to achieving their own goals (Earley and Kanfer, 1985). Long-term assessment of goal setting is difficult, but may be best observed through graduate success. It is this ability to set goals strategically, and follow through with achieving those goals, that leads to a financially successful practice of veterinary medicine.

Basic Accounting and Marketing

Some small business applications such as practice marketing and basic accounting procedures can also be modeled in the clinical education phase of the veterinary curriculum. These topics can be discussed by posing questions regarding the establishment of fair and profitable fees, the cost of giving services away, how to create medical care estimates, and what client-targeted marketing is. Building on the skills learned in personal financial management and budgeting, a direct inference to business practice accounting can be made. The concept of long-term money management with careful recording of income and conscientious expenditure should be stressed.

Accounting methods are reinforced in the clinical setting through group activities targeted at how to determine appropriate fees for clinical services and supplies (Materni and Tumblin, 2013). The purpose of this exercise is then further strengthened by honestly discussing the cost of accidental and intentional "missed" charges within a veterinary practice setting (Opperman, 2010; Tumblin, 2008). This determination of lost revenue always seems to be a revelation to students. An example of a case scenario for a group discussion on fee setting and lost fees is included in Box 30.4.

Marketing can be taught in conjunction with clinical education or as case examples. While it may not initially seem like marketing, providing excellent client education regarding a patient's diagnosis and therapeutic care is a cornerstone on which financial success can be built. Practice tools such as professionally produced hand-outs, brochures, and a clinic website are just a few examples of items that can lend effort to this endeavor. Students may be required to assemble any one of these tools for clinic distribution. The power of marketing can easily be observed clinically with owner compliance and the numerous patient benefits it affords. Likewise, by providing specific examples of applied marketing techniques and data to assess their implementation, students may learn from the success of actual veterinary hospital efforts (Opperman and Grosdidier, 2014; Wutchiett, Tumblin and Associates, 2014).

 Box 30.4: Example of a Case Study for Fee Setting and Lost Fees (Group Activity)

- *Instructor*: "Let's talk about common procedures performed every day in a veterinary practice and how to determine the fee set for each. What are some procedures routinely performed in a small animal practice?"

Generate a list of a dozen or so procedures that generally include such actions as fecal exams, vaccinations, heartworm testing, FeLv/FIV testing, and so on.

Take each procedure and ask the participants how much they would like to charge for it and why. A monetary amount is thrown out and the group comes to a consensus. When prodded further as to why the amount was chosen, the typical answer is one based on the familiarity of what is charged for the procedure in previous places of employment, or what the veterinarian "down the street" charges. This provides the opportunity to discuss a more accurate way to determine fees based on the following information and formula:

$$(\text{cost of materials} + \text{cost of labor})$$
$$\times \text{ overhead and profit factor} = \text{fee}$$

The instructor can then segue into a discussion of lost revenue. This lost revenue is from missed charges that do not make it onto an invoice, lost opportunity charges where a procedure was not recommended or not done due to such factors as time or convenience, or charges that are intentionally not placed on a bill. The latter category is usually at the instruction of the attending veterinarian, and occurs because of guilt over providing inaccurate estimates, assumption of how much the owner can afford, or the feeling of enticing the owner to "like" them by giving away their time. Whatever the reason for this missed opportunity revenue, it can be financially crippling for a veterinary practice.

- *Instructor*: "Let's take each item and honestly discuss the missed opportunity for each. Would it be fair to say that you will either give away (i.e., perform but not charge for) or not recommend (i.e., best practices would indicate the need for the procedure) a fecal exam on five patients a day?"

Once agreement has been reached on the number of missed opportunities for each item on the list, have the group calculate this revenue by multiplying the fee they chose by the number of missed opportunities per day by 5 days per week by 50 working weeks per year. After the missed opportunity revenue for each procedure has been calculated, add these numbers together to get the total revenue "lost" by this small list. Next, explain how this can be extrapolated to the entire fee list and all procedures that a veterinarian would perform throughout the year. One can readily see this number reach tens of thousands of dollars annually.

Economics

Introspection regarding the impact that the national economic health has on our profession continues to be discussed extensively in the United States. Investment by the American Veterinary Medical Association in its Veterinary Economics Division has been observed and is producing much-needed insight into the relationship that free business markets have on the profession. Influence or control over a global economy is impractical, if not impossible, but the ability to plan and prepare strategically in order to respond to changes positively is imperative for the profession's success. It is for this reason that students must understand basic economic principles, especially the law of supply and demand. By definition, demand is the quantity of product (services) that buyers desire, and supply is the amount of product (services) that producers are willing to provide (Sowell, 2008). The relationship of these two factors influences the cost of that product. In its simplest form, supply will increase with higher prices and demand will decrease as prices rise. It is this theoretical concept of equilibrium – the point at which goods produced equal the amount of goods desired – within an economy, and the many factors that influence it, which students should understand.

Assessment of Learning

Veterinary business SKAs may be assessed through formative and summative assessment tools.

Formative Assessment

Formative assessment is defined as ongoing monitoring of student learning by the instructor that allows for improvement of their teaching and consequently better learning by the student. Formative assessment may be further divided into informal and formal techniques. Informal formative assessment is usually observational and done spontaneously during the teaching process, thereby allowing for immediate further explanation or offering of examples. Formal formative assessment generally comprises standardized tests that have been utilized in the past with proven results. Informal formative techniques such as oral or written reflections allow the instructor to guide the lecture or discussion so that it is tailored to the students' level of understanding and ensures comprehension of key concepts (University of Texas, 2015). This seems especially helpful early in the learning process, when concepts, ideas, and terminology are new to the student. It allows appropriate repetition when needed to assist with learning the material. More formal techniques such as individual projects (e.g., online learning modules, student budget) and group projects (e.g., new graduate contract evaluation) allow additional formative evaluation and instructional adaptation during the learning process to confirm that the material is understood.

Summative Assessment

Summative assessment evaluates how well the student learned from the instruction and is done at the end of instruction. It can be measured and is compared to previous benchmarks. Summative assessment of business skills can be more challenging. Summative assessment of business knowledge may be obtained through any of the traditional testing methods. Exams, papers, projects, and presentations are methods that allow the student to demonstrate their grasp of the material. Typical examples may include creation of a first-year graduate budget, a professional cover letter and résumé, or client handouts.

More problematic can be the assessment of life skills learning (UNESCO International Bureau of Education, 2006). In fact, there are several areas of medical education in which assessment is in its early stages and continues to prove difficult (Epstein, 2007). However, the evaluation of the relationship between student learning and life skills pedagogy is the foundation to ensure that a positive influence actually occurs. The teaching evaluation of some of the business SKAs and their impact on student lives can be determined immediately, while others

Table 30.1 Example of a business and ethics curriculum.

Year	Semester	Component name taught
1	1	AVMA available health and life insurance
1	1	Ethics of animals in research
1	1	Ethics of cosmetic surgery
1	1	Ethics of pain management in animals
1	1	Organized veterinary medicine
1	1	Production animal models
1	1	Veterinary workforce (career options in veterinary medicine)
1	2	Cruelty to animals and interpersonal violence
1	2	Ethics of cosmetic surgery 2
1	2	Military careers and scholarships
1	2	Pet overpopulation and early spay/neuter programs
1	2	Public health veterinarians
1	2	US government careers
2	1	Apply decision-making tools to complex problems
2	1	Apply ethical assessment tools to complex problems
2	1	Describe current global issues influencing One Health
2	1	Identify social, political, and economic effects of foreign animal disease incursions
2	1	List key issues that affect poverty and food security
2	1	Recognize and understand a multicultural environment and cross-cultural differences
2	1	State requirements to enter the international veterinary working environment
2	1	Understand the role of animals and livestock in developed and developing countries
2	2	Become familiar with common negotiation tactics
2	2	Develop knowledge of legal issues in practice
2	2	Identify common problems encountered in transition to practice
2	2	Identify critical interpersonal skills required in practice
2	2	Identify important communication techniques used in delivery of veterinary service
2	2	Identify important points to consider in developing a successful financial plan
2	2	Understand how student loan debt can be managed
2	2	Understand important steps in conducting a successful employment search
3/4	2	Action plan to grow a business
3/4	2	Ask the expert – panel discussion
3/4	2	Building successful relationships
3/4	2	Can I afford to buy a practice?
3/4	2	Capturing revenue – do you charge for all you do?
3/4	2	Common human resources mistakes and how to avoid them
3/4	2	Compensation and benefits – determining the total package value
3/4	2	Compensation methods
3/4	2	Contract negotiation
3/4	2	Determinants of a well-managed practice
3/4	2	Determining a practice's value (net cash flow)

(Continued)

Table 30.1 (Continued)

Year	Semester	Component name taught
3/4	2	Essentials of veterinary finance (personal and business value determination)
3/4	2	Etiquette – does it matter?
3/4	2	Fee schedules – charging fair and reasonable professional fees
3/4	2	Formulation of a professional résumé/curriculum vitae
3/4	2	How to attract and keep clients
3/4	2	Importance of client loyalty and retention
3/4	2	Improving compliance – the greatest opportunity of all
3/4	2	Ingredients of a contract
3/4	2	Insurance facts and needs
3/4	2	Inventory control – measuring product profitability
3/4	2	Life as a new graduate
3/4	2	Managing loans and negotiating the best deals with a bank/lender
3/4	2	Managing student debt (basics and options)
3/4	2	Mock interviews
3/4	2	Options for nonowners in practice
3/4	2	Partnering with an industry representative
3/4	2	Passive income – are you positioned to leverage and delegate?
3/4	2	Personal financial planning
3/4	2	Planning for the future
3/4	2	Preparation of a cover letter
3/4	2	Production-based compensation (production salary or ProSal)
3/4	2	Promoting what you bring to the position/practice
3/4	2	Retirement planning
3/4	2	Successful and profitable organization in an initial practice (business)
3/4	2	Terms of financing
3/4	2	The interview – dos and don'ts
3/4	2	The role of computerized medical records in business management
3/4	2	Understanding the average charge per transaction
3/4	2	Value perception determination of veterinary medicine
3/4	2	Veterinary career paths

may take years to appreciate fully. Some of the more immediate successes that can be gathered through surveys are market demand for graduates, new graduate starting salary comparisons, amount of accumulated student debt for graduates, and overall job-hunting outcomes (Cake, Rhind, and Baillie, 2014). Other analyses can be obtained from external outcomes assessment of employers of new graduates. What attributes do they expect of new graduates

and are these expectations met? Ultimately, the lifelong financial success of veterinary graduates is the true measure of a business program.

Conclusion

The veterinary profession has determined that business education is a core competency required of new graduates. Numerous challenges are faced with the instruction of business SKAs and have been identified in this chapter. One such challenge is where to place this instruction due to the diversity in veterinary educational curricula. Additionally, instruction by those with education and/or experience in the given area is crucial. An example of such a curriculum is given in Table 30.1.

With many veterinarians earning less than their potential due to a deficiency in financial and business management expertise (Cron *et al.*, 2000), it is our job as veterinary educators to ensure that our graduates receive this essential training. It is with an encompassing knowledge base that these graduates will become an influential part of the veterinary profession. The learning of business SKAs, like all knowledge associated with veterinary medicine, is constantly changing and must become a lifelong endeavor if the profession is to remain viable.

References

AAHA (2015) *Financial Planning*. American Animal Hospital Association. https://www.aaha.org/professional/resources/financial_planning.aspx#gsc.tab=0 (accessed July 18, 2015).

Australia Learning and Teaching Council (2009) *Enhancing Communication and Life Skills in Veterinary Students*. www.academia.edu/19436949/Enhancing_Communication_and_Life_Skills_in_Veterinary_Students (accessed November 20, 2016).

AVMA (2014) *COE Accreditation Policies and Procedures: Requirements*. American Veterinary Medical Association. https://www.avma.org/ProfessionalDevelopment/Education/Accreditation/Colleges/Pages/coe-pp-requirements-of-accredited-college.aspx (accessed April 15, 2015).

AVMA (2015a) *Veterinary Training*. American Veterinary Medical Association. https://www.avma.org/public/YourVet/Pages/training.aspx (accessed April 17, 2015).

AVMA (2015b) *Personal Financial Planning Tool*. American Veterinary Medical Association. https://www.avma.org/PracticeManagement/BusinessIssues/Pages/personal-financial-planning-tool.aspx (accessed July 20, 2015).

Bridges, D.R., Davidson, R.A., Odegard, P.S., *et al.* (2011) Interprofessional collaboration: Three best practice models of interprofessional education. *Medical Education Online*, **16**, 6035.

Cake, M.A., Rhind, S.M., and Baillie, S. (2014) The need for business skills in veterinary education: Perceptions versus evidence, in *Veterinary Business and Enterprise Theoretical Foundations and Practical Cases* (ed. C. Henry), Saunders Elsevier, Philadelphia, PA, pp. 9–23.

Chadwick, R.F., and Schroeder, D. (2002) *Applied Ethics: Critical Concepts in Philosophy*, Vol. **2**, Routledge, New York.

Cron, W.L., Slocum, J.V., Goodnight, D.B., and Volk, J.O. (2000) Executive summary of the Brakke management and behavior study. *Journal of the American Veterinary Medical Association*, **217**, 332–338.

Danielson, J.A., Wu, T., Fales-Williams, A.J., *et al.* (2012) Predictors of employer satisfaction: Technical and non-technical skills. *Journal of Veterinary Medical Education*, **39** (**1**), 62–70.

Drake, P.P., and Fabozzi, F.J. (2009) *Foundations and Applications of the Time Value of Money*, John Wiley & Sons, Inc., Hoboken, NJ.

DVM360.com Staff (2014) VHMA survey: The best way to attract new veterinary clients. *Veterinary Economics*, October 1. http://veterinarybusiness.dvm360.com/vhma-survey-best-way-attract-new-veterinary-clients (accessed November 18, 2016).

Earley, P.C., and Kanfer, R. (1985) The influence of component participation and role models on goal acceptance, goal satisfaction and performance. *Organizational Behavior and Human Decision Process*, **36**, 378–390.

Epstein, R.M. (2007) Assessment in medical education. *New England Journal of Medicine*, **356**, 387–396.

Harris, D.L. (2012) *Association of American Veterinary Medical Colleges Student Debt Initiative Report.* https://www.aavmc.org/data/files/other%20publications/aavmcharrisstudentdebtreport_2012_07_31.pdf (accessed June 30, 2015).

Klinger, E. (1977) *Meaning and Void: Inner Experience and the Incentives in People's Lives,* University of Minnesota Press, Minneapolis, MN.

Liss, D. (2012) Technician utilization. *Exceptional Veterinary Team,* January/February, 39–32.

Materni, C., and Tumblin, D. (2013) Score big with the right service prices. *Veterinary Economics,* October 1, 24–25.

Molhoek, A.W., and Endenburg, N. (2009) The effectiveness of marketing concepts in veterinary practices. *Tijdschr Dergeneeskd,* **134** (**1**), 4–10.

National Research Council of the National Academies of Sciences (2015) *Workforce Needs in Veterinary Medicine,* National Academies Press, Washington, DC.

NAVMEC (2011) *Roadmap for Veterinary Medical Education in the 21st Century: Responsive, Collaborative, Flexible.* North American Veterinary Medical Education Consortium. http://www.aavmc.org/data/files/navmec/navmec_roadmapreport_web_booklet.pdf (accessed April 16, 2015).

OIE (2013) *Veterinary Education Core Curriculum: OIE Guidelines.* World Organisation for Animal Health. http://www.oie.int/Veterinary_Education_Core_Curriculum.pdf (accessed April 12, 2015).

Opperman, M. (2010) Veterinary practices miss $64,000 in fees each year. *Veterinary Economics,* August 30. http://veterinarybusiness.dvm360.com/veterinary-practices-miss-64000-fees-each-year (accessed November 16, 2016).

Opperman, M., and Grosdidier, S. (2014) *The Art of Veterinary Practice Management,* 2nd edn, Advanstar, Lenexa, KS.

Richardson, F., and Osborne, D. (2006) Veterinary practice management – veterinary manager. *Canadian Veterinary Journal,* **47**, 702–706.

Self, D.J., Baldwin, D.C., Jr., and Wolinsky, F.D. (2009) Evaluation of teaching medical ethics by an assessment of moral reasoning. *Medical Education,* **26**, 178–184.

Shaw, J.R., Adams, C.L., and Bonnett, B.N. (2004) What can veterinarians learn from studies of physician-patient communication about veterinarian-client-patient communication? *Journal of the American Veterinary Medical Association,* **224**, 676–684.

Sowell, T. (2008) *Basic Economics: A Citizen's Guide to the Economy,* Basic Books, New York.

Tassava, B. (2014) *Social Media for Veterinary Professionals,* Halow Tassava Consulting, New York.

Tumblin, D. (2008) Top tips for reducing missed charges. *Veterinary Economics,* August 21. http://veterinarybusiness.dvm360.com/top-tips-reducing-missed-charges (accessed November 20, 2016).

Turkay, S. (2014) Setting goals: Who, why, how? *Harvard Initiative for Learning and Teaching.* https://hilt.harvard.edu/files/hilt/files/settinggoals.pdf (accessed November 18, 2016).

UNESCO International Bureau of Education (2006) *Manual for Integrating HIV and AIDS Education in School Curricula: Tool 7: Assessment of Learning Outcomes.* http://www.ibe.unesco.org/fileadmin/user_upload/HIV_and_AIDS/publications/Tool_7_Dec06_FINAL.pdf (accessed April 26, 2015).

University of Minnesota College of Veterinary Medicine (2015) *Personal Finance Simulator 2015.* http://www.finsim.umn.edu (accessed July 20, 2015).

University of Texas Center for Teaching and Learning (2015) *Methods of Assessment.* http://ctl.utexas.edu/teaching/assess-learning/methods-overview (accessed August 10, 2015).

Veterinary Business Advisors (2013) *Utilizing an Underused Resource: Veterinary Technicians.* http://veterinarybusinessadvisors.com/wp-content/uploads/2016/07/Utilizing_Veterinary_Technicians_11_2013.pdf (accessed November 18, 2016).

Walsh, D.A., Osburn, B.I., and Schumacher, R.L. (2002) Defining the attributes expected of graduating veterinary medical students, Part 2: External evaluation and outcomes assessment. *Journal of Veterinary Medical Education*, **29** (**1**), 36–42.

Wilson, J.F. (2010) *The resume and CV. Personal, Professional, Financial and Career Growth and Development Seminar*, Priority Press, Yardley, PA.

Wilson, J. F., Rollin, B.E., and Garbe, A.L. (2008) *Law and Ethics of the Veterinary Profession*. Priority Press, Yardley, PA.

Wutchiett, Tumblin and Associates (2014) *Benchmarks 2014: A Study of Well-Managed Practices*. https://wellmp.com/wutchiett-tumblin-associates-benchmark-studies/benchmark-study-2014.php (accessed November 18, 2016).

Zimmerman, B.J. (1990) Self-regulated learning and academic achievement: An overview. *Educational Psychologist*, **25** (**1**), 3–17.

Part VII

The Educational Environment

31

Student Selection

Jacquelyn M. Pelzer[1] *and Eloise K.P. Jillings*[2]

[1] *Virginia-Maryland College of Veterinary Medicine, Virginia Tech, USA*
[2] *Institute of Veterinary, Animal and Biomedical Sciences, Massey University, New Zealand*

Box 31.1: Key messages

- Veterinary program selection serves as the gateway for entry into the profession.
- The veterinary selection process in many institutions is based more often on historical decisions rather than research-led innovation.
- There is significant variability between the selection processes of different veterinary programs.
- Veterinary programs have been heavily reliant on undergraduate (also known as preveterinary, also known as preapplication) academic performance as a means to select students.

- Nonacademic personal attributes should be considered during the application review process.
- Increasing diversity in the veterinary profession will require a global effort tailored to the local environment of each program.
- There is relatively little research in the area of student selection and its ability to predict clinical competence.
- Review and analysis of admission processes are essential to detect possible barriers to application and ensure defensibility.

Introduction

The topic of veterinary selection usually draws robust debate among veterinarians, since most of them have an opinion on the best way to select students into the veterinary program. Some would suggest that selection should be on entirely academic merit due to its perceived objectivity, while others would favor an entirely subjective assessment, and most would prefer something in between. Everyone knows someone who should, or perhaps more importantly should not, have been admitted to a veterinary program, and the blame generally falls at the feet of the admission committee.

One might argue that the selection assessment process may be the single most important assessment that a school conducts (Eva *et al.*, 2004; Greenhill *et al.*, 2015), since attrition rates in the health professions are generally low, so selected applicants usually graduate (Prideaux *et al.*, 2011). Thus, the selection committees determine not only who becomes a veterinary

Veterinary Medical Education: A Practical Guide, First Edition. Edited by Jennifer L. Hodgson and Jacquelyn M. Pelzer.
© 2017 John Wiley & Sons, Inc. Published 2017 by John Wiley & Sons, Inc.

student, but ultimately who might become a veterinarian.

Because of the high level of competition for places in medical training programs, where applicant numbers greatly exceed available places (Prideaux *et al.*, 2011; Salvatori, 2001), it is increasingly important that the selection processes used are appropriate.

There are multiple stakeholders of healthcare selection, including but not limited to the applicant, the institution, the profession, the public, and in some cases the government (Patterson *et al.*, 2012; Salvatori, 2001). Admission committees of health professions programs have a relatively formidable task to balance their responsibilities to all these respective stakeholders.

For the applicants, admission processes need to be fair and consistently applied, so that there can be confidence that selection decisions reflect the performance of the applicants, rather than the personal preferences of the admission committee members. Admission committees generally aim to select students who are likely to succeed not only in the program, but also in the profession (Salvatori, 2001; Kogan *et al.*, 2009). For programs funded with public funds, there is also responsibility to the public and to the appropriate government funding body to utilize those funds appropriately and judiciously (Salvatori, 2001).

If you accept the idea that veterinary programs are the gateway to the profession (Kogan and McConnell, 2001), and that selection committees have multiple stakeholders to whom they are responsible, then it follows that veterinary admission processes need to be evidence based, with decisions made utilizing reliable and valid tools. In the 2010 Ottawa Conference consensus statement on assessment for selection for the healthcare professions, it states that "selection processes therefore need to be credible, fair, valid and reliable, and above all publicly defensible, and should follow the same quality assurance processes as in course assessment"

(Prideaux *et al.*, 2011). Currently in many institutions, the veterinary selection process is based more on historical decisions rather than research-led and evidence-based decisions.

Global Perspective on Veterinary Admissions

In this chapter, we explore the state of current admissions processes globally, discuss the common selection tools being utilized and highlight their evidence basis, consider diversity from a global perspective, and offer a guide to reviewing the institutional veterinary selection process.

Given the large number of veterinary programs globally, this chapter will focus on those that are accredited by the American Veterinary Medical Association (AVMA, 2015). When assessed against the medical selection literature, there is substantially less published research regarding veterinary selection. As such, this chapter will draw on both medical and veterinary literature.

Prior to proceeding, a brief clarification on terminology is pertinent. Traditionally, selection criteria have been divided into cognitive and noncognitive. Cognitive usually includes measures such as grade point average (GPA) and standardized testing, while the term noncognitive is typically used to encapsulate all the other desired qualities that may be assessed in applicants (Eva *et al.*, 2009; Prideaux *et al.*, 2011). While some authors have disagreed with these terms, they have largely continued to be utilized in the literature (Prideaux *et al.*, 2011; Kreiter, 2016). However, we feel uncomfortable with using the term noncognitive, as it suggests that these other desirable attributes have no cognitive component. In this chapter we will not use these terms, and will instead discuss criteria as measures of academic and nonacademic performance, with the latter including assessments of personal attributes.

Models of Veterinary Student Selection

Just as veterinary selection is not one size fits all, neither is the model of veterinary education. While variable, the pathways to veterinary qualification can largely be categorized as either postgraduate or undergraduate models of professional training. It should be emphasized that while different, both models can lead to AVMA-accredited veterinary degrees and both have respective advantages. The way in which individuals apply for selection also varies, from centralized application services such as the Veterinary Medical College Application Service (VMCAS) to individual, direct application to the desired institutions.

US and Canadian Models

The veterinary programs offered in the United States and Canada operate on the postgraduate model of professional education. Most applicants would complete or almost complete at least a Bachelor's degree prior to applying for a veterinary program. Veterinary programs are four years in length and, depending on curriculum, students may have the option to pursue a dual degree (e.g. DVM/MS, DVM/MPH, or DVM/PhD).

The majority of AVMA/Council on Education (COE) accredited veterinary programs in the United States utilize VMCAS, which is a centralized application service administered by the Association of American Veterinary Medical Colleges (AAVMC). VMCAS allows prospective students to complete one application, which can then be distributed to their choice of participating programs. The VMCAS application is divided into sections that include coursework completed, grade point average (GPA), veterinary experience, animal experience, research experience, work experience, activities and awards, personal statement, and electronic

letters of recommendation. The application cycle is open from May to September each year.

There is significant variation in prerequisites among US and Canadian veterinary programs, as influenced by organizational goals and values. For example, some programs may require knowledge of animal nutrition or genetics, while other programs do not.

Other Models

The veterinary programs in the United Kingdom, Australia, New Zealand, and many countries in the European Union have traditionally been undergraduate, or a dual degree combination, and usually five to six years in length. Students may enter the program following completion of high school, or as part graduates or graduates, depending on the institution. Some programs select on the basis of previous high school or university academic performance. Others accept a larger numbers of students into a preprofessional phase, and then apply a selection process for entry into the professional phase. Yet others employ a weighted lottery selection process, where the number of entries into the lottery is proportional to the level of academic performance in high school.

More recently, changes have been occurring in Australia and the United Kingdom. Several universities in Australia have moved away from a five-year undergraduate veterinary degree to either a four-year postgraduate DVM program, a six-year conjoined Bachelor's and DVM program, or both options. These are available to both domestic and international residents. While UK universities have retained their five-year Bachelor's degree programs, some have developed graduate entry programs that allow completion of the degree in four years rather than five.

Additionally, the program with lottery selection has introduced a secondary selection pathway for applicants intending on a career involving production animals that incorporates an interview process.

The prerequisites for selection into veterinary programs globally are even more varied than in the United States and Canada. Post–high school entry programs may have no prerequisites, while graduate entry programs may require a whole Bachelor's degree.

Outside of the United States and Canada, the domestic applicants for most institutions apply directly to each school of interest, while several institutions offer partial VMCAS applications for US and Canadian applicants.

Consideration of Diversity in Student Selection

The diversity of the members of medical professions and students in medical training is a source of interest globally (Razack *et al.*, 2015), as the benefits of diversity are substantial. On an individual level, interacting with a more diverse peer group increases students' cultural competence (Whitla *et al.*, 2003). Additionally, a more diverse student group may have a direct impact on learning cultural values within a curriculum, preparing students to succeed not only on a local level, but globally as well. To better reflect society and local communities, it is essential to have diverse representation within the veterinary profession. Members of the public feel a greater level of satisfaction when they can choose a medical professional who is ethnically similar to themselves (LaVeist and Nuru-Jeter, 2002). More diverse representation within the veterinary profession that better reflects societal demographics should translate to better outcomes for both people and the animals for which they have stewardship.

US and Canadian Perspectives on Diversity

There continue to be social, racial, and ethnic inequalities relating to veterinary admissions in the United States and Canada, more specifically within the United States, as race-conscious university admissions policies are constitutional only if they meet certain requirements. Several states where there are publicly supported veterinary programs, including California,

Washington, and Oklahoma, have placed bans on race-conscious admissions practices. These bans prohibit a program from selecting a class that would not only be academically successful, but, once graduated, would contribute to both national and global communities based on race or ethnicity. These restrictions on admissions may have a serious impact not only on the ability of veterinary programs to diversify within their individual communities, but on the profession as well.

Defining Diversity within the Veterinary Education Context

Traditionally within US and Canadian veterinary programs, the definition of diversity has varied, but typically included race and ethnicity, and, more recently, gender. In the medical education literature, considerable variation of inclusiveness was observed, and some programs only included African Americans, Native Americans, Mexican Americans, and mainland Puerto Ricans, while others were more comprehensive and included socioeconomic status, sexual orientation, and characteristics underrepresented in the local context (Page *et al.*, 2013). Additionally, Razack *et al.* (2015) reported that medical schools mostly define diversity as a quantifiable, superficially observable commodity, and that equity was a vaguely defined concept.

Due to race-conscious admissions in the United States, it is essential that veterinary programs universally define diversity. This should be done not only to create legally defensible application review processes, but also to give value to diversity by acknowledging that individual differences are an asset. Diversity in veterinary education should be seen as much broader than ethnicity, race, and gender, and as including other demographic characteristics, attributes, and personal characteristics. Diversity may include socioeconomic background, sexual orientation, gender identification, culture, and even abilities, personal aspirations, and attributes (e.g., resilience and entrepreneurship). While diversity should be defined collectively between veterinary programs, this is not to imply that diversity could not be additionally described within a local context, based on an individual veterinary program's goals and missions, and with consideration of the community in which it is located.

Although efforts have been made to improve the presence of underrepresented minorities within veterinary programs, only 16.8% of the total number of students enrolled are from underrepresented minorities, which is not a reflection of the broader society (Greenhill *et al.*, 2015).

Around 1980 there was a gender shift within the student body of US and Canadian veterinary programs, from a predominantly male population to a dominant female population. While the number of available seats has increased over the past 15 years, female applicants still comprise 87% of the applicant pool, with a continuing decline in male applicants (Greenhill *et al.*, 2015). The reasons for the gender shift within veterinary programs are speculative, but three main factors influencing the feminization of veterinary medicine were identified in a 2010 study. These included a decline in men's completion of undergraduate programs, lower male academic performance, and male avoidance of fields dominated by women (Lincoln, 2010).

The lack of underrepresented minorities within veterinary programs in the United States, and the need to better reflect the current diversity of society through changes in current student demographics, has been recognized. Recent reflections on the reasons for the lack of diversity include the lack of diversity in STEM (science, technology, engineering, and mathematics) disciplines at the undergraduate level, lack of role models, poor understanding of opportunities within the profession, and being educationally disadvantaged (Greenhill *et al.*, 2013).

Addressing Veterinary Admissions Biases and Potential Barriers in the United States and Canada

It is reported in the medical education literature that the focus of admissions remains on academic excellence and not on creating diversity. There is no comparative literature within veterinary education, so we can only theorize that there are similar dynamics. In addition to the methods listed in Table 31.1, to address biases a review of the centralized application process should be conducted with the specific focus of identifying barriers that may

Table 31.1 Addressing biases in admissions.

Methods to address biases in admission practices

College mission statements
- Include a commitment to diversity.
- Send a clear message to both stakeholders and prospective students on diversity position.

Program websites
- Mindful selection of images displayed.
- Accurate representation of program community.

Transparency of the admission process
- Clear and explicit instructions of requirements and process on websites.

Annual admission process reviews
- Review for fairness and potential biases.
- Consider implementing multiple measures to assess a broad range of attributes.

Program collaboration
- To make meaningful change, programs should agree on outcomes and act in a unified manner.
- Adhere to evidence-based best practices.

Professional development
- Development of all involved in the application review process.
- Train admission committee on inclusive definitions of excellence.
- Those involves should be aware of the power of their admissions decisions.

exclude those from underrepresented minorities. Many justifications for the lack of diversity have been mainly focused on external factors, rather than reflecting on how the process itself may be affecting those from underrepresented minorities and their ability to gain entry into a veterinary program (Razack *et al.*, 2015).

The lack of underrepresented minorities in the US and Canadian applicant pool is complicated due to the absence of data and the innumerable factors that influence one's decision to apply to veterinary school. While this information is difficult to capture, it would provide significant background for future changes in admission processes.

It is important that programs work together to address the current lack of diversity, since this initiative cannot be managed by one program or one organization. It must be a collaborative endeavor.

Other Perspectives on Diversity

Outside the United States and Canada, diversity has different focuses. In Australia and New Zealand, the ethnic diversity focus revolves around the access of indigenous communities (Prideaux *et al.*, 2011) to not only veterinary education, but higher education in general. Facilitated selection pathways have been developed to assist indigenous entry into programs, often with retention and support programs running alongside. The gender shift seen in the United States and Canada also occurred at a very similar time in the southern hemisphere, but has not yet resulted in the same magnitude of change.

Widening access is the term used in the United Kingdom to encompass efforts to promote student diversity and appropriate representation from all demographic groups (Patterson *et al.*, 2016) in higher education. One underrepresented group receiving attention in the literature is students from lower socioeconomic backgrounds (Prideaux *et al.*, 2011). Facilitated entry pathways have been established at many institutions for applicants of lower socioeconomic status, particularly those who have not attended private high schools.

Selection Methods, Tools, and Assessments

Historically, many medical training programs have weighted academic performance heavily or even relied on it as the sole determinant of selection (Patterson, Zibarras, and Ashworth, 2016). However, it has been identified that personal characteristics other than academic ability are required for veterinary economic and career success (Conlon, Hecker, and Sabatini, 2012). There is general agreement in the literature that in light of this, both cognitive (academic) and noncognitive (nonacademic) characteristics should be included in the assessment of applicants (Salvatori, 2001).

Within the United States and Canada, the application process of most institutions usually includes academic and nonacademic criteria. However, outside of these countries many institutions still focus heavily on academic performance in the selection of veterinary applicants. This will likely change for AVMA-accredited programs over the coming years, as Standard 7 of the AVMA/COE accreditation guidelines states: "factors other than academic achievement must be considered for admission criteria" (AVMA, 2015). However, the question remains as to what the most appropriate "other factors" to consider would be.

One admission process will not fit all institutions, since the goals of every institution vary. So while no selection process is perfect, or could be expected to be, selection decisions need to be made utilizing reliable and valid tools to minimize the level of imperfection. Institutions that desire fair, defensible selection policies need to conduct analyses of their own data. This is also increasingly important for outcomes assessment of admission required for AVMA accreditation.

In this section we discuss the more common application assessments of academic performance, standardized testing, prior experience (veterinary, animal, and/or research), personal statements, references, and interviews. A recent review article succinctly summarized some of the characteristics of the assessment tools that we discuss here, as shown in Box 31.2.

Box 31.2: Where's the evidence?

Patterson *et al.* (2016) conducted a systematic review of selection methods in medical education to determine how effective they were. For the most common selection methods they reported the reliabilty and validity, candidate acceptability, and how well it promoted widening access (diversity). Their findings were as follows:

- Academic record as a selection method is reliable, valid, and highly acceptable to candidates, although it was poor at widening access.
- Structured interviews, such as the multiple mini interview (MMIs), were both reliable and valid, candidates found them acceptable, and they had a moderate impact on widening access.
- Situational judgment tests (SJTs) were highly reliable and valid, had a high candidate

acceptance rate, and had a good impact on widening access.
- Aptitude tests were highly reliable, but their validity was variable. Acceptability by candidates and the impact on widening access were moderate.
- Personality tests, letters of reference, and traditional interviews were selection methods that had low reliability, validity, and widening of access, but that candidates found acceptable.

When considering nonacademic attributes within the selection process, SJTs and MMIs were more valid predictors than the other available methods. However, academic records and aptitude tests were also effective and should be part of the selection process. Evidence is lacking on how these approaches to student selection should be combined and what weight should be specified for each method.

Academic Performance

Preveterinary GPA is the most common criterion utilized by veterinary selection committees (Roush *et al.*, 2014). For postgraduate veterinary programs, the previous GPA may be calculated in various ways, with some common methods including overall undergraduate GPA, science GPA, prerequisite classes GPA, or the GPA from a specified number of credits taken most recently. For undergraduate veterinary programs, calculation of the GPA can be even more variable depending on whether students are selected directly after high school or as part graduates or graduates.

In considering the wider health professions selection literature, numerous studies have demonstrated that the best predictor of academic success within the program is preadmission academic grades. Once this is explored a little more, there is a good consensus that preadmission GPA is the best predictor

of academic performance in the preclinical component of the program. However, there is less consensus on whether is it also predictive of clinical performance (Salvatori, 2001).

In the veterinary literature, several authors have reported undergraduate GPA to be predictive of performance in the veterinary program (Confer, 1990; Fuentealba *et al.*, 2011; Rush, Sanderson, and Elmore, 2005; Zachary and Schaeffer, 1994), while the authors of one recent study reported the contrary (Roush *et al.*, 2014). Again, on closer examination some authors reported differences in the level of association between prior GPA and preclinical and clinical performance within the program. Fuentealba *et al.* (2011) found that preveterinary GPA predicted performance in the preclinical years, but not the clinical years. This lack of predictive value of preveterinary academic performance on performance in the clinical component of the program is supported by other authors (Roush *et al.*, 2014; Molgaard, Rendahl, and Kustritz,

2015). Since these studies were conducted on data collected from various veterinary programs, the lack of agreement may reflect the different methods used to analyze the data and the differing conditions under which the data were collected (e.g., different selection policies). As mentioned, the method of GPA calculation can vary significantly between institutions, and alteration of the method in and of itself could significantly affect the results.

Further influencing GPA interpretation is the grade inflation phenomenon, which diminishes the discriminative power of calculated GPAs. There is also evidence that academic performance assessments may be discriminatory against some demographic groups. As such, an overreliance on high academic performance may have contributed to both the gender shift and the lack of diversity within veterinary programs.

What is not clear is whether applicants who are the highest academic achievers become the most competent veterinarians. While GPA is the best predictor of academic performance within health professional programs, it only explains a small amount of the variance, which suggests that other variables also contribute to program performance (Salvatori, 2001). Therefore, the increased interest in determining valid and reliable assessments of nonacademic selection criteria appears justifiable.

Standardized Testing

Standardized test scores are commonly utilized in the selection of students into the health professions. For medical student selection, the Medical College Admission Test (MCAT) has been shown to be predictive for academic performance in medical programs (Salvatori, 2001; Prideaux *et al.*, 2011). In the 1980s there was some interest in utilizing the MCAT in veterinary student selection, although this did not become commonplace. Instead, the most common standardized test utilized for veterinary student selection, particularly in the United States, is the Graduate Record Examination (GRE). While the GRE has been reported to significantly predict master's and doctoral degree

program performance in multiple disciplines (Kuncel *et al.*, 2010), the veterinary literature is less clear.

Several authors have reported that GRE scores were predictive of performance in the veterinary program (Confer, 1990; Molgaard, Rendahl, and Kustritz, 2015; Fuentealba *et al.*, 2011; Rush, Sanderson, and Elmore, 2005), while others have not found the same association (Danielson *et al.*, 2011; Roush *et al.*, 2014). Like the reported findings for the predictive validity of GPA discussed previously, these studies were conducted on data collected from various veterinary programs, so would have the same associated limitations. This highlights the need for institutions using the GRE in the selection of their students to conduct analyses on their own student data to inform selection policy.

Personal Statements

There is little to no literature published regarding the effectiveness, reliability, and validity of personal statements within veterinary school admissions. The research evidence regarding the use of personal statements in selecting medical students suggests that they lack validity and reliability and are highly susceptible to coaching (Patterson *et al.*, 2016). It is also difficult to determine whether applicants actually wrote the letter themselves. Despite the concerns regarding their use, personal statements are commonly employed in both veterinary and medical student selection; however, there is little evidence to support the continuation of this practice (Salvatori, 2001).

We would recommend that veterinary selection committees critically evaluate their use of personal statements in the student selection process.

References

In a systematic review of the research regarding medical selection from 1997 to 2015, only nine articles regarding the use of references in medical student applications were found. From these, there was a clear consensus that referees' reports (also known as letters of reference) were of limited use in predicting the performance of students at medical school (Patterson *et al.*, 2016). One reason for this may be that in reference letters, referees tend not to focus on the applicant's areas of weakness, and may be overly positive in other respects (Stedman, Hatch, and Shoenfeld, 2009).

There is little research published regarding the use of references in veterinary student selection. Despite this and the lack of evidence from the medical selection literature, many selection committees utilize references. Authors in both the veterinary and medical literature suggest that there is little evidence to support the use of letters of reference (Molgaard, Rendahl, and Kustritz, 2015; Salvatori, 2001; Patterson *et al.*, 2016). We would agree that the use of letters of reference in veterinary student selection is not well founded in evidence, and would recommend that veterinary selection committees evaluate their use of references for reliability, validity, and defensibility.

Previous Experience

Many veterinary programs worldwide have a requirement for applicants to have experience with animals, or in veterinary clinical or research environments. These requirements can vary, from a small number of days seeing clinical practice only, to hundreds of hours across several different areas. While quantifying these experiences may be possible, verifying them is difficult and very time consuming, and comparing the quality of these experiences across applicants is almost impossible. Inflexibility regarding this requirement may have a direct impact on an individual's decision to apply to veterinary school.

There is little to no literature published in this area demonstrating that having these experiences makes a student a better veterinarian. However, a candidate who is exposed to the profession prior to commitment to a professional program is able to make a more informed decision regarding their career choice. A recent study did find that although preprofessional program GPA predicted academic success within the preclinical curriculum, previous

experiences predicted success within clinical rotations (Stegers-Jager *et al.*, 2015). However, there was no determination of how many hours of preplacement experience were necessary to obtain clinical success.

Access to these experiences can vary widely, and strict adherence to a set number of hours required may have a negative impact on diversity. As an example, students from lower socioeconomic backgrounds are unlikely to have the financial freedom to travel outside of their area to obtain experiences if unavailable locally, or to devote significant time to unpaid endeavors.

Interviews

Interviews are a common tool used during the admission process among veterinary programs, although some do not include an interview. The format of the interview varies greatly between programs: it can be either unstructured or structured in nature and range from an individual interviewer to a panel or series of interviewers. Furthermore, each program may have a different reason for interviewing, the interviews may be managed differently, and the number of sessions may vary. There is some conflicting evidence in regard to interviews, but overall evidence suggests that the traditional interview is not a valid or reliable tool to use for admissions decisions (Patterson *et al.*, 2016).

Structured interviews are standardized, with the purpose of providing each candidate with a similar interview experience, and the interview can be quantitatively measured. Structured interview tools, such as multiple mini interviews (MMIs), have more consistent psychometric measures than traditional interviews, and have been shown to be a reliable and valid interview tool (Patterson *et al.*, 2016).

Multiple mini interviews are a series of timed interviews in which each candidate must participate. Each interview station is based on a scenario designed to assess nonacademic attributes that are relevant to the individual program. The interviews are structured, as the interviewer must adhere to a script when asking follow-up questions, which affords a similar experience for each candidate. The process allows for extensive data analysis, including reliability and validity measures.

Unstructured interviews are still widely used in many North American veterinary admissions programs. Unstructured interview formats typically do not consist of a set of predetermined questions that will be asked of each individual candidate. While the process may be formal, the interaction between interviewer(s) and candidate(s) may vary between candidates. It has been demonstrated that unstructured interviews are not reliable and have poor predictive validity. Unstructured interviews are prone to bias and error, and therefore they may not be legally defensible (Patterson *et al.*, 2016).

Prior to implementation of any interview tool, careful consideration should be given to the overall goals and mission of the veterinary program, as well as how the interview format aligns with the curriculum.

Situational Judgment Tests

Since the 1970s, situational judgment tests (SJTs) have been utilized in assessment in a variety of occupations, and in the last decade have been utilized in selection in the medical profession (Patterson, Zibarras, and Ashworth, 2016). In the United Kingdom and Belgium they are a component of the respective centralized application service of each country for selection into its medical programs, and in Australia they are utilized in the selection of applicants into general practitioner (GP) training programs. As of publication of this text, we are only aware of one veterinary institution currently utilizing SJT in its selection process, and one in the development process to commence doing so.

Situational judgment tests are hypothetical scenarios created to assess the reactions and judgments of individuals in relation to specific personal attributes (Patterson, Zibarras, and Ashworth, 2016). The scenarios are created after the development of a test specification that highlights the desired personal attributes based on job or program analysis and in conjunction with subject matter experts. There are multiple

formats, from video to written, and the response options for the questions vary depending on the experience and age of the target applicants.

It is a time-consuming, complex, and multistep process to develop high-quality SJT scenario questions. However, the key advantage of SJT is that once developed, they can be used to assess the personal attributes of large numbers of applicants. The initial research regarding their reliability and validity looks promising, as is the acceptability to candidates (Patterson, Zibarras, and Ashworth, 2016; Lievens, 2013).

While SJTs are not common practice in veterinary selection, they may represent an area of future promise for selection committees to consider.

A Guide to Reviewing the Admission/Selection Process

There should be a mechanism in place to periodically evaluate the success of a program's admissions process. The "success" of an admissions process must be defined by individual programs based on their own goals and mission statements. Many program reviews are accomplished simply through outcomes reporting on rates of attrition, graduation, and passing of board examinations. However, it is recommended that a more intensive review be conducted, since admission decisions have a broader impact then just on an institution. The evaluation should be systematically performed and framed within program outcomes and measures, with the goal of determining the overall impact of student selection decisions on both stakeholders and the workforce. Veterinary programs should safeguard the fairness, transparency, defensibility, and psychometric properties of the student selection process. Additionally, consideration of the cost efficiency must be included in the evaluation.

The types of data collected will be program dependent, but should include both academic and nonacademic correlates. More than likely, all veterinary programs have an annual reporting system, which provides a brief

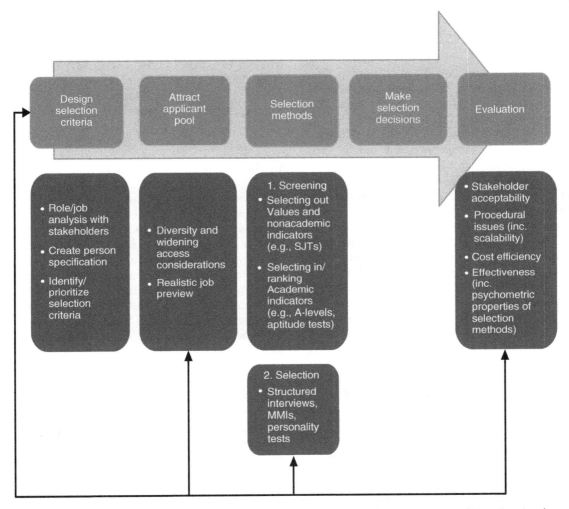

Figure 31.1 Design and evaluation of selection systems. Note: MMIs = multiple mini interviews; SJTs = situational judgment tests. Source: Adapted from Patterson *et al.*, 2016 with permission.

overview of the outcomes of student selection. However, it is our opinion that a detailed review process should occur on a regular basis, to allow for collecting data on a seated class from matriculation to graduation. The review should be completed in a timely manner to allow for implementation of any change. As veterinary programs have different titles for leaders within admission offices, the individuals accountable for the student selection process should be responsible for leading the evaluation process.

The admission committee should be involved, as well as students and perhaps employers. Faculty should be made aware of any proposed changes prior to final implementation.

Figure 31.1 outlines a system for the development of a selection process, but we believe that the same principles apply to a thorough review of existing processes. We encourage selection committees to consider these guidelines in developing or reviewing their selection processes.

Future Considerations

Applicant Numbers

Never before has there been a more pivotal point in veterinary admissions and student selection. Most programs have been, and remain, complacent when it comes to recruitment and student selection, often relying on outdated prerequisites, unreliable standardized testing, and selection based almost exclusively on academic criteria. This is in part due to the fact that, historically, there has always been a large, academically qualified applicant pool.

However, veterinary admissions offices are facing a new reality of a more competitive environment, not from the student perspective, but from that of the colleges themselves. Traditionally, veterinary programs have not experienced difficulty filling their available seats. While this is still currently the case, it may not continue to be the norm, as the applicant to seat ratio has declined dramatically, from 7286 applicants (3.59:1) to 6769 (1.64:1). Some factors contributing to this decline are an annual class size increase of 2% in most accredited US schools, establishment of new veterinary schools in the United States, increased accreditation of programs outside the United States, and an overall decrease in the number of applicants (Greenhill *et al.*, 2015).

There is speculation as to why there has been an overall decline in applicant numbers, with finances cited as the number one issue. However, recent reports indicate that finances have little impact on student decisions regarding whether or where to attend veterinary school. Since 2006, resident tuition has increased, on average, by about 18%, while nonresident tuition has increased by 8% (Greenhill *et al.*, 2015).

Conclusion

In veterinary curricula the value of working in teams rather than as competing individuals is espoused. Perhaps we could apply these lessons to ourselves and, rather than competing, veterinary colleges could work together in teams to review and reform the student selection processes. The combined knowledge and strengths from multiple institutions could have significant impacts on the future of veterinary admission and education. The development of innovative initiatives might lead to improved veterinary education outcomes and student wellbeing, reduce the cost of education, and move student selection into the twenty-first century. If we truly are the gatekeepers to the profession, we have a responsibility to take this role seriously. Cooperation between programs could benefit not only the programs and students, but also the profession and, ultimately, society.

References

AVMA (2015) *Accreditation Policies and Procedures: Requirements*. American Veterinary Medical Association. https://www.avma.org/ProfessionalDevelopment/Education/Accreditation/Colleges/Pages/coe-pp-requirements-of-accredited-college.aspx (accessed December 31, 2015).

Confer, A.W. (1990) Preadmission GRE scores and GPAs as predictors of academic performance in a college of veterinary medicine. *Journal of Veterinary Medical Education*, 17, 56–62.

Conlon, P., Hecker, K., and Sabatini, S. (2012) What should we be selecting for? A systematic approach for determining which personal characteristics to assess for during admissions. *BMC Medical Education*, 12, 105.

Danielson, J.A., Wu, T.-F., Molgaard, L.K., and Preast, V.A. (2011) Relationships among common measures of student performance and scores on the North American Veterinary Licensing Examination. *Journal of the American Veterinary Medical Association*, 38, 454–461.

Eva, K.W., Reiter, H.I., Trinh, K., *et al.* (2009) Predictive validity of the multiple mini-interview for selecting medical trainees. *Medical Education*, **43**, 767–775.

Eva, K.W., Rosenfeld, J., Reiter, H.I., and Norman, G.R. (2004) An admissions OSCE: The multiple mini-interview. *Medical Education*, **38**, 314–326.

Fuentealba, C., Hecker, K.G., Nelson, P.D., *et al.* (2011) Relationships between admissions requirements and pre-clinical and clinical performance in a distributed veterinary curriculum. *Journal of Veterinary Medical Education*, **38**, 52–59.

Greenhill, L., Cipriani, K., Lowrie, P., and Ammass, S. (2013) *Navigating Diversity and Inclusion in Veterinary Medicine*, Purdue University Press, West Lafayette, IN.

Greenhill, L., Elmore, R., Stewart, S., *et al.* (2015) Fifty years in the life of veterinary students. *Journal of Veterinary Medical Education*, **42**, 480–488.

Kogan, L.R., and Mcconnell, S.L. (2001) Gaining acceptance into veterinary school: A review of medical and veterinary admissions policies and practices. *Journal of Veterinary Medical Education*, **28**, 101–110.

Kogan, L.R., Stewart, S.M., Schoenfeld-Tacher, R., and Janke, J.M. (2009) Correlations between pre-veterinary course requirements and academic performance in the veterinary curriculum: Implications for admissions. *Journal of Veterinary Medical Education*, **36**, 158–165.

Kreiter, C.D. (2016) A research agenda for establishing the validity of non-academic assessments of medical school applicants. Advances in Health Science Education. Online ahead of print. doi:10.1007/s10459-016-9672-y

Kuncel, N.R., Wee, S., Serafin, L., and Hezlett, S.A. (2010) The validity of the graduate record examination for master's and doctoral programs: A meta-analytic investigation. *Educational and Psychological Measurement*, **70**, 340–352.

LaVeist, T.A., and Nuru-Jeter, A. (2002) Is doctor-patient race concordance associated with greater satisfaction with care? *Journal of Health and Social Behavior*, **43**, 296–306.

Lievens, F. (2013) Adjusting medical school admission: Assessing interpersonal skills using situational judgement tests. *Medical Education*, **47**, 182–189.

Lincoln, A.E. (2010) The shifting supply of men and women to occupations: Feminization of veterinary education. *Social Forces*, **88**, 1969–1996.

Molgaard, L.K., Rendahl, A., and Kustritz, M.V.R. (2015) Closing the loop: Using evidence to inform refinements to an admissions process. *Journal of Veterinary Medical Education*, **42**, 297–304.

Page, K.R., Castillo-Page, L., Poll-Hunter, N., *et al.* (2013) Assessing the evolving definition of underrepresented minority and its application in academic medicine. *Academic Medicine*, **88**, 67–72.

Patterson, F., Knight, A., Dowell, J., *et al.* (2016). How effective are selection methods in medical education? A systematic review. *Medical Education*, **50**, 36–60.

Patterson, F., Lievens, F., Kerrin, M., *et al.* (2012) Designing selection systems for medicine: The importance of balancing predictive and political validity in high-stakes selection contexts. *International Journal of Selection and Assessment*, **20**, 486–496.

Patterson, F., Zibarras, L., and Ashworth, V. (2016) Situational judgement tests in medical education and training: Research, theory and practice: AMEE guide no. 100. *Medical Teacher*, **38**, 3–17.

Prideaux, D., Roberts, C., Eva, K., *et al.* (2011) Assessment for selection for the health care professions and specialty training: Consensus statement and recommendations from the Ottawa 2010 Conference. *Medical Teacher*, **33**, 215–223.

Razack, S., Hodges, B., Steinert, Y., and Maguire, M. (2015) Seeking inclusion in an exclusive process: Discourses of medical school student selection. *Medical Education*, **49**, 36–47.

Roush, J.K., Rush, B.R., White, B.J., and Wilkerson, M.J. (2014) Correlation of pre-veterinary admissions criteria, intra-professional curriculum measures, AVMA-COE professional competency scores, and the NAVLE. *Journal of Veterinary Medical Education*, **41**, 19–26.

Rush, B.R., Sanderson, M.W., and Elmore, R.G. (2005) Pre-matriculation indicators of academic difficulty during veterinary school. *Journal of Veterinary Medical Education*, **32**, 517–522.

Salvatori, P. (2001) Reliability and validity of admissions tools used to select students for the health professions. *Advances in Health Sciences Education*, **6**, 159–175.

Stedman, J.M., Hatch, J.P., and Schoenfeld, L.S. (2009) Letters of recommendation for the predoctoral internship in medical schools and other settings: Do they enhance decision making in the selection process?

Journal of Clinical Psychology in Medical Settings, **16**, 339–345.

Stegers-Jager, K.M., Themmen, A.P., Cohen-Schotanus, J., and Steyerberg, E.W. (2015) Predicting performance: Relative importance of students' background and past performance. *Medical Education*, **49**, 933–945.

Whitla, D.K., Orfield, G., Silen, W., *et al.* (2003) Educational benefits of diversity in medical school: A survey of students. *Academic Medicine*, **78**, 460–466.

Zachary, J.F., and Schaeffer, D.J. (1994) Correlations between preveterinary admissions variables and academic success in core courses during the first two years of the veterinary curriculum. *Journal of Veterinary Medical Education*, **21**, 56–60.

32

Student Learning Environment

Sue Roff and Sean McAleer

Center for Medical Education, Dundee University Medical School, UK

Box 32.1: Key messages

- Veterinary medical education occurs within social organizations.
- The dynamics of social organizations can be studied using social science methodologies.
- Learning environments are one set of dynamics that have been studied in human health professions education.

- The resources developed from these studies can be adapted for veterinary medical education.
- Guidelines are offered for research in the learning environments of veterinary medical education.

Introduction and Definition of Learning Environments

In the past decade there has been a growing appreciation of the importance of student learning environments in medical education. In 2013, the UK General Medical Council (GMC) developed a discussion paper on Approving Educational Environments (GMC, 2013). As part of the GMC's 2015 revision of this document, it included a definition of an education or learning environment:

> The educational or learning environment can be defined in various ways. At its simplest it can mean the physical surroundings within which learning takes place, such as access to library facilities, seminar rooms or simulation equipment. However, references to the environment generally also encompass broader and less tangible notes of educational "climate", "culture" or "ethos". (GMC, 2015, p. 3)

This GMC paper also points to the American Medical Association (AMA, 2008) definition of the learning environment as:

> A social system that includes the learner (including the external relationships and other factors affecting the learner), the individuals with whom the learner interacts, the setting(s) and purpose(s) of the interaction, and the formal and informal rules/policies/norms governing the interaction. (GMC, 2015, p. 3)

Further, the AMA describes a learning environment as "comprising three broad

Veterinary Medical Education: A Practical Guide, First Edition. Edited by Jennifer L. Hodgson and Jacquelyn M. Pelzer.
© 2017 John Wiley & Sons, Inc. Published 2017 by John Wiley & Sons, Inc.

components in any institution or setting: institutional culture, curriculum (both formal and informal) and educational climate" (GMC, 2015, p. 3).

Some organizations have been more specific in their definition of the learning environment. For example, the GMC's 2015 publication *Promoting Excellence: Standards for Medical Education and Training* devotes the first of its five themes to "Learning Environment and Culture" and includes the following standards:

> Standard 1: The learning environment is safe for patients and supportive for learners and educators. The culture is caring, compassionate and provides a good standard of care and experience for patients, carers and families.

> Standard 2: The learning environment and organisational culture value and support education and training so that learners are able to demonstrate what is expected in good medical practice and to achieve the learning outcomes required by their curriculum. (GMC, 2015, p. 7)

Given these definitions, how can we delineate such a broad and multifaceted aspect of a social organization as its learning environment? Specifically, how can this be done for the learning environments of veterinary medical education?

Social Organizations and Learning Communities

Like all professions, veterinary science is a social organization. In Lave and Wenger's (1991) terminology, it is a community of practice in which veterinarians acquire the learning, meaning, and identity of a specific profession by participating in its learning communities. In veterinary medical education, these learning communities could include preclinical groups, clinical groups in veterinary teaching hospitals, as well as external placements, e-learning groups, or groups formed through continuing education.

Wenger (1999, p. 4) suggests that participation in learning communities such as these "refers not just to local events of engagement in certain activities with certain people, but to a more encompassing process of being active participants in the *practices* of social communities and constructing *identities* in relation to these communities." Merton and Kitt (1950, p. 81) hypothesized more than 60 years ago that learning communities such as medical schools are social structures, and that it should be possible to delineate "the development of relatively precise, statistical indices of social structure" in such a social organization. In his classic study of the "student-physician," Merton suggested in 1957:

> Learning to be a physician, like complex learning of other kinds, is not only a function of intelligence and aptitude, of motivations and self-images; it is also a function of the social *environments* in which learning and performance take place.... Learning and performance vary not as the individual qualities of students vary but also as their social environments vary, with their distinctive *climates* of value and their distinctive organization of relations among students, between students and faculty, and between students and patients. (Merton, 1957, p. 63)

The neo-Mertonian field of analytical social science "endeavours to explicate iterative connections between the properties of a social system and the action of individuals" (Freese, 2009, p. 94). That is, it should be possible to delineate aspects of a social system such as the educational environment or climate through mixed qualitative and quantitative methods in order to describe and analyze them.

Assessment of the Learning Environment

In an effort to apply qualitative and quantitative methods, several psychometric tools have been developed to assess the learning environment. Each of these tools is focused on a specific stage within the professional curriculum.

The Dundee Ready Education Environment Measure (DREEM)

The Dundee Ready Education Environment Measure (DREEM) was developed 20 years ago using a panel of nearly 100 international health professions educators in a grounded theory process, resulting in the generation of 50 items reflecting aspects of the educational environment that the panel considered to be relevant to *preclinical* learning in the health professions. There are more than 200 published reports of DREEM administrations in the human health professions. The psychometrics reported in these studies are consistently good, but there is some weakness in the factor analysis, particularly in social self-perceptions in some of the studies. While factor analysis of DREEM has been reported more than a dozen times in the last decade, seven studies had fewer respondents than the minimum sample size of 300 recommended by Wetzel (2012). Five studies analyzed data from 323 to 586 respondents. The respondents in these studies included German (n=205), Greek (n=323), and New Zealand (n=176) dental students; Irish (n=239), Swedish (n=395), Pakistani (n=419–586), and Greek

(n=487) medical students; Australian (n=245) osteopathy students; and American (n=214) veterinary students. Two studies (one from Germany and one from Spain) had sample sizes of 1119 and 1391, respectively. Yusoff (2012) analyzed four administrations of DREEM to the same cohort of 186 Malaysian medical students. Wetzel (2012, p. 1066) also noted that "Large sample sizes generally produce more stable factor structures and better approximate population parameters," and there are indications of a trend confirming a more stable factor structure for DREEM with larger sample sizes. There may be an opportunity to test this with the data from a nationwide cohort of more than 9000 Korean medical students reported by Park *et al.* (2015).

DREEM has been used in a variety of contexts to evaluate the learning environment (see Box 32.2).

DREEM and Veterinary Medical Education

Two studies have begun to explore the validity and reliability of adapting the widely used DREEM tool to veterinary medical education in the United States and Scotland.

Pelzer, Hodgson, and Werre (2014) administered a slightly adapted version of the 50-item DREEM with its 5 subscales to 224 (53%) of the 419 students in a mostly graduate-entry four-year veterinary medicine program in the

---

 Box 32.2: Focus on uses of the DREEM

- Profile the learning environments of individual schools in a range of health professions in order to understand the students' perceptions of their strengths and weaknesses. The data can be analyzed in relation to variables such as age, route of entry to program, gender, ethnicity, and stage of course.
- Compare perceptions of distributed learning sites.

- Compare perceptions of different stages of curriculum delivery.
- Compare perceptions of different types of curriculum and curriculum change and development.
- Compare perceptions of different teaching and delivery modes.
- Test for correlations between academic performance and perceptions of learning environment.

United States, which comprises three years of preclinical training and a final year of workplace training in a variety of clinical settings, including a veterinary teaching hospital. Cronbach's alpha for the overall score was .93 and for the five subscales was as follows: perceptions of learning .85, perceptions of faculty .79, perceptions of atmosphere .81, academic self-perceptions .68, and social self-perceptions .72. Construct validity was determined to be acceptable (p<0.001) and all items contributed to the overall validity of DREEM. The overall DREEM score was 128.9/200. Four individual items of concern were identified by students, originating from four of the five subscales, but all related to workload. The researchers concluded that in this setting DREEM was a reliable and valid tool to measure veterinary students' perceptions of their learning environment.

Hughes (2015) administered a slightly adapted DREEM (see Box 32.3) to 452 (60%) of 750 students in a UK veterinary school where the curriculum includes a number of transition points when the type of teaching changes. There is also an additional four-year graduate-entry program (GEP) at the school, which presents a combined first and second year in a separate class prior to merging the students into the third year of the program. Statistical analysis of the collected data determined the internal consistency (Cronbach's alpha) for the overall score to be .79, and for the five subscales perceptions of learning .81, perceptions of teachers .76, academic self-perceptions .80, perceptions of atmosphere .80, and social self-perceptions .62. All of these values were interpreted as acceptable to good, indicating a good level of internal consistency. Confirmatory factor analysis of the construct validity also indicated an adequate model fit.

Hughes (2015, p. 2) reported:

> Overall the results of the DREEM were positive from the majority of the students however there was a significant minority of students in all years who held a more negative view of certain aspects of their experience. Additionally, student perceptions were found to be less positive overall in certain areas at key transition points such as entering the first year, moving from pre-clinical to clinical teaching and into final year rotations. In particular the themes "Perceptions of learning" and "Academic self-perception" had up to 30% of respondents in a single year rating them on the negative end of the scale.

A number of results from DREEM allowed this program to make changes to its curriculum. For example, the results

> led to a discussion about the issues students face with transitions and what could be done better to support them. In particular, the teaching staff were surprised at just how unprepared final year students felt for the move from classroom teaching to rotations on clinics and using clinical reasoning. Following this discussion a number of initiatives have been put in place to address this: there will now be a clinical reasoning thread through the earlier years and problem-based learning sessions in other courses; the final year preparation course has been re-structured to help students get ready for final year including a track on problem-based cases, and there will also be tours of the hospital for 4th year students by final years to help them feel more comfortable with what happens there and less intimidated when they start final year. There will also be on-line resources with tasks to undertake on rotation to point to what is important as students go through. In addition to support for the final year transition, there is a pre-entry support project in progress and the school is discussing ways to support the pre-clinical to clinical transition. (Hughes, 2015, p. 7)

Manchester Clinical Placement Index (MCPI)

Dornan *et al.* (2012) developed the Manchester Clinical Placement Index (MCPI) and suggested that its eight items could be sufficient to measure the 50 aspects of educational environment

Box 32.3: Focus on DREEM survey items and subscales

Students' perception of teaching

- I am encouraged to participate in class
- The teaching is often stimulating
- The teaching is student-centred
- The teaching helps to develop my competence
- The teaching is well focused
- The teaching helps to develop my confidence
- The teaching time is put to good use
- **The teaching over-emphasizes factual learning**
- I am clear about the learning objectives of the course
- The teaching encourages me to be an active learner
- Long-term learning is emphasized over short term
- **The teaching is too teacher-centred**

Students' perceptions of teachers

- The teachers are knowledgeable
- The teachers are patient with (clients) and other staff*
- **The teachers ridicule the students**
- **The teachers are authoritarian**
- The teachers have good communications skills*
- The teachers are good at providing feedback to students
- The teachers provide constructive criticism here
- The teachers give clear examples
- **The teachers get angry in class**
- The teachers are well prepared for their classes
- **The students irritate the teachers**

Students' academic self-perceptions

- Learning strategies which worked for me before continue to work for me now
- I am confident about passing this year
- I feel I am being well prepared for my profession

- Last year's work has been a good preparation for this year's work
- I am able to memorize all I need
- I have learned a lot about empathy in my profession
- My problem-solving skills are being well developed here
- Much of what I have to learn seems relevant to a career in veterinary medicine*

Students' perceptions of atmosphere

- The atmosphere is relaxed during the practical class/clinical rotation teaching*
- This school is well timetabled
- **Cheating is a problem in this school**
- The atmosphere is relaxed during lectures
- There are opportunities for me to develop interpersonal skills
- I feel comfortable in class socially
- The atmosphere is relaxed during seminars/tutorials
- **I find the experience disappointing**
- I am able to concentrate well
- The enjoyment outweighs the stress of studying veterinary medicine*
- The atmosphere motivates me as a learner
- I feel able to ask the questions I want

Students' social self-perceptions

- There is a good support system for students who get stressed
- **I am too tired to enjoy this course**
- I am rarely bored on this course
- I have good friends in this school
- My social life is good
- I seldom feel lonely
- My accommodation is pleasant

Notes: Negative items in bold. *Items are modified from the original for veterinary context, adjusting for whether students were experiencing classroom or clinical rotation teaching.

Source: Adapted from Roff, McAleer, and Skinner, 1997.

encompassed by DREEM. However, DREEM is not intended for clinical placement learning but for preclinical environments, as indicated by its item descriptors. Strand *et al.* (2013, p. 1015) comment that MCPI

> consists of eight items mapping out various aspects of experiential learning, support and training in undergraduate clinical placements, complemented by open-ended questions. The tool, a valuable short inventory, is based on experiential learning theory and community of practice theory. However, the eight items are limited in their capacity to address the social and emotional dimensions of the learning climate and the quality of pedagogical strategies, which are aspects of learning emphasized in contemporary workplace learning models.

Undergraduate Clinical Environment Education Measure (UCEEM)

Strand *et al.* (2013, p. 1014) saw the need to develop an Undergraduate Clinical Environment Education Measure (UCEEM), noting that "In medical and health professions education, a significant part of student education takes place in the clinical workplace environment and through workplace experience." UCEEM is a 25-item instrument with two overarching dimensions, experiential learning and social participation, and four subscales that coincide well with theory and empirical findings: opportunities to learn in and through work and quality of supervision; preparedness for student entry; workplace interaction patterns and student inclusion; and equal treatment. Evidence from various sources supports the content validity, construct validity, and reliability of the instrument (see Box 32.4 for the instrument).

Postgraduate Hospital Education Environment Measure (PHEEM)

Over the past decade there has been increased interest in analyzing health professions trainees' perceptions of their learning environment as they begin to move toward clinical autonomy. Quality assurance of medical training programs now commonly includes trainee surveys such as the Veterans Affairs Learners' Perception Survey (US Department of Veterans Affairs, 2016), the Accreditation Council for Graduate Medical Education Resident/Fellow Survey (ACGME, 2016), and the UK General Medical Council's National Trainee Survey (GMC, 2016).

A typical medical resident's contract in the United States states that the program director

> shall be responsible for administering and maintaining an educational environment conducive to educating residents in each of the ACGME competency areas (patient care, medical knowledge, practice-based learning and improvement, interpersonal and communication skills, professionalism, and systems-based practice). This responsibility shall include the provision of a quality didactic and clinical education at all sites that participate in the program, a sufficient number of faculty with documented qualifications to instruct and supervise residents at all locations, formative and summative evaluation of individual resident performance, evaluation of program and faculty performance, and program performance improvement. (University of Washington, Seattle, WA)

The educational environment of a medical resident is understood in this sort of contract to include the affiliated hospitals, which are required to "assure access to appropriate food services at all times; safe and reasonably convenient parking facilities, on-call quarters, hospital and institutional grounds, and related facilities; and safe, quiet, and private call rooms with bathroom facilities. There shall be a sufficient number of call rooms so that on-call residents may sleep and have a secured storage area for personal belongings" (University of Washington, Seattle, WA).

Working with medical education stakeholders in the United Kingdom, we developed the

Box 32.4: Focus on the UCEEM items organized by subscales

Opportunities to learn in and through work including quality of supervision

- My (work) tasks are relevant to the learning objectives
- I am sufficiently occupied with meaningful (work) tasks
- My tasks are suitably challenging for my level of knowledge and skills
- I am encouraged to participate actively in the work here
- I receive useful feedback from my supervisors
- I feel able to ask my supervisors any question I wish
- I get the opportunity to provide a rationale for my actions during supervision sessions
- My problem solving skills are developing well in this placement
- I have the opportunity to put my theoretical knowledge into practice in this placement
- I have the opportunity to learn together with other medical students in this placement
- I feel I have influence over my learning in this placement

Preparedness for student entry

- I received useful induction in this placement
- My supervisors were expecting me when I arrived

- I have a supervisor to whom I know I can turn
- I have sufficient access to supervision
- The supervisors are well prepared for supervising
- It is clear that my supervisors are familiar with the learning objectives

Workplace interaction patterns and student inclusion

- I have adequate access to computers in this placement
- There is sufficient physical space for the number of medical students on placement here
- As a student I am received in a positive way by the staff here
- I feel included in the team of people who work here
- Communication between those working here is good
- I feel welcome in the staff room/lunch room here

Equal treatment

- Everyone is treated equally here regardless of cultural background
- Everyone is treated equally here regardless of gender

Postgraduate Hospital Education Environment Measure (PHEEM; Roff, McAleer, and Skinner, 2005). The grounded theory process generated 40 items, which fell into three domains (see Box 32.5).

In 2007, Boor et al. administered PHEEM to 595 Dutch respondents and reported: "The PHEEM is a questionnaire measuring 1 dimension instead of the hypothesised 3 dimensions. The sample size required to achieve a reliable outcome is feasible. The instrument can be used to evaluate both single and multiple

departments for both clerks and registrars" (Boor et al., 2007, p. 92). Analyzing data from 125 respondents, Riquelme et al. in 2009 suggested that PHEEM is a five-factor instrument. Also in 2009, Wall et al. pooled data from several PHEEM administrations to 1563 respondents and found that the overall Cronbach's alpha was .928 and that the factor analysis supported the postulated domains. In 2014, Shokoohi et al. administered PHEEM in Persian in Iran to 127 respondents and reported five factors. As

Box 32.5: Focus on PHEEM subscales and items

Perceptions of role autonomy

- I have a contract of employment that provides information about hours of work
- I had an informative induction programme
- I have the appropriate level of responsibility in this post
- I have to perform inappropriate tasks
- There is an informative Junior Doctors Handbook
- I am bleeped inappropriately
- There are clear clinical protocols in this post
- My hours conform to the New Deal
- I have the opportunity to provide continuity of care
- I feel part of a team working here
- I have opportunities to acquire the appropriate practical procedures for my grade
- My workload in this job is fine
- The training in this post makes me feel ready to be an SpR/Consultant
- My clinical teachers promote an atmosphere of mutual respect

Perceptions of teaching

- My clinical teachers set clear expectations
- I have protected educational time in this post
- I have good clinical supervision at all times
- My clinical teachers have good communication skills
- I am able to participate actively in educational events
- My clinical teachers are enthusiastic

- There is access to an educational programme relevant to my needs
- I get regular feedback from seniors
- My clinical teachers are well organized
- I have enough clinical learning opportunities for my needs
- My clinical teachers have good teaching skills
- My clinical teachers are accessible
- Senior staff utilize learning opportunities effectively
- My clinical teachers encourage me to be an independent learner
- The clinical teachers provide me with good feedback on my strengths and weaknesses

Perceptions of social support

- There is racism in this post
- There is sex discrimination in this post
- I have good collaboration with other doctors in my grade
- I have suitable access to careers advice
- This hospital has good quality accommodation for junior doctors, especially when on call
- I feel physically safe within the hospital environment
- There is a no-blame culture in this post
- There are adequate catering facilities when I am on call
- My clinical teachers have good mentoring skills
- I get a lot of enjoyment out of my present job
- There are good counselling opportunities for junior doctors who fail to complete their training satisfactorily

Schonrock-Adema and colleagues noted (2009, p. E231), "choices made during data analysis have direct outcomes," not least in factor analysis. As with DREEM, a large national or pooled analysis should make for more robust factor analysis. PHEEM has been found to be reliable in several countries and is used as a quality assurance tool in multisite programs such as the Postgraduate Medical Council in the state of Victoria, Australia (PMCV, 2016).

Finally, it should be noted that the 40 elements of PHEEM map well to other questionnaires for assessing clinical teachers (Fluit *et al.*, 2010), such as the Maastricht Clinical Teaching Questionnaire (Stalmeijer *et al.*, 2010) and the Cleveland Clinic's Clinical Teaching Effectiveness Instrument Rating Scales (Copeland and Hewson, 2000).

Additional Tools for Assessment of the Clinical Learning Environment

Boor *et al.* (2011) worked with Dutch medical trainees to develop the Dutch Residency Educational Climate Test (D-RECT), consisting of 50 items and 11 subscales. However, Silkens *et al.* (2016, p. 477) suggest that individual responses should be aggregated to the level of the department in order to describe a department's learning climate, and this led them to "revisit" D-RECT and conclude: "As a result, the identified structure of the D-RECT may not be the optimal structure for evaluating the learning climate of the department." They suggest nine subscales: educational atmosphere, teamwork, role of specialty tutor, coaching and assessment, formal education, resident peer collaboration, work is adapted to residents' competence, accessibility of supervisors, and patient sign-out.

Tsai *et al.* (2014) worked with 189 Taiwanese medical trainees to develop the 39-item Clinical Learning Environment Questionnaire (CLENQ), which yielded five factors: I: Teaching (13 items), II: Workload (7 items), III: Relationship pressure (9 items), IV: Organisational support (4 items), and V: Mutual trust (6 items). They commented:

> The teaching dimension was mainly adopted from the "teaching subscale" of the PHEEM instrument. We hypothesise that the other dimensions, such as clinical workloads, working and social interactions with patients and medical teams, and organisational culture, may differ between

Taiwan and Western or other countries. Thus, new items of these dimensions of clinical learning environment were constructed in alignment with local medical training settings and the socio-cultural context. (Tsai *et al.*, 2014, p. 228)

In Saudi Arabia, AlHaqwi, Kuntze, and van der Molen (2014) have developed the Clinical Learning Evaluation Questionnaire (CLEQ), consisting of 40 items. The initial factor analysis based on 109 response sets yielded six factors: F1 Cases (8 items), F2 Authenticity of clinical experience (8 items), F3 Supervision (8 items), F4 Organization of the doctor–patient encounter (4 items), F5 Motivation to learn (5 items), and F6 Self-awareness (4 items).

Using the same methodological approaches as generated PHEEM, Cassar (2004) developed the Surgical Theatre Educational Environment Measure (STEEM), and Holt and Roff (2004) developed the Anaesthetic Theatre Educational Environment Measure (ATEEM). The items included in STEEM are outlined in Box 32.6.

Riquelme *et al.* (2013) have developed the Ambulatory Care Learning Education Environment Measure (ACLEEM), which has eight factors: Teachers; Clinical Activities and Patient Care; Protected Time; Infrastructure; Clinical Skills; Assessment and Feedback; Information, Communication and Technology; and Clinical Supervision.

Developing Educational Environment Measures for Veterinary Medical Education

The "utility index" suggested by van der Vleuten (1996) has been widely accepted as a framework for assessment design and evaluation, and its five elements of Education × Validity × Reliability × Cost × Acceptability are, in many ways, a generic formula for constructing and introducing all educational strategies. Therefore, these factors should be included in

Box 32.6: Focus on the Surgical Theatre Educational Environment Measure (STEEM)

- My trainer has a pleasant personality
- I get on well with my trainer
- My trainer is enthusiastic about teaching
- My trainer has a genuine interest in my progress
- I understand what my trainer is trying to teach me
- My trainer's surgical skills are very good
- My trainer gives me time to practise surgical skills in theatre
- My trainer immediately takes the instruments away when I do not perform well
- Before the operation my trainer discusses the surgical technique planned
- Before the operation my trainer discusses what part of the procedure I will perform
- My trainer expects my surgical skills to be as good as his/hers
- My trainer gives me feedback on my performance
- My trainer's criticism is constructive
- On this unit the type of operations performed are too complex for my level
- The elective operating list has the right case mix to suit my training
- There are far too many cases on the elective list to give me the opportunity to operate
- I get enough opportunity to assist
- There are enough theatre sessions per week for me to gain the appropriate experience
- More senior trainees take my opportunities to operate
- The number of emergency procedures is sufficient for me to gain the right operative experience

- The variety of emergency cases gives me the appropriate exposure
- My trainer is in too much of a rush during emergency cases to let me operate
- I miss out on operative experience because of restrictions on working hours
- I have the opportunity to develop the skills required at my stage
- The atmosphere in theatre is pleasant
- In theatre I don't like being corrected in front of medical students, nurses and residents
- The nursing staff dislike it when I operate as the operation takes longer
- The anaesthetists put pressure on my trainer to operate himself to reduce anaesthetic time
- The theatre staff are friendly
- I feel discriminated against in theatre because of my sex
- I feel discriminated against in theatre because of my race
- I feel part of a team in theatre
- I am too busy doing other work to go to theatre
- I am often too tired to get the most out of theatre teaching
- I am so stressed in theatre that I do not learn as much as I could
- I am asked to perform operations alone that I do not feel competent at
- When I am in theatre, there is nobody to cover the ward
- I get bleeped during operations
- The level of supervision in theatre is adequate for my level
- Theatre sessions are too long

the development of educational environment measures for veterinary medical education. The development of such a measure could include the following stages.

Consideration of Current Tools

- Identify elements within medical educational tools that could apply to veterinary medicine and could be identified as core or "generic"

Box 32.7: How to use the DREEM in veterinary medical education

DREEM might be useful in assessing:

- Learners' perceptions of case-based learning, as introduced by Crowther and Baillie (2015) in a UK preclinical veterinary curriculum.
- The perception of the introduction of a peer support program, as reported by Spielman, Hughes, and Rhind (2015).
- The factors influencing veterinary seminar learning and academic achievement reported

by Ruohoniemi *et al.* (2010) and Sprujit *et al.* (2015).
- Possible relationships between resilience, perceptions of educational environment, and quality-of-life measures, as reported in the medical education literature by Tempski *et al.* (2015) and Enns *et al.* (2015).

---

elements. Identify additional elements specific to veterinary education. Use the core and specific elements to open consensus discussions with appropriate stakeholders in veterinary medical education in, for example, an online Delphi process.
- The international success of a tool relies on global collaboration between educators to ensure that components of the learning environment across national cultures are included.

Psychometric Analysis of the Tool

- Reliability usually cannot be confirmed with the development stage of a new tool. The larger the dataset, the greater robustness of a factor analysis.
- Construct validity must also be addressed.

Costs

- The cost of developing, administering, and analyzing the data yielded by the tools should be considered part of a quality assurance program.

Acceptability

- The acceptability of the tool among various stakeholders should be identified.

Potential uses for a tool developed for veterinary medical education are discussed in Box 32.7.

Conclusion

A learning environment is more than the physical makeup of a space – it is a culture. This culture is constituted by the expectations and values of everyone in the learning community, and yes, it does include the physical space. Determining students' perspectives of their learning environment provides invaluable feedback to a program, since the learning environment influences students' academic progress, mental health, and career goals. Identifying the strengths and weaknesses of a program may inform curriculum review and reform. Additionally, issues regarding the culture within the community can be identified, which may lead to improvement of the overall mental wellbeing of students and faculty. Collaboration and sharing of information regarding the learning environment would help establish best practices that veterinary programs could employ.

References

ACGME (2016) *Resident/Fellow and Faculty Surveys*. Accreditation Council for Graduate Medical Education. http://www.acgme.org/Data-Collection-Systems/Resident-Fellow-and-Faculty-Surveys (accessed November 18, 2016).

AlHaqwi, A.I., Kuntze, J., and van der Molen, H.T. (2014) Development of the clinical learning evaluation questionnaire for undergraduate clinical education: Factor structure, validity, and reliability study. *BMC Medical Education*, **14**, 44.

AMA (2008) Initiative to transform medical education. Strategies for transforming the medical education learning environment. Phase 3: Program implementation. Final report of the December 2008 working conference. American Medical Association, Chicago, IL.

Boor, K., Scheele, F., van der Vleuten, C.P.M., *et al.* (2007) Psychometric properties of an instrument to measure the clinical learning environment. *Medical Education*, **41**, 92–99.

Boor, K., van der Vleuten, C., Teunissen. P., *et al.* (2011) Development and analysis of D-RECT, an instrument measuring residents' learning climate. *Medical Teacher*, **33**, 820–827.

Cassar, K. (2004) Development of an instrument to measure the surgical operating theatre learning environment as perceived by basic surgical trainees. *Medical Teacher*, **26** (**3**), 260–264.

Copeland, H.L., and Hewson, M.G. (2000) Developing and testing an instrument to measure the effectiveness of clinical teaching in an academic medical center. *Academic Medicine*, **75**, 161–166.

Crowther, E., and Baillie, S. (2015) A method of developing and introducing case-based learning to a preclinical veterinary curriculum. *Anatomical Sciences Education, May* **7**, 80–89.

Dornan, T., Muijtjens, A., Graham, J., *et al.* (2012) Manchester Clinical Placement Index (MCPI). Conditions for medical students' learning in hospital and community placements. *Advances in Health Sciences Education*, **17** (**5**), 703–716.

Enns, S.C., Perotta, B., Paro, H.B., *et al.* (2015) Medical students' perception of their educational environment and quality of life: Is there a positive association? *Academic Medicine*, **9** (**3**), 409–417.

Fluit, C.R.M.G., Bolhuis, S., Grol, R., *et al.* (2010) Assessing the quality of clinical teachers: A systematic review of content and quality of questionnaires for assessing clinical teachers. *Journal of General Internal Medicine*, **25** (**12**), 1337–1345.

Freese, J. (2009) Preferences, in *The Oxford Handbook of Analytical Sociology* (eds O. Hedstrom and P. Bearman), Oxford University Press, Oxford, pp. 94–114.

GMC (2013) *Approving Educational Environments*. General Medical Council. http://www.gmc-uk.org/Educational_Environments___May_2013.pdf_52096709.pdf (accessed July 6, 2015)/

GMC (2015) *Promoting Excellence: Standards for Medical Education and Training*. General Medical Council. http://www.gmc-uk.org/Promoting_excellence_standards_for_medical_education_and_training_0715.pdf_61939165.pdf (accessed July 6, 2015).

GMC (2016) *National Training Survey*. General Medical Council. http://www.gmc-uk.org/education/surveys.asp (accessed November 18, 2016).

Holt, M.C., and Roff. S. (2004) Development and validation of the Anaesthetic Theatre Educational Environment Measure (ATEEM). *Medical Teacher*, **26** (**6**), 553–558.

Hughes, K. (2015) Transition points in professional degree programmes: Monitoring the student experience to identify enhancement opportunities. Enhancement and Innovation in Higher Education: Student Transitions Conference, Glasgow, June. http://www.enhancementthemes.ac.uk/docs/paper/transition-points-in-professional-degree-programmes-monitoring-the-student-experience-to-identify-enhancement-opportunities.pdf?sfvrsn=6 (accessed November 20, 2016).

Lave, J., and Wenger, E. (1991) *Situated Learning: Legitimate Peripheral Participation*, University of Cambridge Press, Cambridge.

Merton, R.K. (1957) Some preliminaries to a sociology of medical education, in *The Student-Physician* (eds R.K. Merton, G.G. Reader, and P.L. Kendall), Harvard University Press, Cambridge, MA, pp. 3–79.

Merton, R.K., and Kitt, A. (1950) Contributions to the theory of reference group behavior, in *Continuities in Social Research: Studies in the Scope and Method of "The American Soldier"* (eds R.K. Merton and P.F. Lazarsfeld), Free Press, New York, pp. 40–105.

Park, K.H., Park, J.H., Kim, S., *et al.* (2015) Students' perception of the educational environment of medical schools in Korea: Findings from a nationwide survey. *Korean Journal of Medical Education*, **27** (**2**), 117–130.

Pelzer, J.M., Hodgson, J.L., and Werre, S.R. (2014) Veterinary students' perceptions of their learning environment as measured by the Dundee Ready Education Environment Measure. *BMC Research Notes*, **7**, 170.

PMCV (2016) *Victorian PHEEM Program*. Postgraduate Medical Council of Victoria. http://www.pmcv.com.au/education/pheem/victorian-pheemprogram (accessed November 18, 2016).

Riquelme, A., Herrera, C., Aranis, C., *et al.* (2009) Psychometric analyses and internal consistency of the PHEEM questionnaire to measure the clinical learning environment in the clerkship of a medical school in Chile. *Medical Teacher*, **31** (**6**), e221–e225.

Riquelme, A., Padilla, O., Herrera, C., *et al.* (2013) Development of ACLEEM questionnaire, an instrument measuring residents' educational environment in postgraduate ambulatory setting. *Medical Teacher*, **35**, e861–e866.

Roff, S., McAleer, S., and Skinner, A. (2005) Development and validation of an instrument to measure the postgraduate clinical learning and teaching educational environment for hospital-based junior doctors in the UK. *Medical Teacher*, **27**, 326–331.

Ruohoniemi, M., Parpala, A., Lindblom-Ylänne, S., and Katajavuori, N. (2010) Relationships between students' approaches to learning, perceptions of the teaching–learning environment, and study success: A case study of third-year veterinary students. *Journal of Veterinary Medical Education*, **37** (**3**), 282–288.

Schonrock-Adema, J., Heune-Penninga, M., van Hell, E., and Cohen-Schotanus, J. (2009) Necessary steps in factor analysis: Enhancing validation studies of educational instruments. The PHEEM applied to clerks as an example. *Medical Teacher*, **31**, e226–e232.

Shokoohi, S., Hossein Emami, A., Mohammadi, A., *et al.* (2014) Psychometric properties of the postgraduate hospital educational environment measure in an Iranian hospital setting. *Medical Education Online*, **19**, 245–246.

Silkens, M.E., Smirnova, A., Stalmeijer, R.E., *et al.* (2016) Revisiting the D-RECT tool: Validation of an instrument measuring residents' learning climate perceptions. *Medical Teacher*, **38** (**5**), 476–481.

Spielman, S., Hughes, K., and Rhind, S. (2015) Development, evaluation and evolution of a peer support program in veterinary medical education. *Journal of Veterinary Medical Education*, **42** (**3**), 176–183.

Spruijt, A., Leppink, J., Wolfhagen, I., *et al.* (2015) Factors influencing seminar learning and academic achievement. *Journal of Veterinary Medical Education*, **42** (**3**), 259–270.

Stalmeijer, R.E., Dolmans, D.H.J.M., Wolfhagen, I.H.A.P., *et al.* (2010) The Maastricht Clinical Teaching Questionnaire (MCTQ) as a valid and reliable instrument for the evaluation of clinical teachers. *Academic Medicine*, **85**, 1732–1738.

Strand, P., Borg, K.S., Estalmeijer, R., *et al.* (2013) Development and psychometric evaluation of the Undergraduate Clinical Education Environment Measure (UCEEM). *Medical Teacher*, **35**, 1014–1026.

Tempski, P., Santos, I.S., Mayer, F.B., *et al.* (2015) Relationship among medical student resilience, educational environment and quality of life. *PLoS One*, **10**, 6.

Tsai, J., Chen, C., Sun, I., *et al.* (2014) Clinical learning environment measurement for medical trainees at transitions: Relations with socio-cultural factors and mental distress. *BMC Medical Education*, **14**, 226.

US Department of Veterans Affairs (2016) Surveys. http://www.va.gov/oaa/surveys/ (accessed November 18, 2016).

van der Vleuten, C. (1996) The assessment of professional competence: Developments, research and practical implications. *Advances in Health Sciences Education*, **1** (**1**), 41–67.

Wall, D., Clapham, M., Riquelme, A., *et al.* (2009) Is PHEEM a multi-dimensional instrument? An international persective. *Medical Teacher*, **31** (**11**), e521–e527.

Wenger, E. (1999) *Communities of Practice: Learning*, Meaning and Identity, Cambridge University Press, Cambridge.

Wetzel, A. (2012) Factor analysis methods and validity evidence: A review of instrument development across the medical education continuum. *Academic Medicine*, **87** (**8**), 1060–1069.

Yusoff, M.S.B. (2012) Stability of DREEM in a sample of medical students: A prospective study. Education Resesarch International, Article ID 509638.

33

The Hidden Curriculum

Liz Mossop

School of Veterinary Medicine and Science, University of Nottingham, UK

 Box 33.1: Key messages

- Veterinary students must learn to become professionals as well as develop the knowledge and practical skills necessary to become effective clinicians.
- The hidden curriculum exhibits unseen influence over institutional culture, shaping professional identity formation in our students in positive and negative ways.
- The hidden curriculum consists of aspects of informal learning often delivered through the

behavior of role models and organizational strategy and rituals.
- Educators should consider attempting to analyze the hidden curriculum in their institution to try to identify any negative subconscious learning.
- Strategies such as mentoring schemes, professionalism rituals, and faculty development are important considerations in attempts to shape the hidden curriculum.

Introduction

The student journey through veterinary education is a process of professional identity formation. As well as developing the knowledge and skills necessary to become effective clinicians, students are learning how to behave as a member of the veterinary profession. While the teaching of professionalism and professional skills should include formal instruction, there is a significant body of evidence indicating that the hidden curriculum will contribute as much, if not more, to the formation of a professional

identity. This tacit learning can have either a negative or a positive impact on the professionalism of our students. When designing and implementing veterinary curricula, we must consider the presence of this hidden curriculum, which may be difficult to identify and even more challenging to control.

What Is the Hidden Curriculum?

The emergence of discussions around the hidden curriculum in clinical education began in

---

Veterinary Medical Education: A Practical Guide, First Edition. Edited by Jennifer L. Hodgson and Jacquelyn M. Pelzer.
© 2017 John Wiley & Sons, Inc. Published 2017 by John Wiley & Sons, Inc.

Box 33.2: What's the meaning?

Hidden curriculum: The set of influences that function at the level of organizational structure and culture, including implicit rules required to survive the institution, such as rituals, customs, and taken-for-granted aspects (Lempp and Seale, 2004).

the context of teaching medical ethics to trainee doctors. Hafferty and Franks (1994) recognized that while ethical theory and examples of how doctors should behave could be delivered to students in the classroom in a didactic fashion, this may be completely undone by unseen influences in the hospital environment (see Box 33.2). Once students begin interacting with healthcare professionals, their behavior is likely to be significantly influenced by what they see happening around them. Their attitudes are also influenced by the culture of the broader educational environment in which they are trained. The way in which an educational establishment chooses to behave from an ethical perspective leads to tacit learning by students. The hidden curriculum has the potential to undermine even the best teacher of ethics, so when developing a curriculum of

ethics and professionalism this should be a key consideration.

Conceptualizing the Hidden Curriculum within Other Curricular Components

While the terms informal and hidden curriculum are sometimes used interchangeably, it is useful to consider them separately despite overlap between the two. This is considered in Table 33.1.

The hidden curriculum is often described in the context of other aspects of the curriculum. Harden (2009) separates the taught, learned, and declared curricula, with some overlap. He places the hidden curriculum over the taught component, showing how this is delivered by teachers. It could be argued that the hidden curriculum actually overlays all aspects of his model, because it is also reflected in the declared curriculum (e.g., through educational policies) and learned curriculum (e.g., through students actively learning from a role model). A further representation of this is in Figure 33.1 and Table 33.2.

The hidden curriculum is therefore an important consideration for anyone engaging in educational design, particularly when developing a curriculum of professionalism. If sufficient attention is not paid to the hidden curriculum, then the best-intentioned teaching on professionalism is likely to fail.

Table 33.1 A comparison of the formal, informal, and hidden curricula. Note that overlap occurs between these categories, and the terms are often used interchangeably.

Formal curriculum	Informal curriculum	Hidden curriculum
Timetabled, documented learning opportunities such as lectures and scheduled work placements. Attainment demonstrated through assessment of learning outcomes relating primarily to knowledge and skills.	Informal, unscripted learning opportunities such as might occur in a hospital or on a farm. Attainment not always demonstrated through examination, although outcomes are often embedded in formal learning outcomes.	Tacit, subconscious learning that is usually unrecognized by both student and teacher. Influential behavior and policies contributing to the culture of the learning environment shape student behaviors. Attainment not always demonstrated through examination. Some aspects may not be desirable.

Table 33.2 Conceptualization of different aspects of the curriculum.

Intended curriculum	Delivered curriculum	Assessed curriculum	Received curriculum
Formal teaching and learning as described in course documentation.	What is actually delivered "on the day."	Aspects of teaching and learning that are included in examinations.	What students take away from a teaching event. This includes the hidden curriculum.

Source: Thistlethwaite and Spencer, 2008.

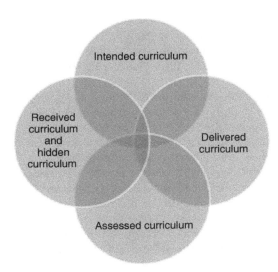

Figure 33.1 Four aspects of the curriculum shown diagrammatically to demonstrate the influence of the hidden curriculum (Thistlethwaite and Spenser, 2008; Harden, 2009).

Development of Ideas about the Hidden Curriculum in Clinical Education

The hidden curriculum was first identified as an important aspect of learning by Jackson (1953), who described the issue in the context of educating children. He recognized that as well as learning knowledge and skills, children went through a process of socialization that strongly influenced their behavior. In other words, they learn their three Rs of "rules, regulation, and routines" as well as reading, writing, and arithmetic. This socialization process is an essential part of a child's development, and the challenge for teachers is ensuring that the outcome is a child who knows how to behave appropriately. This can be difficult, especially when implicit learning conflicts with explicit rules laid out by teachers. The resulting effect can be very challenging to control, as socialization is often a very powerful force in learning.

The classic sociological text *Boys in White* described the hidden curriculum through an ethnographic study of students training in a US medical school during the 1950s (Becker *et al.*, 1961). Much of what was being learned during training was not formally delivered, and these influences were negative as well as positive, shaping the attitudes and behaviors of these future doctors. While the curriculum was attempting formally to encourage proper consideration of ethical dilemmas, the institutional environment and behavior of senior physicians around the students directly conflicted with this learning.

Subsequently there has been a huge amount of publication and discussion around the challenges of the hidden curriculum in medical education. Although there has been less in the context of veterinary education specifically, it is clear that it is no less important in this context, and potentially more so (Whitcomb, 2014). Veterinary practice is often described as a "moral maze," with ethical conflicts regularly occurring in the workplace (Batchelor and McKeegan, 2012). If there is a wish for veterinary students to be able to manage these dilemmas, it is extremely important to consider the

Box 33.3: Where's the evidence for erosion of professional attitudes during clinical training?

Clinical educators will readily identify with the perception of students' attitudes changing during their studies. While it might be hoped that clinical education helps to develop attributes of humanistic professionals, the opposite is certainly true in many educational environments, where the hidden curriculum has a negative impact on students' attitudes. This has been measured in several studies, along with the impact of developing the formal curriculum to try to prevent attitude erosion:

- A cross-sectional study of US medical students in the 1950s found increasing cynicism in fourth-year students compared to freshmen, when assessed using a range of psychometric tests. There was also a suggestion that levels of humanitarianism were decreased in the more advanced cohort surveyed (Eron, 1955).
- Longitudinal testing of medical students' moral reasoning abilities as they progress through a standard curriculum demonstrated a lack of expected improvement that would occur in a standard population of this age (Self *et al.*, 1993).
- The same longitudinal testing was carried out on veterinary students as they progressed

through a standard curriculum with no specific ethics or professionalism teaching. Again, a lack of significant development in moral reasoning skills was recorded (Self *et al.*, 1991).
- A later study of veterinary students undergoing a very short course in veterinary ethics identified a similar lack of development of moral reasoning skills, suggesting that a one-off teaching intervention is not enough to ensure improvement in this aspect of professionalism (Self, Pierce, and Shadduck, 1995).
- Medical students participating in ongoing small-group discussion on ethical issues have, however, been shown to improve their moral reasoning skills at an above-normal rate for their age during progression through the curriculum (Self, Olivarez, and Baldwin, 1998).
- A decline in empathy has been recorded in a longitudinal study of medical students. It was while in their third year of studies that this decline occurred, and the lower levels of empathy were maintained at graduation (Hojat *et al.*, 2009).

hidden curriculum, which will influence their moral development as they learn to become professionals (see Box 33.3).

Situated Learning

When discussing the concept of the hidden curriculum, in effect what we mean is the culture of the environment in which students are learning, and how this may influence their future practice. A useful way to frame this is by consideration of situated learning theory (Lave and Wenger, 1991), which describes how students learn via "legitimate peripheral participation"

in a community of practice such as a hospital. They are learning the "rules of the game" in order that they might fit in seamlessly with the type of behavior happening around them, and be entrusted to carry out tasks. Veterinary students are likely to have to engage with a range of different learning environments, both clinical and nonclinical, encouraging them to, potentially unwittingly, adapt their behaviors accordingly. This may not be a good thing, as the students struggle to establish which of these behaviours is correct. Conflict and stress could be the outcome, leaving educators within the formal curriculum to resolve these difficulties.

The Hidden Curriculum in Workplace Learning

While the hidden curriculum is important in all aspects of veterinary education, veterinary clinics are likely to be the predominant influence on the development of professionalism in students, especially as exposure occurs mostly toward the end of training. The veterinary workplace is a busy, stressful environment, where people make quick decisions and are put under constant pressure to respond to demands from clients and coworkers. Behavior therefore may not always reflect values, and so has the potential to be negative. Resources may also be stretched, or unevenly distributed, and activity like this can further influence the hidden curriculum. It is therefore of particular importance to consider how veterinary students learn in the clinic in order to consider the hidden curriculum and address any issues that it may raise (Scholz, Trede, and Raidal, 2013).

Elements of the Hidden Curriculum

Although it is difficult to define exactly what makes up the hidden curriculum, certain components are frequently considered, particularly when designing a curriculum in its broadest sense. In many ways, the hidden curriculum is the equivalent of an organization's culture, so the model from Johnson (1987) is a useful way to consider its constituent components. This is demonstrated in Figure 33.2.

Role Models

Most veterinary professionals can look back through their career and identify someone who has influenced their choices. Whether this is a charismatic and high-achieving surgeon, or an altruistic shelter veterinarian, their influence may be strong (see Box 33.4). While it may be more challenging to identify someone who has influenced an individual's attitudes to particular situations, learning theories tell us that this is

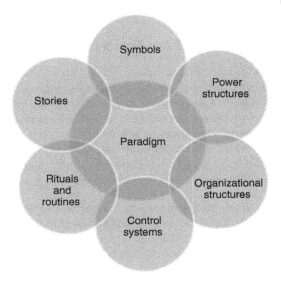

Figure 33.2 The cultural web, a useful way of considering different influential aspects of the educational environment. Source: Johnson, 1987.

almost certainly the case (Lave and Wenger, 1991; Bandura, 1986). As novices develop into experts, they will subconsciously reflect on the attitudes and behaviors of those around them and are very likely to follow their lead, whether their role model is behaving appropriately or not. Positive role models are likely to demonstrate excellence in clinical competence, teaching ability, and their personal attributes (Passi *et al.*, 2013). Negative role models can be failing in one or all of these areas, and are unlikely to recognize the impact that this may have on student development.

The impact of role modeling is therefore clear in many situations. For example, if a resident is judgmental about a certain client who cannot afford to pay for the veterinary treatment offered to them, students may behave this way the next time they see such a client. In contrast, if the resident demonstrates empathy and acts altruistically toward this client, students may be influenced to behave in this more positive fashion in the future. Role models also have the ability to undermine the efforts of the formal curriculum. A good example of this is in the teaching of communication skills.

Box 33.4: Focus on veterinary students' views on role models

Faculty from an Australian veterinary school used a reflective assignment to define attributes of clinical role models (Schull *et al.*, 2012). Final-year students were asked to write a brief account of a positive role model and content analysis was used to identify common themes. While clinical knowledge and skills were commonly cited, communication, teaching skills, and respect towards colleagues and clients were also frequently included. There are many similarities here to attributes established in similar studies in medical education.

Veterinary students may be taught to use the Calgary–Cambridge model of the consultation (Radford *et al.*, 2006), and practice this in role plays with simulated clients. If they then enter the clinical environment and this model is not being implemented, they are likely tacitly to reject this teaching and role model the approach of the clinician they are observing. While this may not necessarily be a poor communication style, it is not helpful for previous teaching that is aimed at novice communicators to be "undone" in this way. Role models therefore influence students not only in career choice, but also in professional behavior and the formation of their professional identity (Passi and Johnson, 2016).

The Role-Modeling Process
While learning theories such as situated learning and social learning help us consider the process of learning from a role model, it is interesting to break down what actually happens during the identification of a role model in order to implement this more formally within the veterinary curriculum. A qualitative study of medical students and senior physicians identified both conscious and subconscious elements to role modeling (Passi and Johnson, 2016). The role-modeling process consists of an exposure phase, where attributes such as communication skills and personality are demonstrated by role models; and an evolution phase, where students observe these behaviors and make a judgment as to whether to engage in them themselves. A model-trialing cycle results, where students experiment with what they have seen and adapt it for their own behavior and attitudes.

Role Modeling and Veterinary Teachers
The daily interactions between veterinary clinicians and veterinary students in the workplace make role modeling an important consideration. Teaching by humiliation and making learners feel embarrassment if they cannot answer questions or perform certain tasks may lead veterinary students to behave in the same way when they become the teacher. If teachers can be encouraged to reflect on their influential position as a role model, then their own teaching skills are likely to improve (Burgess, Oates, and Goulston, 2016). Teacher training is a good way of ensuring that this occurs formally, and veterinary clinicians should be encouraged to engage in programs where reflection is fostered and assessed. Teaching portfolios are an excellent way of helping with this (de Rijdt *et al.*, 2006), and by formally reflecting on their own practice, teachers will prompt students to do the same.

Peer-to-Peer Role Modeling
Role modeling also occurs on a peer-to-peer basis, with students learning about appropriate behavior from each other. If a certain veterinary student is consistently late and rude to teachers, other students may tacitly learn that this is normal behavior, and copy it themselves. It is therefore important that such behavior is not seen to be condoned. The monitoring of this type of low-level unprofessionalism can be

brought into the formal curriculum through systems such as the conscientiousness index (McLachlan, Finn, and MacNaughton, 2009), where students are rated consistently on objectively measurable aspects of their behavior such as timekeeping and communication. Peer mentoring systems are an excellent method of helping students to demonstrate high standards of professional behavior and to encourage peers to do the same.

Moving Role Modeling into the Formal Curriculum

Role modeling has huge potential to have a strong positive influence on students if veterinary educators encourage the concept in a more formal way (Kenny, Mann, and MacLeod, 2003), moving it from the hidden to the informal or formal curriculum. Students can be asked to identify aspects of behavior in the clinicians around them and reflect on both positive and negative attributes. They can also be required within the formal curriculum to identify an individual as a role model and approach them to be a mentor. The mentor–mentee relationship should include discussion about career path, but should also encourage reflection on difficult situations that the student may have experienced.

Institutional Policies

Formal regulations laid out by a veterinary education establishment can unwittingly influence students through the hidden curriculum. While there are many unseen rules to navigate, faculty should seek to ensure that more explicit documents such as codes of conduct and assessment regulations are fair and transparent. If this is not the case, then students could learn to resist authority, which may not be a good thing.

A pertinent example of this is the use of animals in research and teaching by veterinary schools. It is extremely important that students can see that the decision to use animals in this way has been through a robust and transparent ethical review process. If this has not occurred, and students perceive the use of animals as

unnecessary, then they may rebel against the school's authority and lose respect for the leadership. Although this may be necessary to incite change, if the school behaves unethically and students see this as normal, they may do the same in their future career, jeopardizing their position as a veterinarian. A further example of the necessary questioning of authority is in the context of patient safety (Leonard, Graham, and Bonacum, 2004). If the hierarchy is such in a clinical team that a student feels they cannot speak out when they witness an error, this may have a negative impact on animal welfare. The culture of a clinical environment should therefore be conducive to allowing this, which should be reflected in formal rules and regulations.

Language

The "institutional slang" that permeates throughout veterinary schools is considered to be part of the hidden curriculum (Hafferty, 1998). There is certainly a strong inclination for schools to develop their own language, which is often full of acronyms and abbreviations. The same is true of the clinical environment, which can be completely foreign to an outsider such as a new student beginning a clinical placement. The process of learning this language becomes part of the enculturation into this environment, and this can be challenging if no assistance is forthcoming. The tone of this language is also influential: there has been a concern that the marketization of higher education has led to increasing use of business language among faculty, which may deliver the wrong message to students. If students become very consumerist, then they may approach learning in a surface way, and fail to view their education as the partnership it should be (Kahu, 2013). This is concerning, because it could influence students in a nonhumanistic manner (Hafferty, 1998). While students need to learn about the business aspects of veterinary practice, there is an argument that this should be done through the formal curriculum so that negative tacit learning is prevented.

Equally, the overall tone of language can potentially influence student professionalism negatively if challenging issues are made light of. A culture of "gallows humor" – derogatory or cynical language, often seen as a coping mechanism for the management of ongoing interaction with death and the dying – can have a strong negative impact on developing professionals (Piemonte, 2015). It is important to ensure that students can recognize when this type of language may or may not be appropriate, and that it does not cause harm by being misinterpreted (Wear *et al.*, 2009).

Resources

Veterinary schools have to make daily decisions about the allocation of resources. In addition, they may attract sponsors who have a specific stance on a certain ethical issue. Actions taken in this respect will contribute to the hidden curriculum, and care must be taken that this does not influence students in a negative way. For example, a drug company may sponsor a seminar or gift for clinicians. A process should be in place to ensure that such things are declared properly, so that conflicts of interest do not arise (Katz, Caplan, and Merz, 2010). Schools should allocate resources fairly and transparently, so that students do not perceive unfairness and normalize this as a behavior seen in an environment they trust.

Rituals

The importance of professionalism-related rituals such as "white coat ceremonies" has been widely described in medical education (Wear, 1998; Huber, 2003). These events put the focus on the transition to becoming a professional and encourage students to focus on attributes of professionalism, through both the informal and hidden curricula. However, there are other rituals that occur throughout veterinary school that form part of the hidden curriculum. Social and sporting events involving students and faculty are an important aspect of this. Faculty must be aware that even in this environment their

behavior may be role modeled by students, so professionalism must be maintained. Equally, attitudes regarding an appropriate work–life balance can also be demonstrated by engaging in out-of-school social events with students.

Analyzing the Hidden Curriculum

While the elements described in this chapter will almost certainly be present in all veterinary schools and contribute to their hidden curriculum, identifying their exact nature can be extremely challenging. However, this is an important process to carry out in order to consider both positive and negative aspects of the learning environment. There is no established methodology (Tekian, 2009), but any process of discussion of learning and teaching is likely to reveal some parts of the hidden curriculum.

Student narratives, obtained through interview or diary writing, can be an insightful way to reveal their development as a professional, and these have been used in several studies. When students are asked to reflect verbally on an experience related to professionalism from the clinical environment, common themes such as respect, communication, responsibility, and altruism emerge (Karnieli-Miller *et al.*, 2010). When they are asked specifically to focus on negative experiences, issues such as emotional suppression, clinical limitations, hierarchy, and sacrifice are readily identified (Gaufberg *et al.*, 2010). It is also important to involve faculty in collection of this qualitative data, and focus groups have been used in several studies to collect information relating to the hidden curriculum (Doja *et al.*, 2015; Mossop *et al.*, 2013). Observational studies can also be undertaken to attempt to establish what actually occurs during teaching moments, especially within the clinical environment. These studies may identify negative issues such as poor professional behavior, including the way teachers treat students (Shea, Bellini, and Reynolds, 2000), but they can also identify positive attributes such as staying

Box 33.5: How to identify aspects of the hidden curriculum through survey analysis

While qualitative approaches have been used most widely in analysis of the hidden curriculum, these are expensive and time-consuming methods that may not be practical in many veterinary schools. Survey instruments are an alternative method of gaining feedback from students on their educational environment, and although these may not focus specifically on the hidden curriculum, certain aspects can be assessed by inference from the results of using these tools.

Example 1
The Dundee Ready Education Environment Measure (DREEM; Roff *et al.*, 1997) aims to assess the educational climate by asking students to respond to 50 Likert-scale questions covering all aspects of teaching and learning. The questions relating to atmosphere are particularly relevant.

This tool is fully validated and can be a useful preliminary step in uncovering the hidden curriculum in a veterinary school (Pelzer, Hodgson, and Werre, 2014), although normally only students are asked to complete surveys, limiting the scope of the findings.

Example 2
A second survey tool has been developed at a UK veterinary school for analysis of views of professionalism from both faculty and student perspectives (Roder, Whittlestone, and May, 2012). The tool is based on aspects of the veterinary role extracted from Castellani and Hafferty's (2006) medical professionalism roles. By seeking perceptions of professional behavior from veterinary professionals working in one environment, an insight into the hidden curriculum can be achieved.

late with patients when they do not have to (Stern, 1998) (see Box 33.5).

Developing and Utilizing the Hidden Curriculum

The hidden curriculum is a powerful influence on the professional development of students. It therefore makes sense to attempt to harness this influence and ensure that it is a positive one, because the effects are likely to be long-lasting. While identifying the nature of a hidden curriculum is challenging, correcting deficits and ensuring a positive culture are probably even more difficult. That will require a huge amount of institutional time and resource, and very strong leadership (see Boxes 33.6 and 33.8).

A Cautionary Note

Even if it were possible to ensure that the hidden curriculum of an educational environment is

entirely positive in its influences, this may not be a sensible strategy. Veterinary students will enter the workplace on graduation and immediately encounter a huge number of challenges to their professionalism. In order to cope with this transition, it is important that they have previous experience of working with peers and veterinarians where difficult situations arise. Through these situations their reflective skills will develop, an essential component of professionalism (Maudsley and Strivens, 2000). Sterilization of the learning environment should therefore be avoided, and while a positive environment can be encouraged, the focus should be on developing students' reflective skills so that they can recognize and negotiate complex situations.

Faculty Development

When instigating a program of hidden curriculum analysis and development, faculty development is key. There is little point in spending time and money trying to address aspects of the learning environment if faculty do not understand what is being attempted. Education around the teaching and learning of professionalism is therefore essential (Goldie *et al.*, 2007), and in particular recognition of influence over students as a role model must be included. Faculty should be encouraged to develop the attributes of positive role models such as clinical competence, excellent teaching skills, and a positive attitude, meaning that a broad faculty development program is required (Cruess, Cruess, and Steinert, 2008). Training in specific elements of professionalism such as cultural competence – the ability to work with students and clients from all cultural backgrounds – will be helpful (Thistlethwaite and Spencer, 2008). Development of reflective skills is also important to encourage faculty to recognize their personal impact on student behavior and develop their own professionalism. Leadership is key to this type of approach, with a consortium of engaged faculty and students to drive the process forward (Hafferty and Franks, 1994).

Student Engagement

Involving students in analysis and subsequent development of the educational environment is key to the success of such an initiative. Embedding students as partners in their learning means that they must be involved in institutional change, especially around teaching initiatives. Very successful programs using "students as agents of change" are run in many UK higher education establishments (Kay, Dunne, and Hutchinson, 2010). These programs are an excellent way to break down barriers and hierarchies between faculty and students, and engender respect. Students are encouraged to lead projects looking at different aspects of their educational experience, supported by faculty. By doing so they develop key professional skills, and there is a resulting influence on the hidden curriculum through faculty forming new relationships of respect and trust with the change agents.

Student feedback on faculty can also be a helpful way to shape the hidden curriculum. Students can be encouraged to question faculty directly about their behaviors and attitudes, although careful training would be needed to implement this successfully (Doukas, 2004). It may be more appropriate to collate constructive student criticism about faculty members' professional behavior and feed this back in a reflective conversation with a peer, allowing time for discussion and development (Szauter and Turner, 2001).

Mentoring

Mentoring is a method of utilizing positive role models and engaging in a dialog of reflection and

---

Box 33.6: Focus on applying organizational change principles to enhance the hidden curriculum

Principles from studies of organizational culture can be usefully applied in the context of an educational environment in order to consider a change process to positively influence the hidden curriculum of a veterinary school.

- External forces, which can act as barriers or catalysts to change, include student ("customer") requirements of their education, educational competitors, and expectations of society. These require analysis and consideration as

a change process is implemented (Gordon, 1991).

- Three processes needed to bring about organizational change have been described: the creation of a shared vision by faculty and students, a sense of ownership of the change process by all involved, and development of key competencies in individuals implementing the change in culture (Hackett, Lilford, and Jordan, 1999).

Box 33.7: How to develop and implement a mentoring scheme

While role models have the potential to be negative, it is more likely that they will be positive when encouraged through a system of formal mentoring. The following points may be useful for faculty intending to develop a mentoring scheme:

- Development of the scheme should be a joint initiative utilizing enthusiastic faculty and students.
- Mentors should be aware of how influential they can be on their mentees.
- Mentors will require training and potentially debriefing, depending on the scope of the scheme.
- Mentors can be faculty members or peers in a more advanced stage of training.

- Clear boundaries should be defined in an early meeting.
- The aims of the mentoring scheme should be made clear to participants on both sides, as should the amount of time expected to be committed to the scheme.
- As well as face-to-face discussion between mentors and mentees, remote mentoring can also be helpful, for instance via e-mail.
- A basic framework for discussion during meetings can be offered by the scheme leader, including discussion topics around challenging aspects of professionalism, such as altruism.
- Previous mentees often make great mentors in future versions of the scheme.

development. A formal scheme, implemented as a joint initiative between faculty and students, is an excellent way of influencing the hidden curriculum if performed appropriately (Larkin, 2003) (see Box 33.7).

Professionalism-Focused Rituals

Events and formal occasions focusing on humanistic values as part of the formal curriculum have a potential positive influence on the hidden curriculum. While the use of white coat

Box 33.8: Where's the evidence from medical education for developing the hidden curriculum

A case study from Indiana University School of Medicine shows how it is possible to use principles from organizational culture change to reshape an institution's hidden and informal curricula, in order to align these aspects of the educational environment with a newly developed formal curriculum (Cottingham *et al.*, 2008).

- Principles of emergent design were used to encourage an iterative approach to change, involving the project team working with different members of the organization.
- Appreciative inquiry encouraged faculty to focus on success and positive aspects

of the educational culture, motivating the organization for further change.
- A focus on the impact of local small-scale behavior and how this can change large-scale behavior was used to promote contribution and participation in desirable behaviors.
- A range of changes were gradually implemented, covering all aspects of management and teaching within the school. The focus on positive behaviors gathered momentum and student feedback improved greatly.

ceremonies has been criticized because they are not a "quick fix" for a negative hidden curriculum (Wear, 1998), there is certainly value in including formal events such as these, in order to raise the institutional profile of the professionalism aspect of learning to be a clinician (Huber, 2003). It must be made clear to students that anything involving a celebration of their new status as a veterinary student is not a departure from responsibilities, and there should be high-profile inclusion of the importance of humanistic values and a commitment to animal welfare. Other formal events can also be used to highlight the importance of professionalism, such as award ceremonies recognizing these values alongside more traditional achievements such as academic performance.

Formal Professionalism Teaching

Development of a formal curriculum of professionalism and professional skills in an institution with a problematic hidden curriculum will not solve the issue of negative socialization of students, but it is a helpful step and shows that the institution is considering this aspect of learning to become a veterinarian. However, it is important that this learning is held in high regard by students and faculty, and it will therefore need careful planning and almost certainly assessment of attainment (Cruess and Cruess, 2006). The best-intentioned professionalism curriculum will otherwise fail. The hidden curriculum is strongly influenced by the attitude of those implementing the formal curriculum.

Conclusion

There is no doubting the importance of unseen influences on students passing through the veterinary curriculum; the challenge for faculty is identifying this subconscious learning and shaping the teaching where possible. While an entirely positive hidden curriculum should not be the intention, engaging in organizational change strategies can help faculty and students identify and shape their tacit learning. When this is combined with a formal curriculum of professionalism, students should develop into humanistic veterinary professionals who are likely to influence future students in the same way. It is therefore essential that the hidden curriculum is considered during curricular design and review processes – it may be hidden, but it should not become forgotten.

References

Bandura, A. (1986) *Social Foundations of Thought and Action: A Social Cognitive Theory*, Prentice Hall, Englewood Cliffs, NJ.

Batchelor, C., and McKeegan, D. (2012) Survey of the frequency and perceived stressfulness of ethical dilemmas encountered in UK veterinary practice. *Veterinary Record*, **170**, 19.

Becker, H.S., Geer, B., Hughes, E.C., and Strauss, A.L. (1961) *Boys in White*, University of Chicago Press, Chicago, IL.

Burgess, A., Oates, K., and Goulston, K. (2016) Role modelling in medical education: The importance of teaching skills. *Clinical Teacher*, **13** (**2**), 134–137.

Castellani, B., and Hafferty, F.W. (2006) The complexities of medical professionalism: A preliminary investigation, in *Professionalism in Medicine: Critical Perspectives* (eds D. Wear and J.M. Aultman), Springer, New York, pp. 3–23.

Cottingham, A., Suchman, A., Litzelman, D., *et al.* (2008) Enhancing the informal curriculum of a medical school: A case study in organizational culture change. *Journal of General Internal Medicine*, **23**, 715–722.

Cruess, R.L., and Cruess, S.R. (2006) Teaching professionalism: General principles. *Medical Teacher*, **28**, 205–208.

Cruess, S.R., Cruess, R.L., and Steinert, Y. (2008) Role modelling: Making the most of a powerful teaching strategy. *British Medical Journal*, **336**, 718–721.

see Dyrbye *et al.*, 2005), dental (for a review, see Elani *et al.*, 2014), pharmacy (Ford *et al.*, 2014), and veterinary medical training (Kelman, 1978; Elkins, 1984; Gelberg and Gelberg, 2005; Hafen *et al.*, 2008), with findings indicating that students in demanding training programs are at risk of poor mental health outcomes.

Veterinary medical training involves remarkable rewards, but also numerous challenges. It has been described as a rigid, prescriptive program, where coursework is predetermined, credit loads maximized, and students perceive their lives as externally controlled (Zenner *et al.*, 2005). In addition to the information overload, high expectations, and constant evaluations, students also face the challenges of balancing animal and human interests, and the emotional aspects of patient and client care (Williams *et al.*, 2005).

As veterinary students become immersed in training, academic activities become a priority and all significant aspects of students' lives become dependent on program demands. Students lack time to manage their personal needs effectively, and distress may occur as they attempt to balance all aspects of their lives. Such intensity can quickly lead to exhaustion, and for some, veterinary medical training is experienced as a chronic stressor.

Common Stressors for Veterinary Medical Students

Common sources of stress identified by students include academic, intrapersonal, and interpersonal challenges. Academic demands are, as would be expected, the most common student-identified stressor, given the requirements of veterinary medical training, and include the amount of material to study, feeling behind in studies, studying from exam to exam without taking time to learn material, relevance of material to be studied, and unclear instructor expectations (Kelman, 1978; Williams *et al.*, 2005; McLennan and Sutton, 2005; Hafen *et al.*, 2006; Siqueira-Drake *et al.*, 2012; Reisbig *et al.*, 2012).

The rich and challenging academic environment can also create intrapersonal challenges. For instance, Zenner and colleagues (2005) dubbed veterinary students "elite performers," and discussed the challenges of transitioning into elite levels of training, such as veterinary medical training. Veterinary students are commonly a group of individuals who are high-achieving, academically gifted, accustomed to routinely outperforming peers and to having their self-worth heavily associated with performance-based positive social comparison (confidence equals outperforming others). The transition into veterinary training presents a new reality, where students become immersed in a group of academic equals or superiors. This experience is likely to confront their abilities to cope, and lead them to question their abilities and personal worth.

Some students may adjust expectations of themselves and of peers accordingly and cope appropriately when confronted with the transition to professional training. Another possible reaction is experiencing the "impostor phenomenon" (IP; Clance and Imes, 1978), or the internal experience of feeling an intellectual fraud (Bernard, Dollinger, and Ramaniah, 2002), chronically questioning one's abilities (Henning, Ey, and Shaw, 1998), and believing that one's accomplishments were the result of luck, manipulating impressions, or error (Longford and Clance, 1993). IP is associated with trait anxiety, constant fear that others will find out that the student is a fraud, and precarious self-esteem related to achievement, depression, and high neuroticism, and has been found to be common among individuals in professional training such as human medicine, veterinary medicine, dentistry, pharmacy, and nursing (Longford and Clance, 1993; Henning, Ey, and Shaw, 1998; Bernard, Dollinger, and Ramaniah, 2002). Clearly, students' responses to the transition to professional training and the support that they have available can present opportunities for personal growth or for continued challenges.

Interpersonal challenges involve relationships within and outside academic training. As students transition into a professional training program, they also manage life transitions common to young adulthood. These include family stress such as illness, loss, or death of loved ones; relational stress, including personal relationship conflict (Hafen *et al.*, 2013) and difficulty fitting in with peers (Hafen *et al.*, 2006; Sutton, 2007); and transitional stress, such as homesickness (Hafen *et al.*, 2008; Reisbig *et al.*, 2012; Hafen, Ratcliffe, and Rush, 2013). Thus, as students pursue veterinary medical training, they are confronted with difficulties in managing both personal and professional interests. Outcomes will be dependent on students' appraisal of these challenges, the resources they have available, and the coping strategies they use to manage the challenges.

Conducting Research on Veterinary Student Wellbeing: Requirements and Challenges

Social science research, such as investigations regarding veterinary students' wellbeing, is subject to ethical rules for research involving human subjects, including review by an Institutional Review Board (IRB) ensuring that the principles of voluntary participation, harmlessness, anonymity, and confidentiality are preserved (Bhattacherjee, 2012). Self-report surveys are the most common medium for information-gathering in social sciences, and include standardized assessments and/or researcher-constructed assessments. These are completed electronically or in paper–pencil format. In the context of social science research, four common challenges may arise: low response rates, nonselection bias, participants' misrepresentation or omission of information, and timing of data collection.

Low Response Rates

As a general consensus, response rates lower than 50% are considered inadequate (Babbie, 1998), although other writers propose more conservative standards, suggesting that 70% (Bailey, 1987) or even 75% response rates may

more adequately safeguard data from response bias (Schutt, 1999). Thus, high response rates are highly desirable, since representative samples increase the reliability of findings.

Nonselection Bias

Nonselection bias occurs when students who volunteer to complete surveys may exhibit different characteristics compared with those who do not, influencing the results. This is another reason why representative samples are important.

Participants' Omission of Information

Although ethical standards mandate that research participants' identities are protected, students may distrust that researchers will preserve their confidentiality or anonymity. Fear of being identified from survey responses and experiencing stigmatization or repercussions may restrict participants' willingness to participate in research studies and their ability to respond honestly. Thus, research designs that include data-collection methods that safeguard participants' identities can garner better data.

Timing of Data-Gathering Efforts

Students' academic schedules fluctuate in terms of increased versus lower demands, which can also influence research findings. Some planning is necessary to identify a data-collection period that is least likely to be influenced by extenuating circumstances that would mask students' experience, such as the enthusiasm or anxiety of the first week of classes or the pressures of final examinations. Thus, developing research designs that minimize these issues is imperative.

Certain strategies have been put into practice to address common challenges, such as providing a meal at the time of data collection to encourage student participation (Strand, Zaparanick, and Brace, 2005), and following an anonymous survey protocol (Reisbig *et al.*, 2007) intended to promote high response rates and minimize threats to internal validity.

What We Know about Veterinary Student Stress

While the demands of veterinary medical training make stress an ever-present feature of training, not all students experience these challenges and stress in the same manner. Early studies on veterinary student wellbeing focused on documenting students' reports of stressors and their intensity, with variable findings. For instance, three studies found that veterinary students were not under inordinate amounts of stress. Kelman (1978) surveyed over 200 veterinary students from Colorado State University College of Veterinary Medicine (CVM), and concluded that "most students did not appear to experience exorbitant strain" (p. 150). Powers (2002) surveyed over 800 first-year veterinary students from several US CVMs (response rate 38%), finding that only a small number of participants (4%) considered the academic requirements too demanding, and half of the sample indicated perceiving their first year as "not too stressful." Finally, Moore and colleagues (2007) investigated the effects of a student leadership program and leadership activities on student stress and academic performance with a sample of over 200 students from the University of California–Davis CVM. Findings indicate that despite having greater time commitments due to their participation in leadership activities, students experienced fewer stressors (objective stress) and perceived themselves to be under less stress (subjective stress) than the general population. Conversely, a study examining 57 students in the fourth and fifth years of veterinary training at Murdoch University in Australia (response rate 41%) indicated that students experienced a moderate amount of stress: 40% agreed to feeling "overwhelmed" trying to balance study, work, and nonworking life, and two-thirds of the sample agreed or strongly agreed to feeling "panicked about assessments" (Williams *et al.*, 2005). None of these studies reported whether the findings differed by gender.

Early studies investigating the prevalence of stress illustrate the variability of experiences within veterinary training, as well as the challenges in assessing student stress. Low response rates and different measures of stress utilized in studies hinder comparisons, generalizations to the population, and the reliability of findings. However, these studies' findings likely describe the diversity in veterinary medical students' experiences, ranging from "not too stressed" to "panicked" or "overwhelmed."

Beyond Stress

While it is helpful to understand the prevalence and intensity of veterinary students' stress, mixed findings likely reflect the variability in veterinary medical students' experiences (see Box 43.2). It is safe to say that veterinary training is likely to bring a certain level of pressure and strain to students, but the way in which students perceive and cope with the stress varies. More recent studies, however, have shifted the focus from identifying stress to looking into student outcomes that may be associated with stress. For instance, there is a clear association between stressful life events and the onset of depressive symptomology (Kendler, 1999). While not all individuals who face stressful situations develop depression symptoms, it is likely that those who experience depression symptoms after a stressful life event have greater vulnerability to doing so. Current scholarship in mental health and risk factors for psychological distress indicate that stress is a common precursor to psychological distress, particularly depression, substance abuse (Fahlke et al., 2000) , suicide (Feskanitch *et al.*, 2002), and, to a smaller extent, anxiety (Uliasek *et al.*, 2010). Some authors argue that the chronic stress of a rigorous academic training such as medical training – or, possibly, veterinary medical training – may suffice in precipitating the development of psychological distress and psychopathology (Smith *et al.*, 2007).

Depression and Anxiety

Depression is defined as experiencing a lack of interest or enjoyment in daily activities, and may include changes in appetite or weight, alterations in sleep patterns, decreased energy, feelings of worthlessness, difficulty concentrating, and suicidal thoughts (DSM V; APA, 2013). Individuals who are depressed often express feeling sad, hopeless, "down in the dumps," or "blah." In addition to an absence of or blunted feelings, individuals may also experience increased irritability. *Anxiety* is characterized by an "apprehensive anticipation of future danger or misfortune" that is accompanied by emotional disruption or physical tension (DSM V; APA, 2013). An example of this might be a student who fears failing an exam and experiences tension headaches, trouble sleeping, and racing thoughts of worry. Women are more likely to experience depression and anxiety, being one and a half to three times more likely to experience depression, and twice as likely to experience anxiety (DSM V; APA, 2013).

While previous findings regarding the severity of stress experienced by veterinary medical students are varied, often indicating that students' stress is not too intense, studies investigating mental health outcomes associated with stress present a more concerning outlook. For instance, Strand, Zaparanick, and Brace (2005) surveyed a sample of almost 300 students from all four years of veterinary training from the University of Tennessee CVM (response rate 55%). Their findings partially support previous studies on student stress in that, objectively, veterinary students were not managing higher stress than the general population. However, Strand, Zaparanick, and Brace (2005) also found that students experienced greater time pressure and, most importantly, subjective stress and depression symptoms when compared to the general population. They also found that women were more likely to experience higher levels of perceived stress, time pressure, anxiety, and depression than men. While it is reassuring that veterinary students in this study did not experience more objective stress when compared with the general population, it is concerning that students' subjective experience of stress was more pronounced; particularly as subjective

stress can be a superior predictor of distress and psychopathology when compared to objective stress (Solomon, Mikulincer, and Hobfoll, 1987). However, this study's most important contribution is the finding that students' depression rates surpass those found in the general population. This concerning finding has been replicated by several studies since then.

Hafen and colleagues (2006) surveyed a sample of 93 first-year students at Kansas State University (response rate 90%) on their experience of stress, depression, and anxiety symptoms. Their findings were alarming: one-third of their sample of first-year veterinary students were experiencing clinical levels of depression symptoms, as well as elevated anxiety scores. Certain stressors that students identified as "slightly stressful" were more powerful predictors of distress than stressors that students considered "very stressful." Conversely, stressors that students identified as "very stressful" were not necessarily predictive of distress (see Box 34.2). For instance, students endorsed financial concerns, academic performance, time spent studying, and heavy workload as their most important stressors. However, those who perceived their physical health to be poor, or experienced homesickness, unclear instructor expectations, feeling behind in studies, and worried about not being as smart as others, were statistically more likely to experience anxiety and depression symptoms, making these stressors superior predictors of distress. These findings were consistent regardless of gender. This study made two important contributions to the literature examining veterinary medical student wellbeing. First, it was the first time that a study with a representative sample provided prevalence rates for depression symptoms in a sample of veterinary students. Second, it established the difference between student-identified stressors and stressors that are predictive of student distress, based on statistical predictions.

Reisbig and colleagues (2012) utilized the same surveys and procedures as Hafen *et al.* (2006), surveying three cohorts of veterinary students from two CVMs during the first three time points. Students in the first few years of the curriculum do not recognize their own needs in career development and may be unaware or unrealistic about financial considerations (Fish and Griffith, 2014; Carr and Greenhill, 2015). Information regarding career opportunities, career development, and financial planning should be compulsory, regardless of student expectations (Fish and Griffith, 2014). During the final year, most students have a career plan, and seek faculty and administrative support to select electives, identify employment opportunities, prepare application materials, and review position contracts.

Some examples follow of programs or curricula to address students' career development needs implemented by institutions. Many CVMs provide such activities for their students.

Orientation

Family members attend a half-day session designed to strengthen awareness of the rigors of veterinary school and opportunities in the profession. Interactive lectures provide information on traditional and nontraditional careers, expectations for student performance (time commitment, academic standards, attrition), and student services (mental health, financial planning). Data from graduating classes is presented to highlight the range of career paths, average educational debt, and average starting salaries. Family members learn about debt forgiveness programs and expectations for change in career focus.

Year 1: Career Course

Most CVMs deliver a first-semester course that outlines the range of careers in veterinary medicine. Veterinary students often (>50%) reconsider their career plans during the first semester, and career courses appear to contribute to their reassessment (Fish and Griffith, 2014). The range of speakers on these courses changes to meet the needs of the profession. Recently, emphasis has shifted toward careers in public practice (Kedrowicz, Fish, and Hammond, 2015), and lectures to strengthen awareness of financial issues, debt forgiveness programs, and mental health. The final lecture is focused on developing a curriculum vitae (CV) and strategic planning to strengthen employment candidacy at the time of graduation (see Box 34.3). First-year students are asked to construct a CV during winter break to facilitate documentation of their professional school accomplishments. Detailed instructions and a template CV are provided.

 ## Box 34.3: Focus on the Curriculum Vitae

- Veterinary students and employers recognize an increasing need for new graduates to distinguish themselves for candidacy in the workplace (Lord, Brandt, and Newhart, 2013).
- The CV is the cornerstone of every employment application; employers evaluate the CV and cover letter for content and communication skills.
- Absent an in-person interview, candidate CVs and letters of reference are the most important materials evaluated for advanced training programs in most medical professions.

- Errors on an applicant's CV, even unintentional, are judged harshly and have a negative impact on candidate credibility.
- The professional CV should be tailored to highlight professional experiences relevant to the position and discipline of interest.
- The vast majority of students (95%) and recent alumni (93%) agree that on-site CV and cover letter assistance should be available to senior students (Lord, Brandt, and Newhart, 2013).

Mentorship Groups

First-year students are divided into small groups by career interest. Interest groups meet monthly with faculty mentors (usually two) throughout the first year to discuss career planning, current events, and case material. A packed lunch is provided. In addition, all first-year students are paired with a sophomore and senior veterinary student to provide peer support and mentoring.

Years 1–3

Career-focused services for underclassmen continue to be important. Changing career goals is common throughout veterinary school, with one-fifth to one-third of students reconsidering their area of interest during each year of the curriculum (Andrus, Gwinner, and Prince, 2006). During the first three years, students are required to complete one-week mentorships in small animal, large animal, and nontraditional practice to strengthen career awareness. To support research interests, salary funding is provided for 12–14 students per year to complete an independent project in a research laboratory over the summer months. For students interested in specialty training, salary funding is available for 10–14 students per year to participate in scholarly activities with a clinical science faculty member throughout their preclinical years (Barbur *et al.*, 2011).

Informational lectures to promote career development are offered to preclinical students on an annual or biennial basis. Lecture topics include CV preparation, letters of intent, interviewing skills/mock interviews, advanced training programs, and the Veterinary Internship and Residency Matching Program (VIRMP) process. Students are encouraged to identify mentors in their interest areas to provide letters of recommendation, one of the most important discriminators for the matching process in all medical professions (Davidson, 2004; Hillebrand *et al.*, 2015). Early introduction of specialty training is purported to strengthen student candidacy for internship and residency programs (Barbur *et al.*, 2011).

To support academic success, upperclassman tutors are available for all students during the first through third years at no cost. Approximately 30 student tutors are identified each year to serve 50–60 students; funding is provided by the dean's office.

Year 3

Veterinary students and recent graduates rank financial planning/budgeting as the third most important student service during veterinary school (Lord, Brandt, and Newhart, 2013). The management course outlines principles of small business management tailored to private practice. In addition, students are required to submit a budget exercise using genuine values for anticipated debt service, living expenses, and projected income. Additional lecture content reviews personal finances, the time value of money, debt management, debt forgiveness, and income-based repayment.

Year 4

Veterinary students and recent graduates rank online employment services and fourth-year externship opportunities as the two most important student services for career success (Lord, Brandt, and Newhart, 2013). Recent graduates rank attributes taught during communication training (integrity, friendliness, and compassion) as the most important skills for easing the transition from veterinary student to practicing veterinarian (Rhind *et al.*, 2011).

At KSU, communication training consists of lectures in each year of the curriculum, special seminars for interested students, and evaluations of student–client interactions by communication specialists during the fourth year. The details are beyond the scope of this chapter and have been previously published (Hafen, Rush, and Nelson, 2009; Hafen, Ratcliffe, and Rush, 2013; Hafen *et al.*, 2015).

CVM administrators provide a range of employment services designed to strengthen student employment candidacy. Fourth-year student résumés are posted online in a searchable database. Senior students, previous

38

Veterinary Medical Education: Envisioning the Future

Cyril R. Clarke and Jennifer L. Hodgson

Virginia-Maryland College of Veterinary Medicine, Virginia Tech, USA

Box 38.1: Key messages

- Changes in veterinary medical education generally parallel those that have occurred in medical education.
- Veterinary educational programs are differentiated by choices made to optimize the balance between the cost of programs, instructional methodology employed, and the mix of elective and prescriptive coursework.
- To achieve their mission in support of animal and public health, veterinary medical educational programs must pay attention to cross-cutting themes of One Health and global reach, diversity, entrepreneurship, continuing education, and accreditation expectations.

- Further erosion of state-appropriated funding will promote efforts to improve the cost-effectiveness of clinical training programs and focus the work assignments of faculty.
- High expectations for the clinical competence of graduates will drive the disciplinary and species emphasis of individual educational experiences.
- Experiential and collaborative learning will be integrated through the curriculum.
- Educational program development will be driven principally by outcomes assessment of vocational competencies.

Introduction

Higher education is being buffeted by disruptive changes in the way universities are funded, the introduction of new technologies for the delivery of instruction, and raised expectations regarding the outcomes of the educational process. Consequently, the educational debt burdens borne by graduates have escalated, the accountability demanded of universities in regard to the cost-effectiveness of educational programs has increased, and renewed emphasis is being placed on experiential learning opportunities, including those available off campus, to ensure that graduates are well prepared to pursue productive careers.

These developments have not occurred overnight, but are the product of an ongoing process that started over 100 years ago. In many respects, the evolution of veterinary medical education has mirrored that of medical education, with the former often following the latter.

Veterinary Medical Education: A Practical Guide, First Edition. Edited by Jennifer L. Hodgson and Jacquelyn M. Pelzer.
© 2017 John Wiley & Sons, Inc. Published 2017 by John Wiley & Sons, Inc.

Envisioning the future of veterinary medical education, therefore, can be facilitated by analysis of recent and anticipated developments in medical education, as these are likely to have predictive relevance. To build a foundation for understanding the current context of change in health sciences education, this chapter will first review substantive developments in medical education precipitated by the Flexner Report, and then relate these and more recent adaptations in medical education to those occurring in veterinary medical education in response to three important strategic planning initiatives.

The historical context undergirding change in health sciences education, however, serves only as a starting point for predicting the future, as there are many new challenges that must be addressed. Considering the complexity of the many factors driving change in higher education and veterinary medical education in particular, future developments are best understood and envisioned using cognitive frameworks that facilitate analysis of the many interacting factors that collectively determine educational outcomes. The framework employed in this chapter to think about the future is organized around three important intersecting dimensions relating to the cost of education, educational content, and instructional methodology. Each of these dimensions intersects with the others, with the result that educational programs can be tailored to achieve optimal outcomes that best suit a particular educational situation.

Irrespective of the choices made in optimizing the balance across these three domains, there are a number of additional cross-cutting themes that cannot be ignored if veterinary medical education is to remain relevant to its mission. Five of these are discussed, including the veterinary profession's commitment to One Health and global reach, the critical importance of entrepreneurship in the delivery of veterinary services, the relevance of diversity to public service, the need to enable postgraduation career transitions, and the role of accreditation.

Once the historical context for the further development of education has been provided and a cognitive framework for thinking about the problem has been proposed (including a brief discussion of cross-cutting themes), this chapter will then use these as a basis for envisioning the future. The emphasis will be on veterinary medical education in the United States, recognizing that there may be different drivers of change elsewhere in the world.

The History of Change in Health Sciences Education

Flexner Revisited

In 1910, Abraham Flexner authored a report to the Carnegie Foundation for the Advancement of Teaching, entitled *Medical Education in the United States and Canada* (Flexner, 1910). Faced with a landscape of medical education characterized by a lack of consistent admissions, curricular, and graduation standards, and dominated by many stand-alone proprietary colleges, he recommended that the number of colleges be reduced to include only those that were affiliated with universities, employed high admissions standards, and trained physicians to practice evidence-based medicine using the scientific method. With the Johns Hopkins Medical School as a model, he proposed that the curriculum be composed of two years of biomedical science instruction followed by two years of clinical training supervised by university-based clinicians. Within two decades of the report's publication, more than half of the medical colleges in operation at the time of the report had closed and most of those remaining were connected with universities, with a curricular structure and educational philosophy that were very similar to many medical colleges of today.

While the Flexner Report is credited with accelerating much-needed change in medical education, concerns have been expressed that the heavy emphasis placed on the structured and sequential learning of the biomedical and clinical sciences, and the commitment to a "hyper-rational" philosophy, failed to recognize the experiential manner in with adults learn

(Kolb, 1984). As a result, more emphasis was placed on the disease rather than the patient, and on the teacher rather than the student. In their call for the reform of medical education, also commissioned by the Carnegie Foundation and published exactly 100 years after the Flexner Report, Irby, Cooke, and O'Brien (2010) recommended that learning outcomes be standardized, but that the learning process be individualized, knowledge and skills be integrated experientially, habits of inquiry and innovation be inculcated in students, and attention be given to development of a professional identity that recognizes the importance of communication and interpersonal skills, ethical and legal understanding, and aspirational goals in performance excellence, accountability, humanism, and altruism. These recommendations were intended to build on those previously proposed by Flexner and to address concerns that the medical profession was not fully meeting the healthcare needs of the US population.

The system of medical education embraced after publication of the Flexner Report and the need to adapt this to more recent changes in healthcare demands are also reflected in the historical development of veterinary medical education. With few exceptions, most veterinary colleges in the United States and Canada adhere to an educational philosophy that is evidence based, and that assumes that knowledge and skills are best learned by layering clinical training acquired in a teaching hospital on top of preclinical education consisting primarily of lectures and laboratories. Both of these characteristics resonate with Flexner's Germanic system of medical education. Also, most veterinary colleges are now part of large, comprehensive research universities, although a few recently established colleges are affiliated with smaller health sciences institutions.

Recent Initiatives Driving Changes in Veterinary Medical Education

With regard to recent adaptations, there have been a number of initiatives over the last 20 years designed to assess the status of veterinary medical education and develop strategies for future development. Three of these are noteworthy, because they were national in scope and engaged in a broad representation of nonacademic and academic constituents. The first of these, entitled *Future Directions for Veterinary Medicine*, was published by the Pew National Veterinary Education Program in 1988 (Pritchard, 1988). Among its 13 recommendations, those addressed to veterinary colleges advised that research be made a focus, that the basic biological science content of the curriculum be strengthened, and that more emphasis be placed on the achievement of diversity. Furthermore, colleges were encouraged to enable students to elect an area of interest focusing on a single species or class of animal, rather than requiring them to gain experience with many animal species, and to shift the emphasis from an almost exclusive concentration on clinical practice to also include public-sector careers. Recommendations in the Pew report relating to the importance of research and basic sciences reaffirmed Flexner's view, whereas those dealing with diversity and elective opportunity appear to be more in line with more recent trends in medical education in support of providing flexibility to the individual learner and broadening the scope of education beyond the diagnosis and treatment of diseases.

The second major strategic analysis of veterinary medical education employed a process called Foresight Analysis and was published in 2007 under the title *Envisioning the Future of Veterinary Medical Education* (Willis *et al.*, 2007). Using a number of scenarios selected to envision the future, teams of veterinary professionals developed recommendations in support of a flexible educational system that would be able to prepare graduates for opportunities and challenges over a 20–25-year timeframe. A recurring theme that was threaded through the key recommendations arising from this study proposed that colleges select areas of professional focus and then collaborate to provide a collective suite of educational programs broader in scope than could be offered by individual institutions. This approach is conceptually similar to the recommendations of the

Pew report regarding the need to allow students to elect areas of practice emphasis.

The third and most recent strategic initiative was conducted by the North American Veterinary Medical Education Consortium (NAVMEC) and published in 2011 (Shung and Osburn, 2011). The report, entitled *Roadmap for Veterinary Medical Education in the 21st Century: Responsive, Collaborative, Flexible*, built on the previous two reports by recommending that students attain proficiency in an agreed set of core competencies, including multispecies knowledge, clinical competence in a selected species or discipline, One Health knowledge, and professional competencies (communication, collaboration, management, lifelong learning, leadership, diversity and multicultural awareness, and adaptation to changing environments). Veterinary schools were encouraged to collaborate to enable students to access the full range of core competencies. Consistent with its emphasis on core competencies, the NAVMEC report recommended that veterinary curricula be competency driven and delivered in a time-efficient and flexible manner. In addition, the report advised that urgent action be taken to address the economic challenges facing veterinary schools and veterinary students, and it encouraged further development of innovative ways to solve these and other problems.

In summary, the impacts of the Flexner Report on the institutional organization, curricular structure, and evidence-based philosophy of medical education are also reflected in veterinary medical education. Similarly, both medical and veterinary medical educational systems are now changing in response to economic, curricular, and societal drivers that are causing a second revolution, approximately 100 years after the first one precipitated by Flexner.

Differentiating Characteristics of Veterinary Medical Education

While it is clear that there are important parallels between developments in medical education and veterinary medical education, there are nevertheless a number of substantive differences. It can be argued that veterinary medical education is differentiated in the field of health sciences in the breadth of knowledge, skills, and abilities that students must possess on graduation, the length of time available to develop competencies, and the expectation that graduates be ready to practice in a wide range of veterinary medical careers immediately on graduation. For example, newly graduated veterinarians are expected to be competent to perform surgery and anesthesia on multiple animal species, conduct and interpret complex diagnostic tests such as digital radiology and necropsy, and provide information that is essential for the health and safety of individual animals, populations of animals, as well as the general public. Furthermore, the rapid expansion of knowledge and the ease with which it can be accessed in the digital era have presented an additional layer of complexity for veterinary educators. Clearly, these challenges must be met by modern curricula that focus on the core knowledge, skills, and behaviors required of all graduates, and that utilize modern methods grounded in educational theory. Curricula that provide additional opportunities for students in their field of interest may help address the breadth of competencies required of veterinary graduates.

The pervasive use of animals during the educational process is another differentiating feature of veterinary medical education, and has presented a number of challenges over the last 50 years due to evolving societal views and regulatory policies. Veterinary colleges have adapted to these challenges by sharing best practices in training their students in the framework of comparative medicine and the needs of society (Lairmore and Ilkiw, 2015). Furthermore, the emerging use of clinical skills laboratories in veterinary education, with a greater emphasis on models and simulations, will continue to refine the use of live animals.

A Framework for Strategic Planning

Review of the themes and issues addressed in the Flexner Report and subsequent strategic analyses of medical and veterinary medical education reveals the relevance of three important questions that can be used to think about the future (see Figure 38.1). These are: What is the cost? What must students learn? How should students be instructed? Each of these questions captures a domain of choices that intersect with those of the other two questions, providing multiple alternative strategies that can be customized to fit a particular veterinary school and its mission.

What is the Cost?

The medical educational system originally promoted by Flexner, consisting of a structured curriculum overseen by formal faculty dedicated primarily to clinical instruction, was recognized to be expensive, and therefore best situated in a major university that had the financial resources necessary for its sustained support. The budgetary structure of most veterinary colleges is even more challenging, because most of the clinical experiential learning generally occurs in veterinary teaching

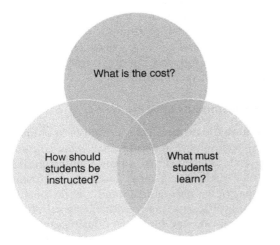

Figure 38.1 Cognitive framework for analysis of veterinary medical educational programs.

hospitals, which seldom are profit centers and which generate much lower service revenues than human hospitals. Attempts to increase the caseload and operational efficiency of these hospitals often carry the risk of diminishing their value as instructional resources, particularly in regard to the development of clinical reflective reasoning skills, which require slower and more deliberate demonstration by experienced faculty. As state allocations to higher education declined over the last decade, veterinary colleges sustained budgets by increasing student enrollment and tuition rates. However, these strategies are no longer viable alternatives for sustaining funding in the future, because of the damaging effects of the resultant educational debt on veterinary graduates and the veterinary profession. Also, while further increases in enrollment will be necessary over the long term to meet the growth in demand for veterinary services, these will be limited in the immediate and intermediate future because of concerns expressed about excess workforce capacity. Considering that other sources of income, such as extramural research grants/contracts and private gifts, generally contribute relatively little to the funding of recurring veterinary medical educational expenses, veterinary schools will have to examine more closely the cost-effectiveness of their educational programs and philosophies. This will involve a reassessment of faculty work expectations, particularly instructional assignments, and a rebalancing of the educational subsidies provided to diagnostic and clinical services that is in line with their instructional value.

What Must Students Learn?

Unlike medical education, which already is highly specialized because of the expectation of establishing a disciplinary focus during the required residencies, the veterinary educational system still assumes that most veterinarians are generalists. However, in reality this is not the experience for a majority of practicing veterinarians. All of the strategic analyses discussed earlier have recommended that the prescriptive attention to comparative biomedical sciences in the curriculum be balanced with elective opportunities to emphasize learning on a single class of animal, species, or nonclinical vocation. Despite these encouragements offered over the last 20 years, most curricula emphasize prescription over election – even tracking curricula generally allow the student to elect only a small portion of their coursework. Concerns have been expressed that a further opportunity for specialization would require segmented licensure, but the experience of physicians who usually specialize but carry general licensure on the basis of their Doctor of Medicine (MD) or Doctor of Osteopathic Medicine (DO) degrees would suggest otherwise.

How Should Students be Instructed?

Research conducted over the last 40 years has laid a firm foundation in support of the merits of student-centered learning as opposed to instructor-centered learning. This style of learning is in alignment with andragogy, as defined by Malcolm Knowles (1970), where the learner is given the opportunity to develop their own educational goals while engaging in learning activities that are directly relevant to their career of interest. This experiential, hands-on, and minds-on approach is best exemplified in the clinical training that occurs in veterinary teaching hospitals and clerkships in nonacademic practices. However, considering that many curricula commit almost all of the first three years to a more instructor-centered approach, as represented by lecture-based courses with little student interaction, veterinary curricula often demonstrate both the best and the worst of instructional methodology, with perhaps all too much emphasis on the latter.

The domains of choices captured by each of these three questions intersect with one another, allowing the selected outcome to be adapted and optimized to fit the particular needs and mission of the veterinary school. For example, a commitment to maximize experiential clinical learning using a student-centered approach has significant cost implications because of the

reliance on teaching hospitals and the high cost of operating these facilities. The cost of clinical training can be managed to some extent by employing nonuniversity clinical facilities, such as private practices, but these distributed learning environments can also be costly because of subsidies provided to secure the commitment of the practices to an academic mission, and the additional administrative support needed to oversee and assess the facilities and student learning. Similarly, a decision to provide more elective opportunities for students to specialize in a particular species or discipline of interest requires the development and maintenance of appropriate areas of strength that align with the respective interest areas, which has cost implications. This challenge could be addressed in part by schools collaborating with one another, each recognizing and taking advantage of its relative areas of strength and need, but there have been few successes in developing and maintaining such partnerships.

Cross-Cutting Themes

Irrespective of the choices made in response to each of the questions dealing with funding, curricular content, and instructional methodology, several cross-cutting themes are preeminently relevant to the future development of veterinary educational programs. These relate to One Health and global reach, entrepreneurship, diversity, postgraduation career transitions, and the role of accreditation.

One Health and Global Reach

Despite the extraordinary advances in biomedical technology, lingering challenges continue to frustrate efforts to advance public health. These include concerns such as healthcare disparities (both animal and public health), chronic diseases (many with microbial etiologies), cancer, emerging infectious diseases, and antimicrobial resistance. In most cases, these challenges involve complex etiologies and interactions in both human and animal populations, living in natural and built environments that are constantly changing in response to factors such as climate change and urban expansion. Solving these health concerns requires the active involvement of veterinarians, who are uniquely trained in principles of comparative biology that are necessary to understand the complicated relationships between animals, people, and their environments. However, to meet this expectation, veterinary educational programs will need to be more intentional in the development and implementation of learning goals addressing population health, the global context of animal and public health, and a basic understanding of data analytics and modeling that goes beyond a superficial review of descriptive epidemiology.

Successful achievement of a One Health approach relies on the implementation of strategies that recruit multiple disciplines and professions in a collaborative effort to understand the involvement of multiple species in disease prevalence from a local to a global scale. Considering the necessity of the experiential context in adult education, access to international experiences is essential.

Entrepreneurship

Given that most graduates for the foreseeable future will earn their living engaging in private practice, and that one of the principal determinants of earning power relates to ownership of a successful practice, it is imperative that graduates be prepared not only to manage these small businesses, but also to compete in the veterinary services market. It is clear from recent analyses of the market for veterinarians and veterinary services that both would benefit from the entrepreneurial development of business models that meet and enhance clients' perceptions of value in regard to the delivery of veterinary services.

Diversity

To meet societal expectations on a global scale, students must acquire a working knowledge of the cultural, racial, ethnic, and other factors that affect a veterinarian's ability to meet the healthcare needs of diverse communities. This imperative goes beyond the compelling benefit of creating a diverse college community capable of exposing students to a variety of perspectives. It also involves placing students in different communities, both local and international, where they can develop an appreciation for the importance of adapting their communication, disease assessment, and disease management approaches to fit the particular context.

Postgraduation Career Transitions

Through the course of a professional career, it is not uncommon for veterinarians to transition from one species emphasis to another, nor to shift between clinical and nonclinical practice. Currently, there are not many formal opportunities to receive training that prepares individuals for such a change, neither are there many credentialing processes to assure the public that such training has been successfully completed. Irrespective of whether segmented licensure is instituted in the future, providing educational opportunities for career transitions will become increasingly important as the profession adapts to new societal needs and business opportunities.

The Role of Accreditation in Promoting Change

The primary role of accreditation is to ensure that professional veterinary education programs implement standards that protect the public interest and serve animal and relevant public health needs. Accreditation is not designed to shape and/or promote any particular strategic direction relevant to sources of educational funding, educational content, or instructional methodology. Instead, it is focused on ensuring that newly minted graduates have the knowledge and skills to engage in general practice, a goal that places increasing emphasis on outcomes assessment. It can be expected, therefore, that all new developments in veterinary medical education will have to occur hand in hand with the creation and application of outcomes assessment systems and measures capable of confirming the success of new initiatives, and supporting the identification and remediation of approaches that are ineffective.

Envisioning the Future of Veterinary Medical Education

A review of strategic analyses conducted over the last approximately 100 years, as well as current trends in education funding and societal needs in the intersecting areas of animal and public health, suggests that a number of changes are likely to emerge or become more common in future, and these are discussed in what follows.

Further Erosion of State-Appropriated Funding, Focusing Increasing Attention on the Cost-Effectiveness of Educational Programs

Veterinary colleges generally rely on a mix of funding sources, including base funding allocated by the parent university and/or state appropriations, student tuition and fees, revenue from clinical and diagnostic services, extramurally funded research, and philanthropic gifts. Considering the limited potential for substantial increases in state-appropriated funding in future and the real risk of this funding declining, colleges will not be able to sustain and grow their programs without substantially increasing income from other funding sources, such as tuition, extramurally funded research, and private gifts. However, as already stated, the capacity to increase tuition income is limited by the risk of aggravating the already high educational debt of graduates and by the concerns of external constituents regarding further increases in enrollment. Diagnostic and clinical services as well as extramurally funded research programs usually require substantial subsidies and are seldom generators of net revenue, at least in regard to their contribution to the veterinary medical educational mission. Private gifts can be transformative in their ability to establish new initiatives, but generally are not a reliable source of the recurring funding necessary to operate a veterinary school. Clearly, strategies to sustain and increase the financial resources available for program development cannot rely

exclusively on the enhancement of income sources, but must be focused also on improving the cost-effectiveness of veterinary education.

To enhance the cost-effectiveness of educational programs, there are multiple functions of a veterinary school that are possible points of intervention, but the two that are most likely to attract attention are the largest cost centers: the veterinary teaching hospital and faculty. Key performance indicators (KPIs) have long been used to assess and improve the efficiency of business enterprises, but have yet to be widely embraced in academia. This is expected to change. In regard to teaching hospitals, the possible benefit of using KPIs, such as net diagnostic and clinical service revenue, patient caseload, and utilization rates of physical space, major equipment, and personnel, will be explored. These KPIs can be applied at the college, unit, and individual faculty levels. In relation to the latter, one can expect that increased scrutiny will be focused on faculty workload guidelines and, where appropriate and necessary, these will be modeled on realistic estimates of time committed to student instruction, with the possibility of reducing the full-time equivalent staff (FTEs) necessary to accomplish this mission. Also, the often unreasonable expectation that faculty have balanced assignments to teaching, research, and service missions will probably be deemphasized in favor of a more differentiated allocation of time to a single major job responsibility. This approach can be expected to have significant impacts on the role of tenure in faculty appointments, especially if tenure continues to carry a significant responsibility for research and scholarship.

Career Specialization, Supported by Institutional Partnerships and Distance Learning

The expectation that veterinarians graduate with Day One skills enabling them to take on sole responsibility for patient care will drive curricula in the direction of providing more opportunities for species and/or disciplinary specialization, because these skills are difficult

Index

Veterinary Medical Education: A Practical Guide, First Edition. Edited by Jennifer L. Hodgson and Jacquelyn M. Pelzer.
© 2017 John Wiley & Sons, Inc. Published 2017 by John Wiley & Sons, Inc.